9th EDITION

CLINICIAN'S POCKET REFERENCE

EDITED BY

LEONARD G. GOMELLA, MD, FACS

The Bernard W. Godwin, Jr., Associate Professor
Department of Urology
Jefferson Medical College
Thomas Jefferson University
Philadelphia, Pennsylvania

WITH

Steven A. Haist, MD, MS, FACP

Professor of Medicine
Division of General Internal Medicine
Department of Internal Medicine
University of Kentucky Medical Center
Lexington, Kentucky

Based on a program originally developed at the
University of Kentucky College of Medicine
Lexington, Kentucky

McGraw-Hill
MEDICAL PUBLISHING DIVISION

New York   Chicago   San Francisco
Lisbon   London   Madrid
Mexico City   Milan   New Delhi   San Juan
Seoul   Singapore   Sydney   Toronto

McGraw-Hill

A Division of The McGraw·Hill Companies

Clinician's Pocket Reference, Ninth Edition

Copyright © 2002 by Leonard G. Gomella. Published by **The McGraw-Hill Companies,** Inc. All rights reserved. Printed in the United States of America. Except as permitted under the United States Copyright Act of 1976, no part of this publication may be reproduced or distributed in any form or by any means, or stored in a data base or retrieval system, without the prior written permission of the publisher.

Previous editions copyright © 1997, 1993, 1989, by Leonard G. Gomella. Copyright © 1986 by Leonard G. Gomella, G. Richard Braen, and Michael Olding. Copyright © 1983 by Capistrano Press, Ltd., Garden Grove, California. Previously published as *So You Want to Be a Scut Monkey: Medical Student's and House Officer's Clinical Handbook,* copyright © 1981, 1980, 1979, by Leonard G. Gomella and Michael J. Olding.

1 2 3 4 5 6 7 8 9 0   DOC/DOC   0 9 8 7 6 5 4 3 2 1

ISBN: 0-8385-1552-5 (domestic)
ISBN: 0-07-112428-4 (international)
ISSN: 1041-1348

Notice

Medicine is an ever-changing science. As new research and clinical experience broaden our knowledge, changes in treatment and drug therapy are required. The authors and the publisher of this work have checked with sources believed to be reliable in their efforts to provide information that is complete and generally in accord with the standards accepted at the time of publication. However, in view of the possibility of human error or changes in medical sciences, neither the authors nor the publisher nor any other party who has been involved in the preparation or publication of this work warrants that the information contained herein is in every respect accurate or complete, and they disclaim all responsibility for any errors or omissions or for the results obtained from use of the information contained in this work. Readers are encouraged to confirm the information contained herein with other sources. For example and in particular, readers are advised to check the product information sheet included in the package of each drug they plan to administer to be certain that the information contained in this work is accurate and that changes have not been made in the recommended dose or in the contraindications for administration. This recommendation is of particular importance in connection with new or infrequently used drugs.

The book was set in Times Roman by Pine Tree Composition, Inc.
The editors were Janet Foltin, Harriet Lebowitz, and Lester A. Sheinis.
The senior production supervisor was Richard C. Ruzycka.
The text designer was Marsha Cohen/Parallelogram Graphics.
The cover designer was Mary McKeon.
The illustration manager was Charissa Baker.
The illustrator was Wendy Beth Jackelow.
The indexer was Alexandra Nickerson.
R. R. Donnelley & Sons was printer and binder.

This book is printed on acid-free paper.

INTERNATIONAL EDITION ISBN 0-07-112428-4
Copyright © 2002. Exclusive rights by The McGraw-Hill Companies, Inc., for manufacture and export. This book cannot be reexported from the country to which it is consigned by McGraw-Hill. The International Edition is not available in North America.

To Tricia, Mom, Dad, Leonard, Patrick, Andrew, Michael
and Aunt Lucy

"We don't drive the trucks, we only load them."

Nick Pavona, MD
UKMC Class of 1980

CONTENTS

	Consulting Editors	vii
	Contributors	viii
	Preface	xiii
	Abbreviations	xv
	"So You Want to Be a Scut Monkey": An Introduction to Clinical Medicine	1
1	History and Physical Examination	9
2	Chartwork	33
3	Differential Diagnosis: Symptoms, Signs, and Conditions	41
4	Laboratory Diagnosis: Chemistry, Immunology, and Serology	53
5	Laboratory Diagnosis: Clinical Hematology	95
6	Laboratory Diagnosis: Urine Studies	109
7	Clinical Microbiology	121
8	Blood Gases and Acid-Base Disorders	161
9	Fluids and Electrolytes	177
10	Blood Component Therapy	193
11	Diets and Clinical Nutrition	205
12	Total Parenteral Nutrition (TPN)	227
13	Bedside Procedures	239
14	Pain Management	315
15	Imaging Studies	325
16	Introduction to the Operating Room	339
17	Suturing Techniques and Wound Care	345
18	Respiratory Care	359
19	Basic ECG Reading	367
20	Critical Care	389
21	Emergencies	445
22	Commonly Used Medications	475
	Appendix	639
	Index	659
	Emergency Medications (inside front and back covers)	

CONSULTING EDITORS

CONTRIBUTORS

Aimee G. Adams, PharmD

Director, Primary Care Pharmacy Practice Residency, University of Kentucky Medical Center; Assistant Professor College of Pharmacy and Department of Medicine, University of Kentucky, Lexington, Kentucky

Marianne Billeter, PharmD, BCPS

Associate Professor of Pharmacy Practice, Division of Distance Education, Bernard J. Dunn School of Pharmacy, Shenandoah University, Winchester, Virginia

Pasquale Casale, MD

Chief Resident, Department of Urology, Thomas Jefferson University, Philadelphia, Pennsylvania

Murray Cohen, MD

Clinical Associate Professor of Surgery, Director, Division of Trauma/Critical Care, Department of Surgery, Jefferson Medical College, Philadelphia, Pennsylvania

Marisa Davis

Doctor of Pharmacy Candidate, Bernard J. Dunn School of Pharmacy, Shenandoah University, Winchester, Virginia

Neil M. Davis, PharmD, FASHP

Professor Emeritus of Pharmacy, Temple University, Philadelphia, Pennsylvania; Director, Safe Medication Practice Consulting, Inc., Huntingdon Valley, Pennsylvania

Ehab A. El Gabry, MD

Fellow, Department of Urology, Thomas Jefferson University, Philadelphia, Pennsylvania

Sue Fosson, MA

Former Associate Dean for Student Affairs, University of Kentucky College of Medicine, Lexington, Kentucky

Leonard G. Gomella, MD, FACS

The Bernard W. Godwin, Jr., Associate Professor, Department of Urology, Jefferson Medical College, Thomas Jefferson University, Philadelphia, Pennsylvania

Steven A. Haist, MD, MS, FACP

Professor of Medicine, Division of General Internal Medicine, Department of Internal Medicine, University of Kentucky Medical Center, Lexington, Kentucky

Sara Maria Haverty, MD

Senior Resident, Department of Obstetrics and Gynecology, Thomas Jefferson University, Philadelphia, Pennsylvania

Mohamed Ismail, MD

Senior Resident, Department of Urology, Thomas Jefferson University, Philadelphia, Pennsylvania

Gregory C. Kane, MD

Clinical Associate Professor of Medicine, Program Director, Internal Medicine Residency, Jefferson Medical College, Philadelphia, Pennsylvania

Matthew J. Killion, MD

Assistant Professor of Medicine, Jefferson Medical College, Philadelphia, Pennsylvania

Alan T. Lefor, MD, MPH, FACS

Director, Division of Surgical Oncology, Director, Surgical Education and Academic Affairs, Department of Surgery, Cedars-Sinai Medical Center, Los Angeles, California; Associate Professor of Clinical Surgery, Department of Surgery, University of California, Los Angeles, Los Angeles, California

Layla F. Makary, MD, MSC, PhD

Lecturer, Department of Anesthesia, Cairo University, Clinical Fellow, Department of Anesthesia, Cleveland Clinic Foundation, Cleveland, Ohio

John Moore, MD

Clinical Associate Professor, Department of Surgery, Division of Plastic Surgery, Jefferson Medical College, Philadelphia, Pennsylvania

Nick A. Pavona, MD

Associate Professor, Department of Surgery, Division of Urology, Benjamin Franklin University Medical Center, Chadds Ford, Pennsylvania

Roger J. Pomerantz, MD, FACP

Professor of Medicine, Biochemistry and Molecular Pharmacology, Division of Infectious Diseases and Center for Human Virology, Jefferson Medical College, Thomas Jefferson University, Philadelphia, Pennsylvania

Ganesh Raj, MD, PhD

Senior Resident, Division of Urology, Department of Surgery, Duke University Medical Center, Durham, North Carolina

Steven Rosensweig, MD

Director, Jefferson Center for Integrative Medicine, Jefferson Medical College,
Philadelphia, Pennsylvania

Paul J. Schenarts, MD

Instructor in Surgery, Section of Surgical Sciences, Vanderbilt University,
Nashville, Tennessee

Francis G. Serio, DMD, MS

Associate Professor and Chairman, Department of Periodontics, University of Mississippi
School of Dentistry, Jackson, Mississippi

Kelly Smith, PharmD

Clinical Associate Professor, Division of Pharmacy Practice & Science, University
of Kentucky College of Pharmacy; Director, Pharmacy Practice Residency,
University of Kentucky Medical Center, Lexington, Kentucky

PREFACE

The *Clinician's Pocket Reference* is based on a University of Kentucky house manual entitled *So You Want to Be a Scut Monkey: Medical Student's and House Officer's Clinical Handbook*. The Scut Monkey Program at the University of Kentucky College of Medicine began in the summer of 1978 and was developed by members of the Class of 1980 to help ease the often frustrating transition from the preclinical to the clinical years of medical school. From detailed surveys at the University of Kentucky College of Medicine and 44 other medical schools, a list of essential information and skills that third-year students should be familiar with at the start of their clinical years was developed. The Scut Monkey Program was developed around this core of material and consisted of reference manuals and a series of workshops conducted at the start of the third year. Presented originally as a pilot program for the University of Kentucky College of Medicine Class of 1981, the program has been incorporated into the third-year curriculum. It is the responsibility of each new fourth-year class to orient the new third-year students. The basis of the program's success is the fact that it was developed and taught by students for other students. This method has allowed us to maintain perspective on those areas that are critical not only for learning while on the wards but also for delivering effective patient care. Information on the Scut Monkey Orientation Program is available from Todd Cheever, MD, Associate Dean for Academic Affairs at the University of Kentucky College of Medicine.

Through the last eight editions, the book has undergone expansion and careful revisions as the practice of medicine and the educational needs of students have changed. Although the book's original mission, providing new clinical clerks with essential patient care information in an easy-to-use format, remains unchanged, our readership has expanded. Residents, practicing physicians, and allied health professionals all use the *Clinician's Pocket Reference* as a "manual of manuals." Even individuals considering careers in medicine have used the book in their decision-making process. An attempt is made to cover the most frequently asked basic management questions that are normally found in many different sources, such as procedure manuals, laboratory manuals, drug references, and critical care manuals, to name a few. It is not meant as a substitute for specialty-specific reference manuals. The core of information presented is a foundation for new medical students as they move through training to more advanced medical studies.

The book is designed to represent a cross section of medical practices around the country. The *Clinician's Pocket Reference* has been translated into six different languages with electronic media versions in development. I was honored to have been asked to grant permission to Warner Brothers, the producers of the TV show "ER," to have the eighth edition of the Scut Monkey book as one of the books used on their series.

I would like to express special thanks to my wife and my family for their long-term support of the Scut Monkey project. Linda Davoli, our extraordinary copy editor, had an exceptional eye for detail in helping create this final work. Janet Foltin, Harriet Lebowitz, Lester

Sheinis, and the team at McGraw-Hill were instrumental in moving the book forward and in giving the ninth edition a fresh, new two-color format. They are also responsible for helping reach our long-term goal of the new companion manual, the *Clinician's Pocket Drug Reference*. A special thanks to my assistant Conchita Ballard, who always kept things organized and flowing smoothly. I am indebted to all of the past contributors and readers who have helped to keep the Scut Monkey book as a useful reference for students and residents worldwide. The original coeditors of this work, G. Richard Braen, MD, and Michael J. Olding, MD, are acknowledged for their early contributions.

Your comments and suggestions for improvement are always welcomed by me personally, since revisions to the book would not be possible if it were not for the ongoing interest of our readers. I hope this book will not only help you learn some of the basics of the art and science of medicine but also allow you to care for your patients in the best way possible.

Leonard G. Gomella, MD
Philadelphia, Pennsylvania
Leonard.Gomella@mail.tju.edu

ABBREVIATIONS

The following are common abbreviations used in medical records and in this edition

÷: divided dose

↓: decrease(d), reduce, downward

×: times for multiplication sign

↑: increase(d), upward (as in titrate upward)

/: per

±: with or without

+: with

<: less than, younger than

>: more than, older than

≅: approximately equal to

AAA: abdominal aortic aneurysm

AaDo₂: difference in partial pressures of oxygen in mixed alveolar gas and mixed arterial blood

A-a gradient: alveolar-to-arterial gradient

AAI: ankle-arm index

AAS: acute abdominal series

AB: antibody, abortion, antibiotic

A&B: apnea and bradycardia

ABD: abdomen

ABG: arterial blood gas

A/B index: ankle-brachial index

ABMT: autologous bone marrow transplantation

ac: before eating (*ante cibum*), assist-controlled

ACCP: American College of Chest Physicians

ACE: angiotensin-converting enzyme

Ach-ase: acetylcholinesterase

ACLS: Advanced Cardiac Life Support

ACS: acute coronary syndrome, American Cancer Society, American College of Surgeons

ACTH: adrenocorticotropic hormone

A.D.C. VAAN DIML: mnemonic for Admit, Diagnosis, Condition, Vitals, Activity, Allergies, Nursing procedures, Diet, Ins and outs, Medications, Labs

A.D.C. VAN DISSEL: mnemonic for Admit, Diagnosis, Condition, Vitals, Activity, Nursing procedures, Diet, Ins and outs, Specific drugs, Symptomatic drugs, Extras, Labs

ADH: antidiuretic hormone

ADHD: attention-deficit hyperactivity disorder

ad lib: as much as needed (*ad libitum*)

AEIOU TIPS: mnemonic for Alcohol, Encephalopathy, Insulin, Opiates, Uremia, Trauma, Infection, Psychiatric, Syncope (diagnosis of coma)

AF: afebrile, aortofemoral, atrial fibrillation

AFB: acid-fast bacilli

AFP: alpha-fetoprotein

A/G: albumin/globulin ratio

AHA: American Heart Association

AHF: antihemophilic factor

AI: aortic insufficiency

AIDS: acquired immunodeficiency syndrome

AJCC: American Joint Committee on Cancer

AKA: above-the-knee amputation

ALAT: alanine aminotransferase

ALL: acute lymphocytic leukemia

ALS: amyotrophic lateral sclerosis

ALT: alanine aminotransferase

AM: morning

amb: ambulate

AMI: acute myocardial infarction

AML: acute myelocytic leukemia, acute myelogenous leukemia

AMMoL: acute monocytic leukemia

amp: ampule

AMP: adenosine monophosphate

ANA: antinuclear antibody

ANC: absolute neutrophil count
ANCA: antineutrophil cytoplasmic antibody
ANLL: acute nonlymphoblastic leukemia
ANS: autonomic nervous system
AOB: alcohol on breath
AODM: adult-onset diabetes mellitus
AP: anteroposterior, abdominal-perineal
APAP: acetaminophen
APL: acute promyelocytic leukemia
aPPT: activated partial thromboplastin time
APSAC: anisoylated plasminogen streptokinase activator complex
APUD: amine precursor uptake (and) decarboxylation
Ara-C: cytarabine
ARD: antibiotic removal device
ARDS: adult respiratory distress syndrome
ARF: acute renal failure
AS: aortic stenosis
ASA: American Society of Anesthesiologists
ASAP: as soon as possible
ASAT: aspartate aminotransferase
ASCVD: atherosclerotic cardiovascular disease
ASD: atrial septal defect
ASHD: atherosclerotic heart disease
ASO: antistreptolysin O
AST: aspartate aminotransferase
ATG: antithymocyte globulin
ATN: acute tubular necrosis
ATP: adenosine triphosphate
AUC: area under the curve
AV: atrioventricular
A-V: arteriovenous
A-Vo₂: arteriovenous oxygen
B I&II: Billroth I and II
BACOD: bleomycin, doxorubicin (Adriamycin), cyclophosphamide, vincristine (Oncovin), dexamethasone
BACOP: bleomycin, doxorubicin (Adriamycin), cyclophosphamide, vincristine (Oncovin), prednisone
BBB: bundle branch block
BC: bone conduction
BCAA: branched-chain amino acid
BCG: bacille Calmette-Guérin
BE: barium enema

BEE: basal energy expenditure
bid: twice a day (*bis in die*)
bili: bilirubin
BKA: below-the-knee amputation
BM: bone marrow, bowel movement
BMR: basal metabolic rate
BMT: bone marrow transplantation
BOM: bilateral otitis media
BP: blood pressure
BPH: benign prostatic hypertrophy
bpm: beats per minute
BR: bed rest
BRBPR: bright red blood per rectum
BRP: bathroom privileges
bs, BS: bowel sounds, breath sounds
BSA: body surface area
BS&O: bilateral salpingo-oophorectomy
BUN: blood urea nitrogen
BW: body weight
Bx: biopsy
c: with (*cum*)
Ca: calcium
CA: cancer
CAA: crystalline amino acid
CABG: coronary artery bypass graft
CAD: coronary artery disease
CAF: cyclophosphamide, doxorubicin (Adriamycin), 5-fluorouracil
CALGB: Cancer and Leukemia Group B
cAMP: cyclic adenosine monophosphate
Cao₂: arterial oxygen content
caps: capsule(s)
CAT: computed axial tomography
CBC: complete blood count
CBG: capillary blood gas
CC: chief complaint
CCI: corrected count increment (platelets)
CCO: continuous cardiac output
Cco₂: capillary oxygen content
CCU: clean-catch urine, cardiac care unit
CCV: critical closing volume
CD: continuous dose
CDC: Centers for Disease Control and Prevention
CEA: carcinoembryonic antigen
CEP/CIEP: counterimmunoelectrophoresis
CF: cystic fibrosis
CFU: colony-forming unit(s)
CGL: chronic granulocytic leukemia

CH$_{50}$: (total serum) hemolytic complement
CHD: coronary heart disease
CHF: congestive heart failure
CHO: carbohydrate
CHOP: cyclophosphamide, doxorubicin, vincristine (Oncovin), prednisone
CI: cardiac index
CIE: counterimmunoelectrophoresis
CIS: carcinoma in situ
CK: creatine phosphokinase
CKI: cyclin-dependent kinase inhibitor
CK-MB: isoenzyme of creatine kinase with muscle and brain subunits
Cl: chlorine
CLL: chronic lymphocytic leukemia
cm: centimeter
CML: chronic myelogenous leukemia
CMV: cytomegalovirus
CN: cranial nerve
CNS: central nervous system
CO: cardiac output
C/O: complaining of
COAD: chronic obstructive airway disease
COLD: chronic obstructive lung disease
COMT: catechol-O-methyltransferase
conc: concentrate
cont inf: continuous infusion
COPD: chronic obstructive pulmonary disease
COX-2: cyclooxygenase-2
CP: chest pain, cerebral palsy
CPAP: continuous positive airway pressure
CPK: creatinine phosphokinase
CPP: central precocious puberty
CPR: cardiopulmonary resuscitation
CR: controlled release
CrCl: creatine clearance
CREST: calcinosis cutis, Raynaud's disease, esophageal dysmotility, syndactyly, telangiectasia
CRF: chronic renal failure
CRH: corticotropin-releasing hormone
CRP: C-reactive protein
C&S: culture and sensitivity
CSF: cerebrospinal fluid, colony-stimulating factor
C-spine: cervical spine
CT: computed tomography
CVA: cerebrovascular accident, costovertebral angle

CVAT: costovertebral angle tenderness
CVH: common variable hypogammaglobulinemia
Cvo$_2$: oxygen content of mixed venous blood
CVP: central venous pressure
CXR: chest x-ray
d: day
D$_5$LR: 5% dextrose in lactated Ringer's solution
D$_5$W: 5% dextrose in water
DAG: diacylglycerol
DAP: diastolic pulmonary artery pressure
DAT: diet as tolerated
DAW: dispense as written
DC: discontinue, discharge, direct current
D&C: dilation and curettage
ddI: dideoxyinosine
DDx: differential diagnosis
DEA: United States Drug Enforcement Administration
DES: diethylstilbestrol
DEXA: dual-energy x-ray absorptiometer
DHEA: dehydroepiandrosterone
DHEAS: dehydroepiandrosterone sulfate
DI: diabetes insipidus
DIC: disseminated intravascular coagulation
DIP: distal interphalangeal joint
DIT: diiodotyrosine
DJD: degenerative joint disease
DKA: diabetic ketoacidosis
dL: deciliter
DM: diabetes mellitus
DMSA: dimercaptosuccinic acid
DNA: deoxyribonucleic acid
DNP: deoxyribonucleic protein
DNR: do not resuscitate
DOA: dead on arrival
DOCA: deoxycorticosterone acetate
DOE: dyspnea on exertion
DOPA: dihydroxyphenylalanine
DP: dorsalis pedis
2,3-DPG: 2,3-diphosphoglycerate
DPL: diagnostic peritoneal lavage
DPT: diphtheria, pertussis, tetanus
DR: delayed release
DRG: diagnosis-related group
DS: double strength
DSA: digital subtraction angiography
DTPA: diethylenetriamine-pentaacetic acid

DTR: deep tendon reflex
DVT: deep venous thrombosis
Dx: diagnosis
EAA: essential amino acid
EBL: estimated blood loss
EBV: Epstein–Barr virus
EC: enteric-coated
ECG: electrocardiogram
ECOG: Eastern Cooperative Oncology Group
ECT: electroconvulsive therapy
EDC: estimated date of confinement
EDTA: ethylenediamine tetraacetic acid
EDVI: end-diastolic volume index
EFAD: essential fatty acid deficiency
ELISA: enzyme-linked immunosorbent assay
EMD: electromechanical dissociation
EMG: electromyelogram
EMS: emergency medical system, eosinophilia-myalgia syndrome
EMV: eyes, motor, verbal response (Glasgow Coma Scale)
ENA: extractable nuclear antigen
ENT: ear, nose, and throat
eod: every other day
EOM: extraocular muscle
EPO: erythropoietin
EPSP: excitatory postsynaptic potential
ER: endoplasmic reticulum, Emergency Room, extended release
ERCP: endoscopic retrograde cholangiopancreatography
ERV: expiratory reserve volume
ESR: erythrocyte sedimentation rate
ESRD: end-stage renal disease
ET: endotracheal
ETOH: ethanol
ETT: endotracheal tube
EUA: examination under anesthesia
ExU: excretory urogram
Fab: antigen-binding fragment
FANA: fluorescent antinuclear antibody
FBS: fasting blood sugar
Fe: iron
FEV$_1$: forced expiratory volume in 1 s
FFP: fresh frozen plasma
FHR: fetal heart rate
FIGO: Fédération Internationale de Gynécologie et d'Obstétrique

Fio$_2$: fraction of inspired oxygen
FRC: functional residual capacity
FSH: follicle-stimulating hormone
FSP: fibrin split product
ft: foot
FTA-ABS: fluorescent treponemal antibody-absorbed
FTT: failure to thrive
FU: follow-up
5-FU: fluorouracil
FUO: fever of unknown origin
FVC: forced vital capacity
Fx: fracture
g: gram
G: gravida
GABA: gamma-aminobutyric acid
GAD: glutamic acid decarboxylase
GC: gonorrhea (gonococcus)
G-CSF: granulocyte colony-stimulating factor
GDP: guanosine diphosphate
GERD: gastroesophageal reflux disease
GETT: general by endotracheal tube (anesthesia)
GFR: glomerular filtration rate
GGT: gamma-glutamyltransferase
GH: growth hormone
GHIH: growth hormone-inhibiting hormone
GI: gastrointestinal
GM-CSF: granulocyte-macrophage colony-stimulating factor
GNID: gram-negative intracellular diplococci
GnRH: gonadotropin-releasing hormone
GOG: Gynecologic Oncology Group
G6PD: glucose-6-phosphate dehydrogenase
gr: grain
GSW: gunshot wound
gt, gtt: drop, drops (*gutta*)
GTP: guanosine triphosphate
GTT: glucose tolerance test
GU: genitourinary
GVHD: graft-versus-host disease
GXT: graded exercise tolerance (cardiac stress test)
HA: headache
HAA: hepatitis B surface antigen (hepatitis-associated antigen)

HAV: hepatitis A virus
HBcAg: hepatitis B core antigen
HBeAg: hepatitis B e antigen
HBP: high blood pressure
HBsAg: hepatitis B surface antigen
HBV: hepatitis B virus
HCG: human chorionic gonadotropin
HCL: hairy cell leukemia
HCT: hematocrit
HCTZ: hydrochlorothiazide
HDL: high-density lipoprotein
HEENT: head, eyes, ears, nose, and throat
HFV: high-frequency ventilation
Hgb: hemoglobin
[Hgb]: hemoglobin concentration
H/H: hemoglobin/hematocrit, Henderson–Hasselbalch equation
HIAA: 5-hydroxyindoleacetic acid
HIDA: hepatic 2,6-dimethyliminodiacetic acid
HIV: human immunodeficiency virus
HJR: hepatojugular reflex
HLA: histocompatibility locus antigen
HO: history of
HOB: head of bed
H&P: history and physical examination
hpf: high-power field
HPI: history of the present illness
HPLC: high-pressure liquid chromatography
HPV: human papilloma virus
HR: heart rate
hs: at bedtime (*hora somni*)
HSG: hysterosalpingogram
HSM: hepatosplenomegaly
HSV: herpes simplex virus
5-HT$_3$: 5-hydroxytryptamine
HTLV-III: human T-lymphotropic virus, type III (AIDS agent, HIV)
HTN: hypertension
Hx: history
IC: inspiratory capacity
ICN: Intensive Care Nursery
ICS: intercostal space
ICSH: interstitial cell-stimulating hormone
ICU: intensive care unit
ID: identification, infectious disease
I&D: incision and drainage
IDDM: insulin-dependent diabetes mellitus
Ig: immunoglobulin

IgG1{k}: immunoglobulin G1 kappa
IHSS: idiopathic hypertrophic subaortic stenosis
IL: interleukin
IM: intramuscular
IMV: intermittent mandatory ventilation
in.: inch
INF: intravenous nutritional fluid
INH: isoniazid
inhal: inhalation
inj: injection
INR: international normalized ratio
I&O: intake and output
IP$_3$: inositol triphosphate
IPPB: intermittent positive pressure breathing
IPSP: inhibitory postsynaptic potential
iPTH: parathyroid hormone by radioimmunoassay
IR: inversion recovery
IRBBB: incomplete right bundle branch block
IRDM: insulin-resistant diabetes mellitus
IRV: inspiratory reserve volume
ISA: intrinsic sympathomimetic activity
IT: intrathecal
ITP: idiopathic thrombocytopenic purpura
IV: intravenous
IVC: intravenous cholangiogram
IVP: intravenous pyelogram
JODM: juvenile-onset diabetes mellitus
JVD: jugular venous distention
K: potassium
katal: unit of enzyme activity
kg: kilogram
KOR: keep open rate
17-KSG: 17-ketogenic steroids
KUB: kidneys, ureters, bladder
KVO: keep vein open
L: left, liter
LAD: left axis deviation, left anterior descending
LAE: left atrial enlargement
LAHB: left anterior hemiblock
LAP: left atrial pressure, leukocyte alkaline phosphatase
LBBB: left bundle branch block
LDH: lactate dehydrogenase
LDL: low-density lipoprotein

LE: lupus erythematosus
LH: luteinizing hormone
LHRH: luteinizing hormone releasing hormone
LIH: left inguinal hernia
liq: liquid
LLL: left lower lobe
LLSB: left lower sternal border
LMP: last menstrual period
LNMP: last normal menstrual period
LOC: loss of consciousness, level of consciousness
LP: lumbar puncture
lpf: low-power field
LPN: licensed practical nurse
LSB: left sternal border
LSD: lysergic acid diethylamide
LUL: left upper lobe
LUQ: left upper quadrant
LV: left ventricle
LVD: left ventricular dysfunction
LVEDP: left ventricular end-diastolic pressure
LVH: left ventricular hypertrophy
m: meter
MAC: *Mycobacterium avium* complex
MACE: methotrexate, doxorubicin (Adriamycin), cyclophosphamide, epipodophyllotoxin
MAG3: mercaptoacetyltriglycine
MAMC: midarm muscle circumference
MAO: monoamine oxidase
MAOI: monoamine oxidase inhibitor
MAP: mean arterial pressure
MAST: military/medical antishock trousers
MAT: multifocal atrial tachycardia
max: maximum
MBC: minimum bactericidal concentration
MBT: maternal blood type
MCH: mean cell hemoglobin
MCHC: mean cell hemoglobin concentration
MCT: medium-chain triglycerides
MCTD: mixed connective tissue disease
MCV: mean cell volume
MEN: multiple endocrine neoplasia
meq: milliequivalent
MESNA: 2-mercaptoethane sulfonate sodium
met-dose: metered-dose

mg: milligram
Mg: magnesium
MHA-TP: microhemagglutination-*Treponema pallidum*
MHC: major histocompatibility complex
MI: myocardial infarction, mitral insufficiency
MIBG: metaiodobenzyl-guanidine
MIC: minimum inhibitory concentration
min: minute, minimum
MIT: monoiodotyrosine
mL: milliliter
MLE: midline episiotomy
mm: millimeter
MMEF: maximal midexpiratory flow
mm Hg: millimeters of mercury
mmol: millimole
MMR: measles, mumps, rubella
mo: month
mol: mole
MOPP: mechlorethamine, vincristine (Oncovin), procarbazine, prednisone
6-MP: mercaptopurine
MPF: M phase-promoting factor
MPGN: membrane-proliferative glomerulonephritis
MPTP: analog of meperidine (used by drug addicts)
MRI: magnetic resonance imaging
mRNA: messenger ribonucleic acid
MRS: magnetic resonance spectroscopy
MRSA: methicillin-resistant *Staphylococcus aureus*
MS: mitral stenosis, morphine sulfate, multiple sclerosis
MSBOS: maximal surgical blood order schedule
MSH: melanocyte-stimulating hormone
MTT: monotetrazolium
MTX: methotrexate
MUGA: multigated (image) acquisition (analysis)
μm: micrometer
MVA: motor vehicle accident
MVI: multivitamin injection
MVV: maximum voluntary ventilation
MyG: myasthenia gravis
Na: sodium
NAACP: mnemonic for *N*eoplasm, *A*llergy, *A*ddison's disease, *C*ollagen-vascular

disease, *Parasites* (causes of
eosinophilia)

NAD: no active disease

Na⁺/K⁺-ATPase: sodium/potassium
adenosine triphosphate

NAPA: *N*-acetylated procainamide,
N-acetylparaaminophenol

NAS: no added sodium

NAVEL: mnemonic for *Nerve, Artery,
Vein, Empty space, Lymphatic*

NCV: nerve conduction velocity

NE: norepinephrine

neb: nebulizer

NED: no evidence of recurrent disease

ng: nanogram

NG: nasogastric

NIDDM: non-insulin-dependent diabetes
mellitus

NK: natural killer

NKA: no known allergies

NKDA: no known drug allergy

nmol: nanomole

NMR: nuclear magnetic resonance

NPC: nuclear pore complex

NPO: nothing by mouth (*nil per os*)

NRM: no regular medicines

NS: normal saline

NSAID: nonsteroidal antiinflammatory
drug

NSILA: nonsuppressible insulin-like
activity

NSR: normal sinus rhythm

NT: nasotracheal

NTG: nitroglycerin

OB: obstetrics

OCD: obsessive-compulsive disorder

OCG: oral cholecystogram

7-OCHS: 17-hydroxycorticosteroids

OD: overdose, right eye (*oculus dexter*)

oint: ointment

OM: otitis media

OOB: out of bed

ophth: ophthalmic

OPV: oral polio vaccine

OR: operating room

OS: opening snap, left eye (*oculus sinister*)

OTC: over-the-counter (medications)

OU: both eyes

p: para

PA: posteroanterior, pulmonary artery

PAC: premature atrial contraction

PAD: diastolic pulmonary artery pressure

PAF: paroxysmal atrial fibrillation

PAL: periarterial lymphatic (sheath)

Pao₂: peripheral arterial oxygen content

PAO₂: alveolar oxygen

PAOP: pulmonary artery occlusion pressure

PAP: pulmonary artery pressure, prostatic
acid phosphatase

PAS: systolic pulmonary artery pressure

PASG: pneumatic antishock garment

PAT: paroxysmal atrial tachycardia

PBM: pharmacy benefit manager

pc: after eating (*post cibum*)

PCA: patient-controlled analgesia

PCI: percutaneous coronary intervention

PCKD: polycystic kidney disease

PCN: percutaneous nephrostomy

pCO₂: partial pressure of carbon dioxide

PCP: *Pneumocystis carinii* pneumonia,
phencyclidine

PCR: polymerase chain reaction

PCWP: pulmonary capillary wedge
pressure

PDA: patent ductus arteriosus

PDGF: platelet-derived growth factor

PDR: *Physicians' Desk Reference*

PDS: polydioxanone

PE: pulmonary embolus, physical examination, pleural effusion

PEA: pulseless electrical activity

PEEP: positive end-expiratory pressure

PEG: polyethylene glycol, percutaneous
gastrostomy

PERRLA: pupils equal, round, reactive to
light and accommodation

PERRLADC: pupils equal, round, reactive
to light and accommodation directly
and consensually

PET: positron emission tomography

PFT: pulmonary function test

pg: picogram

PGE₁: prostaglandin E₁

PI: pulmonic insufficiency (disease)

PICC: peripherally inserted central
catheter

PID: pelvic inflammatory disease

PIE: pulmonary infiltrates with
eosinophilia

PIH: prolactin-inhibiting hormone
PKU: phenylketonuria
PMDD: premenstrual dysphoric disorder
PMH: past medical history
PMI: point of maximal impulse
PMNL: polymorphonuclear leukocyte (neutrophil)
PND: paroxysmal nocturnal dyspnea
PNS: peripheral nervous system
PO: by mouth (*per os*)
pO$_2$: partial pressure of oxygen
POD: postoperative day
postop: postoperative, after surgery
PP: pulsus paradoxus, postprandial
PPD: purified protein derivative
P&PD: percussion and postural drainage
PPN: partial parenteral nutrition
PR: by rectum
PRA: plasma renin activity
PRBC: packed red blood cells
preop: preoperative, before surgery
PRG: pregnancy
PRK: photorefractive keratectomy
PRN: as often as needed (*pro re nata*)
PS: pulmonic stenosis, partial saturation
PSA: prostate-specific antigen
PSV: pressure support ventilation
PSVT: paroxysmal supraventricular tachycardia
Pt: patient
PT: prothrombin time, physical therapy, posterior tibial
PTCA: percutaneous transluminal coronary angioplasty
PTH: parathyroid hormone
PTHC: percutaneous transhepatic cholangiogram
PTT: partial thromboplastin time
PTU: propylthiouracil
PUD: peptic ulcer disease
PVC: premature ventricular contraction
PVD: peripheral vascular disease
PVR: peripheral vascular resistance
PWP: pulmonary wedge pressure
PZI: protamine zinc insulin
q: every (*quaque*)
Q: mathematical symbol for flow
qd: every day
qh: every hour
q{_}h: every {_} hours
qhs: every hour of sleep

qid: four times a day (*quater in die*)
QNS: quantity not sufficient
qod: every other day
Qs: volume of blood (portion of cardiac output) shunted past nonventilated alveoli
Qs/Qt: shunt fraction
Qt: total cardiac output
R: right
RA: rheumatoid arthritis, right atrium
RAD: right axis deviation
RAE: right atrial enlargement
RAP: right atrial pressure
RBBB: right bundle branch block
RBC: red blood cell (erythrocyte)
RBP: retinol-binding protein
RCC: renal cell carcinoma
RDA: recommended dietary allowance
RDS: respiratory distress syndrome (of newborn)
RDW: red cell distribution width
REF: right ventricular ejection fraction
REM: rapid eye movement
RER: rough endoplasmic reticulum
%RH: percentage of relative humidity
RIA: radioimmunoassay
RIH: right inguinal hernia
RIND: reversible ischemic neurologic deficit
RL: Ringer's lactate
RLL: right lower lobe
RLQ: right lower quadrant
RME: resting metabolic expenditure
RML: right middle lobe
RMSF: Rocky Mountain spotted fever
RNA: ribonucleic acid
RNase: ribonuclease
R/O: rule out
ROM: range of motion
ROS: review of systems
RPG: retrograde pyelogram
RPR: rapid plasma reagin
rRNA: ribosomal ribonucleic acid
RRR: regular rate and rhythm
RSV: respiratory syncytial virus
RT: rubella titer, respiratory therapy, radiation therapy
RTA: renal tubular acidosis
RTC: return to clinic
RTOG: Radiation Therapy Oncology Group

RU: resin uptake
RUG: retrograde urethrogram
RUL: right upper lobe
RUQ: right upper quadrant
RV: residual volume
RVEDVI: right ventricular end-diastolic volume index
RVH: right ventricular hypertrophy
Rx: treatment
s: without (*sine*), second
SA: sinoatrial
S&A: sugar and acetone
SAA: synthetic amino acid
Sao₂: arterial oxygen saturation
SBE: subacute bacterial endocarditis
SBFT: small bowel follow-through
SBS: short bowel syndrome
SCr: serum creatinine
segs: segmented cells
SEM: systolic ejection murmur
SER: smooth endoplasmic reticulum
SG: Swan–Ganz
SGA: small for gestational age
SGGT: serum gamma-glutamyl transpeptidase
SGOT: serum glutamic-oxaloacetic transaminase
SGPT: serum glutamic-pyruvic transaminase
SI: Système International (see page 55)
SIADH: syndrome of inappropriate antidiuretic hormone
sig: write on label (*signa*)
SIMV: synchronous intermittent mandatory ventilation
SIRS: systemic inflammatory response syndrome
SKSD: streptokinase-streptodornase
SL: sublingual
SLE: systemic lupus erythematosus
SMA: sequential multiple analysis
SMO: slips made out
SMX: sulfamethoxazole
SOAP: mnemonic for *S*ubjective, *O*bjective, *A*ssessment, *P*lan
SOB: shortness of breath
SOC: signed on chart
soln: solution
SPAG: small-particle aerosol generator
SPECT: single-photon emission computed tomography

SQ: subcutaneous
SR: sustained release
SRP: single recognition particle
SRS-A: slow-reacting substance of anaphylaxis
SSKI: saturated solution of potassium iodide
SSRI: selective serotonin reuptake inhibitor
stat: immediately (*statim*)
STD: sexually transmitted disease
supp: suppository
susp: suspension
SVD: spontaneous vaginal delivery
Svo₂: mixed venous blood oxygen saturation
SVR: systemic vascular resistance
SVT: supraventricular tachycardia
SWOG: Southwest Oncology Group
Sx: symptoms
Ṫ: one, **ṪṪ:** two, etc.
T₃: triiodothyronine
T₃ RU: triiodothyronine resin uptake
T₄: thyroxine
tabs: tablet(s)
TAH: total abdominal hysterectomy
TB: tuberculosis
TBG: thyroxine-binding globulin, total blood gas
TBLC: term birth, living child
T&C: type and cross-match
TC&DB: turn, cough, and deep breathe
TCF: triceps skin fold
TCP: transcutaneous pacer
Td: tetanus-diphtheria toxoid
TD: transdermal
TFT: thyroid function test
6-TG: 6-thioguanine
T&H: type and hold
TIA: transient ischemic attack
TIBC: total iron-binding capacity
tid: three times a day (*ter in die*)
TIG: tetanus immune globulin
TKO: to keep open
TLC: total lung capacity
TMJ: temporal mandibular joint
TMP: trimethoprim
TMP-SMX: trimethoprim-sulfamethoxazole
TNFα: tumor necrosis factor alpha

TNM: tumor-nodes-metastases
TNTC: too numerous to count
TO: telephone order
TOPV: trivalent oral polio vaccine
TORCH: toxoplasma, rubella, cy-
tomegalovirus, herpes virus (*O* = other
[syphilis])
TPA: tissue plasminogen activator
TPN: total peripheral resistance, total par-
enteral nutrition
TRH: thyrotropin-releasing hormone
TSH: thyroid-stimulating hormone
TT: thrombin time
TTP: thrombotic thrombocytopenic pur-
pura
TU: tuberculin units
TUR: transurethral resection
TURBT: TUR bladder tumors
TURP: TUR prostate
TV: tidal volume
TVH: total vaginal hysterectomy
Tx: treatment, transplant, transfer
type 2 DM: noninsulin-dependent diabetes
mellitus, type 2 diabetes mellitus
UA: urinalysis
UAC: uric acid
ud: as directed (*ut dictum*)
UDS: urodynamic studies
UGI: upper gastrointestinal
UPEP: urine protein electrophoresis
URI: upper respiratory infection
US: ultrasonography
USP: United States Pharmacopeia

UTI: urinary infection
UUN: urinary urea nitrogen
V: volt
VAMP: vincristine, doxorubicin
(Adriamycin), methylprednisolone
VC: vital capacity
VCUG: voiding cystourethrogram
VDRL: Venereal Disease Research
Laboratory
VF: ventricular fibrillation
VLDL: very low density lipoprotein
VMA: vanillylmandelic acid
VO: voice order
VP-16: etoposide
V̇/Q̇: ventilation-perfusion
VSS: vital signs stable
VT: ventricular tachycardia
W: watt
WB: whole blood
WBC: white blood cell, white blood cell
count
WD: well developed
WF: white female
wk: week
WM: white male
WN: well nourished
wnl, WNL: within normal limits
WPW: Wolff-Parkinson-White
XRT: x-ray therapy
y: year
YO: years old
ZE: Zollinger–Ellison

"SO YOU WANT TO BE A SCUT MONKEY": AN INTRODUCTION TO CLINICAL MEDICINE*

The transition from the preclinical years to the clinical years of medical school is often a difficult one. Understanding the new responsibilities and a set of ground rules can ease this transition. What follows is a brief introduction to clinical medicine for the new clinical clerk.

THE HIERARCHY

Most services can be expected to have at least one of each of the following physicians on the team.

The Intern

In some programs, the intern is known euphemistically as the first-year resident. This person has the day-to-day responsibilities of patient care. This duty, combined with a total lack of seniority, usually serves to keep the intern in the hospital more than the other members of the team and may limit his or her teaching of medical students. Any question concerning details in the evaluation of the patient, for example, whether Mrs. Pavona gets a complete blood count this morning or this evening, is usually referred first to the intern.

The Resident

The resident is a member of the house staff who has completed at least 1 year of postgraduate medical education. The most senior resident is typically in charge of the overall conduct of the service and is the person you might ask a question such as "What might cause Mrs. Pavona's white blood cell count to be 142,000?" You might also ask your resident for an appropriate reference on the subject or perhaps to arrange a brief conference on the topic for everyone on the service. A surgical service typically has a chief resident, a doctor in the last year of residency who usually runs the service. On medical services the chief resident is

* Adapted, with permission, from Epstein A, Frye T (eds.): *So You Want to Be a Toad.* College of Medicine, Ohio State University, Columbus, OH.

usually an appointee of the chairman of medicine and primarily has administrative responsibilities with limited ward duties.

The Attending Physician

The attending physician is also called simply "The Attending," and on nonsurgical services, "the attending." This physician has completed postgraduate education and is now a member of the teaching faculty. The attending is morally and legally responsible for the care of all patients whose charts are marked with the attending's name. All major therapeutic decisions made about the care of these patients are ultimately passed by the attending. In addition, this person is responsible for teaching and evaluating house staff and medical students. This is the member of the team you might ask, "Why are we treating Mrs. Pavona with busulfan?"

The Fellow

Fellows are physicians who have completed their postgraduate education and elected to do extra study in one special field, such as, nephrology, high-risk obstetrics, or surgical oncology. They may or may not be active members of the team and may not be obligated to teach medical students, but usually they are happy to answer any questions you may ask. You might ask this person to help you read Mrs. Pavona's bone marrow smear.

TEAMWORK

The medical student, in addition to being a member of the medical team, must interact with members of the professional team of nurses, dietitians, pharmacists, social workers, and all others who provide direct care for the patient. Good working relations with this group of professionals can make your work go more smoothly; bad relations with them can make your rotation miserable.

Nurses are generally good-tempered, but overburdened. Like most human beings, they respond very favorably to polite treatment. Leaving a mess in a patient's room after the performance of a floor procedure, standing by idly while a 98-lb licensed practical nurse struggles to move a 350-lb patient onto the chair scale, and obviously listening to three ringing telephones while room call lights flash are acts guaranteed not to please. Do not let anyone talk you into being an acting nurse's aide or ward secretary, but try to help when you can.

You will occasionally meet a staff member who is having a bad day, and you will be able to do little about it. Returning hostility is unwarranted at these times, and it is best to avoid confrontations except when necessary for the care of the patient.

When faced with ordering a diet for your first sick patient, you will no doubt be confronted with the inadequacy of your education in nutrition. Fortunately for your patient, dietitians are available. Never hesitate to call one.

In matters concerning drug interactions, side effects, individualization of dosages, alteration of drug dosages in disease, and equivalence of different brands of the same drug, it never hurts to call the pharmacist. Most medical centers have a pharmacy resident who follows every patient on a floor or service and who will gladly answer any questions you have on medications. The pharmacist or pharmacy resident can very often provide pertinent articles on a requested subject.

YOUR HEALTH AND A WORD ON "AGGRESSIVENESS"

In your months of curing disease both day and night, it becomes easy to ignore your own right to keep yourself healthy. There are numerous bad examples of medical and surgical interns who sleep 3 hours a night and get most of their meals from vending machines. Do not let anyone talk you into believing that you are not entitled to decent meals and sleep. If you offer yourself as a sacrifice, it will be a rare rotation on which you will not become one.

You may have the misfortune someday of reading an evaluation that says a student was not "aggressive enough." This is an enigmatic notion to everyone. Does it mean that the student refused to attempt to start an intravenous line after eight previous failures? Does it mean that the student was not consistently the first to shout out the answer over the mumblings of fellow students on rounds? Whatever constitutes "aggressiveness" must be a dubious virtue at best.

A more appropriate virtue might be **assertiveness in obtaining your education.** Ask **good** questions, have the house staff show you procedures and review your chartwork, read about your patient's illness, review the surgery basics before going to the OR, participate actively in your patient's care, and take an interest in other patients on the service. This approach avoids the need for victimizing your patients and comrades that the definition of *aggression* suggests.

ROUNDS

Rounds are meetings of all members of the service for discussing the care of the patient. These occur daily and are of three kinds.

Morning Rounds

Also known as "work rounds," these take place anywhere from 6:30 to 9:00 AM on most services and are attended by residents, interns, and students. This is the time for discussing what happened to the patient during the night, the progress of the patient's evaluation or therapy or both, the laboratory and radiologic tests to be ordered for the patient, and, last but not least, talking with and evaluating the patient. Know about your patient's most recent laboratory reports and progress—this is a chance for you to look good.

Ideally, differences of opinion and any glaring omissions in patient care are politely discussed and resolved here. Writing new orders, filling out consultations, and making any necessary telephone calls are best done right after morning rounds.

Attending Rounds

These vary greatly depending on the service and on the nature of the attending physician. The same people who gathered for morning rounds will be here, with the addition of the attending. At this meeting, the patients are often seen again (especially on the surgical services); significant new laboratory, radiographic, and physical findings are described (often by the student caring for the patient); and new patients are formally presented to the attending (again, often by the medical student).

The most important priority for the student on attending rounds is to **know the patient.** Be prepared to concisely tell the attending what has happened to the patient. Also be ready to give a brief presentation on the patient's illness, especially if it is unusual. The attending will probably not be interested in minor details that do not affect therapeutic decisions. Additionally, the attending will probably not wish to hear a litany of normal laboratory values, only the pertinent ones, such as, Mrs. Pavona's platelets are still 350,000/μL in spite of her bone marrow disease. You do not have to tell everything you know on rounds, but you must be prepared to do so.

Open disputes among house staff and students are bad form on attending rounds. For this reason, the unwritten rule is that any differences of opinion not previously discussed shall not be initially raised in the presence of the attending.

Check-out or Evening Rounds

Formal evening rounds on which the patients are seen by the entire team a second time are typically done only on surgical services and pediatrics. Other services, such as, medicine, often will have check-out with the resident on call for the service that evening (sometimes called "card rounds"). Expect to convene sometime between 3:00 and 7:00 PM on most days. All new data are presented by the person who collected them (usually the student). Orders are again written, laboratory work desired for early the next day is requested, and those unfortunates on call compile a "scut list" of work to be done that night and a list of patients who need close supervision.

BEDSIDE ROUNDS

Basically, these are the same as any other rounds except that tact is at a premium. The first consideration at the bedside must be for the patient. If no one else on the team says "Good morning" and asks how the patient is feeling, do it yourself; this is not a presumptuous act on your part. Keep this encounter brief and then explain that you will be talking about the patient for a while. If handled in this fashion, the patient will often feel flattered by the attention and will listen to you with interest.

Certain points in a hallway presentation are omitted in the patient's room. The patient's race and sex are usually apparent to all and do not warrant inclusion in your first sentence. The patient must *never* be called by the name of the disease, eg, Mrs. Pavona is not "a 45-year-old CML (chronic myelogenous leukemia)" but "a 45-year-old *with* CML." The patient's general appearance need not be reiterated. Descriptions of evidence of disease must not be prefaced by words such as *outstanding* or *beautiful*. Mrs. Pavona's massive spleen is not beautiful to her, and it should not be to the physician or student either.

At the bedside, keep both feet on the floor. A foot up on a bed or chair conveys impatience and disinterest to the patient and other members of the team. It is poor form to carry beverages or food into the patient's room.

Although you will probably never be asked to examine a patient during bedside rounds, it is still worthwhile to know how to do so considerately. Bedside examinations are often done by the attending at the time of the initial presentation or by one member of a surgical service on postoperative rounds. First, warn the patient that you are about to examine the wound or affected part. Ask the patient to uncover whatever needs to be exposed rather than boldly removing the patient's clothes yourself. If the patient is unable to do so alone, you may do it, but remember to explain what you are doing. Remove only as much clothing as is necessary and then promptly cover the patient again. In a ward room, remember to pull the curtain.

Bedside rounds in the intensive care unit call for as much consideration as they do in any other room. That still, naked soul on the bed might not be as "out of it" as the resident (or anyone else) might believe and may be hearing every word you say. Again, exercise discretion in discussing the patient's illness, plan, prognosis, and personal character as it relates to the disease.

Remember that the patient information you are entrusted with as a health care provider is confidential. There is a time and place to discuss this sensitive information and public areas such as elevators or cafeterias are not the appropriate location for these discussions.

READING

Time for reading is at a premium on many services, and it is therefore important to use that time effectively. Unless you can remember everything you learned in the first 20 months of medical school, you will probably want to review the basic facts about the disease that brought your patient into the hospital. These facts are most often found in the same core texts that got you through the preclinical years. Unless specifically directed to do so, avoid the temptation to sit down with MEDLINE/*Index Medicus* to find all the latest articles on a disease you have not read about for the last 7 months; you do not have the time.

The appropriate time to head for the MEDLINE/*Index Medicus* is when a therapeutic dilemma arises and only the most recent literature will adequately advise the team. You may wish to obtain some direction from the attending, the fellow, or the resident before plunging into the library on your only Friday night off call this month. Ask the residents or fellow students for the pocket manuals or PDA downloads that they found most useful for a given rotation.

THE WRITTEN HISTORY AND PHYSICAL

Much has been written on how to obtain a useful medical history and perform a thorough physical examination, and there is little to add to it. Three things worth emphasizing are your own physical findings, your impression, and your own differential diagnosis.

Trust and record your own physical findings, even if other examiners have written things different from those you found. You just may be right, and, if not, you have learned something from it. Avoid the temptation to copy another examiner's findings as your own when you are unable to do the examination yourself. Still, it would be an unusually cruel resident who would make you give Mrs. Pavona her fourth rectal examination of the day, and in this circumstance you may write "rectal per resident." *Do not do this routinely just to avoid performing a complete physical examination. Check with the resident first.*

Although not always emphasized in physical diagnosis, your clinical impression is probably the most important part of your write-up. Reasoned interpretation of the medical history and physical examination is what separates physicians from the computers touted by the tabloids as their successors. Judgment is learned only by boldly stating your case, even if you are wrong more often than not.

The differential diagnosis, that is, your impression, should include only those entities that you consider when evaluating your patient. Avoid including every possible cause of your patient's ailments. List only those that you are seriously considering, and include in your plan what you intend to do to exclude each one. Save the exhaustive list for the time your attending asks for all the causes of a symptom, syndrome, or abnormal laboratory value.

THE PRESENTATION

The object of the presentation is to *briefly* and *concisely* (usually in a few minutes) describe your patient's reason for being in the hospital to all members of the team who do not know the patient and the story. Unlike the write-up, which contains all the data you obtained, the presentation may include only the pertinent positive and negative evidence of a disease and its course in the patient. It is hard to get a feel for what is pertinent until you have seen and done a few presentations yourself.

Practice is important. Try never to read from your write-up, as this often produces dull and lengthy presentations. Most attendings will allow you to carry note cards, but this method can also lead to trouble unless content is carefully edited. Presentations are given in the same order as a write-up: identification, chief complaint, history of the present illness, past medical history, family history, psychosocial history, review of systems, physical examination, laboratory and x-ray data, clinical impression, and plan. Only pertinent positives and negatives from the review of systems should be given. These and truly relevant items from other parts of the interview often can be added to the history of the present illness. Finally, the length and content of the presentation vary greatly according to the wishes of the attending and the resident, but you will learn quickly what they do and do not want.

RESPONSIBILITY

Your responsibilities as a student should be clearly defined on the first day of a rotation by either the attending or the resident. Ideally, this enumeration of your duties should also include a list of what you might expect concerning teaching, floor skills, presentations, and all the other things you are paying many thousand dollars a year to learn.

On some services, you may feel like a glorified unit secretary (clinical rotations are called "clerkships" for good reason!), and you will not be far from wrong. This is *not* what you are going into hock for. The scut work should be divided among the house staff.

You will frequently be expected to call for a certain piece of laboratory data or to go review an x-ray with the radiologist. You may then mutter under your breath, "Why waste my time? The report will be on the chart in a day or two!" You will feel less annoyed in this situation if you consider that every piece of data ordered is vital to the care of your patient.

Outpatient clinic experiences are incorporated into many rotations today. The same basic rules and skill set necessary for inpatient care can be easily transferred to the outpatient setting.

The student's responsibility may be summarized in three words: **know your patient.** The whole service relies to a great extent on a well-informed presentation by the student. The better informed you are, the more time left for education and the better your evaluation will be. A major part of becoming a physician is learning responsibility.

ORDERS

Orders are the physician's instructions to the nursing and other members of the professional staff on the care of the patient. These may include the frequency of vital signs, medications, respiratory care, laboratory and x-ray studies, and nearly anything else that you can imagine.

There are many formats for writing concise admission, transfer, and postoperative orders. Some rotations may have a precisely fixed set of routine orders, but others will leave you and the intern to your own devices. It is important in each case to avoid omitting instructions critical to the care of the patient. Although you will be confronted with a variety of lists and mnemonics, ultimately it is helpful to devise your own system and commit it to memory. Why memorize? Because when you are an intern and it is 3:30 AM, you may overlook something if you try to think it out. One system for writing admission or transfer orders uses the mnemonic "A.D.C. Vaan Diml" and is discussed in Chapter 2.

The word *stat* is the abbreviation for the Latin word *statim,* which means "immediately." When added to any order, it puts the requested study in front of all the routine work waiting to be done. Ideally, this order is reserved for the truly urgent situation, but in practice it is often inappropriately used. Most of the blame for this situation rests with physicians who either fail to plan ahead or order stat lab results when routine studies would do.

Student orders usually require a co-signature from a physician, although at some institutions students are allowed to order routine laboratory studies. Do not ask a nurse or pharmacist to act on an unsigned student order; it is **illegal** for them to do so.

The intern is usually responsible for most orders. The amount of interest shown by the resident and the attending varies greatly, but ideally you will review the orders on routinely admitted patients with the intern. Have the intern show you how to write some orders on a few patients, then take the initiative and write the orders yourself and review them with the intern.

THE DAY

The events of the day and the effective use of time are two of the most distressing enigmas encountered in making the transition from preclinical to clinical education. For example, there are no typical days on surgical services, as the operating room schedule prohibits making rounds at a regularly scheduled time every day. The following are suggestions that will help on any service.

1. Schedule special studies early in the day. The free time after work rounds is usually ideal for this. Also, call consultants early in the morning. Often, they can see your patient on the same day or at least early the next day.

2. Try to take care of all your business in the radiology department in one trip unless a given problem requires viewing a film promptly. *Do not* make as many separate trips as you have patients.

3. Make a point of knowing when certain services become unavailable, for example, electrocardiograms, contrast-study scheduling, and blood drawing. Be sure to get these procedures done while it is still possible to do so.

4. Make a daily work or "scut"* list, and write down laboratory results as soon as you obtain them. Few people can keep all the daily data in their heads without making errors.

5. Try to arrange your travels around the hospital efficiently. If you have patients to see on four different floors, try to take care of all their needs, such as, drawing blood, removing sutures, writing progress notes, and calling for consultations, in one trip.

6. Strive to work thoroughly but quickly. If you do not try to get work done early, you never will (this is not to say that you will succeed even if you do try). There is no sin in leaving at 5:00 PM or earlier if your obligations are *completed* and the supervising resident has dismissed you.

A PARTING SHOT

The clinical years are when all the years of premed study in college and the first two years of medical school suddenly come together. Trying to tell you adequately about being a clinical clerk is similar to trying to make someone into a swimmer on dry land.

The terms to describe new clinical clerks may vary at different medical centers ("scut monkey," "scut boy," "scut dog," "torpedoes"). These euphemistic expressions describing the new clinical clerk acknowledge that the transition, a sort of rite of passage, into the next phase of physician training has occurred. It is hoped that this "So You Want to Be a Scut Monkey" introduction and the information contained in this book will give you a good start as you enter the "hands on" phase of becoming a successful and respected physician.

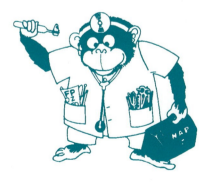

---

* Although the origin of the word *scut* is obscure, it probably represents an acronym for "some common unfinished task" or "some clinically useful training."

HISTORY AND PHYSICAL EXAMINATION

History and Physical Examination
Psychiatric History and Physical
   Psychiatric Mental Status
      Examination
   Mini Mental Status Examination
Heart Murmurs and Extra Heart Sounds
Blood Pressure Guidelines

Dental Examination
Dermatologic Descriptions
Dermatome and Cutaneous Innervation
Physical Symptoms and Eponyms
Example of a Written History and
   Physical Examination

HISTORY AND PHYSICAL EXAMINATION

An example of a complete H&P write-up can be found on page 28. The details provided and length of the written H&P can vary with the particular problem and with the service to which the patient is admitted.

History

Identification: Name, age, sex, referring physician, and the informant (eg, patient, relative, old chart) and the informant's reliability.

Chief Complaint: State, in patient's own words, the current problem.

History of the Present Illness (HPI):   Defines the present illness by quality; quantity; setting; anatomic location and radiation; time course, including when it began; whether the complaint is progressing, regressing, or steady; of constant or intermittent frequency; and aggravating, alleviating, and associated factors. The information should be in chronologic order, including diagnostic tests done prior to admission. Related history, including previous treatment for the problem, risk factors, and pertinent negatives should be included. Any other significant ongoing problems should be included in the HPI in a separate section or paragraph. For instance, if a patient with poorly controlled diabetes mellitus comes to the emergency room because of chest pain, the HPI would first include information regarding the chest pain followed by a detailed history of the diabetes mellitus. If the diabetes mellitus was well controlled or diet-controlled, the history of the diabetes mellitus is placed in the past medical history.

Past Medical History (PMH):   Current medications, including OTC medications, vitamins, and herbals; allergies (drugs and other—include how allergies are manifested); surgeries; hospitalizations; blood transfusions, include when and how many units and the type of blood product; trauma; stable current and past medical problems unrelated to the HPI. Specific illnesses to inquire about include diabetes mellitus, hypertension, MI, stroke, peptic ulcer disease, asthma, emphysema, thyroid and kidney disease, bleeding disorders, cancer,

TB, hepatitis, and STDs. Also inquire about routine health maintenance. This category depends on the age and sex of the patient but could include last Pap smear and pelvic exam, breast exam, whether the patient does self breast examination, date of last mammogram, diphtheria/tetanus immunization, pneumococcal and flu vaccine, stool samples for hemoccult, sigmoidoscopy, cholesterol, HDL cholesterol, and use of seat belts. **Pediatric patients:** Include prenatal and birth history, feedings, food intolerance, and immunization history.

Family History: Age, status (alive, dead) of blood relatives and medical problems for any blood relatives (inquiry about cancer, especially breast, colon, and prostate; TB, asthma; MI; HTN; thyroid disease; kidney disease; peptic ulcer disease; diabetes mellitus; bleeding disorders; glaucoma, and macular degeneration). Can be written out or use family tree.

Psychosocial (Social) History: Stressors (financial, significant relationships, work or school, health) and support (family, friends, significant other, clergy); life-style risk factors, (alcohol, drugs, tobacco, and caffeine use; diet; and exposure to environmental agents; and sexual practices); patient profile (may include marital status and children; present and past employment; financial support and insurance; education; religion; hobbies; beliefs; living conditions); for veterans, include military service history. **Pediatric patients:** Include grade in school, sleep, and play habits.

Review of Systems (ROS)

General. Weight loss, weight gain, fatigue, weakness, appetite, fever, chills, night sweats

Skin. Rashes, pruritus, bruising, dryness, skin cancer or other lesions

Head. Trauma, headache, tenderness, dizziness, syncope

Eyes. Vision, changes in the visual field, glasses, last prescription change, photophobia, blurring, diplopia, spots or floaters, inflammation, discharge, dry eyes, excessive tearing, history of cataracts or glaucoma

Ears. Hearing changes, tinnitus, pain, discharge, vertigo, history of ear infections

Nose. Sinus problems, epistaxis, obstruction, polyps, changes in or loss of sense of smell

Throat. Bleeding gums; dental history (last checkup, etc); ulcerations or other lesions on tongue, gums, buccal mucosa

Respiratory. Chest pain; dyspnea; cough; amount and color of sputum; hemoptysis; history of pneumonia, influenza, pneumococcal vaccinations, or positive PPD

Cardiovascular. Chest pain, orthopnea, dyspnea on exertion, paroxysmal nocturnal dyspnea, murmurs, claudication, peripheral edema, palpitations

Gastrointestinal. Dysphagia, heartburn, nausea, vomiting, hematemesis, indigestion, abdominal pain, diarrhea, constipation, melena (hematochezia), hemorrhoids, change in stool shape and color, jaundice, fatty food intolerance

Gynecologic. Gravida/para/abortions; age at menarche; last menstrual period (frequency, duration, flow); dysmenorrhea; spotting; menopause; contraception; sexual history, including history of venereal disease, frequency of intercourse, number of partners, sexual orientation and satisfaction, and dyspareunia

Genitourinary. Frequency, urgency, hesitancy; dysuria; hematuria; polyuria; nocturia; incontinence; venereal disease; discharge; sterility; impotence; polyuria; polydipsia; change in urinary stream; and sexual history, including frequency of intercourse, number of partners, sexual orientation and satisfaction, and history of venereal disease

Endocrine. Polyuria, polydipsia, polyphagia, temperature intolerance, glycosuria, hormone therapy, changes in hair or skin texture

Musculoskeletal. Arthralgias, arthritis, trauma, joint swelling, redness, tenderness, limitations in ROM, back pain, musculoskeletal trauma, gout

Peripheral Vascular. Varicose veins, intermittent claudication, history of thrombophlebitis

Hematology. Anemia, bleeding tendency, easy bruising, lymphadenopathy

Neuropsychiatric. Syncope; seizures; weakness; coordination problems; alterations in sensations, memory, mood, sleep pattern; emotional disturbances; drug and alcohol problems

Physical Examination

General: Mood, stage of development, race, and sex. State if patient is in any distress or is assuming an unusual position, such as, sitting up leaning forward (position often seen in patients with acute exacerbation of COPD or pericarditis)

Vital Signs: Temperature (note if oral, rectal, axillary), pulse, respirations, blood pressure (may include right arm, left arm, lying, sitting, standing), height, weight. Blood pressure and heart rate supine and after standing 1 min should always be included if volume depletion is suspected, such as in GI bleeding, diarrhea, dizziness, or syncope

Skin: Rashes, eruptions, scars, tattoos, moles, hair pattern (See page 20 for definitions of dermatologic lesions.)

Lymph Nodes: Location (head and neck, supraclavicular, epitrochlear, axillary, inguinal), size, tenderness, motility, consistency

Head, Eyes, Ears, Nose, and Throat (HEENT)

Head. Size and shape, tenderness, trauma, bruits. **Pediatric patients:** Fontanels, suture lines

Eyes. Conjunctiva; sclera; lids; position of eyes in orbits; pupil size, shape, reactivity; extraocular muscle movements; visual acuity (eg, 20/20); visual fields; fundi (disc color, size, margins, cupping, spontaneous venous pulsations, hemorrhages, exudates, A-V ratio, nicking)

Ears. Test hearing, tenderness, discharge, external canal, tympanic membrane (intact, dull or shiny, bulging, motility, fluid or blood, injected)

Nose. Symmetry; palpate over frontal, maxillary, and ethmoid sinuses; inspect for obstruction, lesions, exudate, inflammation. **Pediatric patients:** Nasal flaring, grunting

Throat. Lips, teeth, gums, tongue, pharynx (lesions, erythema, exudate, tonsillar size, presence of crypts)

Neck: ROM, tenderness, JVD, lymph nodes, thyroid examination, location of larynx, carotid bruits, HJR. JVD should be reported in relationship to the number of centimeters above or below the sternal angle, such as "1 cm above the sternal angle," rather than "no JVD."

Chest: Configuration and symmetry of movement with respiration; intercostal retractions; palpation for tenderness, fremitus, and chest wall expansion; percussion (include diaphragmatic excursion); breath sounds; adventitious sounds (rales, rhonchi, wheezes, rubs). If indicated: vocal fremitus, whispered pectoriloquy, egophony (found with consolidation)

Heart: Rate, inspection, and palpation of precordium for point of maximal impulse and thrill; auscultation at the apex, LLSB, and right and left second intercostal spaces with diaphragm and apex and LLSB with bell. Heart murmurs are reviewed on pages 16 to 18.

Breast: Inspection for nipple discharge, inversion, excoriations and fissures, and skin dimpling or flattening of the contour; palpation for masses, tenderness; gynecomastia in males

Abdomen: Note shape (scaphoid, flat, distended, obese); examine for scars; auscultate for bowel sounds and bruits; percussion for tympani and masses; measure liver size (span in midclavicular line); note costovertebral angle tenderness; palpate for tenderness (if present, check for rebound tenderness), note hepatomegaly, splenomegaly; guarding, inguinal adenopathy

Male Genitalia: Inspect for penile lesions, scrotal swelling, testicles (size, tenderness, masses, varicocele), and hernia, and observe for transillumination of testicular masses
Pelvic: See Chapter 13, page 289.
Rectal: Inspect and palpate for hemorrhoids, fissures, skin tags, sphincter tone, masses, prostate (size [grade from small 1+ to massively enlarged 4+], note any nodules, tenderness); note presence or absence of stool; test stool for occult blood
Musculoskeletal: Note amputations, deformities, visible joint swelling, and ROM; also palpate joints for swelling, tenderness, and warmth
Peripheral Vascular: Note hair pattern; color change of skin; varicosities; cyanosis; clubbing; palpation of radial, ulnar, brachial, femoral, popliteal, posterior tibial, dorsalis pedis pulses; simultaneous radial pulses; calf tenderness; Homans's sign; edema; auscultate for femoral bruits
Neurologic
Mental Status Examination. (If appropriate, see sections "Psychiatric History and Physical," and "Psychiatric Mental Status Examination," page 13.)
Cranial Nerves. There are 12 cranial nerves, the functions of which are as follows:

- **I** Olfactory—Smell
- **II** Optic—Vision, visual fields, and fundi; afferent limb of pupillary response
- **III, IV, VI** Oculomotor, trochlear, abducens—Efferent limb pupillary response, ptosis, volitional eye movements, pursuit eye movements
- **V** Trigeminal—Corneal reflex (afferent), facial sensation, masseter and temporalis muscle tested by biting down
- **VII** Facial—Raise eyebrows, close eyes tight, show teeth, smile, or whistle, corneal reflex (efferent)
- **VIII** Acoustic—Test hearing by watch tick, finger rub, Weber–Rinne test (see also page 27) to be done if hearing loss noted on history or by gross testing. (Air conduction lasts longer than bone conduction in a normal person.)
- **IX, X** Glossopharyngeal and vagus—Palate moves in midline; gag; speech
- **XI** Spinal accessory—Shoulder shrug, push head against resistance.
- **XII** Hypoglossal—Stick out tongue. Strength can be tested by having the patient press tongue against the buccal mucosa on each side and the examiner can press a finger against the patient's cheek. Also look for fasciculations.

Motor. Strength should be tested in upper and lower extremities proximally and distally. (Grading system: 5 active motion against full resistance; 4 active motion against some resistance; 3 active motion against gravity; 2 active motion with gravity eliminated; 1 barely detectable motion; 0 no motion or muscular contraction detected)
Cerebellum. Romberg's test (see page 27)—heel to shin (should not be with assistance from gravity), finger to nose, heel and toe walking, rapid alternating movements upper and lower extremities
Sensory. Pain (sharp) or temperature distal and proximal upper and lower extremities, vibration using either a 128- or 256-Hz tuning fork or position sense distally upper and lower extremities, and stereognosis or graphesthesia. Identify any deficit using the dermatome and cutaneous innervation diagrams (see Figure 1–3).
Reflexes. Brachioradialis and biceps C5–6, triceps C7–8, abdominal (upper T8–10, lower T10–12), quadriceps (knee) L3–4–5, ankle S1–2, (Grading system: 4+ Hyperactive with clonus; 3+ brisker than usual; 2+ normal or average; 1+ decreased or less than normal; 0 absent). Check for pathologic reflexes: Babinski's sign, Hoffmann's sign, snout, others (see pages 21 to 27). **Pediatric patients:** Moro's reflex (startle) and suck reflexes

Database

Laboratory tests, x-rays ordered as indicated by the history and physical

Problem List

(See example page 31.) Should include entry date of problem, date of problem onset, problem number. (With initial problem list, the more severe problems are numbered first. After the initial list is generated, problems are added chronologically.) List problem by status: active or inactive.

Assessment (Impression)

A discussion and evaluation of the current problems with a differential diagnosis.

Plan: Additional laboratory tests, medical treatment, consults, etc.
Note: The history and physical examination should be legibly signed and your title noted. Each entry should be dated and timed.

PSYCHIATRIC HISTORY AND PHYSICAL

The elements of the psychiatric history and physical are identical to those of the basic history and physical outlined earlier. The main difference involves attention to the past psychiatric history and more detailed mental status examination as described in the following section.

Psychiatric Mental Status Examination

The following factors are evaluated as part of the psychiatric status examination.

- **Appearance:** Gestures, mannerisms, and so on
- **Speech:** Coherence, flight of ideas, and so on
- **Mood and Affect:** Depression, elation, anger, and so on
- **Thought Process:** Blocking, evasion, and so on
- **Thought Content:** Worries, hypochondriasis, lack of self-confidence, delusions, hallucinations, and so on
- **Motor Activity:** Slow, rapid, purposeful, and so on
- **Cognitive Functions:**
  Attention and concentration
  Memory (immediate, recent, and remote recall)
  Calculations
  Abstractions
  Judgment

Mini Mental Status Examination

A thorough mental status exam should be done on every geriatric patient, every patient with AIDS, and any patient suspected of having dementia. The mini mental status exam is a simple, practical test that takes only a few minutes and can be followed over time. It may show progression, improvement, or no changes in the underlying process. The mini mental status exam developed by Folstein, Folstein, and McHugh is discussed in detail in the *Journal of Psychiatric Research*, 1975, Vol. 12, pages 189–198. The test is divided into two sections: one assessing orientation, memory, and attention and the other testing the patient's ability to write a sentence and to copy a diagram (usually two intersecting pentagons whose intersect forms a four-sided figure. Table 1–1 is the "Mini Mental State" Examination as outlined by Folstein and associates.

HEART MURMURS AND EXTRA HEART SOUNDS

Table 1–2 and Figure 1–1 describe the various types of heart murmurs and extra heart sounds.

BLOOD PRESSURE GUIDELINES

There is a clear association between hypertension and coronary artery and cerebrovascular disease.

Hypertension is defined as systolic BP >140 mm Hg or a diastolic BP >90 mm Hg in adults. Measure the BP after 5 min of rest with patient seated and arm at heart level. Use the bell of the stethoscope, the last sounds heard are the Korotkoff sounds, which are low-pitched. Take the average of two readings separated by 2 min. Elevated readings on three separate days should be obtained prior to diagnosing hypertension. Classification and follow-up recommendations for adults are shown in Table 1–3.

In children from age 1 to 10 years, systolic blood pressure can be calculated as follows:

Lower limits (5th percentile): 70 mm Hg + (child's age in years × 2)
Typical (50th percentile): 90 mm Hg + (child's age in years × 2)

DENTAL EXAMINATION

The dental examination is an often overlooked part of the history and physical. Many times, the patient may have some intraoral problem that is contributing to the overall medical condition (ie, the inability to eat due to a toothache, abscess, or ill-fitting denture in a poorly controlled diabetic) for which a dental consult may be necessary. Loose dentures can compromise the ability to manually maintain an open airway. In addition, in an emergency situation when intubation is necessary, complications may occur if the clinician is unfamiliar with the oral structures.

The patient may be able to give some dental history, including recent toothaches, abscesses, and loose teeth or dentures. Be sure to ask if the patient is wearing a removable partial denture (partial plate), which should be removed before intubation. As lost dentures are a chief dental complaint of hospitalized patients, care must be taken not to misplace the removed prosthesis.

A brief dental examination may be performed with gloved hand, two tongue blades, and a flashlight. Look for any obvious inflammation, erythema, edema, or ulceration of the gingiva (gums) and oral mucosa. Gently tap on any natural teeth to test for sensitivity. Place each tooth between two tongue blades and push gently to check for looseness. This is especially important for the maxillary anterior teeth, which serve as the fulcrum for the laryngoscope blade. Any abnormal dental findings should be noted and the appropriate consults obtained. Many diseases, including AIDS, STDs, pemphigus, pemphigoid, allergies, uncontrolled diabetes, leukemia, and others, may first manifest themselves in the mouth.

Hospitalized patients often have difficulty cleaning their teeth or dentures. This care should be added to the daily orders if indicated. Patients who will be receiving head and neck radiation must be examined and treated for any tooth extractions or dental infections before the initiation of the radiation therapy. Extractions after radiation to the maxilla and particularly the mandible may lead to osteoradionecrosis, a condition that may be impossible to control.

(*text continues on page 17*)

TABLE 1-1
The Mini Mental State Examination

Patient _____
Examiner _____
Date _____

"Mini Mental State"

Maximum Score	Score	

Orientation

5
What is the (year) (season) (date) (day) (month)?

5
Where are we? (state) (county) (town) (hospital) (floor)

Registration

3
Name 3 objects: 1 second to say each. Then ask the patient all 3 after you have said them. Give 1 point for each correct answer. Then repeat until he learns all 3. Count trials and record.
Trials _____

Attention and Calculation

5
Serial 7's: One point for each correct. Stop after 5 answers. Alternatively, spell "world" backward.

Recall

3
Ask for the 3 objects repeated above. Give 1 point for each correct answer.

Language

9
Point to a pencil, and watch and ask the patient to name it. (2 points)
Repeat the following: "No if's, and's, or but's." (1 point)
Follow a 3-stage command: "Take a paper in your right hand, fold it in half, and put it on the floor." (3 points)
Read and obey the following:

Close your eyes	(1 point)
Write a sentence	(1 point)
Copy design	(1 point)

_____ Total Score

Assess level of consciousness along the following continuum

Alert	Drowsy	Stupor	Coma

Source: Based on data from Folstein, Folstein, and McHugh: *J Psychiatr Res* 1975; **12:**189–198, 1975.

TABLE 1–2
Heart Murmurs and Extra Heart Sounds*

Type†	Description
A. Aortic stenosis (AS)	Heard best at second intercostal space. Systolic (medium-pitched) crescendo–decrescendo murmur with radiation to the carotid arteries. A_2 decreased, ejection click and S_4 often heard at apex. Paradoxical splitting of S_2. Narrow pulse pressure and delayed carotid upstroke and left ventricular hypertrophy (LVH) with lift at apex.
B. Aortic insufficiency (AI)	Heard best at left lower sternal border third and fourth interspace with patient sitting up, leaning forward and fully exhaled. Diastolic (high-pitched) decrescendo murmur. Often with LVH. Widened pulse pressure, bisferious pulse, Traube's sign, Quincke's sign, and Corrigan's pulse may be seen with chronic aortic insufficiency. S_3 and pulsus alternans often present with acute aortic insufficiency.
C. Pulmonic stenosis (PS)	Heard best at left second intercostal space. Systolic crescendo–decrescendo murmur. Louder with inspiration. Click often present. P_2 delayed and soft if severe. Right ventricular hypertrophy (RVH) with parasternal lift.
D. Pulmonic insufficiency (PI)	Heard best at left second intercostal space. Diastolic decrescendo or crescendo–decrescendo murmur. Louder with inspiration. RVH usually present.
E. Mitral stenosis (MS)	Localized at the apex. Diastolic (low-pitched rumbling sound) murmur heard best with the bell in the left lateral decubitus position. With increased or decreased S_1. Opening snap (OS) heard best at apex with diaphragm. Increased P_2, right-sided S_4, left-sided S_3 often present. RVH with parasternal lift may be present.
F. Mitral insufficiency (MI)	Heard best at apex. Holosystolic (high-pitched) murmur with radiation to axilla. Soft S_1, may be masked by murmur. S_3 and LVH often present. Midsystolic click suggests mitral valve prolapse.
G. Tricuspid insufficiency (TI)	Heard best at left lower sternal border. Holosystolic (high-pitched) murmur. Increases with inspiration. Right-sided S_3 often present. Large V wave in jugular venous pulsations.

(continued)

**TABLE 1–2
(Continued)**

Type[†]	Description
H. Atrial septal defect (ASD)	Heard best at left upper sternal border. Systolic (medium-pitched) murmur. Fixed splitting of S_2 and RVH, often with left- and right-sided S_4.
I. Ventricular septal defect (VSD)	Heard best at left lower sternal border. Harsh holosystolic (high-pitched) murmur with midsystolic peak. S_1 and S_2 may be soft.
J. Patent ductus arteriosus (PDA)	Heard best at left first and second intercostal space. Continuous, machinery (medium-pitched) murmur. Increased P_2 and ejection click may be present.
K. Third heard sound (S_3)	Early diastolic sound caused by rapid ventricular filling. Heard best with bell. Left-sided S_3 heard at apex, right-sided S_3 heard at left lower sternal border. Left-sided S_3 seen normally in young people, also pregnancy, thyrotoxicosis, mitral regurgitation, and congestive heart failure.
L. Fourth heart sound (S_4)	Late diastolic sound caused by a noncompliant ventricle. Heard best with bell. Left-sided S_4 heard at apex, right-sided S_4 heard at left lower sternal border. Left-sided S_4 seen with hypertension, aortic stenosis, and myocardial infarction. Right-sided S_4 seen with pulmonic stenosis and pulmonary hypertension.

*Refer to Figure 1–1 for graphic representations of murmurs.
[†]Capital letters preceding type of murmur refer to graphs in Figure 1–1.

Eruption of Teeth

The eruption of teeth may be of great concern to new parents. Often, parents think something is developmentally wrong with their child if teeth have not appeared by a certain age. The timing of tooth eruption varies tremendously. Factors contributing to this variation include family history, ethnic background, vitality during fetal development, position of teeth in the arch, size and shape of the dental arch itself, and, in the case of the eruption of permanent teeth, when the primary tooth was lost. Radiographs of the maxilla and mandible can determine whether or not the teeth are present. Figure 1–2 serves as a guide to the chronology of tooth eruption. Remember that variations may be greater than 1 year in some cases.

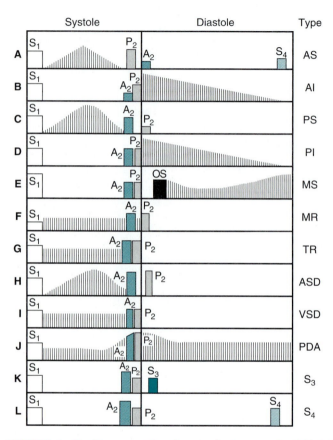

FIGURE 1-1 Graphic representation of common heart murmurs. See Table 1-2 for abbreviations and descriptions of murmurs.

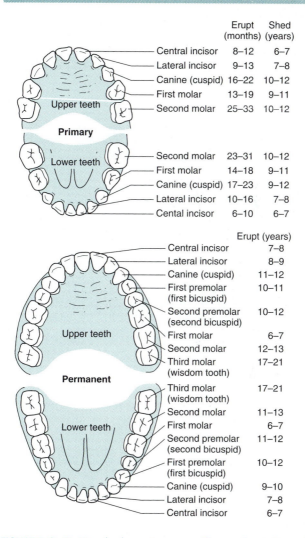

	Erupt (months)	Shed (years)
Primary — Upper teeth		
Central incisor	8–12	6–7
Lateral incisor	9–13	7–8
Canine (cuspid)	16–22	10–12
First molar	13–19	9–11
Second molar	25–33	10–12
Primary — Lower teeth		
Second molar	23–31	10–12
First molar	14–18	9–11
Canine (cuspid)	17–23	9–12
Lateral incisor	10–16	7–8
Cental incisor	6–10	6–7

	Erupt (years)
Permanent — Upper teeth	
Central incisor	7–8
Lateral incisor	8–9
Canine (cuspid)	11–12
First premolar (first bicuspid)	10–11
Second premolar (second bicuspid)	10–12
First molar	6–7
Second molar	12–13
Third molar (wisdom tooth)	17–21
Permanent — Lower teeth	
Third molar (wisdom tooth)	17–21
Second molar	11–13
First molar	6–7
Second premolar (second bicuspid)	11–12
First premolar (first bicuspid)	10–12
Canine (cuspid)	9–10
Lateral incisor	7–8
Central incisor	6–7

FIGURE 1–2 Dentition development sequences. The age when teeth are shed and erupt varies widely. (Based on data from: McDonald RE and Avery DR [eds]: *Dentistry for the Child and Adolescent*, Mosby, St. Louis, 1994. Used with permission.)

TABLE 1–3
Guidelines for Blood Pressure Management in Adults

CLASSIFICATION SYSTEM

Category	Systolic (mm Hg)	Diastolic (mm Hg)
Desired	<120	<80
Normal	<130	<85
High normal	130–139	85–89
Hypertension		
Stage 1	140–159	90–99
Stage 2	160–179	100–109
Stage 3	>180	>110

FOLLOW-UP RECOMMENDATIONS
INITIAL SCREENING BP
(MM HG)

Systolic	Diastolic	Action
<130	<85	Recheck in 2 years
130–139	85–89	Recheck in 1 yr
140–159	90–99	Confirm within 2 months
160–179	100–109	Evaluate or refer within 1 month
>180	>110	Evaluate or refer immediately or within 1 wk depending on the clinical situation

DERMATOLOGIC DESCRIPTIONS

Atrophy: Thinning of the surface of the skin with associated loss of normal markings. Examples: Aging, striae associated with obesity, scleroderma

Bulla: A superficial, well-circumscribed, raised, fluid-filled lesion greater than 1 cm in diameter. Examples: Bullous pemphigoid, pemphigus, dermatitis herpetiformis

Burrow: A subcutaneous linear track made by a parasite. Example: Scabies

Crust: A slightly raised lesion with irregular border and variable color resulting from dried blood, serum, or other exudate. Examples: Scab resulting from an abrasion, or impetigo

Ecchymoses: A flat, nonblanching, red-purple-blue lesion that results from extravasation of red blood cells into the skin. Differs from purpura in that ecchymoses are large purpura. Examples: Trauma, long-term steroid use

Erosion: A depressed lesion resulting from loss of epidermis due to rupture of vesicles or bullae. Example: Rupture of herpes simplex blister

Excoriation: A linear superficial lesion, which may be covered with dried blood. Early lesions with surrounding erythema. Often self-induced. Example: Scratching associated with pruritus from any cause

Fissure: A deep linear lesion into the dermis. Example: Cracks seen in athlete's foot

Keloid: Irregular, raised lesion resulting from scar tissue that is hypertrophied. Examples: Often seen with burns, and African-Americans are more prone to keloid formation.

Lichenification: A thickening of the skin with an increase in skin markings resulting from chronic irritation and rubbing. Example: Atopic dermatitis

Macule: A circumscribed nonpalpable discoloration of the skin less than 1 cm in diameter. Examples: Freckles, rubella, petechiae

Nodule: A solid, palpable, circumscribed lesion larger than a papule and smaller than a tumor. Examples: Erythema nodosum, gouty tophi

Papule: A solid elevated lesion less than 1 cm. Examples: Acne, warts, insect bites

Patch: A nonpalpable discoloration of the skin with an irregular border, greater than 1 cm in diameter. Example: Vitiligo

Petechiae: A flat pinhead-sized, nonblanching, red-purple lesion caused by hemorrhage into the skin. Example: Seen in DIC, ITP, SLE, meningococcemia (*Neisseria meningitidis*)

Plaque: A solid, flat, elevated lesion greater than 1 cm in diameter. Examples: Psoriasis, discoid lupus erythematosus, actinic keratosis

Purpura: A flat, nonblanching, red-purple lesion larger than petechiae caused by hemorrhage into the skin. Examples: Henoch–Schönlein purpura, TTP.

Pustule: A vesicle that is filled with purulent fluid. Examples: Acne, impetigo

Scales: Partial separation of the superficial layer of skin. Examples: Psoriasis, dandruff

Scar: Replacement of normal skin with fibrous tissue, often resulting from injury. Examples: Surgical scar, burn

Telangiectasia: Dilatation of capillaries resulting in red, irregular, clustered lines that blanch. Examples: Seen in scleroderma, Osler–Weber–Rendu disease, cirrhosis

Tumor: A solid, palpable, circumscribed lesion that is greater than 2 cm in diameter. Example: Lipoma

Ulcer: A depressed lesion resulting from loss of epidermis and part of the dermis. Examples: Decubitus ulcers, primary lesion of syphilis, venous stasis ulcer

Vesicle: A superficial, well-circumscribed, raised, fluid-filled lesion that is less than 1 cm in diameter. Examples: Herpes simplex, varicella (chickenpox)

Wheal: Slightly raised, red, irregular lesions that are transient and secondary to edema of the skin. Examples: Urticaria (hives), allergic reaction to injections or insect bites

DERMATOME AND CUTANEOUS INNERVATION

The diagrams (Figures 1–3A and B) demonstrate dermatome levels and cutaneous innervation distribution useful in the physical examination.

PHYSICAL SYMPTOMS AND EPONYMS

Allen's Test: (See Chapter 13, page 246.)

Apley's Test: Determination of meniscal tear in the knee by grinding the joint manually

Argyll–Robertson Pupil: Bilaterally small, irregular, unequal pupils that react to accommodation but not to light. Seen with tertiary syphilis

Austin Flint Murmur: Late diastolic mitral murmur; associated with aortic insufficiency with a normal mitral valve

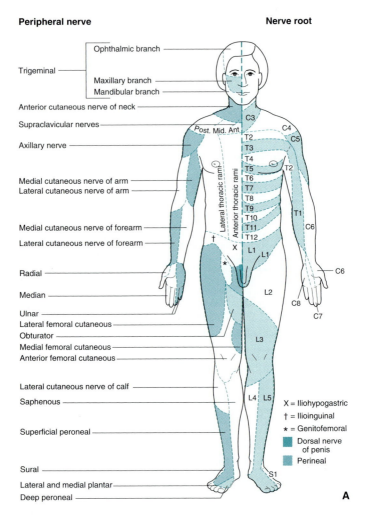

Peripheral nerve

Nerve root

Trigeminal
- Ophthalmic branch
- Maxillary branch
- Mandibular branch

Anterior cutaneous nerve of neck

Supraclavicular nerves

Axillary nerve

Medial cutaneous nerve of arm
Lateral cutaneous nerve of arm

Medial cutaneous nerve of forearm
Lateral cutaneous nerve of forearm

Radial

Median

Ulnar
Lateral femoral cutaneous
Obturator
Medial femoral cutaneous
Anterior femoral cutaneous

Lateral cutaneous nerve of calf
Saphenous

Superficial peroneal

Sural
Lateral and medial plantar
Deep peroneal

Post. Mid. Ant

Lateral thoracic rami

Anterior thoracic rami

C3
C4
C5
T2
T3
T4
T5
T6
T7
T8
T9
T10
T11
T12
L1
L2
L3
L4 L5
S1

T2
T1
C6
C6
C8
C7

X = Iliohypogastric
† = Ilioinguinal
★ = Genitofemoral

Dorsal nerve
of penis

Perineal

A

FIGURE 1–3 A: Dermatomes and cutaneous innervation patterns, anterior view. (Reprinted, with permission, from: Aminoff MJ et al [eds]: *Clinical Neurology*, 3rd ed, Appleton & Lange, Stamford CT, 1996.)

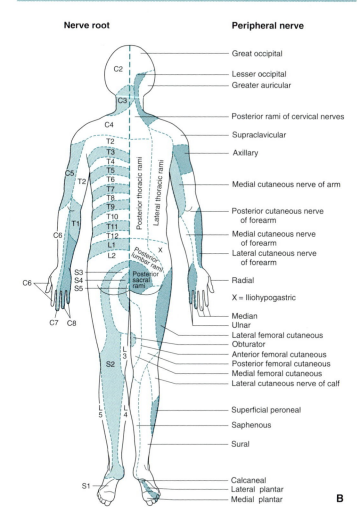

Nerve root   **Peripheral nerve**

Great occipital
Lesser occipital
Greater auricular
Posterior rami of cervical nerves
Supraclavicular
Axillary
Medial cutaneous nerve of arm
Posterior cutaneous nerve of forearm
Medial cutaneous nerve of forearm
Lateral cutaneous nerve of forearm
Radial
X = Iliohypogastric
Median
Ulnar
Lateral femoral cutaneous
Obturator
Anterior femoral cutaneous
Posterior femoral cutaneous
Medial femoral cutaneous
Lateral cutaneous nerve of calf
Superficial peroneal
Saphenous
Sural
Calcaneal
Lateral plantar
Medial plantar

FIGURE 1–3 B: Dermatomes and cutaneous innervation patterns, posterior view. (Reprinted, with permission, from: Aminoff MJ et al [eds]: *Clinical Neurology,* 3rd ed, Appleton & Lange, Stamford CT, 1996.)

Babinski's Sign: Extension of the large toe with stimulation of the plantar surface of the foot instead of the normal flexion; indicative of upper motor neuron disease (normal in neonates)

Bainbridge's Reflex: Increased heart rate due to increased right atrial pressure

Battle's Sign: Ecchymosis behind the ear associated with basilar skull fractures.

Beau's Lines: Transverse depressions in nails due to previous systemic disease

Beck's Triad: JVD, diminished or muffled heart sounds, and decreased blood pressure associated with cardiac tamponade

Bell's Palsy: Lower motor neuron lesion of the facial nerve affecting muscles of upper and lower face. Easily distinguished from upper motor lesions, which affect predominately muscles of lower face since upper motor neurons from each side innervate muscles on both sides of the upper face

Bergman's Triad: Altered mental status, petechiae, and dyspnea associated with fat embolus syndrome

Biot's Breathing: Seen with brain injury; abruptly alternating apnea and equally deep breaths

Bisferious Pulse: A double-peaked pulse seen in severe chronic aortic insufficiency

Bitot's Spots: Small scleral white patches suggesting vitamin A deficiency

Blumberg' Sign: Pain felt in the abdomen when steady constant pressure is quickly released. Seen with peritonitis

Blumer's Shelf: Hardness palpable on rectal examination due to metastatic cancer of the rectouterine (pouch of Douglas) or rectovesical pouch

Bouchard's Nodes: Hard, nontender, painless nodules in the dorsolateral aspects of the proximal interphalangeal joints associated with osteoarthritis. Results from hypertrophy of the bone

Branham's Sign: With large AV fistulas, abrupt slowing of the heart rate with compression of the feeding artery

Brudzinski's Sign: Flexion of the neck causing flexion of the hips in meningitis

Chadwick's Sign: Bluish color of cervix and vagina, seen with pregnancy

Chandelier's Sign: Extreme pain elicited with movement of the cervix during bimanual pelvic examination. Indicates PID

Charcot's Triad: Right upper quadrant pain, fever (chills), and jaundice associated with cholangitis

Cheyne–Stokes Respiration: Repeating cycle of a gradual increase in depth of breathing followed by a gradual decrease to apnea; seen with CNS disorders, uremia, some normal sleep patterns

Chvostek's Sign: Tapping over the facial nerve causes facial spasm in hypocalcemia (tetany). May be normal finding in some patients

Corrigan's Pulse: A palpable hard pulse immediately followed by sudden collapse, seen in aortic regurgitation

Cullen's Sign: Ecchymosis around the umbilicus associated with severe intraperitoneal bleeding. Seen with ruptured ectopic pregnancy and hemorrhagic pancreatitis

Cushing's Triad: Hypertension, bradycardia, and irregular respiration associated with increased intracranial pressure

Darier's Sign: Stroking of the skin causes erythema and edema in mastocytosis

Doll's Eyes: Conjugated movement of eyes in one direction as head is briskly turned in the other direction in comatose patients. Tests oculocephalic reflex indicating intact brain stem

Drawer Sign: Forward (or backward) movement of the tibia with pressure, indicating laxity or a tear in the anterior (or posterior) cruciate ligament

Dupuytren's Contracture: Proliferation of fibrosis tissue of the palmar fascia resulting in contracture of the fourth and/or fifth digits, which is often bilateral. May be hereditary or seen in patients with chronic alcoholic liver disease or seizures

Duroziez's Sign: Found in aortic regurgitation a "to and fro" murmur when stethoscope is pressed over the femoral artery

Electrical Alternans: Beat to beat variation in the electrical axis, seen in large pericardial effusions, suggests impending hemodynamic compromise

Ewart's Sign: Dullness to percussion, increased fremitus and bronchial breathing beneath the angle of the left scapula found with pericardial effusion

Fong Lesion/Syndrome: Autosomal-dominant anomalies of the nails and patella associated with renal abnormalities

Frank's Sign: Fissure of the ear lobe; may be associated with CAD, diabetes, and hypertension

Gibbus: Angular convexity of the spine due to vertebral collapse; associated with osteoporosis or metastasis

Gregg's Triad: Cataracts, heart defects, and deafness with congenital rubella

Grey Turner's Sign: Ecchymosis in the flank associated with retroperitoneal hemorrhage

Grocco's Sign: Triangular area of paravertebral dullness, opposite side of a pleural effusion

Heberden's Nodes: Hard, nontender, painless nodules on the dorsolateral aspects of the distal interphalangeal joints associated with osteoarthritis. Results from hypertrophy of the bone

Hegar's Sign: Softening of the distal uterus. Reliable early sign of pregnancy

Hellenhorst's Plaque: A cholesterol plaque on retina seen on funduscopic examination associated with amaurosis fugax

Hill's Sign: Femoral artery pressure 20 mm Hg greater than brachial pressure seen in severe aortic regurgitation

Hoffmann's Sign/Reflex: Flicking of the volar surface of the distal phalanx causing fingers to flex; associated with pyramidal tract disease

Homans' Sign: Calf pain with forcible dorsiflexion of the foot, associated with venous thrombosis

Horner's Syndrome: Unilateral miosis, ptosis, and anhidrosis (absence of sweating). From destruction of ipsilateral superior cervical ganglion often from lung carcinoma, especially squamous cell carcinoma

Janeway's Lesion: Erythematous or hemorrhagic lesion seen on the palm or sole with subacute bacterial endocarditis

Joffroy's Reflex: Inability to wrinkle the forehead when patient asked to bend head and look up, seen in hyperthyroidism

Kayser–Fleischer Ring: Brown pigment lesion due to copper deposition seen in Wilson's disease

Kehr's Sign: Left shoulder and left upper quadrant pain associated with splenic rupture

Kernig's Sign: When the thigh is flexed at a right angle, complete extension of the leg is not possible because of inflammation of the meninges; seen with meningitis

Koplik's Spots: White papules on buccal mucosa opposite molars seen in measles

Korotkoff's Sounds: Low-pitched sounds resulting from vibration of the artery, detected when obtaining a blood pressure using the bell of the stethoscope. The last Korotkoff sound may be a more accurate estimate of the true diastolic blood pressure than the diastolic blood pressure obtained using the diaphragm.

Kussmaul's Respiration: Deep, rapid respiratory pattern seen in coma or DKA

Kussmaul's Sign: Paradoxical rise in the jugular venous pressure on inspiration in constrictive pericarditis or COPD

Kyphosis: Excessive rounding of the thoracic spinal convexity, associated with aging, especially in women

Lasègue's Sign/Straight-Leg-Raising Sign: The patient is extended in the supine position and raises the leg gently. Pain in the distribution of nerve root suggests sciatica.

Levine's Sign: Clenched fist over the chest while describing chest pain; associated with angina and AMI

Lhermitte's Sign: In MS, neck flexion results in a "shock sensation."

List: Lateral tilt of the spine, frequently associated with herniated disk and muscle spasm

Lordosis: Accentuated normal concavity of the lumbar spine, normal in pregnancy

Louvel's Sign: Coughing or sneezing causes pain in the leg with DVT

Marcus–Gunn Pupil: Dilation of pupils with swinging flashlight test. Results from unilateral optic nerve disease. Normal pupillary response is elicited when light is directed from the normal eye and a subnormal response when light is quickly directed from the normal eye into the abnormal eye. When light is directed into the abnormal eye, both pupils dilate rather than maintain the previous degree of miosis.

McBurney's Point/Sign: Point located one-third of the distance from the anterior superior iliac spine to the umbilicus on the right; tenderness at the site is associated with acute appendicitis.

McMurray's Test: External rotation of the foot produces a palpable or audible click on the joint line, suggesting medial meniscal injuries

Möbius' Sign: Weakness of convergence seen in thyrotoxicosis

Moro's Reflex (Startle Reflex): Abduction of hips and arms with extension of arms when infant's head and upper body is suddenly dropped several inches while being held. Normal reflex in early infancy

Murphy's Sign: Severe pain and inspiratory arrest with palpation of the right upper quadrant during deep inspiration; associated with cholecystitis

Musset's or de Musset's Sign: Rhythmic nodding or movement of the head with each heart beat caused by blood flow back into the heart in aortic insufficiency

Obturator Sign: Flexion and internal rotation of the thigh elicits hypogastric pain in cases of inflammation of the obturator internus; positive with pelvic abscess and appendicitis

Ortolani's Test/Sign: Sign is hip click that suggests congenital hip dislocation. With the infant supine, point the legs toward you and flex the legs to 90 degrees at the hips and knees.

Osler's Node: Tender, red, raised lesions on the hands or feet seen with SBE.

Pancoast's Syndrome: Carcinoma involving apex of lung, resulting in arm and or shoulder pain from involvement of brachial plexus and Horner's syndrome from involvement of the superior cervical ganglion

Pastia's Lines: Linear striations of confluent petechiae in axillary folds are antecubital fossa seen in scarlet fever

Phalen's Test: Prolonged maximum flexion of wrists while opposing dorsum of each hand against each other. A positive test results in pain and tingling in the distribution of the median nerve, indicating carpal tunnel syndrome

Psoas Sign (Iliopsoas Test): Flexion against resistance or extension of the right hip, producing pain; seen with inflammation of the psoas muscle; positive with appendicitis.

Pulsus Alternans: Fluctuation of pulse pressure with every other beat. Seen in aortic stenosis and CHF

Queckenstedt's Test: Tests patency of the subarachnoid space; compression of the internal jugular vein during lumbar puncture; should normally immediately raise CSF pressure

Quincke's Sign: Alternating blushing and blanching of the fingernail bed following light compression; seen in chronic aortic regurgitation

Radovici's Sign: A frontal release sign, scratching palm causes chin contractions

Raynaud's Phenomenon/Disease: Pain and tingling in fingers after exposure to cold with characteristic color changes of white to blue and then often red. May be seen with scleroderma, and SLE

Romberg's Test: Used to test position sense or cerebellar function. The patient stands with heels and toes together. Arms may be outstretched with palms facing upward or down or arms can be at the patient's side. The patient may be lightly tapped by the examiner with the eyes open and then closed. A positive test is a loss of balance. A loss of balance with the eyes open indicates cerebellar dysfunction. Normal balance with eyes open and loss of balance with eyes closed indicates loss of position sense.

Roth's Spots: Oval retinal hemorrhages with a pale central area occurring in patients with bacterial endocarditis

Rovsing's Sign: Pain in the right lower quadrant with deep palpation of the left lower quadrant. Seen in acute appendicitis

Schmorl's Node: Degeneration of the intervertebral disk resulting in herniation into the adjacent vertebral body

Scoliosis: Lateral curvature of the spine

Sentinel Loop: A single dilated loop of small or large bowel, usually occurs localized inflammation such as pancreatitis

Sister Mary Joseph's Sign/Node: Metastatic cancer to umbilical lymph node

Stellwag's Sign: Infrequent ocular blinking

Tinel's Sign: Radiation of an electric shock sensation in the distal distribution of the median nerve elicited by percussion of the flexor surface of the wrist when fully extended. Seen in carpal tunnel syndrome

Traube's Sign: Booming or pistol shot sounds heard over the femoral arteries in chronic aortic insufficiency

Trendelenburg's Test: Observe patient from behind while patient shifts weight from one leg to the other; a pelvis tilt to opposite side suggests hip disease and weakness of the gluteus medius muscle. If normal, pelvis will not tilt.

Trousseau's Sign: Carpal spasm produced by inflating a blood pressure cuff above the systolic pressure for 2–3 min, indicates hypocalcemia; also migratory thrombophlebitis associated with cancer

Turner's Sign: See Grey Turner's sign

Virchow's Node (Signal or Sentinel Node): A palpable, left supraclavicular lymph node; often first sign of a GI neoplasm, such as pancreatic or gastric carcinoma

von Graefe's Sign: Lid lag associated with thyrotoxicosis

Weber–Rinne Test: For the Weber test a 512- or 1024-Hz tuning fork is placed on the middle of the skull to determine if the sound lateralizes. For the Rinne test, the tuning fork is held against the mastoid process (BC) with the opposite ear covered. The patient indicates when the sound is gone. The tuning fork is then held next to the ear and the patient indicates whether the sound is present and when the sound (AC) disappears. Normally AC is better than BC. With sensorineural hearing loss, the Weber test lateralizes to the less affected ear and AC > BC; with conduction hearing loss, the Weber test lateralizes to the more affected ear and BC > AC.

Whipple's Triad: Hypoglycemia, CNS, and vasomotor symptoms (ie, diaphoresis, syncope); relief of symptoms with glucose; associated with insulinoma

EXAMPLE OF A WRITTEN HISTORY AND PHYSICAL EXAMINATION

(Adult Admitted to a Medical Service)

- 7/10/01 5:30 PM

Identification: Mr. Robert Jones is a 50-year-old male referred by Dr. Harry Doyle from Whitesburg, Kentucky. The informant is the patient, who seems reliable, and a photocopy of the ER records from Whitesburg Hospital accompanies the patient.

Chief Complaint: "Squeezing chest pain for 10 h, 4 d ago"

HPI: Mr. Jones awoke at 6 AM 3 d ago with squeezing substernal chest pain that felt "like a ton of bricks" sitting on his chest. The chest pain was a 9 on a 10-point scale, with 10 being pain from a kidney stone. The pain was progressively worse after its onset and decreased in intensity after going to the Whitesburg ER. The pain radiated to his left neck and elbow and was associated with dyspnea and diaphoresis. He denies experiencing any associated nausea. He notes the pain seemed to get worse with any movement, and nothing seemed to alleviate it.

He presented to the Whitesburg ER 10 h after the onset of pain and was given 3 NTG tablets SL and 2 mg morphine sulfate. ECG revealed 3 mm ST depression in leads V_1 through V_4. He was admitted to the ICU at Whitesburg Hospital and had an uneventful course. CPK increased to 850 at 24 h. He has been on aspirin 325 mg/d PO, isosorbide dinitrate 20 mg PO q6h, and diltiazem 60 mg PO q8h. He was transferred for possible cardiac catheterization.

He notes a similar chest pain that was less intense and occurred intermittently over the last 3 mo. The pain was precipitated by exercise and relieved with rest. He denies seeking medical attention in the past. He denies a history of orthopnea, paroxysmal nocturnal dyspnea, dyspnea on exertion, or pedal edema.

He has smoked two packs of cigarettes per day for 35 years, notes a 2-y history of hypertension for which he has been taking HCTZ 25 mg/d and denies a history of hypercholesterolemia or diabetes.

The patient's father died of an MI at age 54, and his brother underwent coronary artery bypass graft surgery last year at age 48.

PMH

Medications. As above and ranitidine 300 mg PO qhs. Occasional ibuprofen 200 mg two to three tablets PO for back pain and acetaminophen 500 mg PO for headache

Vitamins. One-a-day
Herbals. None
Allergies. Penicillin, rash entire body 20 years of age
Surgeries. Appendectomy age 20, Dr. Smith, Whitesburg
Hospitalization. See above.
Trauma. Roof fall in mine accident 10 years ago, injured back. Notes occasional pain, which is relieved with ibuprofen 200 mg two or three tablets at a time
Transfusions. None
Illnesses. Denies asthma, emphysema, thyroid disease, kidney disease, peptic ulcer disease, cancer, bleeding disorders, tuberculosis, or hepatitis. He notes a several-year history of water brash/heartburn and has been on ranitidine for 1 year

Routine Health Maintenance. Last diphtheria/tetanus immunization 3 years ago. Stools for guaiac were negative times 3. Refused sigmoidoscopy. He has been seen by Dr. Doyle every 3–4 months for the last 2 years for hypertension.

Family History

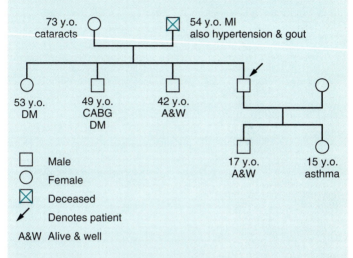

☐	Male
○	Female
☒	Deceased
✓	Denotes patient
A&W	Alive & well

Psychosocial History: Mr. Jones has been married for 25 years and has three children. He and his family live in a home on 3 acres about three miles from Whitesburg. He worked in a coal mine until 10 years ago when he was injured in a "roof fall." He is currently employed in a local chair factory. He graduated from high school. He is Baptist and attends church regularly. Hobbies include woodworking and gardening. He eats breakfast and supper every day and has a soft drink and crackers for lunch. He currently works 8 h/d Monday through Friday. He notes going to bed every day by 10:00 PM and awakens at 5:30 AM. He drinks one to two cups of coffee per day and denies drinking any alcohol. He denies drug use but smokes as noted earlier. He denies exposure to environmental toxins. He denies any financial problems but is concerned about how his illness will affect his income. He has "good" health insurance. He denies any other stressor in his life. His sources of support are his wife, minister, and a sister who lives near the patient.

ROS: Negative unless otherwise noted.

Eyes. Has worn reading glasses since 1995; notes blurred vision for 1 year; last eye appointment 1996. Denies loss of vision, double vision, or history of cataracts.

Respiratory. Notes cough every morning and has produced 1 teaspoon of gray sputum for years. Denies hemoptysis or pleuritic chest pain. Last chest x-ray prior to today was 3 years ago. All other ROS negative.

PHYSICAL EXAMINATION

General: Mr. Jones is a pleasant male lying comfortably supine in bed. He appears to be the stated age.

Vital Signs: Temp 98.6°F orally. Resp 16, HR 88 and regular, BP 110/70 left arm supine

Skin: Tattoo left arm, otherwise no lesions

Node: 1×1 left axillary node, nontender and mobile. No other lymphadenopathy

HEENT

Head. Normocephalic, atraumatic, nontender, no lesions

Eyes. Visual acuity 20/40 left and right corrected. External structures normal, without lesions, PERRLA. EOM intact. Visual fields intact. Funduscopic examination disks sharp bilaterally, moderate arteriolar narrowing and A-V nicking.

Ears. Hearing intact to watch tick at 3 ft bilaterally. Tympanic membranes intact with good cone of light bilaterally

Nose. Symmetrical. No lesions. Sinuses nontender

Mouth. Several dental fillings, otherwise normal dentition. No lesions

Neck. Full ROM without tenderness. No masses or lymphadenopathy. Carotids +2/4 bilaterally, no bruits. Internal jugular vein visible 2 cm above the sternal angle, patient at 30 degrees.

Chest: Symmetrical expansion. Fremitus by palpation bilaterally equal. Diaphragm moves 5.5 cm bilaterally by percussion. Lung fields clear to percussion. Breath sounds normal except end-inspiratory crackles heard at both bases that do not clear with coughing.

Breast: Normal to inspection and palpation

Heart: No cardiac impulse visible. Apical impulse palpable at the sixth intercostal space 2 cm lateral to the midclavicular line. Normal S_1, physiologically split S_2. S_4 heard at apex. No murmurs, rub, or S_3.

Abdomen: Flat, no scars. Positive bowel sounds. No bruits. Liver 10 cm midclavicular line. No CVA tenderness. No hepatomegaly or splenomegaly by palpation. No tenderness or guarding. No inguinal lymphadenopathy

Genital: Normal circumcised male, both testes descended without masses or tenderness

Rectal: Normal sphincter tone. No external lesions. Prostate smooth without tenderness or nodules. No palpable masses. Stool present, stool for occult blood negative

Musculoskeletal: Lumbar spine decreased flexion to 75 degrees, extension to 5 degrees, decreased rotary and lateral movement. Otherwise full ROM of all joints, no erythema, tenderness, or swelling. No clubbing cyanosis or edema

Peripheral Vascular: Radial, ulnar, brachial, femoral, dorsalis pedis, and posterior tibial pulses +2/4 bilaterally. Popliteal pulses nonpalpable. No femoral bruits

Neurologic: Cranial nerves: I through XII intact. Motor: +5/5 upper and lower extremity, proximally and distally. Sensory intact to pinprick upper and lower extremities proximally and distally. Vibratory sense intact in great toes and thumbs bilaterally. Stereognosis intact

Reflexes. Biceps, triceps, brachioradialis, quadriceps, and ankles +2/4 bilaterally. Toes down going bilaterally

Cerebellum. Romberg's sign negative. Intact finger-to-nose and heel-to-shin bilaterally; gait normal—normal heel-and-heel, toe-and-toe, and heel-to-toe gaits. Rapid alternating movements intact upper and lower extremities bilaterally

DATABASE

ECG. HR 80, NSR inverted T waves V_1 through V_5

CXR. Cardiomegaly, otherwise clear
UA. Normal
PT, PTT. Normal
Chemistry Profile. Normal. Except elevated CPK
CBC. 6700 WBC; 49 Hct; HBG 16; 40 S, 5 B, 44 L, 5 M, 6 E

ASSESSMENT AND PLAN

Coronary Artery Disease: Mr. Jones presented with a classic history for MI. The CPK and electrocardiogram support the diagnosis. The ST depression without evolving Q waves was consistent with a nontransmural MI. Mr. Jones is at risk for further MI since it was a nontransmural MI, and he will require further evaluation before discharge.

- Continue aspirin 325 mg/d PO and diltiazem 60 mg/d PO.
- Change isosorbide to tid prior to discharge.
- Monitor by telemetry unit for next 24–48 h.
- Stress test by modified Bruce protocol prior to discharge.
- Consider cardiac catheterization especially if any further pain or if an early positive stress test.
- Continue cardiac rehabilitation.

Hypertension: In view of the patient's age, sex, and degree of hypertension, and the fact that there is no evidence of a secondary cause, the hypertension is most likely primary in nature. It is important that blood pressure be well controlled after this infarct. Mr. Jones' blood pressure has been well controlled on diltiazem alone.

- Continue diltiazem.
- Dietary consult to instruct patient on low-sodium as well as low-fat diet prior to discharge.
- Continue discussion of other problems as shown earlier.

Signature: _____
Title: _____

Date Entered	Date of Onset	Problem	Active	Inactive	Date Inactive
7-10-01	4-01	1	Coronary artery disease		
7-10-01	7-7-01	1a	Subendocardial MI—anterior		
7-10-01	1998	2	Hypertension		
7-10-01	1997	3	Bronchitis		
7-10-01	1999	4	Heartburn/reflux esophagitis		
7-10-01	1990	5	Back injury		
7-10-01	7-10-01	6	Eosinophilia		
7-10-01	2000	7	Blurred vision		
7-10-01	1970	8		Appendicitis	1970

2

CHARTWORK

How to Write Orders
Problem-Oriented Progress Note
Discharge Summary/Note
On-Service Note
Off-Service Note
Bedside Procedure Note

Preoperative Note
Operative Note
Night of Surgery Note (Postop Note)
Delivery Note
Outpatient Prescription Writing
Shorthand for Laboratory Values

HOW TO WRITE ORDERS

The following format is useful for writing concise admission, transfer, and postoperative orders. It involves the mnemonic "A.D.C. VAAN DIML," which stands for **A**dmit/Attending, **D**iagnosis, **C**ondition, **V**itals, **A**ctivity, **A**llergies, **N**ursing procedures, **D**iet, **I**ns and outs, **M**edications, and **L**abs.

A.D.C. Vaan Diml

Admit: Admitting team, room number
Attending: The name of the attending physician, the person legally responsible for the patient's care. Also include the resident's and intern's names.
Diagnosis: List admitting diagnosis or procedure if postop orders.
Condition: Stable, critical, etc
Vitals: Determine frequency of vital signs (temperature, pulse, blood pressure, central venous pressure, pulmonary capillary wedge pressure, weight, etc)
Activity: Specify bedrest, up ad lib, ambulate qid, bathroom privileges, etc
Allergies: Note any drug reactions or food or environmental allergies.
Nursing Procedures
Bed Position. Elevate head of bed 30 degrees, etc
Preps. Enemas, scrubs, showers
Respiratory Care. P&PD. TC&DB, etc
Dressing Changes, Wound Care. Change dressing bid, etc
Notify House Officer If. Temperature >101°F, BP <90 mm Hg, etc
Diet: NPO, clear liquid, regular, etc
Ins and Outs: Refers to all "tubes" a patient may have.
Record Daily I&O.
IV Fluids. Specify type and rate.
Drains. NG to low wall suction, Foley to gravity, etc

Endotracheal Tubes, Arterial Lines, Pulmonary-Artery Catheters. Specify care desired.

Medications: Write orders for specific medications (eg, diuretic, antibiotics, hormones, etc) and symptomatic drugs as needed (eg, pain medications, laxatives, "sleepers"). Include dose frequency and special instructions, ie, take with food.

Labs: Indicate studies and specify times desired if applicable. This includes ECGs, x-rays, nuclear scans, consultation requests, etc.

PROBLEM-ORIENTED PROGRESS NOTE

(See Chapter 20 for a sample ICU progress note.)

1. List each medical, surgical, psychiatric problem separately: pneumonia, pancreatitis, congestive heart failure, etc.
2. Give each problem a call number: 1, 2, 3, ... (as on page 31).
3. Retain the number of each problem throughout the hospitalization.
4. When the problem is resolved, mark it as such and delete it from the daily progress note.
5. Evaluate each problem by number in the following SOAP format. Or, you may do a separate assessment and plan for each problem

Soap

Subjective
- How the patient feels, any complaints

Objective
- How the patient looks
- Vital signs
- Physical examination
- Laboratory data, etc

Assessment: (for each problem)
- Evaluation of the data and any conclusions that can be drawn

Plan: (for each problem)
- Any new lab tests or medications
- Changes or additions to orders
- Discharge or transfer plans

DISCHARGE SUMMARY/NOTE

A formal discharge note is usually required for any admission that is longer than 24 h at most hospitals. This note provides a framework for the complete dictated note as well as providing a reference, if needed, before the dictated note is transcribed and filed. The following skeleton includes most of the information needed for a discharge note.

Date of Admission:
Date of Discharge:
Admitting Diagnosis:
Discharge Diagnosis:
Attending Physician and Service Caring for Patient:
Referring Physician: Provide address if available.
Procedures: Include surgery and any invasive diagnostic procedures, eg, lumbar punctures, arteriograms.

Brief History, Pertinent Physical and Lab Data: Briefly review the main points of the history, physical, and admission lab tests. Do not repeat what is available in the admission note; summarize the most important points about the patient's admission.

Hospital Course: Briefly summarize the evaluation, treatment, and progress of the patient during the hospitalization.

Condition at Discharge: Note if improved, unchanged, etc.

Disposition: Where was the patient discharged to (eg, home, another hospital, nursing home)? Try to give specific address if transferred to another medical institution, and note who will be assuming responsibility for the patient.

Discharge Medications: List medications, dosing, refills.

Discharge Instructions and Follow-up: Clinic return date, diet instructions, activity restrictions, etc

Problem List: List active and past medical problems.

ON-SERVICE NOTE

Also known as a "pick-up note," the on-service note is written by a new member of the team taking over the care of a patient who has been on the service for some time. The note should be brief and summarize the hospital course to date as well as demonstrate that the new team member has reviewed the patient's care to date. The following skeleton includes most of the information needed in an on-service note.

Date of Admission:
Admitting Diagnosis:
Procedures (with Results) to Date:
Hospital Course to Date: This should be briefly summarized.
Brief Physical Examination: Pertinent to the patient's problems.
Pertinent Lab Data:
Problem List:
Assessment:
Plan:

OFF-SERVICE NOTE

This is written by the team member who is rotating off the service but who was primarily responsible for the patient before the patient is ready for discharge. The components are identical to the "On-Service" note in the previous section.

BEDSIDE PROCEDURE NOTE

Procedure: (eg, LP, thoracentesis, etc)
Indications: (eg, R/O meningitis, symptomatic pleural effusion)
Permit: Note risks and benefits explained and indicate signed and on chart
Physicians: Note physicians present and responsible for procedure
Description of Procedure: Indicate type of positioning, prep, anesthesia, and amount. Briefly describe technique and instruments used.
Complications: List.
EBL: List.
Specimens/Findings Obtained: (eg, opening pressure for LP, CSF appearance, and tubes sent to lab, etc)
Disposition: Describe patient's status after procedure (eg, Patient alert and oriented with no complaints; BP stable)

PREOPERATIVE NOTE

2

The specific items in the preoperative note depend on institutional guidelines, the nature of the procedure, and the age and health of the patient. For example, an ECG and blood set-up may not be necessary for a 2-year-old child being treated for a hernia but essential for a 70-year-old scheduled for vascular surgery. The following list includes most of the information needed in a preoperative note.

Preop Diagnosis: Such as "acute appendicitis"
Procedure: The planned procedure, eg, "exploratory laparotomy"
Labs: Results of CBC, electrolytes, PT, PTT, urinalysis, etc
CXR: Note results.
ECG: Note results.
Blood: T&C 2 units PRBC, blood not needed, etc
History and Physical: Should be "on chart."
Orders: Note any special preop orders, such as preop colon preps, vaginal douches, prophylactic antibiotics.
Permit: If completed, write "signed and on chart"; if not, indicate plans for obtaining permit.

OPERATIVE NOTE

The operative note is written immediately after surgery to summarize the operation for those who were not present and is meant to complement the formal operative summary dictated by the surgeon. The following list includes most of what is needed in an operative note.

Preop Diagnosis: Reason for the surgery, eg, "acute appendicitis"
Postop Diagnosis: Based on the operative findings, eg, "mesenteric lymphadenitis"
Procedure: Surgery performed, eg, "exploratory laparotomy"
Surgeons: List the attending physicians, residents, and students who scrubbed on the case, including their titles (MD, CCIV, MSII, etc). It is often helpful to identify the dictating surgeon.
Findings: Briefly note operative findings, eg, "normal appendix with marked lymphadenopathy."
Anesthesia: Specify the type of anesthesia, eg, local, spinal, general, endotracheal, etc.
Fluids: Amount and type of fluid administered during case, eg, 1500 mL NS, 1 unit PRBC, 500 mL albumin. This is usually obtained from the anesthesia records.
EBL: Usually obtained from the anesthesia or nursing records.
Drains: State location and type of drain, eg, "Jackson–Pratt drain in left upper quadrant," "T-tube in midline," etc.
Specimens: State any samples sent to pathology and the results of examination of any intraoperative frozen sections.
Complications: Note any complications during or after the surgery.
Condition: Note where the patient is taken immediately after surgery and the patient's condition. Example: "Transferred to the recovery room in stable condition."

NIGHT OF SURGERY NOTE (POSTOP NOTE)

This type of progress note is written several hours after or the night of surgery.

Procedure: Indicate the operation performed.
Level of Consciousness: Note if the patient is alert, drowsy, etc.

Vital Signs: BP, pulse, respiration.

I&O: Calculate amount of IV fluids, blood, urine output, and other drainage, and attempt to assess fluid balance.

Physical Examination: Examine and note the findings of the chest, heart, abdomen, extremities, and any other part of the physical examination pertinent to the surgery; examine the dressing for bleeding.

Labs: Review lab results if any were obtained since surgery.

Assessment: Evaluate the postop course thus far (stable, etc).

Plan: Note any changes in orders.

DELIVERY NOTE

__ -year-old (married or single) G __ now para __, AB __, clinic (note if patient received prenatal clinic care) patient with EDC __, and a prenatal course (uncomplicated or describe any problems). Any comments concerning labor (eg, Pitocin-induced, premature rupture) and draped in the usual sterile fashion. Under controlled conditions delivered a __ lb __ oz (__ g) viable male or female infant under __ (general, spinal, pudendal, none) anesthesia. Delivery was via SVD with midline episiotomy (or forceps or cesarean section). Apgars were __ at 1 min and __ at 5 min (for Apgar scoring, see Appendix). State delivery date and time. Cord blood sent to lab and placenta expressed intact with trailing membranes. Lacerations of the __ degree repaired by standard method with good hemostasis and restoration of normal anatomy.

- EBL:
- MBT:
- HCT (predelivery and postdelivery):
- RT:
- VDRL test:
- Condition of mother:

OUTPATIENT PRESCRIPTION WRITING

The format for outpatient prescription writing is outlined in the following list and illustrated in Figure 2–1. Controlled substances, such as narcotics, require a DEA number on the prescription and in some states may require that the controlled substance be written on a special type of prescription paper (see Chapter 22 for controlled drugs indicated by a [C]). For security, the DEA number should never be preprinted on a prescription pad but written by hand at the time the prescription is written.

Elements of an outpatient prescription include:

Patient's Name, Address, and Age: Print clearly where indicated.

Date: State requirements vary, but most prescriptions must be filled within 6 months.

Rx: Drug name, strength, and type (usually listed as the generic name); if you specifically want a brand name you must designate "no substitution." Rx is an abbreviation from the Latin for "recipe." List the strength of the product (usually in mg) and the form (eg, tablets, capsule, suspension, transdermal, etc).

Dispense: Amount of drug (number of capsules), or time period (1 month supply, etc).

Sig: Short for the Latin "signa," which means "mark through" on patient instructions. This part can be written out or noted in shorthand. Shorthand use is generally discouraged, however, because writing out the prescription decreases the likelihood of errors. Frequently used abbreviations are noted here with a more complete listing provided at the front of the book.

2

NICK PAVONA, MD
BENJAMIN FRANKLIN UNIVERSITY MEDICAL CENTER
CHADDS FORD, PA 19317

LICENSE PA MD 685-488-194   **DEA** NP–3612982

NAME NICK PAVONA, Sr.   **AGE** 84

ADDRESS 34-10 75th Street   **DATE** 10/24/2001

Wilmington, DE

> Rx: minoxidil (Rogaine) 2% topical solution
> DISP: 60 mL
> SIG: Apply BID to scalp
>   Brand medically necessary

REFILL X5

SUBSTITUTION PERMISSIBLE ☐   *Nick Pavona* M.D.

TO ENSURE BRAND NAME DISPENSING, PRESCRIBER MUST
SPECIFY "DISPENSE AS WRITTEN" ON THE PRESCRIPTION.*

*This can vary by state; some require that you write "Brand Medically
Necessary" to specify a brand name and not a generic.

FIGURE 2–1 Example of an outpatient prescription. As a safety feature DEA numbers should **never** be preprinted on a prescription form. The "Dispense as Written"
statement can vary by state requirements; this statement requests that the pharmacist
fill the prescription as requested and not substitute a generic equivalent.

ad lib = freely at pleasure
PO = by mouth
PR = by rectum
OS = left eye
OD = right eye
qd = daily (this is a dangerous abbreviation and **should not be used;** see "Dangerous Prac-
    tices," page 39)
PRN = as needed
$\dot{T}$ = one
$\ddot{T}$ = two
$\dddot{T}$ = three
qhs = every night at bedtime
bid = twice a day
tid = three times a day
q6h = every 6 h

qid = four times a day. (Note that qid and q6h are NOT the same orders: qid means that the
medication is given four times a day while awake (eg, 8 AM, 12 noon, 6 PM, and 10 PM);
q6h means that the medication is given four times a day but by the clock (eg, 6 AM, 12
noon, 6 PM, 12 midnight).

Refills: Indicate how many times this prescription can be refilled.

Substitution: Can a generic drug be used instead of the one prescribed?

Tips for Safe Prescription Writing

Legibility

1. Take time to write legibly.
2. Print if this would be more legible than handwriting.
3. Use a typewriter or computer if necessary. In the near future, physicians will generate
   all prescriptions by computer to eliminate legibility problems.
4. When prescribing a new or rarely used drug, carefully print the order to avoid mis-
   reading.

Dangerous Practices

1. NEVER use a trailing zero.
   Correct: 1 mg
   Dangerous: 1.0 mg. If the decimal is not seen, a 10-fold overdose can occur.
2. NEVER leave a decimal point "naked."
   Correct: 0.5 mL
   Dangerous: .5 mL. If the decimal point is not seen, a 10-fold overdose can occur.
3. NEVER abbreviate a drug name because the abbreviation may be misunderstood or
   have multiple meanings.
4. NEVER abbreviate U for units as it can easily be read as a zero, thus "6 U regular insulin" can be misread as 60 units. The order should be written as "6 units regular insulin."
5. NEVER use qd (abbreviation for once a day). When poorly written, the tail of the "q"
   can make it read qid or four times a day.

SHORTHAND FOR LABORATORY VALUES

(See Figure 2–2)

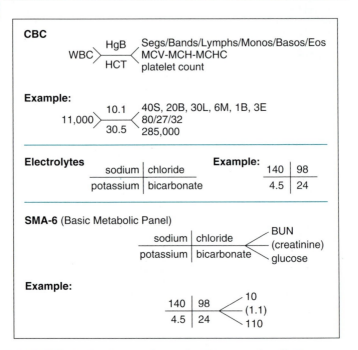

FIGURE 2–2   Shorthand notation for recording laboratory values. The basic metabolic panel is similar to the SMA-6 except that the creatinine is also listed.

DIFFERENTIAL DIAGNOSIS: SYMPTOMS, SIGNS, AND CONDITIONS

Abdominal Distention
Abdominal Pain
Adrenal Mass
Alopecia
Amenorrhea
Anorexia
Anuria
Arthritis
Ascites
Back Pain
Breast Lump
Chest Pain
Chills
Clubbing
Coma
Constipation
Cough
Cyanosis
Delirium
Dementia
Diarrhea
Diplopia
Dizziness
Dysphagia
Dyspnea
Dysuria
Earache
Edema
Epistaxis
Failure to Thrive
Fever
Fever of Unknown Origin (FUO)
Flatulence

Frequency
Galactorrhea
Gynecomastia
Headache
Heartburn (Pyrosis)
Hematemesis and Melena
Hematochezia
Hematuria
Hemoptysis
Hepatomegaly
Hiccups (Singultus)
Hirsutism
Impotence (Erectile Dysfunction)
Incontinence (Urinary)
Jaundice
Lymphadenopathy and Splenomegaly
Melena
Nausea and Vomiting
Nystagmus
Oliguria and Anuria
Pleural Effusion
Pruritus
Seizures
Splenomegaly
Syncope
Tremors
Vaginal Bleeding
Vaginal Discharge
Vertigo
Vomiting
Weight Loss
Wheezing

This chapter provides a general guide to commonly encountered symptoms and conditions and their frequent causes. Remember: "There are more uncommon presentations of common diseases than common presentations of uncommon diseases."

ABDOMINAL DISTENTION

Ascites, intestinal obstruction, cysts (ovarian or renal), tumors, hepatosplenomegaly, aortic aneurysm, uterine enlargement (pregnancy), bladder distention, inflammatory mass

ABDOMINAL PAIN

Diffuse: Intestinal angina, early appendicitis, colitis, diabetic ketoacidosis, hereditary angioedema, gastroenteritis, mesenteric thrombosis, mesenteric lymphadenitis, peritonitis, porphyria, sickle cell crisis, uremia, renal colic, renal infarct, pancreatitis

Right Upper Quadrant: Dissecting aneurysm, gallbladder disease (cholecystitis, cholangitis, choledocholithiasis), hepatitis, hepatomegaly, pancreatitis, peptic ulcer disease, pneumonia, PE, pyelonephritis, renal colic, renal infarct, appendicitis (retroperitoneal)

Left Upper Quadrant: Dissecting aneurysm, esophagitis, hiatal hernia, esophageal rupture, gastritis, pancreatitis, peptic ulcer disease, MI, pericarditis, pneumonia, PE, pyelonephritis, renal colic, renal infarct, splenic rupture or infarction

Lower Abdomen: Aortic aneurysm, colitis, diverticulitis including Meckel's, intestinal obstruction, hernias, perforated viscus, pregnancy, ectopic pregnancy, dysmenorrhea, endometriosis, mittelschmerz (ovulation), ovarian cyst or tumor (especially with torsion), PID, renal colic, UTI, rectal hematoma, bladder distention.

Right Lower Quadrant Specific: Appendicitis, ectopic pregnancy, ovarian cyst or tumor, salpingitis, mittelschmerz, cholecystitis, perforated duodenal ulcer, Crohn's disease

ADRENAL MASS

Adrenal adenoma, adrenal hyperplasia (unilateral or bilateral), adrenal metastasis (solid tumors, lymphoma, leukemia), adrenocortical carcinoma, pheochromocytoma, adrenal myelolipoma, adrenal cyst, Wolman's disease, adrenal varices, hemorrhage, congenital adrenal hyperplasia, ganglioneuroma, micronodular adrenal disease

ALOPECIA

Male pattern baldness (alopecia, androgenic type in both men and women), trauma and hair pulling, congenital, tinea capitis, bacterial folliculitis, telogen arrest, anagen arrest (chemotherapy/radiation therapy), alopecia areata, discoid lupus

AMENORRHEA

Pregnancy, menopause (physiologic or premature), severe illness, weight loss, stress, athletic training, "physiologically delayed puberty," anatomic (imperforate hymen, uterine agenesis, etc), gonadal dysgenesis (Turner's syndrome, etc), hypothalamic and pituitary tumors, virilizing syndromes (polycystic ovaries, idiopathic hirsutism, etc). Amenorrhea is categorized as primary (never had menses) or secondary (cessation of menses).

ANOREXIA

Hepatitis, carcinoma (most types, especially advanced), anorexia nervosa, generalized debilitating diseases, digitalis toxicity, uremia, depression, CHF, pulmonary failure, radiation exposure, chemotherapy

ANURIA

See Oliguria, page 49

ARTHRITIS

Osteoarthritis, bursitis, tendonitis, connective tissue disease (RA, SLE, rheumatic fever, scleroderma, gout, pseudogout, rheumatoid variants [ankylosing spondylitis, psoriatic arthritis, Reiter's syndrome]), infection (bacterial, viral, TB, fungal Lyme disease), trauma, sarcoidosis, sickle cell anemia, hemochromatosis, amyloidosis, coagulopathy

ASCITES

(See Chapter 13, page 296, under "Peritoneal Paracentesis" for more details.) CHF, tricuspid insufficiency, constrictive pericarditis, venous occlusion (including Budd–Chiari syndrome), cirrhosis, pancreatitis, peritonitis (ruptured viscus, TB, bile leak, spontaneous bacterial), tumors (most common ovarian, gastric, uterine, unknown primary, breast, lymphoma), trauma, Meigs' syndrome (ovarian fibroma associated with hydrothorax and ascites), myxedema, anasarca (hypoalbuminemia)

BACK PAIN

Herniated disk, spinal stenosis, ankylosing spondylitis, metastatic tumor, multiple myeloma, mechanical back sprain, referred pain (visceral, vascular), vertebral body fracture, osteoporosis induced fracture, infectious processes (diskitis, osteomyelitis, epidural abscess

BREAST LUMP

Cancer, fibroadenoma, fibrocystic breast disease, fat necrosis, gynecomastia (males, alcoholics)

CHEST PAIN

Deep, Dull, Poorly Localized: Angina, variant angina, unstable angina, AMI, aortic aneurysm, PE, tumor, gallbladder disease, pulmonary hypertension

Sharp, Well Localized: PE, pneumothorax, epidemic pleurodynia, pericarditis, atypical MI, hyperventilation, hiatal hernia, esophagitis, esophageal spasm, herpes zoster, aortic aneurysm, breast lesions, variety of bony and soft tissue abnormalities (rib fractures, costochondritis, muscle damage), perforated ulcer, acute cholecystitis, pancreatitis

CHILLS

Infection (bacterial with bacteremia, viral, TB, fungal), neoplasm (Hodgkin's disease), drug and transfusion reactions, hypothermia, malaria

CLUBBING

Pulmonary causes (bronchiectasis, lung abscesses, tuberculosis, neoplasms, fibrosis), AV malformations, cardiac (congenital cyanotic heart diseases, bacterial endocarditis), GI (ulcerative and regional enteritis, cirrhosis), hereditary, thyrotoxicosis

COMA

Use the mnemonic **AEIOU TIPS: A**lcohol; **E**ncephalitis (other CNS causes—epilepsy, hemorrhage, mass), **I**nsulin (hypoglycemia, hyperglycemia), **O**piates (drugs), **U**remia (and other metabolic conditions, such as hypernatremia, hyponatremia, hypercalcemia, hepatic failure, and thiamine deficiency), **T**rauma, **I**nfection, **P**sychiatric causes, **S**yncope (or decreased cardiac output such as from arrhythmias).

CONSTIPATION

Dehydration, lack of exercise, bedrest, medications (narcotics, anticholinergics, antidepressants, calcium channel blockers—verapamil, diuretics, clonidine, aluminum- or calcium-containing antacids), laxative abuse, megacolon, spastic colon, chronic suppression of the urge to defecate, fecal impaction (often with paradoxical diarrhea), neoplasm, intestinal obstruction, vascular occlusion to the bowel, inflammatory lesions (diverticulitis, proctitis), hemorrhoids, anal fissures, neurological disorders, depression, porphyria, hypothyroidism, hypercalcemia

COUGH

Acute: Tracheobronchitis, pneumonia, sinusitis, pulmonary edema, foreign body, toxic inhalation, allergy, pharyngitis (viral or bacterial), asthma, GERD ACE inhibitors, impacted cerumen or foreign body in ear

Chronic: Bronchitis (smoker), chronic sinusitis, emphysema, cancer (bronchogenic, head and neck, and esophageal), TB, sarcoidosis, fungal infection, bronchiectasis, mediastinal lymphadenopathy, thoracic aneurysm, GERD, ACE inhibitors

CYANOSIS

Peripheral: Arterial occlusion and insufficiency, vasospasm/Raynaud's disease, venous stasis, venous obstruction
Central: Hypoxia, congenital heart disease (right to left shunt), PE, pseudo-cyanosis (eg, polycythemia vera), methemoglobinemia

DELIRIUM

Metabolic: Hypoglycemia, hypoxia, sodium and calcium disorders, hypercarbia, uremia

Neurologic: Stroke, subdural and epidural hematoma, subarachnoid hemorrhage, postictal, concussion and contusion, meningitis, encephalitis, brain tumor

Drug or Toxin-Induced: Lithium intoxication, ethanol, steroids, anticholinergics, sympathomimetics, poisons (eg, mushrooms, carbon monoxide), drugs of abuse

DEMENTIA

Chronic CNS disease: Alzheimer's, senile dementia, Pick's disease, Parkinson's, chronic demyelinating disease (MS), ALS, brain tumor, normal pressure hydrocephalus, Wilson's disease, Huntington's disease, lipid storage diseases (eg, Tay–Sachs)

Metabolic: Usually chronic (hypoxia, hypoglycemia, hypocalcemia), hyperammonemia, dialysis, heavy-metal intoxication, pernicious anemia (B_{12} deficiency), niacin and thiamine

deficiency (usually chronic alcoholic) posthepatic coma, medications (barbiturates, phenothiazines, lithium, benzodiazepines, many others)

Infectious: AIDS encephalopathy, brain abscess, chronic meningoencephalitis (eg, fungal neurosyphilis), encephalitis, Jakob–Creutzfeldt disease

Vascular: Vasculitis, multicerebral/cerebellar infarcts

Traumatic: Contusion, hemorrhage, subdural hematoma

Psychiatric: Sensory deprivation, depression (pseudodementia)

DIARRHEA

Acute: Infections (bacterial, viral, fungal, protozoan, parasitic), toxic (food poisoning,
chemical), drugs (antibiotics, cholinergic agents, lactulose, magnesium-containing antacids,
quinidine, reserpine, guanethidine, metoclopramide, bethanechol), appendicitis, diverticular
disease, GI bleeding, ischemic colitis, food intolerance, fecal impaction (paradoxical diarrhea), pseudomembranous colitis

Chronic: After gastrectomy or vagotomy, ZE syndrome, regional enteritis, ulcerative colitis, malabsorption, diverticular disease, carcinoma, villous adenoma, gastrinomas, lymphoma of the bowel, functional bowel disorders (irritable colon, mucous colitis),
pseudomembranous colitis, endocrine disease (carcinoid, hyperthyroidism, Addison's disease), radiation enteritis, drugs, Whipple's disease, amyloidosis, AIDS

DIPLOPIA

Problems with the third, fourth, or sixth cranial nerve, such as from vascular disturbances,
meningitis, tumor, demyelination, orbital blow-out fracture, hyperthyroid ocular myopathy

DIZZINESS

Hyperventilation, depression, hypoglycemia, anemia, volume depletion, hypoxia, trauma,
Ménière's disease, benign positional vertigo, aminoglycoside toxicity, vestibular neuronitis,
MS, brain stem ischemia or stroke, posterior fossa lesions, cerebellar ischemia or stroke, ar-
rhythmias, aortic stenosis, carotid sinus hypersensitivity

DYSPHAGIA

Loss of tongue function, pharyngeal dysfunction (myasthenia gravis), Zenker's diverticulum, tumors (bronchogenic, head and neck, and esophageal), stricture, esophageal web,
Schatzki's ring, lower esophageal sphincter spasm, foreign body, aortic aneurysm, achalasia,
scleroderma, diabetic neuropathy, amyloidosis, infection (especially candidiasis), dermato-
myositis, polymyositis, MS, brain stem infarctions

DYSPNEA

Laryngeal and tracheal infections and foreign bodies, tumors (both intrinsic and extrinsic),
COPD, asthma, pneumonia, lung carcinoma, atelectasis, pneumothorax, pleural effusion,
hemothorax, PE, pulmonary infarction, carbon monoxide poisoning, any cause of pain from
respiratory movements, cardiac and noncardiac pulmonary edema, AMI, pericardial tamponade, anemia, abdominal distention, anxiety

DYSURIA

Urethral stricture, stones, blood clot, tumor (bladder, prostate, urethral), prostatic enlarge-ment, infection (urethritis, cystitis, vaginitis, prostatitis), trauma, bladder spasm, dehydra-tion

EARACHE

Otitis media and externa, mastoiditis, serous otitis, otic barotrauma, foreign body, impacted cerumen, referred pain (dental or TMJ)

EDEMA

CHF, constrictive pericarditis, liver disease (cirrhosis), nephrotic syndrome, nephritic syn-drome, hypoalbuminemia, malnutrition, myxedema, hemiplegia, volume overload, throm-bophlebitis, lymphatic obstruction, medications (nifedipine), venous stasis

EPISTAXIS

Trauma (nose picking, blunt trauma), neoplasm, polyps, foreign body, desiccation, coagu-lopathy, medications (use of cocaine, nasal sprays), infections (sinusitis), uremia, hyperten-sion (more often a result rather than a cause of epistasis)

FAILURE TO THRIVE

Environmental: Social deprivation, decreased food intake

Organic: CNS disorder, intestinal malabsorption, CF, parasites, cleft palate, heart fail-ure, endocrine diseases, hypercalcemia, Turner's syndrome, renal disease, chronic infection, malignancies

FEVER

Based on adult population studies an AM temperature above 98.8°F (37.2°C) or PM above 99.9°F (37.7°C) is generally defined as a fever. Rectal temperatures are generally 1°F (0.6°C) higher and reflect core temperature

Infections (viral, bacterial, mycobacterial, fungal, parasitic), neoplasm (lymphoma, leukemia, renal and hepatic carcinoma), connective tissue disease (SLE, vasculitis, RA, adult Still's disease, temporal arteritis), heat stroke, malignant hyperthermia, thyroid storm, adrenal insufficiency, PE, MI, atrial myxoma, inflammatory bowel disease, factitious, drugs (most common offenders: amphotericin, bleomycin, barbiturates, cephalosporins, methyl-dopa, penicillins, phenytoin, procainamide, sulfonamides, quinidine, cocaine, LSD, phency-clidine and amphetamines)

FEVER OF UNKNOWN ORIGIN (FUO)

Defined as a temperature of 101°F (38.3°C) or greater for at least 3 weeks and for which a diagnosis is not established after 1 week of hospitalization. In children, the minimum dura-tion is 2 weeks and the temperature is at least 101.3°F (38.5°C): TB, fungal infection, endo-carditis, abscess (especially hepatic), neoplasm (lymphoma, renal cell, hepatoma, preleukemia), atrial myxoma, connective tissue disease, drugs (see Fever, previous listing), PE, Crohn's disease, ulcerative colitis, hypothalamic injury, factitious; in elderly, temporal arteritis

FLATULENCE

Aerophagia, food intolerance, disturbances in bowel motility (diabetes, uremia), lactose intolerance, gallbladder disease, peptic ulcer fiber, cholestyramine

FREQUENCY

Infection (bladder, prostate), excessive fluid intake, use of diuretics (also coffee, tea, or colas), diabetes mellitus, diabetes insipidus, prostatic obstruction, bladder stones, bladder tumors, pregnancy, psychogenic bladder syndrome, neurogenic bladder, interstitial cystitis

GALACTORRHEA

Hyperprolactinemia, prolonged breast feeding, major stress, pituitary tumors, breast lesions (benign, cancer, inflammatory), idiopathic with menses and after oral contraceptive use

GYNECOMASTIA

Normal (Physiologic):   Newborn, adolescence, aging

Pathologic: Medications or drug use(cimetidine, spironolactone, estrogens, gonadotropins, antiandrogens, marijuana), decreased testosterone (Klinefelter's syndrome, testicular failure or absence), increased estrogen production (hermaphroditism, testicular or lung cancers, adrenal and liver diseases)

HEADACHE

Includes cluster, tension, and migraine (classic or simple), benign exertional, headache associated with sexual activity, benign cough headache, ice-pick (idiopathic stabbing), vascular (menstruation, hypertension), eye strain, acute glaucoma, sinusitis, dental problems, TMJ dysfunction, trauma, subarachnoid hemorrhage, intracranial mass, fever, meningitis, pseudo-tumor cerebri, trigeminal neuralgia, temporal arteritis (especially in elderly), hypoglycemia, toxin exposure (carbon monoxide poisoning), drugs (vasodilators—nifedipine [Procardia]), vasculitis

HEARTBURN (PYROSIS)

GERD, esophagitis, hiatal hernia, peptic ulcer, gallbladder disease, medications, tumors, scleroderma, food intolerance. Myocardial ischemia maybe mistaken for heartburn.

HEMATEMESIS AND MELENA

Melena generally means that the bleeding site is in the upper GI tract (ie, proximal to the ligament of Treitz), but occasionally can be as distal as the right colon.) Swallowed blood (eg, epistaxis), esophageal varices, esophagitis, Mallory–Weiss syndrome, hiatal hernia, gastritis, peptic ulcer, duodenitis, carcinoma of the stomach, tumors (both small and large bowel), ischemic colitis, aortoenteric fistula, bleeding diathesis, anticoagulation (may unmask GI tract pathology)

HEMATOCHEZIA

Massive upper GI bleeding, hemorrhoids, diverticular disease, angiodysplasia, polyps, carcinoma, inflammatory bowel disease, ischemic colitis

3

HEMATURIA (see also page 111)

First rule out false-positives: myoglobinuria, hemoglobinuria, porphyria. GU neoplasms (malignant and benign), polycystic kidneys, trauma, infection (urethral, bladder, prostate, etc), stones, glomerulonephritis, renal infarction, renal vein thrombosis, anticoagulation (may unmask GU tract pathology), bleeding diathesis, enterovesical fistula, sickle cell anemia, vigorous exercise ("runners' hematuria"), accelerated hypertension, factitious, and vaginal and rectal bleeding

HEMOPTYSIS

Infection (pneumonia, bronchitis, fungal, TB), bronchiectasis, cancer (usually bronchogenic), PE, arteriovenous malformations, Wegener's granulomatosis, Goodpasture's syndrome, SLE, pulmonary hemosiderosis, foreign body, trauma, bleeding diatheses, excessive anticoagulation (may unmask respiratory tract pathology), pulmonary edema, mitral stenosis

HEPATOMEGALY

CHF, hepatitis (viral, alcoholic, drug-induced, autoimmune), cirrhosis (alcoholic, etc), tumors (primary and metastatic), amyloid, biliary obstruction, hemochromatosis, chronic granulomatous disease, infections (schistosomiasis, liver abscess). Riedel's lobe is a normal variant, elongated right lobe of the liver with normal liver volume.

HICCUPS (SINGULTUS)

Uremia, electrolyte disorders, diabetes, medications (benzodiazepines, barbiturates, others), emotionally induced (excitement, fright), gastric distention, CNS disorders, psychogenic, thoracic and diaphragmatic disorders (pneumonia, MI, diaphragmatic irritation), alcohol ingestion

HIRSUTISM

Idiopathic, familial, adrenal causes (Cushing's disease, congenital adrenal hyperplasia, virilizing adenoma or carcinoma), polycystic ovaries, medications (minoxidil, androgens)

IMPOTENCE (ERECTILE DYSFUNCTION)

Psychogenic, vascular, neurologic (cord injury, radical prostatectomy, rectal surgery, aortic bypass), pelvic radiation, medications (some common drugs: antihypertensives, thiazide diuretics, beta-blockers, methyldopa; antidepressants especially the SSRIs, anticholinergics; addictive medications: alcohol, narcotics; antipsychotics; antiandrogens: histamine H_2 blockers, finasteride, LHRH analogues, spironolactone, others; history of priapism, Peyronie's disease, testicular failure, hyperprolactinemia

INCONTINENCE (URINARY)

Cystitis, dementia and delirium, stroke, prostatic hypertrophy, fecal impaction, peripheral or autonomic neuropathy, medications (diuretics, sedatives, alpha blockers), diabetes, spinal cord trauma or lesions, MS, childbirth, surgery (prostate, rectal), aging, acute and chronic medical conditions, estrogen deficiency

JAUNDICE

Hepatitis (alcoholic, viral, drug-induced, autoimmune), Gilbert's disease, Crigler–Najjar syndrome, Dubin–Johnson syndrome, Wilson's disease, drug-induced cholestasis (phenothiazines and estrogen), gallbladder and biliary tract disease (including inflammation, infection, obstruction, and tumors—primary hepatic and metastatic), hemolysis, neonatal jaundice, cholestatic jaundice of pregnancy, total parenteral nutrition

LYMPHADENOPATHY AND SPLENOMEGALY

Infection (bacterial, fungal, viral, parasitic), benign neoplasm (histiocytosis), malignant neoplasm (primary lymphoma, metastatic), sarcoid, connective tissue disease, drugs (phenytoin, etc), AIDS, splenomegaly without lymphadenopathy (cirrhosis, hereditary spherocytosis, hemoglobinopathies, ITP, hairy cell leukemia, and amyloidosis)

MELENA

(See Hematemesis, page 47.)

NAUSEA AND VOMITING

Appendicitis, acute cholecystitis, chronic gallbladder disease, peptic ulcer disease, gastritis (especially alcoholic), pancreatitis, gastric distention (diabetic atony, pyloric obstruction), intestinal obstruction, peritonitis, food intolerance, intestinal infection (bacterial, viral, parasitic), acute systemic infections (especially in children), hepatitis, toxins (food poisoning), CNS disorders ([increased intracranial pressure often cause vomiting without headache], tumor, hemorrhagic stroke, hydrocephalus, meningitis, labyrinthitis, Ménière's disease, migraine headaches) AMI, CHF, endocrine disorders (DKA, adrenal crisis), hypercalcemia, hyperkalemia, hypokalemia, pyelonephritis, nephrolithiasis, uremia, hepatic failure, pregnancy, PID, drugs (opiates, digitalis, chemotherapeutic agents, L-dopa, NSAIDs), psychogenic vomiting, porphyria, radiation therapy

NYSTAGMUS

Congenital, vision loss early in life, MS, neoplasms, infarction, toxic or metabolic encephalopathy, alcoholic cerebellar degeneration, medications (anticonvulsants, barbiturates, phenothiazines, lithium, others), encephalitis, vascular brainstem lesions, Arnold– Chiari malformation, nonpathologic (extreme lateral gaze), opticokinetic nystagmus (attempt to fix gaze on rapidly moving object, eg, train)

OLIGURIA AND ANURIA

(See also Urinary Indices, page 119.)

    Oliguria is <500 mL urine/24 h; **anuria** is <100 mL urine/24 h in adults.

Prerenal: Volume depletion, shock, heart failure, fluids in the third space, renal artery compromise

Renal: Glomerular disease, acute tubular necrosis, bilateral cortical necrosis, interstitial disease (acute and chronic interstitial nephritis, urate or hypercalcemic nephropathy), transfusion reaction, myoglobulinuria, radiographic contrast media (especially in diabetics, dehydration, multiple myeloma and elderly), ESRD, drugs (aminoglycosides, amphotericin B, vancomycin, NSAIDs, cephalosporins, penicillins, and sulfonamides), emboli, thrombosis, and DIC

Postrenal: Bilateral ureteral obstruction, prostatic obstruction, neurogenic bladder

PLEURAL EFFUSION

(See Chapter 13, page 304, Thoracentesis, for more details.)

Transudate: (Pleural to serum protein ratio <0.5, and pleural to serum LDH ratio <0.6 and pleural LDH <$\frac{2}{3}$ the upper limits of normal for serum LDH), CHF, cirrhosis, nephrotic syndrome, peritoneal dialysis

Exudate: (Pleural to serum protein ratio >0.5, or pleural to serum LDH ratio >0.6, or pleural LDH >$\frac{2}{3}$ the upper limits of normal for serum LDH), bacterial or viral pneumonia, pulmonary infarction, TB, RA, SLE, malignancy (most common, breast, lung lymphoma, leukemia, ovarian, unknown primary, GI, mesothelioma, others), pancreatitis, pneumothorax, chest trauma, uremia

Chylothorax: Traumatic or postoperative complication

Empyema: Bacteria, fungi, TB, trauma, surgery

Hydrothorax: Usually iatrogenic (central venous catheter complication)

PRURITUS

Skin lesions (papulosquamous, vesicobullous, contact dermatitis, infestations [scabies, etc], infections), dry skin (especially in winter), liver disease, uremia, diabetes, gout, Hodgkin's disease, leukemias, polycythemia vera, intestinal parasites, drug reactions, pregnancy, psychosomatic, neurologic, or circulatory disturbances

SEIZURES

Types

Generalized: Grand mal and petit mal (absence), febrile

Partial Seizures: Partial motor, partial sensory, partial complex (psychomotor or temporal lobe, déjà vu, automatisms)

Causes: Primary, CNS tumors (primary, metastatic), trauma, metabolic (hypoglycemia, hyponatremia, hypernatremia, acidosis, alkalosis, porphyria, uremia, etc), fever (especially in children), infection (meningitis, encephalitis, and abscess), anoxia (arrhythmias, stroke, carbon monoxide poisoning), drugs (alcohol or barbiturate withdrawal, cocaine, amphetamines), collagen-vascular disease (SLE), chronic renal failure, trauma, hypertensive encephalopathy, toxemia of pregnancy, psychogenic

SPLENOMEGALY

(See Lymphadenopathy and Splenomegaly, page 49)

SYNCOPE

Includes vasovagal (simple faint), orthostatic (volume depletion, sympathectomy [either functional or surgical], diabetes, Shy–Drager [idiopathic], tricyclic antidepressants and diuretics) and hysterical. Cardiac syncope (Adams–Stokes attack), paroxysmal atrial tachycardia, atrial fibrillation, ventricular tachycardia, sinoatrial or atrioventricular block, pacemaker malfunction, aortic stenosis, IHSS, primary pulmonary hypertension, atrial myxoma, cough syncope, hypoglycemia, seizure disorder, subclavian steal syndrome, cerebrovascular accident, AMI, alcohol-related

TREMORS

Resting (decrease with movement):   Parkinson's disease, Wilson's disease, brain tumors (rare), medications (SSRI antidepressants, metoclopramide, phenothiazines [tardive dyskinesia])

Action (present with movement):   Benign essential tremor (familial and senile), cerebellar diseases, withdrawal syndromes (alcohol, benzodiazepines, opiates), normal/physiologic (induced by anxiety, fatigue)

Ataxic (worse at end of voluntary movement):   MS, cerebellar diseases

Others: Medication-induced (caffeines [coffee, tea], steroids, valproic acid, bronchodilators) febrile, hypoglycemic, hyperthyroidism, pheochromocytoma

VAGINAL BLEEDING

Normal menstrual period, dysfunctional uterine bleeding (premenopausal bleeding, oral contraceptives, luteal phase defect), anovulatory abnormal uterine bleeding (hypothalamic/pituitary disorders, stress, thyroid and adrenal disease, endometriosis), pregnancy-related (ectopic pregnancy, threatened/spontaneous abortion, retained products of gestation), neoplasia (uterine fibroids; cervical polyps; and endometrial, cervical, ovarian, and vulvar carcinoma)

VAGINAL DISCHARGE

Vaginitis due to *Candida albicans, Trichomonas vaginalis, Gardnerella vaginalis, Neisseria gonorrhoeae, Chlamydia trachomatis, Mycoplasma,* herpesvirus, chronic cervicitis, tumors, irritants, foreign bodies, estrogen deficiency

VERTIGO

Ménière's disease (recurrent vertigo, deafness and tinnitus), labyrinthitis, aminoglycoside toxicity, benign positional vertigo, vestibular neuronitis, brainstem ischemia and infarction, basilar artery migraine, cerebellar infarction, acoustic neuroma motion sickness, excess of ethanol, quinine, and salicylic acid

VOMITING

(See Nausea and Vomiting page 49)

WEIGHT LOSS

Normal or Increased Appetite: Diabetes, hyperthyroidism, anxiety, drugs (thyroid), carcinoid, sprue, pancreatic deficiency, parasites

Decreased Appetite: Depression, anorexia nervosa, GI obstruction, neoplasm, liver disease, severe infection, severe cardiopulmonary disease, uremia, adrenal insufficiency, hypercalcemia, hypokalemia, intoxication (alcohol, lead), old age, drugs (amphetamines, digitalis, SSRIs, such as fluoxetine [Prozac]), AIDS

WHEEZING

Large airway difficulty (laryngeal stridor, tracheal stenosis, foreign body), endobronchial tumor, asthma, bronchitis, emphysema, pulmonary edema, PE, anaphylactic reactions, myocardial ischemia

LABORATORY DIAGNOSIS: CHEMISTRY, IMMUNOLOGY, AND SEROLOGY

Acetoacetate
Acid Phosphatase
ACTH
ACTH Stimulation Test
Albumin
Albumin/Globulin Ratio
Aldosterone
Alkaline Phosphatase
Alpha-fetoprotein (AFP)
ALT
Ammonia
Amylase
ASO Titer
AST
Autoantibodies
Base Excess/Deficit
Bicarbonate
Bilirubin
Blood Urea Nitrogen (BUN)
BUN/Creatinine Ratio
C-Peptide
C-Reactive Protein
CA 15-3
CA 19-9
CA-125
Calcitonin
Calcium, Serum
Captopril Test
Carbon Dioxide
Carboxyhemoglobin
Carcinoembryonic Antigen (CEA)
Catecholamines, Fractionated Serum
Chloride, Serum
Cholesterol
Clostridium difficile Toxin Assay, Fecal
Cold Agglutinins
Complement (C3, C4, CH$_{50}$)

Cortisol, Serum
Counterimmunoelectrophoresis
Creatine Phosphokinase
Creatinine, Serum
Cryoglobulins, Serum
Cytomegalovirus Antibodies
Dehydroepiandrosterone
Dehydroepiandrosterone Sulfate
Dexamethasone Suppression Test
Erythropoietin
Estradiol, Serum
Estrogen/Progesterone Receptors
Ethanol
Fecal Fat
Ferritin
Folic Acid
Follicle-Stimulating Hormone (FSH)
FTA-ABS
Fungal Serologies
Gastrin, Serum
GGT
Glucose
Glucose Tolerance Test, Oral
Glycohemoglobin
Haptoglobin
Helicobacter pylori Antibody Titers
Hepatitis Testing
High-Density Lipoprotein Cholesterol
HLA
Homocysteine, Serum
Human Chorionic Gonadotropin (HCG)
Human Immunodeficiency Antibody Testing (HIV)
Immunoglobulins, Quantitative
Iron
Iron-Binding Capacity, Total
Lactate Dehydrogenase (LDH)

4

Lactic Acid
LAP Score
LE Preparation
Lead, Blood
Legionella Antibody
Lipase
Lipid Profile
Low-Density Lipoprotein-
   Cholesterol
Luteinizing Hormone
Lyme Disease Serology
Magnesium
Metyrapone Test
MHA-TP
β_2-Microglobulin
Monospot
Myoglobin
5'-Nucleotidase
Oligoclonal Banding, CSF
Osmolality, Serum
Oxygen
P-24 Antigen (HIV Antigen)
Parathyroid Hormone
Phosphorus
Potassium, Serum
Progesterone, Serum
Prolactin
Prostate-Specific Antigen (PSA)
Protein Electrophoresis, Serum
   and Urine
Protein, Serum

Renin
   Plasma
   Renal Vein
Retinol-Binding Protein
Rheumatoid Factor
Rocky Mountain Spotted Fever
   Antibodies
Semen Analysis
SGGT
SGOT
SGPT
Sodium, Serum
Stool for Occult Blood
Sweat Chloride
T_3 RU
Testosterone
Thyroglobulin
Thyroid-Stimulating Hormone
Thyroxine
Thyroxine-Binding Globulin
Thyroxine Index, Free
TORCH Battery
Transferrin
Triglycerides
Triiodothyronine
Troponin, Cardiac-Specific
Uric Acid
VDRL Test
Vitamin B_{12}
Zinc

This chapter outlines commonly ordered blood chemistry, immunology, and serology tests with normal values and a guide to the diagnosis of common abnormalities. Other laboratory tests can be found in the following chapters: Hematology, Chapter 5; Urine Studies, Chapter 6; Microbiology, Chapter 7; and Blood Gases, Chapter 8.

With the institution of DRGs, it becomes imperative to understand appropriate, as well as economical, laboratory testing patterns. Laboratory testing should be guided by, but not a substitute for, an effective history, physical, and careful clinical assessment.

Most laboratories offer AMA recommended "panel" tests, whereby multiple determinations are performed on a single sample. Although your lab may vary, some common chemistry panels include:

Basic Metabolic Panel: BUN, calcium, creatinine, electrolytes (Na, K, Cl, CO_2), glucose
Cardiac Enzymes: CK-MB (if total CK >150 IU/L), troponin
Chem-7 Panel/SMA-7: BUN, creatinine, electrolytes (Na, K, Cl, CO_2),glucose

Comprehensive Metabolic Panel: Albumin, alkaline phosphatase, ALT (SGPT), AST (SGOT), bilirubin (total), BUN, calcium, creatinine, electrolytes (Na, K, Cl, CO_2), glucose, protein (total)

Electrolytes: Sodium, potassium, chloride, CO_2, (Na, K, Cl, CO_2)

Health Screen-12/SMA-12: Albumin, alkaline phosphatase, AST (SGOT), bilirubin (total), calcium, cholesterol, creatinine, glucose, LDH, phosphate, protein (total), uric acid

Hepatic Function Panel: Albumin, alkaline phosphatase, ALT (SGPT), AST (SGOT), bilirubin (total & direct), protein

Lipid Panel: Cholesterol, HDL cholesterol, LDL cholesterol (calculated), triglycerides

The Système International (SI) is a metric-based laboratory data-reporting system that is used internationally. The mole is the unit used most extensively in the system. The SI unit for expressing enzymatic activity is the "katal"; however, most countries have adopted units per liter (U/L) as an alternative measure of enzymatic activity. For most lab values, representative SI units have been included; however, each individual laboratory should be consulted for its "normal" values.

If an increased or decreased value is not clinically useful, it is usually not listed. Because each laboratory has its own set of normal reference values, the normals given should only be used as a guide. The range for common normal values is given in parentheses. Unless specified, values reflect normal adult levels. This section includes the method of collection since laboratories have attempted to standardize collection methods; however, be aware that some labs may have alternative collection methods. Blood specimen tubes are listed in Chapter 13, page 311.

ACETOACETATE (KETONE BODIES, ACETONE)

• Normal = negative • Collection: Red top tube

Positive: DKA, starvation, emesis, stress, alcoholism, infantile organic acidemias, isopropanol ingestion

ACID PHOSPHATASE (PROSTATIC ACID PHOSPHATASE, PAP)

• <3.0 ng/mL by RIA, or <0.8 IU/L by enzymatic • Collection: Tiger top tube
   Not a useful screening test for cancer; most useful as a marker of response to therapy or in confirming metastatic disease. PSA is more sensitive in diagnosis of cancer.

Increased: Carcinoma of the prostate (usually outside of prostate), prostatic surgery or trauma (including prostatic massage), rarely in infiltrative bone disease (Gaucher's disease, myeloid leukemia), prostatitis, or BPH

ACTH (ADRENOCORTICOTROPIC HORMONE)

• 8 AM 20–140 pg/mL (SI: 20–140 ng/L), midnight, approximately 50% of AM value • Collection: Tiger top tube

Increased: Addison's disease (primary adrenal hypofunction), ectopic ACTH production (small [oat] cell lung carcinoma, pancreatic islet cell tumors, thymic tumors, renal cell carcinoma, bronchial carcinoid), Cushing's disease (pituitary adenoma), congenital adrenal hyperplasia (adrenogenital syndrome)

Decreased: Adrenal adenoma or carcinoma, nodular adrenal hyperplasia, pituitary insufficiency, corticosteroid use

ACTH STIMULATION TEST (CORTROSYN STIMULATION TEST)

• Collection: Tiger top tube

Used to help diagnose adrenal insufficiency. Cortrosyn (an ACTH analogue) is given at a dose of 0.25 mg IM or IV in adults or 0.125 mg in children <2 years. Collect blood at time 0, 30, and 60 min for cortisol and aldosterone.

Normal Response: Three criteria are required: basal cortisol of at least 5 mg/dL, an incremental increase after cosyntropin (Cortrosyn) injection of at least 7 mg/dL, and a final serum cortisol of at least 16 mg/dL at 30 or 18 mg/dL at 60 min or cortisol increase of >10 mg/dL. Aldosterone increases >5 ng/dL over baseline.

Addison's Disease (Primary Adrenal Insufficiency):   Neither cortisol nor aldosterone increase over baseline.

Secondary Adrenal Insufficiency: Caused by pituitary insufficiency or suppression by exogenous steroids, cortisol does not increase, but aldosterone does.

ALBUMIN

• Adult 3.5–5.0 g/dL (SI: 35–50 g/L), child 3.8–5.4 g/dL (SI: 38–54 g/L) • Collection: Tiger top tube; part of SMA-12

Decreased: Malnutrition (see page 211), overhydration, nephrotic syndrome, CF, multiple myeloma, Hodgkin's disease, leukemia, metastatic cancer, protein-losing enteropathies, chronic glomerulonephritis, alcoholic cirrhosis, inflammatory bowel disease, collagen-vascular diseases, hyperthyroidism

ALBUMIN/GLOBULIN RATIO (A/G RATIO)

• Normal >1

A calculated value (Total protein minus albumin = globulins. Albumin divided by globulins = A/G ratio). Serum protein electrophoresis is a more informative test (see page 85).

Decreased: Cirrhosis, liver diseases, nephrotic syndrome, chronic glomerulonephritis, cachexia, burns, chronic infections and inflammatory states, myeloma

ALDOSTERONE

• Serum: Supine 3–10 ng/dL (SI: 0.083–0.28 nmol/L) early AM, normal sodium intake [3 g sodium/d] • Upright 5–30 ng/dL (SI: 0.138–0.83 nmol/L); urinary 2–16 mg/24 h (SI: 5.4–44.3 nmol/d) • Collection: Green or lavender top tube

Discontinue antihypertensives and diuretics 2 wk prior to test. Upright samples should be drawn after 2 h. Primarily used to screen hypertensive patients for possible Conn's syndrome (adrenal adenoma producing excess aldosterone).

Increased: Primary hyperaldosteronism, secondary hyperaldosteronism (CHF, sodium depletion, nephrotic syndrome, cirrhosis with ascites, others), upright posture

Decreased: Adrenal insufficiency, panhypopituitarism, supine posture

ALKALINE PHOSPHATASE

• Adult 20–70 U/L, child 20–150 U/L • Collection: Tiger top tube; part of SMA-12

A fractionated alkaline phosphatase was formerly used to differentiate the origin of the enzyme in the bone from that in the liver. Replaced by the GGT and 5′-nucleotidase determinations

Increased: Increased calcium deposition in bone (hyperparathyroidism), Paget's disease, osteoblastic bone tumors (metastatic or osteogenic sarcoma), osteomalacia, rickets, pregnancy, childhood, healing fracture, liver disease such as biliary obstruction (masses, drug therapy), hyperthyroidism

Decreased: Malnutrition, excess vitamin D ingestion

ALPHA-FETOPROTEIN (AFP)

• (<16 ng/mL (SI: <16 mL) • third trimester of pregnancy maximum 550 ng/mL (SI: 550 mL) • Collection: Tiger top tube

Increased: Hepatoma (hepatocellular carcinoma), testicular tumor (embryonal carcinoma, malignant teratoma), neural tube defects (in mother's serum [spina bifida, anencephaly, myelomeningocele]), fetal death, multiple gestations, ataxia–telangiectasia, some cases of benign hepatic diseases (alcoholic cirrhosis, hepatitis, necrosis)

Decreased: Trisomy 21 (Down syndrome) in maternal serum

ALT (ALANINE AMINOTRANSFERASE, ALAT) OR SGPT

• 0–35 U/L (SI: 0–0.58 mkat/L), higher in newborns • Collection: Tiger top tube

Increased: Liver disease, liver metastasis, biliary obstruction, pancreatitis, liver congestion (ALT is more elevated than AST in viral hepatitis; AST elevated more than ALT in alcoholic hepatitis.)

AMMONIA

• Adult 10–80 mg/dL (SI: 5–50 mmol/L) • To convert mg/dL to mmol/L, multiply by 0.5872 • Collection: Green top tube, on ice, analyze immediately

Increased: Liver failure, Reye's syndrome, inborn errors of metabolism, normal neonates (normalizes within 48 h of birth)

AMYLASE

• 50–150 Somogyi units/dL (SI: 100–300 U/L) • Collection: Tiger top tube

Increased: Acute pancreatitis, pancreatic duct obstruction (stones, stricture, tumor, sphincter spasm secondary to drugs), pancreatic pseudocyst or abscess, alcohol ingestion, mumps, parotiditis, renal disease, macroamylasemia, cholecystitis, peptic ulcers, intestinal obstruction, mesenteric thrombosis, after surgery

Decreased: Pancreatic destruction (pancreatitis, cystic fibrosis), liver damage (hepatitis, cirrhosis), normal newborns in the first year of life

ASO (ANTISTREPTOLYSIN O/ANTISTREPTOCOCCAL O) TITER (STREPTOZYME)

• <200 IU/mL (Todd units) school-age children • <100 IU/mL preschool and adults • varies with lab • Collection: Tiger top tube

Increased: Streptococcal infections (pharyngitis, scarlet fever, rheumatic fever, poststreptococcal glomerulonephritis), RA, and other collagen diseases

AST (ASPARTATE AMINOTRANSFERASE, ASAT) OR SGOT

- 8–20 U/L (SI: 0–0.58 mkat/L) • Collection: Tiger top tube; part of SMA-12
  Generally parallels changes in ALT in liver disease.

Increased: AMI, liver disease, Reye's syndrome, muscle trauma and injection, pancreatitis, intestinal injury or surgery, factitious increase (erythromycin, opiates), burns, cardiac catheterization, brain damage, renal infarction

Decreased: Beriberi (vitamin B_6 deficiency), severe diabetes with ketoacidosis, liver disease, chronic hemodialysis

AUTOANTIBODIES

- Normal = negative • Collection: Tiger top tube

Antinuclear Antibody (ANA, FANA)

A useful screening test in patients with symptoms suggesting collagen–vascular disease, especially if titer is >1:160.

Positive: SLE, drug-induced lupus-like syndromes (procainamide, hydralazine, isoniazid, etc), scleroderma, MCTD, RA, polymyositis, juvenile RA (5–20%). Low titers are also seen in non-collagen–vascular disease.

Specific Immunofluorescent ANA Patterns

Homogenous. Nonspecific, from antibodies to DNP and native double-stranded DNA. Seen in SLE and a variety of other diseases. Antihistone is consistent with drug-induced lupus.

Speckled. Pattern seen in many connective tissue disorders. From antibodies to ENA, including anti-RNP, anti-Sm, anti-PM-1, and anti-SS. Anti-RNP is positive in MCTD and SLE. Anti-Sm is very sensitive for SLE. Anti-SS-A and anti-SS-B are seen in Sjögren's syndrome and subacute cutaneous lupus. The speckled pattern is also seen with scleroderma.

Peripheral Rim Pattern. From antibodies to native double-stranded DNA and DNP. Seen in SLE

Nucleolar Pattern. From antibodies to nucleolar RNA. Positive in Sjögren's syndrome and scleroderma

Anticentromere: Scleroderma, Raynaud's disease, CREST syndrome

Anti-DNA (Antidouble-stranded DNA): SLE (but negative in drug-induced lupus), chronic active hepatitis, mononucleosis

Antimitochondrial: Primary biliary cirrhosis, autoimmune diseases such as SLE

Antineutrophil Cytoplasmic: Wegener's granulomatosis, polyarteritis nodosa, and other vasculitides

Anti-SCL 70: Scleroderma

Antismooth Muscle: Low titers are seen in a variety of illnesses; high titers (>1:100) are suggestive of chronic active hepatitis.

Sjögren Syndrome Antibody (SS-A): Sjögren syndrome, SLE, RA

Antimicrosomal: Hashimoto's thyroiditis

BASE EXCESS/DEFICIT

• −2 to +2 • See Chapter 8, page 162

BICARBONATE (OR "TOTAL CO$_2$")

• 23–29 mmol/L • See CARBON DIOXIDE, page 61

BILIRUBIN

• Total, 0.3–1.0 mg/dL (SI: 3.4–17.1 mmol/L) • direct, <0.2 mg/dL (SI: <3.4 mmol/L) • indirect, <0.8 mg/dL (SI: <3.4 mmol/L) • To convert mg/dL to mmol/L, multiply by 17.10 • Collection: Tiger top tube

Increased Total: Hepatic damage (hepatitis, toxins, cirrhosis), biliary obstruction (stone or tumor), hemolysis, fasting.

Increased Direct (Conjugated): *Note:* Determination of the direct bilirubin is usually unnecessary with total bilirubin levels <1.2 mg/dL (SI: 21 mmol/L) Biliary obstruction/cholestasis (gallstone, tumor, stricture), drug-induced cholestasis, Dubin–Johnson and Rotor's syndromes

Increased Indirect (Unconjugated): *Note:* This is calculated as total minus direct bilirubin. So-called hemolytic jaundice caused by any type of hemolytic anemia (transfusion reaction, sickle cell, etc), Gilbert's disease, physiologic jaundice of the newborn, Crigler–Najjar syndrome

Bilirubin, Neonatal("Baby Bilirubin")

• Normal levels dependent on prematurity and age in days • "panic levels" usually >15–20 mg/dL (SI: >257–342 mmol/L in full-term infants) • Collection: Capillary tube

Increased: Erythroblastosis fetalis, physiologic jaundice (may be due to breast-feeding), resorption of hematoma or hemorrhage, obstructive jaundice, others

BLOOD UREA NITROGEN (BUN)

• Birth–1 year: 4–16 mg/dL (SI: 1.4–5.7 mmol/L) • 1–40 years 5–20 mg/dL (SI: 1.8–7.1 mmol/L)]] • Gradual slight increase with age • To convert mg/dL to mmol/L, multiply by 0.3570 • Collection: Tiger top tube

Less useful measure of GFR than creatinine because BUN is also related to protein metabolism

Increased: Renal failure (including drug-induced from aminoglycosides, NSAIDs), pre-renal azotemia (decreased renal perfusion secondary to CHF, shock, volume depletion), postrenal (obstruction), GI bleeding, stress, drugs (especially aminoglycosides)

Decreased: Starvation, liver failure (hepatitis, drugs), pregnancy, infancy, nephrotic syndrome, overhydration

BUN/CREATININE RATIO (BUN/CR)

• Mean 10, range 6–20

Calculated based on serum levels

Increased: Prerenal azotemia (renal hypoperfusion), GI bleeding, high-protein diet, ileal conduit, drugs (steroids, tetracycline)

Decreased: Malnutrition, pregnancy, low-protein diet, ketoacidosis, hemodialysis, SIADH, drugs (cimetidine)

4 C-PEPTIDE, INSULIN ("CONNECTING PEPTIDE")

• Fasting, <4.0 ng/mL (SI: <4.0 mg/L) • Male >60 years, 1.5–5.0 ng/mL (SI: 1.5–5.0 mg/L) • Female 1.4–5.5 ng/mL (SI: 1.4–5.5 mg/L) • Collection: Tiger top tube
     Differentiates between exogenous and endogenous insulin production/administration. Liberated when proinsulin is split to insulin; levels suggest endogenous production of insulin

Decreased: Diabetes (decreased endogenous insulin), insulin administration (factitious or therapeutic), hypoglycemia

C-REACTIVE PROTEIN (CRP)

• Normal = none detected • Collection: Tiger top tube
     A nonspecific screen for infectious and inflammatory diseases, correlates well with ESR. In the first 24 h, however, ESR may be normal and CRP elevated.

Increased: Bacterial infections, inflammatory conditions (acute rheumatic fever, acute RA, MI, transplant rejection, embolus, inflammatory bowel disease), last half of pregnancy, oral contraceptives, some malignancies

CA 15-3

Used to detect breast cancer recurrence in asymptomatic patients and monitor therapy. Levels related to stage of disease

Increased: Progressive breast cancer, benign breast disease and liver disease

Decreased: Response to therapy (25% change considered significant)

CA 19-9

• <37 U/ml (SI:<37 kU/L) • Collection: Tiger top tube
     Primary used to determine resectability of pancreatic cancers (ie, >1000U/mL 95% unresectable)

Increased: GI cancers such as pancreas, stomach, liver, colorectal, hepatobiliary, some cases of lung and prostate, pancreatitis

CA-125

• <35 U/mL (SI: <35 kU/L) • Collection: Tiger top tube
     Not a useful screening test for ovarian cancer when used alone; best used in conjunction with ultrasound and physical examination. Rising levels after resection predictive for recurrence

Increased: Ovarian, endometrial, and colon cancer; endometriosis; inflammatory bowel disease; PID; pregnancy; breast lesions; and benign abdominal masses (teratomas)

CALCITONIN (THYROCALCITONIN)

• <19 pg/mL (SI: <19 ng/L) • Collection: Tiger top tube

Increased: Medullary carcinoma of the thyroid, C-cell hyperplasia (precursor of medullary carcinoma), small (oat) cell carcinoma of the lung, newborns, pregnancy, chronic renal insufficiency, Zollinger–Ellison syndrome, pernicious anemia.

CALCIUM, SERUM

• Infants to 1 month: 7–11.5 mg/dL (SI: 1.75–2.87 mmol/L) • 1 month to 1 year: 8.6–11.2 mg/dL (SI: 2.15–2.79 mmol/L) • >1 year and adults: 8.2–10.2 mg/dL (SI: 2.05–2.54 mmol/L) • Ionized: 4.75–5.2 mg/dL (SI: 1.19–1.30 mmol/L) • To convert mg/dL to mmol/L, multiply by 0.2495 • Collection: Tiger top tube; ionized requires green or red tube

When interpreting a total calcium value, albumin must be known. If it is not within normal limits, a corrected calcium can be roughly calculated by the following formula. Values for ionized calcium need no special corrections.

$$\text{Corrected total Ca} = 0.8 \, (\text{Normal albumin} - \text{Measured albumin}) + \text{Reported Ca}$$

Increased: (*Note:* Levels >12 mg/dL [2.99 mmol/L] may lead to coma and death) Primary hyperparathyroidism, PTH-secreting tumors, vitamin D excess, metastatic bone tumors, osteoporosis, immobilization, milk-alkali syndrome, Paget's disease, idiopathic hypercalcemia of infants, infantile hypophosphatasia, thiazide diuretics, chronic renal failure, sarcoidosis, multiple myeloma

Decreased: (*Note:* Levels <7 mg/dL [<1.75 mmol/L] may lead to tetany and death.) Hypoparathyroidism (surgical, idiopathic), pseudo-hypoparathyroidism, insufficient vitamin D, calcium and phosphorus ingestion (pregnancy, osteomalacia, rickets), hypomagnesemia, renal tubular acidosis, hypoalbuminemia (cachexia, nephrotic syndrome, CF), chronic renal failure (phosphate retention), acute pancreatitis, factitious decrease because of low protein and albumin

CAPTOPRIL TEST

• See Aldosterone, page 56, and renin (plasma renin), page 88, for normal values

Used in the evaluation of renovascular hypotension, the drug is an ACE inhibitor that blocks angiotensin II. Captopril is administered (25 mg IV at 8AM). Aldosterone decreases 2 h later from baseline in normals or essential hypertension, but does not suppress in patients with aldosteronism. For renovascular hypertension, the PRA increases >12 ng/mL/h and an absolute increase of 10 ng/mL/h plus a 400% increase in PRA if pretest level <3 ng/mL/h and >150% over baseline if the pretest PRA was >3 ng/mL/h. Test now also combined with nuclear renal scan to identify renal artery stenosis

CARBON DIOXIDE ("TOTAL CO₂" OR BICARBONATE)

• Adult 23–29 mmol/L, child 20–28 mmol/L • (See Chapter 8 for pCO_2 values • Collection: Tiger top tube, do not expose sample to air

Increased: Compensation for respiratory acidosis (emphysema) and metabolic alkalosis (severe vomiting, primary aldosteronism, volume contraction, Bartter's syndrome)

Decreased: Compensation for respiratory alkalosis, and metabolic acidosis (starvation, diabetic ketoacidosis, lactic acidosis, alcoholic ketoacidosis, toxins [methanol, ethylene glycol, paraldehyde], severe diarrhea, renal failure, drugs [salicylates, acetazolamide], dehydration, adrenal insufficiency)

CARBOXYHEMOGLOBIN (CARBON MONOXIDE)

• Nonsmoker <2%; smoker <9%; toxic >15%• Collection: Gray or lavender top tube; confirm with lab

Increased: Smokers, smoke inhalation, automobile exhaust inhalation, normal newborns

CARCINOEMBRYONIC ANTIGEN (CEA)

• Nonsmoker <3.0 ng/mL (SI: <3.0 μg/L) • smoker <5.0 ng/mL (SI: <5.0 μg/L) • Collection: Tiger top tube

   Not a screening test; useful for monitoring response to treatment and tumor recurrence of adenocarcinomas of the GI tract

Increased: Carcinoma (colon, pancreas, lung, stomach), smokers, nonneoplastic liver disease, Crohn's disease, and ulcerative colitis

CATECHOLAMINES, FRACTIONATED SERUM

• Collection: Green or lavender tube; check with lab

   Values vary and depend on the lab and method of assay used. Normal levels shown here are based on a HPLC technique. Patient must be supine in a nonstimulating environment with IV access to obtain sample.

Catecholamine	Plasma (Supine) Levels
Norepinephrine	70–750 pg/mL (SI: 414–4435 pmol/L)
Epinephrine	0–100 pg/mL (SI: 0–546 pmol/L)
Dopamine	<30 pg/mL (SI: 196 pmol/L)

Increased: Pheochromocytoma, neural CREST tumors (neuroblastoma), with extra-adrenal pheochromocytoma, norepinephrine may be markedly elevated compared with epinephrine.

CHLORIDE, SERUM

• 97–107 mEq/L (SI: 97–107 mmol/L) • Collection: Tiger top tube

Increased: Diarrhea, renal tubular acidosis, mineralocorticoid deficiency, hyperalimentation, medications (acetazolamide, ammonium chloride)

Decreased: Vomiting, diabetes mellitus with ketoacidosis, mineralocorticoid excess, renal disease with sodium loss

CHOLESTEROL

• Total • Normal, see Table 4–1; see also LIPID PROFILE/CHOLESTEROL SCREENING, page 79, and Figure 4–4, see page 80.• To convert mg/dL to mmol/L, multiply by 0.02586 • Collection: Tiger top tube

TABLE 4–1
Normal Total Cholesterol Levels by Age

Age	Standard Units (mg/dL)	SI Units (mmol/L)
<29	<200	<5.20
30–39	<225	<5.85
40–49	<245	<6.35

Increased: Idiopathic hypercholesterolemia, biliary obstruction, nephrosis, hypothyroidism, pancreatic disease (diabetes), pregnancy, oral contraceptives, hyperlipoproteinemia (types IIb, III, V)

Decreased: Liver disease (hepatitis, etc), hyperthyroidism, malnutrition (cancer, starvation), chronic anemias, steroid therapy, lipoproteinemias, AMI

High-Density Lipoprotein Cholesterol (HDL, HDL-C)

• Fasting 30–70 mg/dL (SI: 0.8–1.80 mmol/L) • Female 30–90 mg/dL (SI: 0.80–2.35)
   HDL-C has the best correlation with the development of CAD; decreased HDL-C in males leads to an increased risk. Levels <45 mg/dL associated with increased risk of CAD

Increased: Estrogen (females), regular exercise, small ethanol intake, medications (nicotinic acid, gemfibrozil, others)

Decreased: Males, smoking, uremia, obesity, diabetes, liver disease, Tangier disease

Low-Density Lipoprotein Cholesterol (LDL, LDL-C)

• 50–190 mg/dL (SI: 1.30–4.90 mmol/L)

Increased: Excess dietary saturated fats, MI, hyperlipoproteinemia, biliary cirrhosis, endocrine disease (diabetes, hypothyroidism)

Decreased: Malabsorption, severe liver disease, abetalipoproteinemia

CLOSTRIDIUM DIFFICILE TOXIN ASSAY, FECAL

• Normal negative
   Majority of patients with pseudomembranous colitis have positive *C. difficile* assay. Often positive in antibiotic associated diarrhea and colitis. Can be seen in some normals and neonates

COLD AGGLUTININS

• <1:32 • Collection: Lavender or blue top tube
   Most frequently used to screen for atypical pneumonias.

Increased: Atypical pneumonia (mycoplasmal pneumonia), other viral infections (especially mononucleosis, measles, mumps), cirrhosis, parasitic infections, Waldenström's macroglobulinemia, lymphomas and leukemias, multiple myeloma

COMPLEMENT

- Collection: Tiger or lavender top tube
  Complement describes a series of sequentially reacting serum proteins that participate in pathogenic processes and lead to inflammatory injury.

Complement C3

- 85–155 mg/dL, (SI: 800–1500 ng/L)
  Decreased levels suggest activation of the classical or alternative pathway, or both.

Increased: RA (variable finding), rheumatic fever, various neoplasms (gastrointestinal, prostate, others), acute viral hepatitic, MI, pregnancy, amyloidosis

Decreased: SLE, glomerulonephritis (poststreptococcal and membranoproliferative), sepsis, SBE, chronic active hepatitis, malnutrition, DIC, gram-negative sepsis

Complement C4

- 20–50 mg/dL (SI: 200–500 ng/L)

Increased: RA (variable finding), neoplasia (gastrointestinal, lung, others)

Decreased: SLE, chronic active hepatitis, cirrhosis, glomerulonephritis, hereditary angioedema (test of choice).

Complement CH50 (Total)

- 33–61 mg/mL (SI: 330–610 ng/L)
  Tests for complement deficiency in the classical pathway.

Increased: Acute-phase reactants (tissue injury, infections, etc)

Decreased: Hereditary complement deficiencies

CORTISOL, SERUM

- 8 AM, 5.0–23.0 mg/dL (SI: 138–365 nmol/L) • 4 PM, 3.0–15.0 mg/dL (SI: 83–414 nmol/L) • Collection: Green or red top tube

Increased: Adrenal adenoma, adrenal carcinoma, Cushing's disease, nonpituitary ACTH-producing tumor, steroid therapy, oral contraceptives

Decreased: Primary adrenal insufficiency (Addison's disease), congenital adrenal hyperplasia, Waterhouse-Friderichsen syndrome, ACTH deficiency

COUNTERIMMUNOELECTROPHORESIS (CIEP, CEP)

- Normal = negative
  An immunologic technique that allows for rapid identification of infecting organisms from fluids, including serum, urine, CSF, and other body fluids. Organisms identified in-

clude *Neisseria meningitidis, Streptococcus pneumoniae, Haemophilus influenzae,* and group B *Streptococcus.*

CREATINE PHOSPHOKINASE (KINASE) (CP, CPK)

• 25–145 mU/mL (SI: 25–145 U/L) • Collection: Tiger top tube
Used in suspected MI or muscle diseases. Heart, skeletal muscle, and brain have high levels

Increased: Muscle damage (AMI, myocarditis, muscular dystrophy, muscle trauma [including injections], after surgery), brain infarction, defibrillation, cardiac catheterization and surgery, rhabdomyolysis, polymyositis, hypothyroidism

CPK Isoenzymes

MB: (Normal <6%, heart origin) increased in AMI (begins in 2–12 h, peaks at 12–40 h, returns to normal in 24–72 h), pericarditis with myocarditis, rhabdomyolysis, crush injury, Duchenne's muscular dystrophy, polymyositis, malignant hyperthermia, and cardiac surgery

MM: (Normal 94–100%, skeletal muscle origin) increased in crush injury, malignant hyperthermia, seizures, IM injections

BB: (Normal 0%, brain origin) brain injury (CVA, trauma), metastatic neoplasms (prostate), malignant hyperthermia, colonic infarction

CREATININE, SERUM

• Adult male <1.2 mg/dL (SI: 106 mmol/L) • Adult female <1.1 mg/dL (SI: 97 mmol/L)
• Child 0.5–0.8 mg/dL (SI: 44–71 mmol/L) • To convert mg/dL to μmol/L, multiply by 88.40 • Collection: Tiger top tube
A clinically useful estimate of GFR. As a rule of thumb, serum creatinine doubles with each 50% reduction in the GFR. Creatine clearance is discussed in Chapter 6.

Increased: Renal failure (prerenal, renal, or postrenal obstruction or medication-induced [aminoglycosides, NSAIDs, others]), gigantism, acromegaly, ingestion of roasted meat, false-positive with DKA

Decreased: Pregnancy, decreased muscle mass, severe liver disease

CRYOGLOBULINS (CRYOCRIT)

<0.4% (or negative if qualitative) {·}
Collection: Tiger top tube, process immediately
These abnormal proteins precipitate out of serum at low temperatures. Cryocrit, a quantitative measure, is preferred over the qualitative method. Should be collected in nonanticoagulated tubes and transported at body temperature. Positive samples can be analyzed for immunoglobulin class, and light-chain type on request.

Monoclonal: Multiple myeloma, Waldenström's macroglobulinemia, lymphoma, CLL

Mixed Polyclonal or Mixed Monoclonal: Infectious diseases (viral, bacterial, parasitic), such as SBE or malaria; SLE; RA; essential cryoglobulinemia; lymphoproliferative diseases; sarcoidosis; chronic liver disease (cirrhosis)

CYTOMEGALOVIRUS (CMV) ANTIBODIES

• IgM <1:8, IgG <1:16 • Collection: Tiger top tube

Used in neonates (CMV is the most common intrauterine infection), posttransfusion CMV infection, and organ donors and recipients. Most of adults will have detectable titers.

Increased: Serial measurements 10–14 days apart with a 4× increase in titers or a single IgM >1:8 is suspicious for acute infection. Universally increased titers in AIDS. IgM most useful in neonatal infections

DEHYDROEPIANDROSTERONE (DHEA)

• Male 2.0–3.4 ng/mL (SI: 5.2–8.7 mmol/L) • Female, premenopausal 0.8–3.4 ng/mL (SI: 2.1–8.8 mmol/L) • Postmenopausal 0.1–0.6 ng/mL (SI: 0.3–1.6 mmol/L) • Collection: Tiger top tube

Increased: Anovulation, polycystic ovaries, adrenal hyperplasia, adrenal tumors

Decreased: Menopause

DEHYDROEPIANDROSTERONE SULFATE (DHEAS)

• Male 1.7–4.2 ng/mL (SI: 6–15 mmol/L) • Female 2.0–5.2 ng/mL (SI: 7–18 mmol/L) • Collection: Tiger top tube

Increased: Hyperprolactinemia, adrenal hyperplasia, adrenal tumor, polycystic ovaries, lipoid ovarian tumors

Decreased: Menopause

DEXAMETHASONE SUPPRESSION TEST

Used in the differential diagnosis of Cushing's syndrome (elevated cortisol)

Overnight Test: In the "rapid" version of this test, a patient takes 1 mg of dexamethasone PO at 11 PM and a fasting 8 AM plasma cortisol is obtained. Normally the cortisol level should be <5.0 mg/dL [138 nmol/L]. A value that is >5 mg/dL [138 nmol/L] usually confirms the diagnosis of Cushing's syndrome; however, obesity, alcoholism, or depression may occasionally show the same result. In these patients, the best screening test is a 24-h urine for free cortisol.

Low-Dose Test: After collection of baseline serum cortisol and 24-h urine-free cortisol levels, dexamethasone 0.5 mg is administered PO every 6 h for eight doses. Serum and urine cortisol are repeated on the second day. Failure to suppress to a serum cortisol of <5.0 mg/dL [138 nmol/L] and a urine-free cortisol of <30 μg/dL (82 nmol/L) confirms Cushing's syndrome.

High-Dose Test: After the low-dose test, dexamethasone, 2 mg PO every 6 h for eight doses will cause a fall in urinary-free cortisol to 50% of the baseline value in bilateral adrenal hyperplasia (Cushing's disease) but not in adrenal tumors or ectopic ACTH production.

ERYTHROPOIETIN (EPO)

• 5–36 mU/L (5–36 IU/L) • Collection: Tiger top tube

EPO is a renal hormone that stimulates RBC production.

Increased: Pregnancy, secondary polycythemia (high altitude, COPD, etc), tumors (renal cell carcinoma, cerebellar hemangioblastoma, hepatoma, others), PCKD, anemias with bone marrow unresponsiveness (aplastic anemia, iron deficiency, etc)

Decreased: Bilateral nephrectomy, anemia of chronic disease (ie, renal failure, nephrotic syndrome), primary polycythemia (*Note:* The determination of EPO levels before administration of recombinant EPO for renal failure is not usually necessary.)

ESTRADIOL, SERUM

• Collection: Tiger top tube

Serial measurements useful in assessing fetal well-being, especially in high-risk pregnancy. Also useful in evaluation of amenorrhea and gynecomastia in males.

Female	**Normal Values**
Follicular phase	25–75 pg/mL
Midcycle peak	200–600 pg/mL
Luteal phase	100–300 pg/mL
Pregnancy 1st trimester	1–5 ng/mL
2nd trimester	5–15 ng/mL
3rd trimester	10–40 ng/mL
Postmenopause	5–25 pg/mL
Oral contraceptives	<50 pg/mL
Male	
Prepubertal	2–8 pg/mL
Adult	10–60 pg/mL

ESTROGEN/PROGESTERONE RECEPTORS

These are typically determined on fresh surgical (breast cancer) specimens. The presence of the receptors is associated with a longer disease-free interval, survival from breast cancer, and increased likelihood of responding to endocrine therapy. Fifty to seventy-five percent of breast cancers are estrogen-receptor-positive.

ETHANOL (BLOOD ALCOHOL)

• 0 mg/dL (0 mmol/L) • Collection: Tiger top tube; do not use alcohol to clean venipuncture site, use povidone-iodine

Physiologic changes can vary with degree of alcohol tolerance of an individual.

• <50 mg/dL [<10.85 mmol/L]: Limited muscular incoordination
• 50–100 [10.85–21.71]: Pronounced incoordination
• 100–150 [21.71–32.57]: Mood and personality changes; legally intoxicated in most states
• 150–400 [32.57–87]: Nausea, vomiting, marked ataxia, amnesia, dysarthria
• ≥400: Coma, respiratory insufficiency and death

FECAL FAT

• 2–6 g/d on an 80–100 g/d fat diet • 72-h collection time • Sudan III stain, random <60 droplets fat/hpf

Increased: CF, pancreatic insufficiency, Crohn's disease, chronic pancreatitis, sprue

FERRITIN

- Male 15–200 ng/mL (SI: 15–200 mg/L) • Female 12–150 ng/mL (SI: 12–150 mg/L)
- Collection: Tiger top tube

Increased: Hemochromatosis, hemosiderosis, sideroblastic anemia

Decreased: Iron deficiency (earliest and most sensitive test before red cells show any morphologic change), severe liver disease

FOLIC ACID

Serum Folate
- >2.0 ng/mL (SI: >5 nmol/L)

RBC

- 125–600 ng/mL (283–1360 nmol/L) • Collection: Lavender top tube

   Serum folate can fluctuate with diet. RBC levels are more indicative of tissue stores. Vitamin B_{12} deficiency can result in the RBC unable to take up folate in spite of normal serum folate levels.

Increased: Folic acid administration

Decreased: Malnutrition/malabsorption (folic acid deficiency), massive cellular growth (cancer) or cell turnover, ongoing hemolysis, medications (trimethoprim, some anticonvulsants, oral contraceptives), vitamin B_{12} deficiency (low RBC levels), pregnancy

FOLLICLE-STIMULATING HORMONE (FSH)

- Males: <22 IU/L • Females: nonmidcycle <20 IU/L, midcycle surge <40 IU/L (Midcycle peak should be two times basal level • Postmenopausal 40–160 IU/L • Collection: Tiger top tube

   Used in the workup of impotence, infertility in men, and amenorrhea in women

Increased: (Hypergonadotropic >40 IU/L) postmenopausal, surgical castration, gonadal failure, gonadotropin-secreting pituitary adenoma

Decreased: (Hypogonadotropic <5 IU/L) prepubertal, hypothalamic and pituitary dysfunction, pregnancy

FTA-ABS (FLUORESCENT TREPONEMAL ANTIBODY ABSORBED)

- Normal = nonreactive • Collection: Tiger top tube

   FTA-ABS may be negative in early primary syphilis and remain positive in spite of adequate treatment.

Positive: Syphilis (test of choice to confirm diagnosis after a reactive VDRL test), other treponemal infections can cause false-positive (Lyme disease, leprosy, malaria)

FUNGAL SEROLOGIES

- Negative <1:8 • Collection: Tiger top tube

   This is a screening technique for complement-fixed fungal antibodies, which usually detects antibodies to *Histoplasma capsulatum, Blastomyces dermatitidis, Cryptococcus neoformans, Aspergillus* species, *Candida* species, and *Coccidioides immitis.*

GASTRIN, SERUM

• Fasting <100 pg/mL (SI: 47.7 pmol/L) • Postprandial 95–140 pg/mL (SI: 45.3–66.7 pmol/L) • Collection: Tiger top tube, freeze immediately

Make sure patient is not on H_2 blockers or antacids.

Increased: Zollinger–Ellison syndrome, medications (antacids, cimetidine, others) pyloric stenosis, pernicious anemia, atrophic gastritis, ulcerative colitis, renal insufficiency, and steroid and calcium administration

Decreased: Vagotomy and antrectomy

GGT (SERUM GAMMA-GLUTAMYL TRANSPEPTIDASE, SGGT)

• Male 9–50 U/L • Female 8–40 U/L • Collection: Tiger top tube

Generally parallels changes in serum alkaline phosphatase and 5'-nucleotidase in liver disease. Sensitive indicator of alcoholic liver disease

Increased: Liver disease (hepatitis, cirrhosis, obstructive jaundice), pancreatitis.

GLUCOSE

• Fasting, 70–105 mg/dL (SI: 3.89–5.83 nmol/L) • 2 h postprandial <140 mg/dL (SI: <7.8 nmol/L) • To convert mg/dL to nmol/L, multiply by 0.05551 • Collection: Tiger top tube

American Diabetes Association Diagnostic Criterion for Diabetes: normal fasting <110, Impaired fasting 110–126, diabetes >126 or any random level >200 when associated with other symptoms. Confirm with repeat testing.

Increased: Diabetes mellitus, Cushing's syndrome, acromegaly, increased epinephrine (injection, pheochromocytoma, stress, burns, etc), acute pancreatitis, ACTH administration, spurious increase caused by drawing blood from a site above an IV line containing dextrose, elderly patients, pancreatic glucagonoma, drugs (glucocorticoids, some diuretics)

Decreased: Pancreatic disorders (pancreatitis, islet cell tumors), extrapancreatic tumors (carcinoma of the adrenals, stomach), hepatic disease (hepatitis, cirrhosis, tumors), endocrine disorders (early diabetes, hypothyroidism, hypopituitarism), functional disorders (after gastrectomy), pediatric problems (prematurity, infant of a diabetic mother, ketotic hypoglycemia, enzyme diseases), exogenous insulin, oral hypoglycemic agents, malnutrition, sepsis

GLUCOSE TOLERANCE TEST (GTT), ORAL (OGTT)

A fasting plasma glucose level >126 mg/dl (7.0 mmol/L) or a casual plasma glucose –200 mg/dL (11.1 mmol/L) meets the threshold for the diagnosis of diabetes, if confirmed on a subsequent day, and precludes the need for any glucose challenge. GTT is usually unnecessary to diagnose asymptomatic diabetes mellitus; it may be useful in gestational diabetes. The GTT is unreliable in the presence of severe infection, prolonged fasting, or after the injection of insulin. After an overnight fast, a fasting blood glucose is drawn, and the patient is given a 75-g oral glucose load (100 g for gestational diabetes screening, 1.75 mg/kg ideal body weight in children up to a dose of 75 g). Plasma glucose is then drawn at 30, 60, 120, and 180 min.

Interpretation of GTT

Adult-Onset Diabetes: Any fasting blood sugar >126, or >200 at both 120 min and one other time interval measured

Gestational Diabetes: Any fasting blood sugar >126, 60 min >180, 120 min >155, 180 min >140

GLYCOHEMOGLOBIN (GHB, GLYCATED HEMOGLOBIN, GLYCOHEMOGLOBIN, HBA₁C, HBA₁ HEMOGLOBIN A₁C, GLYCOSYLATED HEMOGLOBIN)

• 4.6–7.1% or new standard: Nondiabetic <6, near normal 6–7 • Excellent glucose control 7–8 • Good control 8–9 • Fair control 9–10 • Poor control >10 • Collection: Lavender top tube

Useful in long-term monitoring control of blood sugar in diabetics; reflects levels over preceding 3–4 months. Glycated serum protein (GSP) under study and may reflect serum glucose over the preceding 1–2 weeks

Increased: Diabetes mellitus (uncontrolled), lead intoxication

Decreased: Chronic renal failure, hemolytic anemia, pregnancy, chronic blood loss

HAPTOGLOBIN

• 40–180 mg/dL (SI: 0.4–1.8 g/L) • Collection: Tiger top tube

Increased: Obstructive liver disease, any cause of increased ESR (inflammation, collagen-vascular diseases)

Decreased: Any type of hemolysis (transfusion reaction, etc), liver disease, anemia, oral contraceptives, children and infants

HELICOBACTER PYLORI ANTIBODY TITERS

• IgG <0.17 = negative

Most patients with gastritis and ulcer disease (gastric or duodenal) have chronic *H. pylori* infection that should be treated. Positive in 35–50% asymptomatic patients (increases with age). Use in dyspepsia controversial. Four diagnostic methods are available to test for *H. pylori,* the organism associated with gastritis and ulcers. These include noninvasive (serology and a ^{13}C breath test) and invasive (gastric mucosal biopsy and the *Campylobacter*-like organism test). The IgG subclass is found in all patient populations; occasionally only IgA antibodies can be detected. Serology is most useful in the evaluation of newly diagnosed *H. pylori* infection or in monitoring response to therapy. IgG levels decrease slowly after treatment, but can remain elevated after clearing infection.

Positive: Active or recent *H. pylori* infection, some asymptomatic carriers

HEPATITIS TESTING

Recommended hepatitis panel tests based on clinical settings is shown in Table 4–2. Interpretation of testing patterns is shown in Table 4–3. Profile patterns of hepatitis A and B are shown in Figures 4–1 and 4–2, respectively.

Hepatitis Tests (Collection: Tiger top tube)

TABLE 4-2
Hepatitis Panel Testing to Guide the Ordering of Hepatitis Profiles for Given Clinical Settings

Clinical Setting	Test	Purpose
SCREENING TESTS		
Pregnancy	HBsAg*	All expectant mothers should be screened during third trimester
High-risk patients on admission (homosexuals, dialysis patients)	HBsAg	To screen for chronic or active infection
Percutaneous inoculation		
Donor	HBsAg Anti-HBc IgM Anti-Hep C	To test patient's blood (esp. dialysis and HIV patients) for infectivity with hepatitis B and C if a health care worker is exposed
Victim	HBsAg Anti-HBc Anti-Hep C	To test exposed health care worker for immunity or chronic infection
Pre-HBV vaccine	Anti-HBc Anti-HBs	To determine if an individual is infected or has antibodies to HBV
Screening blood donors	HBsAg Anti-HBc Anti-Hep C	Used by blood banks to screen donors for hepatitis B and C
DIAGNOSTIC TESTS		
Differential diagnosis of acute jaundice, hepatitis, or fulminant liver failure	HBsAg Anti-HBc IgM Anti-HAV IgM Anti-Hep C	To differentiate between HBV, HAV, and hepatitis C in an acutely jaundiced patient with hepatitis or fulminant liver failure
Chronic hepatitis	HBsAg HBeAg Anti-HBe Anti-HDV (total + IgM)	To diagnose HBV infection: if positive for HBsAg to determine infectivity If HBsAg patient worsens or is very ill, to diagnose concomitant infection with hepatitis delta virus
MONITORING		
Infant follow-up	HBsAg Anti-HBc	To monitor the success of vaccination and passive

(continued)

**TABLE 4–2
(Continued)**

Clinical Setting	Test	Purpose
	Anti-HBs	immunization for perinatal transmission of HBV 12–15 mo after birth
Postvaccination screening	Anti-HBs	To ensure immunity has been achieved after vaccination (CDC recommends "titer" determination, but usually qualitative assay is adequate)
Sexual contact	HBsAg Anti-HBc Anti-Hep C	To monitor sexual partners of a patient with chronic HBV or hepatitis C

*See text for abbreviations.

**TABLE 4–3
Interpretation of Viral Hepatitis Serologic Testing Patterns**

Anti-HAV (IgM)	HBsAg	Anti-HBc (IgM)	Anti-HBc (Total)	Anti-C (ELISA)	Interpretation
+	–	–	–	–	Acute hepatitis A
+	+	–	+	–	Acute hepatitis A in hepatitis B carrier
–	+	–	+	–	Chronic hepatitis B*
–	–	+	+	–	Acute hepatitis B
–	+	+	+	–	Acute hepatitis B
–	–	–	+	–	Past hepatitis B infection
–	–	–	–	+	Hepatitis C†
–	–	–	–	–	Early hepatitis C or other cause (other virus, toxin)

*Patients with chronic hepatitis B (either active hepatitis or carrier state) should have HBeAg and anti-HBe checked to determine activity of infection and relative infectivity. Anti-HBs is used to determine response to hepatitis B vaccination.
†Anti-C often takes 3–6 mo before being positive. PCR may allow earlier detection.

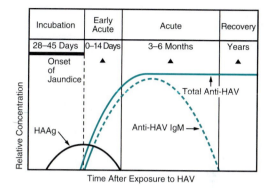

FIGURE 4–1   Hepatitis A diagnostic profile. (Courtesy of Abbott Laboratories, Diagnostic Division, North Chicago, Illinois.)

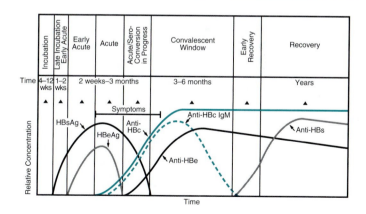

FIGURE 4–2   Hepatitis B diagnostic profile. (Courtesy of Abbott Laboratories, Diagnostic Division, North Chicago, Illinois.)

Hepatitis A

Anti-HAV Ab: Total antibody to hepatitis A virus; confirms previous exposure to hepatitis A virus, elevated for life.

Anti-HAV IgM: IgM antibody to hepatitis A virus; indicative of recent infection with hepatitis A virus; declines typically 1–6 months after symptoms

Hepatitis B

HBsAg: Hepatitis B surface antigen. Earliest marker of HBV infection. Indicates either chronic or acute infection with hepatitis B virus. Used by blood banks to screen donors; vaccination does not affect this test

Anti-HBc-Total: IgG and IgM antibody to hepatitis B core antigen; confirms either previous exposure to hepatitis B virus (HBV) or ongoing infection. Used by blood banks to screen donors

Anti-HBc IgM: IgM antibody to hepatitis B core antigen. Early and best indicator of acute infection with hepatitis B

HBeAg: Hepatitis Be antigen; when present, indicates high degree of infectivity. Order only when evaluating for chronic HBV infection

HBV-DNA: Most sensitive and specific for early evaluation of hepatitis B and may be detected when all other markers are negative

Anti-HBe: Antibody to hepatitis Be antigen; associated with resolution of active inflammation

Anti-HBs: Antibody to hepatitis B surface antigen; when present, typically indicates immunity associated with clinical recovery from HBV infection or previous immunization with hepatitis B vaccine. Order only to assess effectiveness of vaccine and request titer levels

Anti-HDV: Total antibody to delta hepatitis; confirms previous exposure. Order only in patients with known acute or chronic HBV infection.

Anti-HDV IgM: IgM antibody to delta hepatitis; indicates recent infection. Order only in cases of known acute or chronic HBV infection

Hepatitis C

Anti-HCV: Antibody against hepatitis C. Indicative of active viral replication and infectivity. Used by blood banks to screen donors. Many false-positives

HCV-RNA: Nucleic acid probe detection of current HCV infection

HIGH-DENSITY LIPOPROTEIN CHOLESTEROL

- See CHOLESTEROL, page 62.

HLA (HUMAN LEUKOCYTE ANTIGENS; HLA TYPING)

- Collection: Green top tube

This test identified a group of antigens on the cell surface that are the primary determinants of histocompatibility and useful in assessing transplantation compatibility. Some are associated with specific diseases but are not diagnostic of these diseases.

HLA-B27:   Ankylosing spondylitis, psoriatic arthritis, Reiter's syndrome, juvenile RA

HLA-DR4/HLA DR2:   Chronic Lyme disease arthritis

HLA-DRw2:   MS

HLA-B8:   Addison's disease, juvenile-onset diabetes, Grave's disease, gluten-sensitive enteropathy

HOMOCYSTEINE, SERUM

• Normal fasting 5 and 15 µmol/L • Fasting target <10 µmol/L

Under investigation as a risk factor for CAD and atherosclerosis. Moderate, intermediate, and severe hyperhomocystinemia refer to concentrations between 16 and 30, between 31 and 100, and >100 µmol/L, respectively. May be useful to screen high-risk patients and recommend strategies to obtain target of <10 (ie, dietary, lifestyle changes, vitamin supplementation)

Increased: Vitamin B_{12}, B_6 and folate deficiency, kidney and renal failure, medications (nicotinic acid, theophylline, methotrexate, L-dopa, anticonvulsants) advanced age, hypothyroidism, impaired kidney function, SLE, and certain medications

HUMAN CHORIONIC GONADOTROPIN, SERUM (HCG, BETA SUBUNIT)

• Normal, <3.0 mIU/mL • 10 days after conception, >3 mIU/mL • 30 days, 100–5000 mIU/mL • 10 weeks, 50,000–140,000 mIU/mL • >16 weeks, 10,000–50,000 mIU/mL • Thereafter, levels slowly decline (SI units IU/L equivalent to mIU/mL) • Collection: Tiger top tube

Increased: Pregnancy, some testicular tumors (nonseminomatous germ cell tumors, but not seminoma), trophoblastic disease (hydatidiform mole, choriocarcinoma levels usually >100,000 mIU/mL)

HUMAN IMMUNODEFICIENCY VIRUS (HIV) TESTING

See Figure 4–3 CDC guidelines. Any HIV-positive person over 13 years of age with a CD4[+] T-cell level <200/mL or an HIV-positive patient with a series of CDC-defined indicator conditions (eg, pulmonary candidiasis, disseminated histoplasmosis, HIV wasting, Kaposi's sarcoma, TB, various lymphomas, PCP, and others) is considered to have AIDS.

HIV Antibody

• Normal = negative • Collection: Tiger top tube

Assay kits recognize both HIV-1 and HIV-2 antibodies. Used in the diagnosis of AIDS and to screen blood for use in transfusion. Antibodies appear in blood 1–4 mo after infection in most cases.

HIV Antibody, ELISA

• Normal = negative

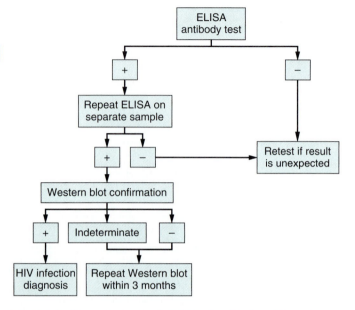

FIGURE 4–3 Diagnostic algorithm for HIV infection. (Courtesy of Burroughs-Wellcome Company, Research Triangle Park, North Carolina.)

Initial screen to detect HIV antibody; a positive test is often repeated or confirmed by Western blot.

Positive: AIDS, asymptomatic HIV infection

False-Positive: Flu vaccine within 3 months, hemophilia, rheumatoid factor, alcoholic hepatitis, dialysis patients

HIV Western Blot

• Normal = negative

The technique is used as the reference procedure for confirming the presence or absence of HIV antibody, usually after a positive

HIV Antibody by ELISA Determination

Positive: AIDS, asymptomatic HIV infection (if indeterminate, repeat in 1 mo or perform PCR for HIV-1 DNA or RNA)

False-Positive: Autoimmune or connective tissue diseases, hyperbilirubinemia, HLA antibodies, others

HIV DNA PCR

• Normal = negative

Performed on peripheral blood mononuclear cells. Preferred test to diagnose HIV infection in children <18 months of age

HIV RNA PCR

• Normal = <400 copies/mL

Used to quantify plasma "viral load." Establishes the diagnosis before antibody production begins or when HIV antibody test is indeterminate. Obtained at baseline diagnosis, serves as an important parameter to initiate or modify HIV therapy (see the following details of viral load). Not recommended for routine testing of children <18 months

HIV VIRAL LOAD

• Normal <50 copies/mL

Single best predictor of progression to AIDS and death among HIV-infected individuals. Also used as a baseline and for initiation and modification of HIV therapy, but not for diagnosis. For example, antiretroviral therapy is uniformly initiated when the viral load is >20,000 copies/mL RNA or RT PCR.

HIV Antigen (P-24 antigen)

• Normal = negative

Detects early HIV infection before antibody conversion, used along with PCR testing

IMMUNOGLOBULINS, QUANTITATIVE

• **IgG:** 65–1500 mg/dL or 6.5–15 g/L • **IgM:** 40–345 mg/dL or 0.4–3.45 mg/L • **IgA:** 76–390 mg/dL or 0.76–3.90 g/L • **IgE:** 0–380 IU/mL or KIU/L • **IgD:** 0–8 mg/dL or 0–80 mg/L • Collection: Tiger top tube

Levels are determined in the evaluation of immunodeficiency diseases, during replacement therapy, and to evaluate humoral immunity.

Increased: Multiple myeloma (myeloma immunoglobulin increased, other immunoglobulins decreased); Waldenström's macroglobulinemia (IgM increased, others decreased); lymphoma; carcinoma; bacterial infection; liver disease; sarcoidosis; amyloidosis; myeloproliferative disorders

Decreased: Hereditary immunodeficiency, leukemia, lymphoma, nephrotic syndrome, protein-losing enteropathy, malnutrition

IRON

• Males 65–175 mg/dL (SI: 11.64–31.33 mmol/L) • Females 50–170 mg/dL (SI: 8.95–30.43 mmol/L) • To convert mg/dL to mmol/L, multiply by 0.1791 • Collection: Tiger top tube

Increased: Hemochromatosis, hemosiderosis caused by excessive iron intake, excess destruction or decreased production of erythrocytes, liver necrosis

Decreased: Iron deficiency anemia, nephrosis (loss of iron-binding proteins), normochromic anemia of chronic diseases and infections

IRON-BINDING CAPACITY, TOTAL (TIBC)

• 250–450 mg/dL (SI: 44.75–80.55 mmol/L) • Collection: Tiger top tube
   The normal iron/TIBC ratio is 20–50%. Decreased ratio (<10%) is almost diagnostic of iron deficiency anemia. Increased ratio is seen with hemochromatosis.

Increased: Acute and chronic blood loss, iron deficiency anemia, hepatitis, oral contraceptives

Decreased: Anemia of chronic diseases, cirrhosis, nephrosis/uremia, hemochromatosis, iron therapy overload, hemolytic anemia, aplastic anemia, thalassemia, megaloblastic anemia

LACTATE DEHYDROGENASE (LD, LDH)

• Adults <230 U/L, (<3.82 mkat/L) • Higher levels in childhood • Collection: Tiger top tube; carefully avoid hemolysis because this can increase LDH levels

Increased: AMI, cardiac surgery, prosthetic valve, hepatitis, pernicious anemia, malignant tumors, pulmonary embolus, hemolysis (anemias or factitious), renal infarction, muscle injury. megaloblastic anemia, liver disease

LDH Isoenzymes (LDH 1 to LDH 5)

Normally, the ratio LDH 1/LDH 2 is <0.6–0.7. If the ratio becomes >1 (also termed "flipped"), suspect a recent MI (change in ratio can also be seen in pernicious or hemolytic anemia). With an AMI, the LDH will begin to rise at 12–48 h, peak at 3–6 days, and return to normal at 8–14 days. LDH 5 is >LDH 4 in liver diseases. (Largely replaced by troponin.)

LACTIC ACID (LACTATE)

• 4.5–19.8 mg/dL (SI: 0.5–2.2 mmol/L) • Collection: Gray top tube on ice
   Suspect lactic acidosis with elevated anion gap in the absence of other causes (renal failure, ethanol or methanol ingestion)

Increased: Lactic acidosis due to hypoxia, hemorrhage, shock, sepsis, cirrhosis, exercise, ethanol, DKA, regional ischemia (extremity, bowel) spurious (prolonged use of a tourniquet)

LAP SCORE (LEUKOCYTE ALKALINE PHOSPHATASE SCORE/STAIN)

• 50–150 • Collection: Finger stick blood sample directly on slide; air dry
   Used to differentiate among various hematologic conditions

Increased: Leukemoid reaction, acute inflammation, Hodgkin's disease, pregnancy, liver disease

Decreased: Chronic myelogenous leukemia, nephrotic syndrome

LE (LUPUS ERYTHEMATOSUS) PREPARATION

• Normal = no cells seen

Positive: SLE, scleroderma, RA, drug-induced lupus (procainamide, others)

LEAD, BLOOD

• Adult <40 mg/dL (1.93 mmol/L) • Child <25 mg/dL (1.21 mmol/L) • Collection: Lavender, navy, or green top tube; lab-specific

Neurologic findings can be detected at 15 mg/dL in children and 30 mg/dL in adults; severe symptoms (lethargy, ataxia, coma) are present >60 mg/dL.

Increased: Lead poisoning, occupational exposure

LEGIONELLA ANTIBODY

• <1:32 titers

Obtain two sera, acute (within 2 wk of onset) and convalescent (at least 3 wk after onset of fever). A fourfold rise in titers or a single titer of 1:256 is diagnostic.

Increased: *Legionella* infection; false-positives with *Bacteroides fragilis*, *Francisella tularensis*, *Mycoplasma pneumoniae*.

LIPASE

• 0–1.5 U/mL (SI: 10–150 U/L) by turbidimetric method • Collection: Tiger top tube

Increased: Acute or chronic pancreatitis, pseudo-cyst, pancreatic duct obstruction (stone, stricture, tumor, drug-induced spasm), fat embolus syndrome, renal failure, dialysis (usually normal in mumps) gastric malignancy, intestinal perforation, diabetes (usually in DKA only)

LIPID PROFILE/LIPOPROTEIN PROFILE/LIPOPROTEIN ANALYSIS

• See also CHOLESTEROL, page 62, and TRIGLYCERIDES, page 91.

Usually includes cholesterol, HDL cholesterol, LDL cholesterol (calculated), triglycerides. Useful in the evaluation of CAD and allows classification of dyslipoproteinemias to direct treatment. Initial screening for cardiac risk includes total cholesterol and HDL as outlined in Figure 4–4 (page 80). The main lipids in the blood are cholesterol and triglycerides. These lipids are carried by lipoproteins. Lipoproteins are further classified by density (least dense to most dense):

- **Chylomicrons** (least dense, rise to surface of unspun serum) and are normally found only after a fatty meal is eaten (a "lipemic specimen" on a lab report usually refers to these chylomicrons).
- **VLDL** consist mainly of triglycerides.
- **LDL** in the fasting state; the LDL carry most cholesterol.
- **HDL** are the densest and consist of mostly apoproteins and cholesterol.

Table 4–4 (see page 81) indicates the dyslipoproteinemias based on the lipid profile.

LOW-DENSITY LIPOPROTEIN-CHOLESTEROL (LDL, LDL-C)

• See CHOLESTEROL, page 62.

LUTEINIZING HORMONE, SERUM (LH)

• Male 7–24 IU/L • Female 6–30 IU/L, midcycle peak increase two- to threefold over baseline, postmenopausal >35 IU/L • Collection: Tiger top tube

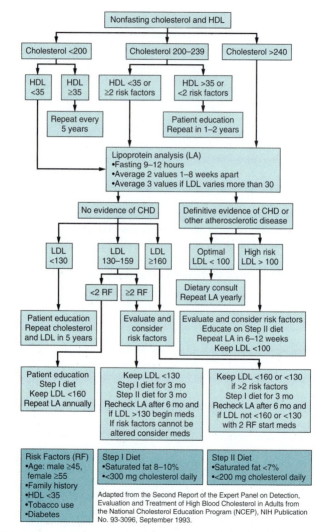

FIGURE 4–4 Cholesterol and lipoprotein screening. (Reprinted, with permission, from: Gordon JD [ed]: *Obstetrics, Gynecology, and Infertility*, 4th ed. Scub Hill Press, Menlo Park CA, 1995.)

TABLE 4-4
Lipoproteins

Fredrickson Classification System	Type I (Rare)	Type IIa (Common)	Type IIb (Common)	Type III (Uncommon)	Type IV (Uncommon)	Type V (Uncommon)
Cholesterol	N or slightly ⇑	Very ⇑	Very ⇑	Very ⇑	N or slightly ⇑	⇑
LDL	N	⇑	⇑	⇑	N	N
HDL	N or ⇓	N or ⇓	N or ⇓	N or ⇓	N or ⇓	N or ⇑
Triglycerides	Very ⇑	N	⇑	Very ⇑	Very ⇑	⇑
Increased lipoproteins	Chylomicrons	LDL	LDL, VLDL	IDL	VLDL	VLDL and chylomicrons
Atherogenesis risk	No increase	Very ⇑	⇑	⇑	No increase	No increase

Increased: (Hypergonadotropic >40 IU/L) postmenopausal, surgical or radiation castration, ovarian or testicular failure, polycystic ovaries

Decreased: (Hypogonadotropic <40 IU/L prepubertal) hypothalamic, and pituitary dysfunction, Kallmann's syndrome, LHRH analogue therapy

LYME DISEASE SEROLOGY

• Normal varies with assay, ELISA <1:8 • Western blot nonreactive

   Most useful when comparing acute and convalescent serum levels for relative titers. Normal values differ among labs. IgM antibody becomes detectable 2–4 weeks after onset of rash; IgG rises in 4–6 weeks and peaks up to 6 mo after infection and may stay elevated for months to years.

Positive: Infection with *Borrelia burgdorferi,* syphilis, and other rickettsial diseases

Negative: After antibiotic therapy or during first few weeks of disease

MAGNESIUM

• 1.6–2.6 mg/dL (SI: 0.80–1.20 mmol/L) • Collection: Tiger top tube

Increased: Renal failure, hypothyroidism, magnesium-containing antacids, Addison's disease, diabetic coma, severe dehydration, lithium intoxication

Decreased: Malabsorption, steatorrhea, alcoholism and cirrhosis, hyperthyroidism, aldosteronism, diuretics, acute pancreatitis, hyperparathyroidism, hyperalimentation, NG suctioning, chronic dialysis, renal tubular acidosis, drugs (cisplatin, amphotericin B, aminoglycosides), hungry bone syndrome, hypophosphatemia, intracellular shifts with respiratory or metabolic acidosis

METYRAPONE TEST

• See Chapter 22, page 570

MHA-TP (MICROHEMAGGLUTINATION, *TREPONEMA PALLIDUM*)

• Normal <1:160 • Collection: Tiger top tube

   Confirmatory test for syphilis, similar to FTA-ABS. Once positive, remains so, therefore cannot be used to judge effect of treatment. False-positives with other treponemal infections (pinta, yaws, etc), mononucleosis, and SLE

B$_2$-MICROGLOBULIN

• 0.1–0.26 mg/dL)1–2.6 mg/L) • Collection: Tiger top tube

   A portion of the class I MHC antigen. A useful marker to follow the progression of HIV infections

Increased: HIV infection, especially during periods of exacerbation, lymphoid malignancies, renal diseases (diabetic nephropathy, pyelonephritis, ATN, nephrotoxicity from medications), transplant rejection, inflammatory conditions

Decreased: Treatment of HIV with AZT (zidovudine)

MONOSPOT

• Normal = negative   • Collection: Tiger top tube

Positive: Mononucleosis, rarely in leukemia, serum sickness, Burkitt's lymphoma, viral hepatitis, RA

MYOGLOBIN

• 30–90 ng/mL   • Collection: Tiger top tube

Increased: Skeletal muscle injury (crush, injection, surgical procedures), delirium tremens, rhabdomyolysis (burns, seizures, sepsis, hypokalemia, others)

5′-NUCLEOTIDASE

• 2–15 U/L
    Used in the workup of increased alkaline phosphatase and biliary obstruction

Increased: Obstructive or cholestatic liver disease, liver metastasis, biliary cirrhosis

OLIGOCLONAL BANDING, CSF

• Normal = negative   • Collection: Serum tiger top tube and simultaneous CSF sample collected in a plain tube by LP
    This is performed simultaneously on CSF and serum samples when MS is clinically suspected. Agarose gel electrophoresis will reveal multiple bands in the IgG region not seen in the serum. Oligoclonal banding is present in up to 90% of patients with MS. Occasionally seen in other CNS inflammatory conditions and CNS syphilis

OSMOLALITY, SERUM

• 278–298 mOsm/kg (SI: 278–298 mmol/kg)   • Collection: Tiger top tube
    A rough estimation of osmolality is [2(Na) + BUN/2.8 + glucose/18]. Measured value is usually less than calculated value. If measured value is 15 mOsm/kg less than calculated, consider methanol, ethanol, or ethylene glycol ingestion.

Increased: Hyperglycemia; ethanol, methanol, mannitol, or ethylene glycol ingestion; increased sodium because of water loss (diabetes, hypercalcemia, diuresis)

Decreased: Low serum sodium, diuretics, Addison's disease, SIADH (seen in bronchogenic carcinoma, hypothyroidism), iatrogenic causes (poor fluid balance)

OXYGEN

• See Chapter 8, Table 8–1, page 162

P-24 ANTIGEN (HIV CORE ANTIGEN)

• Normal = negative   • Collection: Tiger top tube   • See also Human Immunodeficiency Virus Testing, page 75
    Used to diagnose recent acute HIV infection; becomes positive earlier than HIV antibodies. Decreases "window" period. Can be positive as early as 2–4 weeks but becomes undetectable during antibody seroconversion (periods of latency). With progression of disease, P-24 usually becomes evident again. Used to screen blood donors

PARATHYROID HORMONE (PTH)

- Normal based on relationship to serum calcium, usually provided on the lab report
- Also, reference values vary depending on the laboratory and whether the N-terminal, C-terminal or midmolecule is measured. • PTH midmolecule: 0.29– –0.85 ng/mL (SI: 29–85 pmol/L) • With calcium: 8.4–10.2 mg/dL (SI: 2.1–2.55 mmol/L) • Collection: Tiger top tube

Increased: Primary hyperparathyroidism, secondary hyperparathyroidism (hypocalcemic states, such as chronic renal failure, others)

Decreased: Hypercalcemia not due to hyperparathyroidism, hypoparathyroidism

PHOSPHORUS

- Adult 2.5–4.5 mg/dL (SI: 0.81–1.45 mmol/L) • Child 4.0–6.0 mg/dL (SI: 1.29–1.95 mmol/L) • To convert mg/dL to mmol/L, multiply by 0.3229 • Collection: Tiger top tube

Increased: Hypoparathyroidism (surgical, pseudo-hypoparathyroidism), excess vitamin D, secondary hyperparathyroidism, renal failure, bone disease (healing fractures), Addison's disease, childhood, factitious increase (hemolysis of specimen)

Decreased: Hyperparathyroidism, alcoholism, diabetes, hyperalimentation, acidosis, alkalosis, gout, salicylate poisoning, IV steroid, glucose or insulin administration, hypokalemia, hypomagnesemia, diuretics, vitamin D deficiency, phosphate-binding antacids

POTASSIUM, SERUM

- 3.5–5 mEq/L (SI: 3.5–5 mmol/L) • Collection: Tiger top tube

Increased: Factitious increase (hemolysis of specimen, thrombocytosis), renal failure, Addison's disease, acidosis, spironolactone, triamterene, ACE inhibitors, dehydration, hemolysis, massive tissue damage, excess intake (oral or IV), potassium-containing medications, acidosis

Decreased: Diuretics, decreased intake, vomiting, nasogastric suctioning, villous adenoma, diarrhea, Zollinger–Ellison syndrome, chronic pyelonephritis, renal tubular acidosis, metabolic alkalosis (primary aldosteronism, Cushing's syndrome)

PREALBUMIN

- See Chapter 11, page 211

PROGESTERONE

- Collection: Tiger top tube

 Used to confirm ovulation and corpus luteum function

Sample Collection	Normal Values (female)
Follicular phase	<1 ng/mL
Luteal phase	5–20 ng/mL
Pregnancy	
1st trimester	10–30 ng/mL
2nd trimester	50–100 ng/mL
3rd trimester	100–400 ng/mL
Postmenopause	–1 ng/mL

PROLACTIN

• Males 1–20 ng/mL (SI: 1–20 mg/L) • Females 1–25 ng/mL (SI: 1–25 mg/L) • Collection: Tiger top tube

Used in the workup of infertility, impotence, hirsutism, amenorrhea, and pituitary neoplasm

Increased: Pregnancy, nursing after pregnancy, prolactinoma, hypothalamic tumors, sarcoidosis or granulomatous disease of the hypothalamus, hypothyroidism, renal failure, Addison's disease, phenothiazines, haloperidol

PROSTATE-SPECIFIC ANTIGEN (PSA)

• <4 ng/dL by monoclonal, eg, Hybritech assay

Most useful as a measure of response to therapy of prostate cancer; approved for screening for prostate cancer. Although any elevation increases suspicion of prostate cancer, levels >10.0 ng/dL are frequently associated with carcinoma. Age corrected levels gaining popularity (40–50 y 2.5 ng/dL; 50–60 y 3.5 ng/dL; 60–70 years 4.5 ng/dL; >70 years 6.5 ng/dL.)

Increased: Prostate cancer, acute prostatitis, some cases of BPH, prostatic infarction, prostate surgery (biopsy, resection), vigorous prostatic massage (routine rectal exam does not elevate levels), rarely postejaculation

Decreased: Radical prostatectomy, response to therapy of prostatic carcinoma (radiation or hormonal therapy)

PSA Velocity

A rate of rise in PSA of 0.75 ng/mL or greater per year is suspicious for prostate cancer based on at least three separate assays 6 mo apart.

PSA Free and Total

Patients with prostate cancer tend to have lower free PSA levels in proportion to total PSA. Measurement of the free/total PSA can improve the specificity of PSA in the range of total PSA from 2.0–10.0 ng/mL. Some recommend prostate biopsy only if the free PSA percentage is low. Threshold for biopsy is controversial, ranging from a ratio of less than 15% to less than 25%, with a higher threshold having improved sensitivity and lower threshold having improved specificity.

PROTEIN ELECTROPHORESIS, SERUM AND URINE (SERUM PROTEIN ELECTROPHORESIS, SPEP) (URINE PROTEIN ELECTROPHORESIS, UPEP)

Qualitative analysis of the serum proteins is often used in the workup of hypoglobulinemia, macroglobulinemia, α_1-antitrypsin deficiency, collagen disease, liver disease, myeloma, and occasionally in nutritional assessment. Serum electrophoresis yields five different bands (Figure 4–5 and Table 4–5, pages 86 and 87). If a monoclonal gammopathy or a low globulin fraction is detected, quantitative immunoglobulins should be ordered.

Urine protein electrophoresis can be used to evaluate proteinuria and can detect Bence Jones protein (light chain) that is associated with myeloma, Waldenström's macroglobulinemia, and Fanconi's syndrome.

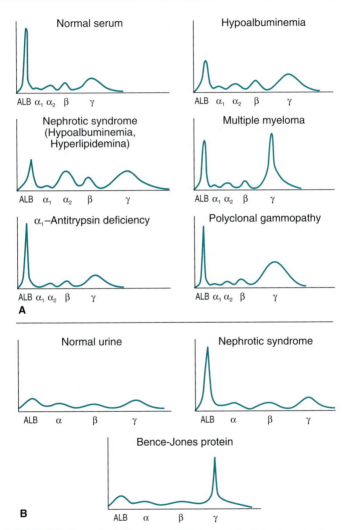

FIGURE 4–5 Examples of (**A**) serum and (**B**) urine protein electrophoresis patterns. See also Table 4–5. (Courtesy of Dr. Steven Haist.)

TABLE 4–5
Normal Serum Protein Components and Fractions as Determined by Electrophoresis, Along with Associated Conditions*

Protein Fraction	Percentage of Total Protein	Constituents	Increased	Decreased
Albumin	52–68	Albumin	Dehydration (only known cause)	Nephrosis, malnutrition, chronic liver disease
Alpha-1 (α_1) globulin	2.4–4.4	Thyroxine-binding globulin, antitrypsin, lipoproteins, glycoprotein, transcortin	Inflammation, neoplasia	Nephrosis, α_1-antitrypsin deficiency (emphysema related)
Alpha-2 (α_2) globulin	6.1–10.1	Haptoglobin, glycoprotein, macroglobulin, ceruloplasmin	Inflammation, infection, neoplasia, cirrhosis	Severe liver disease, acute hemolytic anemia
Beta (β) globulin	8.5–14.5	Transferrin, glycoprotein, lipoprotein	Cirrhosis, obstructive jaundice	Nephrosis
Gamma (γ) globulins (immunoglobulins)	10–21	IgA, IgG, IgM, IgD, IgE	Infections, collagen vascular diseases, leukemia, myeloma	Agammaglobulinemia, hypogammaglobulinemia, nephrosis

*(See also Figure 4–5).

PROTEIN, SERUM

• 6.0–8.0 g/dL • See also Serum Protein Electrophoresis, page 85. • Collection: Tiger top tube

Increased: Multiple myeloma, Waldenström's macroglobulinemia, benign monoclonal gammopathy, lymphoma, chronic inflammatory disease, sarcoidosis, viral illnesses

Decreased: Malnutrition, inflammatory bowel disease, Hodgkin's disease, leukemias, any cause of decreased albumin

RENIN

Plasma (Plasma Renin Activity [PRA])

• Adults, Normal sodium diet, upright 1–6 ng/mL/h (SI: 0.77–4.6 nmol/L/h) • Renal vein renin: L & R should be equal)

Useful in the diagnosis of hypertension associated with hypokalemia. Values highly dependent on salt intake and position. Stop diuretics, estrogens for 2–4 wk before testing.

Increased: Medications (ACE inhibitors, diuretics, oral contraceptives, estrogens), pregnancy, dehydration, renal artery stenosis, adrenal insufficiency, chronic hypokalemia, upright posture, salt-restricted diet, edematous conditions (CHF, nephrotic syndrome), secondary hyperaldosteronism

Decreased: Primary aldosteronism (renin will not increase with relative volume depletion, upright posture)

Renal Vein

• Normal L & R should be equal

A ratio of >1.5 (affected/nonaffected) suggestive of renovascular hypertension

RETINOL-BINDING PROTEIN (RBP)

• Adults 3–6 mg/dL • Children 1.5–3.0 mg/dL • Collection: Tiger top tube

Decreased: Malnutrition, vitamin A deficiency, intestinal malabsorption of fats, chronic liver disease

RHEUMATOID FACTOR (RA LATEX TEST)

• <15 IU by Microscan kit or <1:40 • Collection: Tiger top tube

Increased: Collagen-vascular diseases (RA, SLE, scleroderma, polyarteritis nodosa, others), infections (TB, syphilis, viral hepatitis), chronic inflammation, SBE, some lung diseases, MI

ROCKY MOUNTAIN SPOTTED FEVER ANTIBODIES (RMSF)

• Normal: <4(times) increase in paired acute and convalescent sera • IgG <1:64 • IgM <1:8 • Collection: Tiger top tube acute and convalescent

The diagnosis of RMSF is made by acute and convalescent titers that demonstrate a 4× rise or a single convalescent titer >1:64 in the clinical setting of RMSF. Occasional false-positives in late pregnancy

SEMEN ANALYSIS

• Volume 2–5 mL • Sperm count >20-40 × 10^6/mL • Motility >60% • Forward migration • Morphology >60% normal

Specimen must be collected after 48–72 h abstinence and analyzed within 1–2 h. Test may not be valid after a recent illness or high fever. Verify abnormal analysis by serial tests.

Decreased: After vasectomy (should be 0 sperm after 3 mo), varicocele, primary testicular failure (ie, Klinefelter's syndrome), secondary testicular failure (chemotherapy, radiation, infections),varicocele, after recent illness, congenital obstruction of the vas, retrograde ejaculation, endocrine causes (hyperprolactinemia, low testosterone, others)

SGGT (SERUM GAMMA-GLUTAMYL TRANSPEPTIDASE)

• See GGT, page 69.

SGOT (SERUM GLUTAMIC-OXALOACETIC TRANSAMINASE)

• See AST, page 58.

SGPT SERUM (GLUTAMIC-PYRUVIC TRANSAMINASE)

• See ALT, page 57.

SODIUM, SERUM

• 136–145 mmol/L • Collection: Tiger top tube
    In factitious hyponatremia due to hyperglycemia, for every 100 mmol/L blood glucose above normal, serum sodium decreases 1.6. For example, a blood glucose of 800 and a sodium of 129 would factitiously lower the sodium value by about 7×1.6, or 11.6. Corrected serum sodium would therefore be $129 + 11 = 140$.

Increased: Associated with low total body sodium (glycosuria, mannitol, or lactulose use urea, excess sweating), normal total body sodium (diabetes insipidus [central and nephrogenic], respiratory losses, and sweating), and increased total body sodium (administration of hypertonic sodium bicarbonate, Cushing's syndrome, hyperaldosteronism)

Decreased: Associated with excess total body sodium and water (nephrotic syndrome, CHF, cirrhosis, renal failure), excess body water (SIADH, hypothyroidism, adrenal insufficiency), decreased total body water and sodium (diuretic use, renal tubular acidosis, use of mannitol or urea, mineralocorticoid deficiency, vomiting, diarrhea, pancreatitis), and pseudo-hyponatremia (hyperlipidemia, hyperglycemia, and multiple myeloma)

STOOL FOR OCCULT BLOOD (HEMOCCULT TEST)

Normal-Negative: Apply small amount of stool to test site on Hemoccult card and close. Open test panel on other side of card and apply 2–3 drops developer to the test and the positive control panels; read in 30 s. Blue color is positive. Detects >5 mg hemoglobin/g feces. Repeat three times for maximum yield. (A positive test more informative than a negative test)

Positive: Any GI tract ulcerated lesion (ulcer, carcinoma, polyp, diverticulosis, inflammatory bowel disease), hemorrhoids, telangiectasias, drugs that cause GI irritation (eg, NSAIDs) swallowed blood, ingestion of rare red meat, certain foods (horseradish, turnips) (vitamin C [>500 mg/d], antacids may result in false-negative test)

SWEAT CHLORIDE

• 5–40 mEq/L (SI: 5–40 mmol/L) • Collection: 100–200 mg sweat on filter paper after electrical stimulation of sweating by pilocarpine iontophoresis on an extremity

Increased: CF (not valid on children <3 wk); Addison's disease, meconium ileus, and renal failure can occasionally raise levels.

T₃ RU (RESIN UPTAKE; THYROXINE-BINDING GLOBULIN RATIO)

• 30–40%

This test is used in conjunction with a T_4 to yield the Free T_4 Index [FTI]), an estimate of the free T_4.

Increased: Hyperthyroidism, medications (phenytoin [Dilantin], steroids, heparin, aspirin, others), nephrotic syndrome

Decreased: Hypothyroidism, medications (iodine, propylthiouracil, others), any cause of increased TBG, such as oral estrogen or pregnancy

TESTOSTERONE

• Male free: 9–30 ng/dL, total 300–1200 ng/dL • Female, see following table

Sample Collection	Normal Values (female)
Follicular phase	20–80 ng/dL
Midcycle peak	20–80 ng/dL
Luteal phase	20–80 ng/dL
Postmenopause	10–40 ng/dL

Increased: Adrenogenital syndrome, ovarian stromal hyperthecosis, polycystic ovaries, menopause, ovarian tumors.

Decreased: Some cases of impotence, hypogonadism, hypopituitarism, Klinefelter's syndrome

THYROGLOBULIN

• 1–20 ng/mL (mg/L) • Collection: Tiger top tube

Useful for following patients with nonmedullary thyroid carcinomas

Increased: Differentiated thyroid carcinomas (papillary, follicular), Graves' disease, nontoxic goiter

Decreased: Hypothyroidism, testosterone, steroids, phenytoin

THYROID-STIMULATING HORMONE (TSH)

• 0.7–5.3 mU/mL • Collection: Tiger top tube

Excellent screening test for hyperthyroidism as well as hypothyroidism. Differentiates between a low normal and a decreased TSH

Increased: Hypothyroidism

Decreased: Hyperthyroidism. Less than 1% of hypothyroidism is from pituitary or hypothalamic disease resulting in a decreased TSH.

THYROXINE (T₄ TOTAL)

• 5–12 mg/dL (SI: 65–155 nmol/L) • Males: >60 years, 5–10 mg/dL (SI: 65–129 nmol)
• Females: 5.5–10.5 µg/dL (SI: 71–135 nmol/L) • Collection: Tiger top tube

Good screening test for hyperthyroidism. Measures both bound and free T_4, therefore, can be affected by TBG levels.

Increased: Hyperthyroidism, exogenous thyroid hormone, estrogens, pregnancy, severe illness, euthyroid sick syndrome

Decreased: Hypothyroidism, euthyroid sick syndrome, any cause of decreased TBG

THYROXINE-BINDING GLOBULIN (TBG)

• 21–52 mg/dL (270–669 nmol/L) • Collection: Tiger top tube

Increased: Hypothyroidism, pregnancy, oral contraceptives, estrogens, hepatic disease, acute porphyria

Decreased: Hyperthyroidism, androgens, anabolic steroids, prednisone, nephrotic syndrome, severe illness, surgical stress, phenytoin, hepatic disease

THYROXINE INDEX, FREE (FTI)

• 6.5–1.25

Practically speaking, the FTI is equivalent to the free thyroxine. Useful in patients with clinically suspected hyper- or hypothyroidism. Determined as follows:

$$\text{Thyroxine (Total } T_4) \times T_3 \text{ RU}$$

Increased: Hyperthyroidism, high-dose beta-blockers, psychiatric illnesses

Decreased: Hypothyroidism, phenytoin (Dilantin)

TORCH BATTERY

• Normal = negative • Collection: Tiger top tube

Serial determinations best (acute and convalescent titers).

Test is based on serologic evidence of exposure to toxoplasmosis, rubella, cytomegalovirus, and herpesviruses.

TRANSFERRIN

• 220–400 mg/dL (SI: 2.20–4.0 g/L) • Collection: Tiger top tube, avoid hemolysis

Used in the workup of anemias; transferrin levels can also be assessed by the total iron-binding capacity.

Increased: Acute and chronic blood loss, iron deficiency, hemolysis, oral contraceptives, pregnancy, viral hepatitis

Decreased: Anemia of chronic disease, cirrhosis, nephrosis, hemochromatosis, malignancy

TRIGLYCERIDES

• Recommended values: • Males: 40–160 mg/dL (SI: 0.45–1.81 mmol/L) • Females: 35–135 mg/dL (SI: 0.40–1.53 mmol/L) • Can vary with age. • Collection: Tiger top tube • Fasting preferred • See also LIPID PROFILE page 79

Increased: Nonfasting specimen, hyperlipoproteinemias (types I, IIb, III, IV, V), hypothyroidism, liver diseases, poorly controlled diabetes mellitus, alcoholism, pancreatitis,

AMI, nephrotic syndrome, familial, medications (oral contraceptives, estrogens, beta-blockers, cholestyramine)

Decreased: Malnutrition, malabsorption, hyperthyroidism, Tangier disease, medications (nicotinic acid, clofibrate, gemfibrozil) congenital abetalipoproteinemia

TRIIODOTHYRONINE (T_3 RIA)

- 120–195 ng/dL (SI: 1.85–3.00 nmol/L) • Collection: Tiger top tube
    Useful when hyperthyroidism is suspected, but T_4 is normal; not useful in the diagnosis of hypothyroidism

Increased: Hyperthyroidism, T_3 thyrotoxicosis, pregnancy, exogenous T_4, any cause of increased TBG, such as oral estrogen or pregnancy

Decreased: Hypothyroidism and euthyroid sick state, any cause of decreased TBG

TROPONIN, CARDIAC-SPECIFIC

- Troponin 1 (cTn1) <0.35 ng/mL • Troponin T cTnT <0.2 µg/L
    Used to diagnose AMI; increases rapidly 3–12 h, peak at 24 h and may stay elevated for several days (cTn1 5–7 days, cTnT up to 14 days). More cardiac-specific than CK-MB

Positive: Myocardial damage, including MI, myocarditis (false-positive: renal failure)

URIC ACID (URATE)

- Males: 3.4–7 mg/dL (SI: 202–416 mmol/L) • Females: 2.4–6 mg/dL (SI: 143–357 mmol/L) • To convert mg/dL to mmol/L, multiply by 59.48 • Collection: Tiger top tube
    Increased uric acid is associated with increased catabolism, nucleoprotein synthesis, or decreased renal clearing of uric acid (ie, thiazide diuretics or renal failure).

Increased: Gout, renal failure, destruction of massive amounts of nucleoproteins (leukemia, anemia, chemotherapy, toxemia of pregnancy), drugs (especially diuretics), lactic acidosis, hypothyroidism, PCKD, parathyroid diseases

Decreased: Uricosuric drugs (salicylates, probenecid, allopurinol), Wilson's disease, Fanconi's syndrome

VDRL TEST (VENEREAL DISEASE RESEARCH LABORATORY) OR RAPID PLASMA REAGIN (RPR)

- Normal = nonreactive • Collection: Tiger top tube
    Good screening for syphilis. Almost always positive in secondary syphilis, but frequently becomes negative in late syphilis. Also, in some patients with HIV infection, the VDRL can be negative in primary and secondary syphilis.

Positive (Reactive):   Syphilis, SLE, pregnancy and drug addiction. If reactive, confirm with FTA-ABS (false-positives with bacterial or viral illnesses).

VITAMIN B_{12} (EXTRINSIC FACTOR, CYANOCOBALAMIN)

- >100–700 pg/mL (SI: 74–516 pmol/L) • Collection: Tiger top tube

Increased: Excessive intake, myeloproliferative disorders

Decreased: Inadequate intake (especially strict vegetarians), malabsorption, hyperthyroidism, pregnancy

ZINC

• 60–130 mg/dL (SI: 9–20 mmol/L) • Collection: Check with lab; special collection to limit contamination

Increased: Atherosclerosis, CAD

Decreased: Inadequate dietary intake (parenteral nutrition, alcoholism); malabsorption; increased needs, such as pregnancy or wound healing; acrodermatitis enteropathica; dwarfism

LABORATORY DIAGNOSIS: CLINICAL HEMATOLOGY

Blood Collection
Blood Smears: Wright's Stain
Normal CBC Values
Normal CBC Variations
Hematocrit
Three-Cell Differential Count
The "Left Shift"
Reticulocyte Count

CBC Differential Diagnosis
Lymphocyte Subsets
RBC Morphology Differential Diagnosis
WBC Morphology Differential
    Diagnosis
Coagulation and Other Hematologic
    Tests

BLOOD COLLECTION

Venipuncture is discussed in detail in Chapter 13, page 39. The best CBC sample is venous blood drawn with at least a 22-gauge or larger needle. For a routine CBC, venous blood needs to be placed in a special hematology lab tube, usually a purple top tube, that has an anticoagulant (EDTA) and that is mixed gently. Blood for a CBC should be fresh, less than 3 h old. Most coagulation studies are submitted in a blue top (citrate) tube. (See page 311 for detailed description of blood collection tubes.)

If a **capillary fingerstick** or **heelstick** (see page 274) is used, the hematocrit may be falsely low. If the finger needs to be "milked," sludging of the RBCs can create a falsely high hematocrit. In practice, you can draw the blood up in a capillary tube, seal an end with clay, and spin a tube on the hematocrit centrifuge for 2–3 min and rapidly determine a hematocrit. Wright's staining can also be done and viewed as outlined in the next section.

BLOOD SMEARS: WRIGHT'S STAIN
Making the Blood Smear

In some clinical situations a quick interpretation of a smear can be useful.

1. Place a small drop of blood from the anticoagulated lab sample tube (usually purple top) in the center of a clean glass slide, about 1–2 cm from the end.
2. Place the spreading slide (a glass slide with a perfectly smooth edge) at a 45-degree angle on the slide with the blood sample and slowly move it back to make contact with the drop. The drop should spread out quickly along the line of contact between the two slides. The moment this occurs, spread the film by a rapid, smooth forward movement of the spreader (Figure 5–1).
3. The drop of blood should result in a film about 3 cm long. The faster a film is spread, the more even it is and the better the slide it produces. The ideal thickness shows some overlap by the RBCs throughout much of the film's length with separation and lack of distortion toward the feathered edge of the film. Leukocytes should be easily recognizable throughout the length of the film.

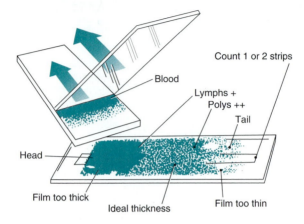

FIGURE 5–1   The technique of preparing a blood smear for staining and the distribution of white blood cells on the standard smear.

Staining the Blood Smear (Wright's stain)

Make sure that all reagents are fresh, or the slide may not turn out properly.

1. Let the slide air dry, and mark the patient's name and date in pencil on the blood film itself. It will not be removed by staining. An alternative method is to bring the slide to the hematology lab where instruments can automatically stain the slides.
2. Fix the slide in methanol for 1 min.
3. Shake off excess methanol from the slide, but do not rinse or dry it.
4. Flood the slide with Wright's stain, and allow the slide to stand for 3–5 min. (This time can vary with the batch of stain.)
5. Flood the slide with Wright's buffer (pH 6.4) until about 50% of the Wright's stain is washed off. Blow air gently over the top of the slide to mix the fluids, and look for a greenish copper sheen that appears on the surface. Let the slide stand for about 8 min.
6. Rinse the slide with tap water, wipe the back of the slide with methanol, and air dry it.

Viewing the Film: The Differential WBC

1. The film should not be so thick that the leukocytes in the body of the film shrink. Examine the smear in an area where the red cells approximate but do not overlap.
2. If the film is too thin or if a rough-edged spreader is used, up to 50% of the WBCs may accumulate in the edges and tail (See Fig. 5–1).
3. WBCs are NOT randomly dispersed even in a well-made smear. Polys and monos predominate at the margins and tail, and lymphs are prevalent in the middle of the film. To overcome this problem, use the "high dry" or oil immersion objective, and count cells in a strip running the whole length of the film. Avoid the lateral edges of the film.

TABLE 5–1
Estimated WBC Based on Cells Counted in a Blood Smear

WBC/hpf (high dry or 40×)	Estimated WBC (per mm³)
2–4	4000–7000
4–6	7000–10,000
6–10	10,000–13,000
10–20	13,000–18,000

Abbreviations: WBC = white blood cell; hpf = high-power field.

4. If fewer than 200 cells are counted in a strip, count another strip until at least 200 are seen. The special white cell counter found in most labs is ideal for this purpose. In patients receiving chemotherapy, the total count may be so small that only a 25–50 cell differential is possible.

5. In smears of blood from patients with very high white counts, such as those with leukemia, count the cells in any well-spread area where the different cell types are easy to identify. Table 5–1 shows the correlation between the number of cells in a smear and the estimated white cell count. A platelet count can be estimated by averaging the number of platelets seen in 10 hpf (oil immersion) and multiplying by 20,000.

NORMAL CBC VALUES

A CBC panel generally includes WBC count, RBC count, hemoglobin, hematocrit, MCH, MCHC, MCV, and the RDW and platelets. The differential is usually ordered separately. Normal CBC, differential, and platelet values are outlined in Tables 5–2 and 5–3.

NORMAL CBC VARIATIONS

Hemoglobin and hematocrit are highest at birth (20 g/100 mL and 60%, respectively). The values fall steeply to a minimum at 3 mo (9.5 g/100 mL and 32%). Then they slowly rise to near adult levels at puberty, and thereafter both values are higher in males. A normal decrease occurs in pregnancy. The number of WBCs is highest at birth (mean of 25,000/mm³) and slowly falls to adult levels by puberty. Lymphs predominate (up to 60% from the second week of life until age 5–7 y when polys begin to predominate.

HEMATOCRIT

The hematocrit is a simple screening test and can be performed on the medical floor as described previously (page 95). Always remember that because an equal amount of plasma and red cells are lost in acute blood loss, the hematocrit will not reflect the loss until sometime later (sometimes 2–3 h). If an anemia is suspected, the red cell indices and reticulocyte count should be checked.

THREE-CELL DIFFERENTIAL COUNT

Instead of a manual differential count of WBCs, many labs now rely on a **three-cell differential count** that is automatically performed by newer instruments. White cells are separated on the basis of three sizes: **small cells** (mostly normal lymphocytes), **middle cells**

TABLE 5-2
Normal CBC for Selected Age Ranges

Age	WBC Count (cells/mm³) [SI: 10^9/L]	RBC Count (10^6/µL) [SI: 10^{12}/L]	Hemoglobin (g/dL) [SI: g/L]	Hematocrit (%)	MCH (pg) [SI: pg]	MCHC (g/dL) [SI: g/L]*	MCV (µm³) [SI: fL]	RDW
Adult ♂	4500-11,000 [4.5-11.0]	4.73-5.49 [4.73-5.49]	14.40-16.60 [144-166]	42.9-49.1	27-31	33-37	76-100	11.5-14.5
Adult ♀	As above	4.15-4.87	12.2-14.7	37.9-43.9	As above	As above	As above	As above
		[4.15-5.49]	[122-147]					
11-15 years	4500-13,500	4.8	13.4	39	28	34	82	
6-10 years	5000-14,500	4.7	12.9	37.5	27	34	80	
4-6 years	5500-15,500	4.6	12.6	37.0	27	34	80	
2-4 years	6000-17,000	4.5	12.5	35.5	25	32	77	
4 mo-2 y	6000-17,500	4.6	11.2	35.0	25	33	77	
1 wk-4 mo	5500-18,000	4.7±0.9	14.0±3.3	42.0±7.0	30	33	90	
24 hr-1 wk	5000-21,000	5.1	18.3±4.0	52.5	36	35	103	
First day	9400-34,000	5.1±1.0	19.5±5.0	54.0±10.0	38	36	106	

*To convert standard reference value to SI units, multiply by 10.

Abbreviations: WBC = white blood cell; RBC = red blood cell; MCH = mean cell hemoglobin; MCHC = mean cell hemoglobin concentration; MCV = mean cell volume; RDW = red cell distribution width.

TABLE 5–3
Normal CBC for Selected Age Ranges

Age	Platelet Count (10³/µL) [SI: 10⁹/L]	Lymphocytes, Total (% WBC count)	Neutrophils, Band (% WBC count)	Neutrophils, Segmented (% WBC count)	Eosinophils (% WBC count)	Basophils (% WBC count)	Monocytes (% WBC count)
Adult ♀	238±49	34	3.0	56	2.7	0.5	4.0
Adult ♂	270±58	As above	As above	As above	As above	As above	As above
11–15 years	282±63	38	3.0	51	2.4	0.5	4.3
6–10 years	351±85	39	3.0	50	2.4	0.6	4.2
4–6 years	357±70	42	3.0	39	2.8	0.6	5.0
2–4 years	357±70	59	3.0	30	2.6	0.5	5.0
4 mo–2 y	As above	61	3.1	28	2.6	0.4	4.8
1 wk–4 mo	As above	56	4.5	30	2.8	0.5	6.5
24 hr–1 wk	240–380	24–41	6.8–9.2	39–52	2.4–4.1	0.5	5.8–9.1
First day	As above	24	10.2	58	2.0	0.6	5.8

Abbreviations: CBC = complete blood count; WBC = white blood cell.

(monocytes, eosinophils, large lymphocyte variants), and **large cells** (neutrophils [stabs and band cells]). Each lab sets its own reference ranges based on "normal" populations. If one of the three cell populations falls outside the reference range, the sample is made into a slide, and a microscopic differential count is performed. With the anticipated shortage of health care workers and the expense of manual counting, these types of determinations will become more widely used.

As an example of the three-cell count, a patient with sepsis may have a large-cell count of 95% and a small-cell count of 5% with no middle cells. On manual examination of the slide, there may be 70% segmented neutrophils and 25% stabs, for a total of 95%.

THE "LEFT SHIFT"

The degree of nuclear lobulation of PMNs is thought to give some indication of cell age. A predominance of immature cells with only one or two nuclear lobes separated by a thick chromatin band is called a "**shift to the left.**" Conversely, a predominance of cells with four nuclear lobes is called a "**shift to the right.**" (For historical information, left and right designations come from the formerly used manual lab counters, in which the keys for entering the stabs were located on the left of the keyboard.)

As a general rule, 40–50% of PMNs have three lobes, approximately 5% have two lobes, and 15–25% have four lobes. More than 20 five-lobed cells/100 WBCs suggest incipient megaloblastic anemia, and a six-lobed or seven-lobed poly is virtually diagnostic.

"**Bands**" or "**stabs,**" the more immature forms of PMNs (the more mature are called "**segs**"), are identified by the fact that the connections between ends or lobes of a nucleus are greater than one-half the width of the hypothetical round nucleus. In bands or stabs, the connection between the lobes of the nucleus is by a thick band; in segs, by a thin filament. A band is defined as a connecting strip wide enough to reveal two distinct margins with nuclear material in between. A filament is so narrow that no intervening nuclear material is present. When in doubt if a cell is a band or seg, call it a seg.

For practical purposes, **a left shift is present in the CBC when more than 10–12% bands are seen or when the total PMN count (segs plus bands) is greater than 80.**

Left Shift: Bacterial infection, toxemia, hemorrhage

Right Shift: Liver disease, megaloblastic anemia, iron deficiency anemia

RETICULOCYTE COUNT

• Collection: Lavender top tube

The reticulocyte count is not a part of the routine CBC. The count is used in the initial workup of anemia (especially unexplained) and in monitoring the effect of hematinic or erythropoietin therapy, monitoring the recovery from myelosuppression or monitoring engraftment following bone marrow transplant. Reticulocytes are juvenile RBCs with remnants of cytoplasmic basophilic RNA. These are suggested by **basophilia** of the RBC cytoplasm on Wright's stain; however, confirmation requires a special reticulocyte stain. The result is reported as a percentage, and you should calculate the **corrected reticulocyte count** for interpretation of the results

$$\text{Corrected reticulocyte count} = \frac{\text{Reported count} \times \text{Patient's HCT}}{\text{Normal HCT}}$$

This corrected count is an excellent indicator of erythropoietic activity. The **normal corrected reticulocyte count is <1.5.**

Normal bone marrow responds to a decrease in erythrocytes (shown by a decreased hematocrit) with an increase in the production of reticulocytes. Lack of increase in a reticulocyte count with an anemia suggests a chronic disease, a deficiency disease, marrow replacement, or marrow failure.

CBC DIFFERENTIAL DIAGNOSIS

- See Tables 5–2 and 5–3 for normal age and sex-specific ranges.

Basophils

- 0–1%

Increased: Chronic myeloid leukemia, after splenectomy, polycythemia, Hodgkin's disease, and, rarely, in recovery from infection and from hypothyroidism

Decreased: Acute rheumatic fever, pregnancy, after radiation, steroid therapy, thyrotoxicosis, stress

Eosinophils

- 1–3%

Increased: Allergy, parasites, skin diseases, malignancy, drugs, asthma, Addison's disease, collagen–vascular diseases (handy mnemonic **NAACP: N**eoplasm, **A**llergy, **A**ddison's disease, **C**ollagen–vascular diseases, **P**arasites), pulmonary diseases including Löffler's syndrome and PIE

Decreased: Steroids, ACTH, after stress (infection, trauma, burns), Cushing's syndrome

Hematocrit (Male 40–54%; Female 37–47%)

Decreased: Megaloblastic anemia (folate or B_{12} deficiency); iron deficiency anemia; sickle cell anemia; acute or chronic blood loss; hemolysis; anemia due to chronic disease, dilution, alcohol, or drugs

Increased: Primary polycythemia (polycythemia vera), secondary polycythemia (reduced fluid intake or excess fluid loss, congenital and acquired heart disease, lung disease, high altitudes, heavy smoking, tumors [renal cell carcinoma, hepatoma], renal cysts)

Lymphocytes

- 24–44% • See also Lymphocyte Subsets, page 103

Increased: Virtually any viral infection (AIDS, measles, rubella, mumps, whooping cough, smallpox, chickenpox, influenza, hepatitis, infectious mononucleosis), acute infectious lymphocytosis in children, acute and chronic lymphocytic leukemias

Decreased: (Normal finding in 22% of population) Stress, burns, trauma, uremia, some viral infections, AIDS, AIDS-related complex, bone marrow suppression after chemotherapy, steroids, MS

Atypical Lymphocytes

>20%: Infectious mononucleosis, CMV infection, infectious hepatitis, toxoplasmosis

<20%: Viral infections (mumps, rubeola, varicella), rickettsial infections, TB

MCH (Mean Cellular [Corpuscular] Hemoglobin)

- 27–31 pg (SI: pg)

    The weight of hemoglobin of the average red cell. Calculated by

$$MCH = \frac{\text{Hemoglobin (g / L)}}{\text{RBC } (10^6 / \mu L)}$$

Increased: Macrocytosis (megaloblastic anemias, high reticulocyte counts)

Decreased: Microcytosis (iron deficiency, sideroblastic anemia, thalassemia)

MCHC (Mean Cellular [Corpuscular] Hemoglobin Concentration)

- 33–37 g/dL (SI:330–370 g/L)

    The average concentration of hemoglobin in a given volume of red cells. Calculated by the formula

$$MCHC = \frac{\text{Hemoglobin (g / dL)}}{\text{Hematocrit}}$$

Increased: Very severe, prolonged dehydration; spherocytosis

Decreased: Iron deficiency anemia, overhydration, thalassemia, sideroblastic anemia

MCV (Mean Cell [Corpuscular] Volume)

- 76–100 cu μm (SI: fL)

    The average volume of red blood cells. Calculated by the formula

$$MCV = \frac{\text{Hematocrit} \times 1000}{\text{RBC } (10^6 / \mu L)}$$

Increased/Macrocytosis: Megaloblastic anemia (B_{12}, folate deficiency), macrocytic (normoblastic) anemia, reticulocytosis, myelodysplasias, Down syndrome, chronic liver disease, treatment of AIDS with AZT, chronic alcoholism, cytotoxic chemotherapy, radiation therapy, Dilantin use, hypothyroidism, newborns

Decreased/Microcytosis: Iron deficiency, thalassemia, some cases of lead poisoning or polycythemia

Monocytes

- 3–7%

Increased: Bacterial infection (TB, SBE, brucellosis, typhoid, recovery from an acute infection), protozoal infections, infectious mononucleosis, leukemia, Hodgkin's disease, ulcerative colitis, regional enteritis

Decreased: Lymphocytic leukemia, aplastic anemia, steroid use

Platelets

- 150–450,000 μL

    Platelet counts may be normal in number, but abnormal in function as occurs in aspirin therapy. Abnormalities of platelet function are assessed by bleeding time.

Increased: Sudden exercise, after trauma, bone fracture, after asphyxia, after surgery (especially splenectomy), acute hemorrhage, polycythemia vera, primary thrombocytosis, leukemias, after childbirth, carcinoma, cirrhosis, myeloproliferative disorders, iron deficiency

Decreased: DIC, ITP, TTP, congenital disease, marrow suppressants (chemotherapy, alcohol, radiation), burns, snake and insect bites, leukemias, aplastic anemias, hypersplenism, infectious mononucleosis, viral infections, cirrhosis, massive transfusions, eclampsia and preeclampsia, prosthetic heart valve, more than 30 different drugs (NSAIDs, cimetidine, aspirins, thiazides, others)

PMNs (Polymorphonuclear Neutrophils) (Neutrophils)

- 40–76% • See also the "Left Shift" page 100.

Increased

    Physiologic (Normal). Severe exercise, last months of pregnancy, labor, surgery, newborns, steroid therapy

    Pathologic. Bacterial infections, noninfective tissue damage (MI, pulmonary infarction, pancreatitis, crush injury, burn injury), metabolic disorders (eclampsia, DKA, uremia, acute gout), leukemias

Decreased: Pancytopenia, aplastic anemia, PMN depression (a mild decrease is referred to as **neutropenia,** severe is called **agranulocytosis**), marrow damage (x-rays, poisoning with benzene or antitumor drugs), severe overwhelming infections (disseminated TB, septicemia), acute malaria, severe osteomyelitis, infectious mononucleosis, atypical pneumonias, some viral infections, marrow obliteration (osteosclerosis, myelofibrosis, malignant infiltrate), drugs (more than 70, including chloramphenicol, phenylbutazone, chlorpromazine, quinine), B_{12} and folate deficiencies, hypoadrenalism, hypopituitarism, dialysis, familial decrease, idiopathic causes

RDW (Red Cell Distribution Width)

- 11.5–14.5

    RDW is a measure of the degree of anisocytosis (variation in RBC size) and measured by the automated hematology counters.

Increased: Many anemias (iron deficiency, pernicious, folate deficiency, thalassemias), liver disease

LYMPHOCYTE SUBSETS

Specific monoclonal antibodies are used to identify specific T and B cells. Lymphocyte subsets (also called lymphocyte marker assays, or T- and B-cell assay) are useful in the diagnosis of AIDS and various leukemias and lymphomas. The designation **CD ("clusters of differentiation")** has largely replaced the older antibody designations (eg, Leu 3a or OKT3). Results are most reliable when reported as an absolute number of cells/μL rather than a percentage of cells. A CD4/CD8 ratio < 1 is seen in patients with AIDS. Absolute CD4 count is used to initiate therapy with antiretrovirals or prophylaxis for PCP (see page 75). The CDC includes in the category of AIDS any patient with a CD4 count < 200 who is HIV-positive.

Normal Lymphocyte Subsets

- Total lymphocytes 0.66–4.60 thousand/μL
- T cell 644–2201 μL (60–88%)
- B cell 82–392 μL (3–20%)
- T helper/inducer cell (CD4, Leu 3a, OKT4) 493–1191 μL (34–67%)
- Suppressor/cytotoxic T cell (CD8, Leu 2, OKT8) 182–785 μL (10–42%)
- CD4/CD8 ratio > 1

RBC MORPHOLOGY DIFFERENTIAL DIAGNOSIS

The following lists some erythrocyte abnormalities and the associated conditions. General terms include **poikilocytosis** (irregular RBC shape such as sickle or burr) and **anisocytosis** (irregular RBC size such as microcytes and macrocytes).

Basophilic Stippling: Lead or heavy-metal poisoning, thalassemia, severe anemia

Burr Cells (Acanthocytes):   Severe liver disease; high levels of bile, fatty acids, or toxins

Helmet Cells (Schistocytes):   Microangiopathic hemolysis, hemolytic transfusion reaction, transplant rejection, other severe anemias, TTP

Howell–Jolly Bodies: After splenectomy, some severe hemolytic anemias, pernicious anemia, leukemia, thalassemia

Nucleated RBCs: Severe bone marrow stress (hemorrhage, hemolysis, etc), marrow replacement by tumor, extramedullary hematopoiesis

Polychromasia (Basophilia):   The appearance of a bluish gray red cell on routine Wright's stain suggests reticulocytes.

Sickling: Sickle cell disease and trait

Spherocytes: Hereditary spherocytosis, immune or microangiopathic hemolysis, severe burns, ABO transfusion reactions

Target Cells (Leptocytes):   Thalassemia, hemoglobinopathies, obstructive jaundice, any hypochromic anemia, after splenectomy

WBC MORPHOLOGY DIFFERENTIAL DIAGNOSIS

The following gives conditions associated with certain changes in the normal morphology of WBCs.

Auer Rods: AML

Döhle's Inclusion Bodies: Severe infection, burns, malignancy, pregnancy

Hypersegmentation: Megaloblastic anemias

Toxic Granulation: Severe illness (sepsis, burn, high temperature)

COAGULATION AND OTHER HEMATOLOGIC TESTS

The coagulation cascade is shown in Figure 5–2. A variety of coagulation-related and other blood tests follow.

Activated Clotting Time (ACT)

• 114–186 s • Collection: Black top tube from instrument manufacturer
    This is a bedside test used in the operating room, dialysis unit, or other facility to document neutralization of heparin (ie, after coronary artery bypass, heparin is reversed.)

Increased: Heparin, some platelet disorders, severe clotting factor deficiency

Antithrombin-III (AT-III)

• 17–30 mg/dL or 80–120% of control • Collection: Blue top tube, patient must be off heparin for 6 h
    Used in the evaluation of thrombosis. Heparin must interact with AT-III to produce anticoagulation effect.

Decreased: Autosomal-dominant familial AT-III deficiency, PE, severe liver disease, late pregnancy, oral contraceptives, nephrotic syndrome, heparin therapy (>3 days)

Increased: Coumadin, after MI

Bleeding Time

• Duke, Ivy <6 min; Template <10 min • Collection: Specialized bedside test performed by technicians. A small incision is made, and the wound is wicked with filter paper every 30 s until the fluid is clear.
    In vivo test of hemostasis that tests platelet function, local tissue factors, and clotting factors. Nonsteroidal medications should be stopped 5–7 d before the test because these agents can affect platelet function.

Increased: Thrombocytopenia (DIC, TTP, ITP), von Willebrand's disease, defective platelet function (NSAIDs such as aspirin)

Coombs' Test, Direct (Direct Antiglobulin Test)

• Normal = negative • Collection: Purple top tube
    Uses patient's erythrocytes; tests for the presence of antibody on the patient's cells and used in the screening for autoimmune hemolytic anemia.

Positive: Autoimmune hemolytic anemia (leukemia, lymphoma, collagen–vascular diseases), hemolytic transfusion reaction, some drug sensitizations (methyldopa, levodopa, cephalosporins, penicillin, quinidine), hemolytic disease of the newborn (erythroblastosis fetalis)

Coombs' Test, Indirect (Indirect Antiglobulin Test/Autoantibody Test)

• Normal = negative • Collection: Purple top tube
    Uses serum that contains antibody, usually from the patient. Used to check cross-match prior to blood transfusion in the blood bank.

5

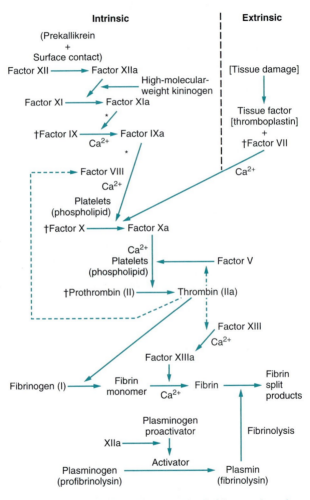

FIGURE 5–2 Blood coagulation cascade. Nearly all of the coagulation factors apparently exist as inactive proenzymes (Roman numeral) that, when activated (Roman numeral + a), serve to activate the next proenzyme in the sequence. *Symbol key:* * = Heparin acts to inhibit. Ü = Plasma content decreased by Coumadin. (Reprinted, with permission, from: Krupp MA [ed]: *The Physician's Handbook.* Lange Medical Publications, Los Angeles CA, 1985.)

Positive: Isoimmunization from previous transfusion, incompatible blood due to improper cross-matching or medications such as methyldopa.

Fibrin D-Dimers

• Negative or <0.5 µg/mL • Collection: Blue, green, or purple top tube
Fibrin broken into various D-dimer fragments by plasmin.

Increased: DIC, thromboembolic diseases (PE, arterial or venous thrombosis)

Fibrin Degradation Products (FDP), Fibrin Split Products (FSP)

• <10 µg/mL • Collection: Blue top tube
Generally replaced by the fibrin D-dimer as a screen for DIC

Increased: DIC (usually >40 µg/mL), any thromboembolic condition (DVT, MI, PE), hepatic dysfunction

Fibrinogen

• 200–400 mg/dL (SI:2.0–4.0 g/L) • Collection: Blue top tube
Most useful in the diagnosis of DIC and congenital hypofibrinogenemia. Fibrinogen is cleaved by thrombin to form insoluble fragments that polymerize to form a stable clot.

Increased: Inflammatory reactions, oral contraceptives, pregnancy, cancer (kidney, stomach, breast)

Decreased: DIC (sepsis, amniotic fluid embolism, abruptio placentae), surgery (prostate, open heart), neoplastic and hematological conditions, acute severe bleeding, burns, venomous snake bite, congenital

Lee-White Clotting Time

• 5–15 min • Collection: Draw into plain plastic syringe; clotting time measured in separate tube

Increased: Heparin therapy, plasma–clotting factor deficiency (except Factors VII and XIII). (*Note:* This is not a sensitive test and so is therefore not considered a good screening test.)

Partial Thromboplastin Time (Activated Partial Thromboplastin Time, PTT, APTT)

• 27–38 s • Collection: Blue top tube
Evaluates the intrinsic coagulation system (See Figure 5–2). Most commonly used to monitor heparin therapy

Increased: Heparin and any defect in the **intrinsic coagulation system** (includes Factors I, II, V, VIII, IX, X, XI, and XII), prolonged use of a tourniquet before drawing a blood sample, hemophilia A and B

Prothrombin Time (PT)

• 11.5–13.5 s • Figure 5–2, page 106 • Collection: Blue top tube

PT evaluates the **extrinsic coagulation system** that includes Factors I, II, V, VII, and X. The use of **INR** instead of the Patient/Control ratio to guide anticoagulant (Coumadin) therapy is becoming standard. **INR provides a more universal and standardized result because it measures the control against a WHO standard reference reagent.** Therapeutic INR levels are 2–3 for DVT, PE, TIAs, and atrial fibrillation. Recurrent DVT on adequate treatment requires an INR of 3–4.5. Mechanical heart valves require an INR of 3–4.5 (See also Chapter 22, Table 22–10 [page 637].)

Increased: Drugs (sodium warfarin [Coumadin]), vitamin K deficiency, fat malabsorption, liver disease, prolonged use of a tourniquet before drawing a blood sample, DIC

Sedimentation Rate (Erythrocyte Sedimentation Rate, ESR)

• Collection: Lavender top tube

The ESR is a very nonspecific test with a high sensitivity and a low specificity. Most useful in serial measurement to follow the course of disease (eg, polymyalgia rheumatica or temporal arteritis). ZETA rate is not affected by anemia. ESR correlates well with C-reactive protein levels.

Wintrobe Scale: Males, 0–9 mm/h, females, 0–20 mm/h

ZETA Scale: 40–54% normal, 55–59% mildly elevated, 60–64% moderately elevated, >65% markedly elevated

Westergren Scale: Males <50 years 15 mm/h, >50 years 20 mm/h; female <50 years 20 mm/h, >50 years 30 mm/h

Increased: Any type of infection, inflammation, rheumatic fever, endocarditis, neoplasm, AMI

Thrombin Time

• 10–14 s • Collection: Blue top tube

A measure of the rate of conversion of fibrinogen to fibrin and fibrin polymerization. Used to detect the presence of heparin and hypofibrinogenemia and as an aid in the evaluation of prolonged PTT

Increased: Systemic heparin, DIC, fibrinogen deficiency, congenitally abnormal fibrinogen molecules

LABORATORY DIAGNOSIS: URINE STUDIES

Urinalysis Procedure
Urinalysis, Normal Values
Differential Diagnosis for Routine Urinalysis
Urine Sediment
Spot or Random Urine Studies
Creatinine and Creatinine Clearance

24-Hour Urine Studies
Other Urine Studies
Urinary Indices in Renal Failure
Urine Output
Urine Protein Electrophoresis

URINALYSIS PROCEDURE

For a routine screening urinalysis, a fresh (less than 1-h old), clean-catch urine is acceptable. If it cannot be interpreted immediately, it should be refrigerated (urine standing at room temperature for long periods causes lysis of casts and red cells and becomes alkalinized.) See Chapter 13 under Urinary Tract Procedures, page 306, for the different ways to collect the sample.

1. Pour about 5–10 mL of well-mixed urine into a centrifuge tube. Check the specific gravity with a urinometer or optic refractory urinometer (refractometer) on the remaining sample.
2. Check for appearance (color, turbidity, odor).
3. Spin the capped sample at 3000 rpm (450 g) for 3 min.
4. While the sample is in the centrifuge and using the dipstick (Chemstrip, etc) supplied by your lab, perform the dipstick evaluation on the remaining portion of the sample. Read the results according to the color chart and instructions on the bottle. Make sure to allow the time noted before reading the test because reading before the time (up to 60 s) may yield false results. Record glucose, ketones, blood, protein, pH, nitrite, and leukocyte esterase if available. Be sure to recap the bottle tightly after use. Agents that color the urine (phenazopyridine [Pyridium]) may interfere with the results of the dipstick.
5. Decant and discard the supernatant. Mix the remaining sediment by flicking it with your finger and pour or pipette one or two drops on a microscope slide. Cover with a coverslip. If a urine sample looks very grossly cloudy, it is sometimes advisable to examine an unspun sample. If an unspun sample is used, note this on the report. In general, for routine urinalysis, a spun sample is more desirable.
6. Examine 10 lpf (10× objective) for epithelial cells, casts, crystals, and mucus. Casts are usually reported per low-power field. Casts tend to collect around the periphery of the coverslip.
7. Examine several high-power fields (40× objective) for epithelial cells, crystals, RBCs, WBCs, bacteria, and parasites (trichomonads). RBCs, WBCs, and bacteria are usually reported per high-power field. Two reporting systems are commonly used:

System One	**System Two**
Rare = <2 per field	Trace = <¼ of field
Occasional = 3–5 per field	1+ = ¼ of field
Frequent = 5–9 per field	2+ = ½ of field
Many = "large number" per field	3+ = ¾ of field
TNTC = too numerous to count	4+ = field is full

URINALYSIS, NORMAL VALUES

1. **Appearance:** "Yellow, clear," or "straw-colored, clear"
2. **Specific Gravity**
   a. Neonate: 1.012
   b. Infant: 1.002–1.006
   c. Child and Adult: 1.001–1.035 (with normal fluid intake 1.016–1.022)
3. **pH**
   a. Newborn/Neonate: 5–7
   b. Child and Adult: 4.6–8.0
4. **Negative for:** Bilirubin, blood, acetone, glucose, protein, nitrite, leukocyte esterase, reducing substances
5. **Trace:** Urobilinogen
6. **RBC:** Male 0–3/hpf, female 0–5/hpf
7. **WBC:** 0–4/hpf
8. **Epithelial Cells:** Occasional
9. **Hyaline Casts:** Occasional
10. **Bacteria:** None
11. **Crystals:** Some limited crystals based on urine pH (see below)

DIFFERENTIAL DIAGNOSIS FOR ROUTINE URINALYSIS

Appearance

Colorless: Diabetes insipidus, diuretics, excess fluid intake

Dark: Acute intermittent porphyria, malignant melanoma

Cloudy: UTI (pyuria), amorphous phosphate salts (normal in alkaline urine), blood, mucus, bilirubin

Pink/Red:
   Heme-positive. Blood, hemoglobin, sepsis, dialysis, myoglobin
   Heme-negative. Food coloring, beets, sulfa drugs, nitrofurantoin, salicylates

Orange/Yellow: Dehydration, phenazopyridine (Pyridium), rifampin, bile pigments

Brown/Black: Myoglobin, bile pigments, melanin, cascara, iron, nitrofurantoin, alkaptonuria

Green: Urinary bile pigments, indigo carmine, methylene blue

Foamy: Proteinuria, bile salts

pH

Acidic: High-protein (meat) diet, ammonium chloride, mandelic acid and other medications, acidosis, (due to ketoacidosis [starvation, diabetic], COPD)

Basic: UTI, renal tubular acidosis, diet (high-vegetable, milk, immediately after meals), sodium bicarbonate therapy, vomiting, metabolic alkalosis

Specific Gravity

Usually corresponds with osmolarity except with osmotic diuresis. Value >1.023 indicates normal renal concentrating ability. Random value 1.003–1.030

Increased: Volume depletion; CHF; adrenal insufficiency; diabetes mellitus; SIADH; increased proteins (nephrosis); if markedly increased (1.040–1.050), suspect artifact or excretion of radiographic contrast media

Decreased: Diabetes insipidus, pyelonephritis, glomerulonephritis, water load with normal renal function

Bilirubin

Positive: Obstructive jaundice (intrahepatic and extrahepatic), hepatitis. (*Note:* False-positives occur with stool contamination.)

Blood

Note: If the dipstick is positive for blood, but no red cells are seen, free hemoglobin from trauma may be present; a transfusion reaction may have occurred, from lysis of RBCs (RBCs will lyse if the pH is <5 or >8); or myoglobin may be present because of a crush injury, burn, or tissue ischemia.

Positive: Stones, trauma, tumors (benign and malignant, anywhere in the urinary tract), urethral strictures, coagulopathy, infection, menses (contamination), polycystic kidneys, interstitial nephritis, hemolytic anemia, transfusion reaction, instrumentation (Foley catheter, etc)

Glucose

Positive: Diabetes mellitus, pancreatitis, pancreatic carcinoma, pheochromocytoma, Cushing's disease, shock, burns, pain, steroids, hyperthyroidism, renal tubular disease, iatrogenic causes. (*Note:* Glucose oxidase technique in many kits is specific for glucose and will not react with lactose, fructose, or galactose.)

Ketones

Detects primarily acetone and acetoacetic acid and not β-hydroxybutyric acid.

Positive: Starvation, high-fat diet, DKA, vomiting, diarrhea, hyperthyroidism, pregnancy, febrile states (especially in children)

Nitrite

Many bacteria will convert nitrates to nitrite. (See also the section on Leukocyte Esterase, page 112.)

Positive: Infection (A negative test does not rule out infection because some organisms, such as *Streptococcus faecalis* and other gram-positive cocci, do not produce nitrite, and the urine must also be retained in the bladder for several hours to allow the reaction to take place.)

Protein

Indication by dipstick of persistent proteinuria should be quantified by 24-h urine studies.

Positive: Pyelonephritis, glomerulonephritis, Kimmelstiel–Wilson syndrome (diabetes), nephrotic syndrome, myeloma, postural causes, preeclampsia, inflammation and malignancies of the lower tract, functional causes (fever, stress, heavy exercise), malignant hypertension, CHF

Leukocyte Esterase

Test detects ≥5 WBC/hpf or lysed WBCs. When combined with the nitrite test, it has a predictive value of 74% for UTI if both tests are positive and a value of >97% if both tests are negative.

Positive: UTI (false-positive with vaginal contamination)

Reducing Substances

Positive: Glucose, fructose, galactose, false-positives (vitamin C, salicylates, antibiotics, etc)

Urobilinogen

Positive: Cirrhosis, CHF with hepatic congestion, hepatitis, hyperthyroidism, suppression of gut flora with antibiotics

URINE SEDIMENT

Many labs no longer do microscopic examinations unless specifically requested or if evidence exists for an abnormal finding on dipstick test (such as positive leukocyte esterase). Figure 6–1 is a pictorial representation of materials found in urine sediments.

Red Blood Cells (RBCs):   Trauma, pyelonephritis, genitourinary TB, cystitis, prostatitis, stones, tumors (malignant and benign), coagulopathy, and any cause of blood on dipstick test (See previous section on blood pH, page 111.)

White Blood Cells (WBCs):   Infection anywhere in the urinary tract, TB, renal tumors, acute glomerulonephritis, radiation, interstitial nephritis (analgesic abuse)

Epithelial Cells: ATN, necrotizing papillitis. (Most epithelial cells are from an otherwise unremarkable urethra.)

Parasites: *Trichomonas vaginalis, Schistosoma haematobium* infection

Yeast: *Candida albicans* infection (especially in diabetics, immunosuppressed patients, or if a vaginal yeast infection is present)

Spermatozoa: Normal in males immediately after intercourse or nocturnal emission

Crystals
 Abnormal. Cystine, sulfonamide, leucine, tyrosine, cholesterol
 Normal. Acid urine: Oxalate (small square crystals with a central cross), uric acid. *Alkaline urine:* Calcium carbonate, triple phosphate (resemble coffin lids)

Contaminants: Cotton threads, hair, wood fibers, amorphous substances (all usually unimportant)

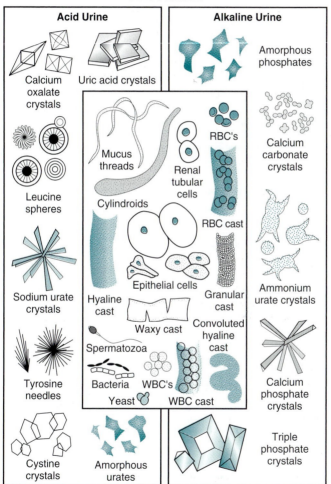

Urine Sediment

Acid Urine	Alkaline Urine

Calcium oxalate crystals
Uric acid crystals
Leucine spheres
Sodium urate crystals
Tyrosine needles
Cystine crystals
Amorphous urates

Mucus threads
Cylindroids
RBC's
Renal tubular cells
RBC cast
Epithelial cells
Hyaline cast
Granular cast
Waxy cast
Convoluted hyaline cast
Spermatozoa
Bacteria
WBC's
Yeast
WBC cast

Amorphous phosphates
Calcium carbonate crystals
Ammonium urate crystals
Calcium phosphate crystals
Triple phosphate crystals

FIGURE 6-1   Urine sediment as seen under the microscope. (Reprinted, with permission, from: Greene MG [ed]: *The Harriet Lane Handbook: A Manual for Pediatric House Officers,* 12th ed,. Yearbook Medical Publishers, Chicago IL, 1991.)

Mucus: Large amounts suggest urethral disease (normal from ileal conduit or other forms of urinary diversion)

Glitter Cells: WBCs lysed in hypotonic solution

Casts: The presence of casts in a urine localizes some or all of the disease process to the kidney itself.

Hyaline Casts. (Acceptable unless they are "numerous"), benign hypertension, nephrotic syndrome, after exercise

RBC Casts. Acute glomerulonephritis, lupus nephritis, SBE, Goodpasture's disease, after a streptococcal infection, vasculitis, malignant hypertension

WBC Casts. Pyelonephritis

Epithelial (Tubular) Casts. Tubular damage, nephrotoxin, virus

Granular Casts. Breakdown of cellular casts, leads to waxy casts; "dirty brown granular casts" typical for ATN

Waxy Casts. (End stage of granular cast). Severe chronic renal disease, amyloidosis

Fatty Casts. Nephrotic syndrome, diabetes mellitus, damaged renal tubular epithelial cells

Broad Casts. Chronic renal disease

SPOT OR RANDOM URINE STUDIES

The so-called spot urine, which is often ordered to aid in diagnosing various conditions, relies on only a small sample (10–20 mL) of urine.

Spot Urine for β_2-microglobulin

- <0.3 mg/L
  A marker for renal tubular injury

Increased: Diseases of the proximal tubule (ATN, interstitial nephritis, pyelonephritis), drug-induced nephropathy (aminoglycosides), diabetes, trauma, sepsis, HIV, lymphoproliferative and lymphodestructive diseases

Spot Urine for Electrolytes

The usefulness of this assay is limited because of large variations in daily fluid and salt intake, and the results are usually indeterminate if a diuretic has been given.

1. **Sodium <10 mEq/L (mmol/L)**: Volume depletion, hyponatremic states, prerenal azotemia (CHF, shock, etc), hepatorenal syndrome, glucocorticoid excess
2. **Sodium >20 mEq/L (mmol/L)**: SIADH, ATN (usually >40 mEq/L), postobstructive diuresis, high salt intake, Addison's disease, hypothyroidism, interstitial nephritis
3. **Chloride <10 mEq/L (mmol/L)**: Chloride-sensitive metabolic alkalosis (vomiting, excessive diuretic use), volume depletion
4. **Potassium <10 mEq/L (mmol/L)**: Hypokalemia, potassium depletion, extrarenal loss

Spot Urine for Erythrocyte Morphology

The morphology of red blood cells in a sample of urine that tests positive for blood may give some indication of the nature of the hematuria. **Eumorphic red cells** are typically seen in cases of postrenal, nonglomerular bleeding. **Dysmorphic red cells** are more likely associated with glomerular causes of bleeding. Each reference lab has standards, but as a general rule, the presence of >90% dysmorphic erythrocytes in patients with asymptomatic hematuria indicates a renal glomerular source of bleeding, especially if associated with proteinuria and or casts (ie, IgA nephropathy, poststreptococcal glomerular, sickle cell disease or trait, etc). If ≥90% eumorphic erythrocytes or even "mixed" results (10–90% eumorphic erythrocytes) indicates a postrenal cause of hematuria requiring a complete urologic evaluation (ie, hypercalciuria, urolithiasis, cystitis, trauma, tumors, hemangioma, exercise induced, BPH, etc).

Spot Urine for Microalbumin

• Normal <30 μg albumin/mg creatinine

Used to determine which patients with diabetes are at risk for nephropathy. Clinical albuminuria occurs at >300 μg albumin/mg creatinine. Base test on two or three separate determinations over 6 mo. Diabetic patients with levels between 30–300 μg have microalbuminuria and are usually initiated on ACE inhibitor or angiotensin receptor blocker.

Spot Urine for Myoglobin

• Qualitative negative

Positive: Skeletal muscle conditions (crush injury, electrical burns, carbon monoxide poisoning, delirium tremens, surgical procedures, malignant hyperthermia), polymyositis.

Spot Urine for Osmolality

• 75–300 mOsm/kg (mmol/kg) • Varies with water intake

Patients with normal renal function should concentrate >800 mOsm/kg (mmol/kg) after a 14-h fluid restriction; <400 mOsm/kg (mmol/kg) is a sign of renal impairment.

Increased: Dehydration, SIADH, adrenal insufficiency, glycosuria, high-protein diet

Decreased: Excessive fluid intake, diabetes insipidus, acute renal failure, medications (acetohexamide, glyburide, lithium)

Spot Urine for Protein

• Normal <10 mg/dL (0.1 g/L) or <20 mg/dL (0.2 g/L) for a sample taken in the early AM

See page 112 for the differential diagnosis of protein in the urine.

CREATININE AND CREATININE CLEARANCE

Normal

Adult Male. Total creatinine 1–2 g/24 h (8.8–17.7 mmol/d); clearance 85–125 mL/min/1.73 m^2

Adult Female. Total creatinine 0.8–1.8 g/24 h (7.1–15.9 mmol/d); clearance 75–115 mL/min 1.73 m^2 (1.25–1.92 mL/s/1.73 m^2)

Child. Total creatinine (>3 years) 12–30 mg/kg/24 h; clearance 70–140 mL/min/1.73 m^2 (1.17–2.33 mL/s/1.73 m^2)

Decreased: A decreased creatinine clearance results in an increase in serum creatinine usually secondary to renal insufficiency. See Chapter 4, page 65, for differential diagnosis of increased serum creatinine.

Increased: Early diabetes mellitus, pregnancy

Creatinine Clearance Determination

Creatinine clearance is one of the most sensitive indicators of early renal insufficiency. Clearances are ordered for patients with suspected renal disease and are useful for following patients who are taking nephrotoxic medications, (eg, gentamicin). Clearance normally decreases with age. A creatinine clearance of 10–20 mL/min indicates severe renal failure, and a clearance of <10 mL/min usually indicates the need for dialysis.

To determine a creatinine clearance, order a concurrent serum creatinine and a 24-h urine creatinine. A shorter time interval can be used, for example, 12 h, but remember that the formula must be corrected for this change and that a 24-h sample is less prone to collection error.

6

Example: (A quick formula is also found under "Aminoglycoside Dosing," page 620.) The following are calculations of (a) the creatinine clearance from a 24-h urine sample with a volume of 1000 mL, (b) a urine creatinine of 108 mg/100 mL, and (c) a serum creatinine of 1 mg/100 mL (1 mg/dL).

$$\text{Clearance} = \frac{\text{Urine creatinine} \times \text{Total urine volume}}{\text{Plasma creatinine} \times \text{Time}}$$

where time = 1440 min if 24-h collection.

$$\text{Clearance} = \frac{(108 \text{ mg} / 100 \text{ mL}) (1000 \text{ mL})}{(1 \text{ mg} / 100 \text{ mL}) (1440 \text{ min})} = 75 \text{ mL} / \text{min}$$

To see if the urine sample is valid, some clinicians advocate a preliminary evaluation by determining first if the sample contains at least 18–25 mg/kg/24 h of creatinine for adult males or 12–20 mg/kg/24 h for adult females. This preliminary test is not a requirement, but can confirm if a 24–h sample was collected or if some of the sample was lost.

If the patient is an adult (150 lb = body surface area of 1.73 m^2), adjustment of the clearance for body size is not routinely done. Adjustment for pediatric patients is a necessity. If the values in the previous example were for a 10-year-old boy who weighed 70 lb (1.1 m^2), the clearance would be:

$$75 \text{ mL} / \text{min} \times \frac{1.73 \text{ m}^2}{1.1 \text{ m}^2} = 118 \text{ mL} / \text{min}$$

24-HOUR URINE STUDIES

A wide variety of diseases, most of them endocrine, can be diagnosed by assays of 24-h urine samples. The following information gives the normal values for certain agents and the conditions associated with changes in these values.

Calcium, Urine

Normal: On a calcium-free diet <150 mg/24 h (3.7 mmol/d), average calcium diet (600–800 mg/24 h) 100–250 mg/24 h (2.5–6.2 mmol/d)

Increased: Hyperparathyroidism, hyperthyroidism, hypervitaminosis D, distal renal tubular acidosis (type I), sarcoidosis, immobilization, osteolytic lesions (bony metastasis, multiple myeloma), Paget's disease, glucocorticoid excess, immobilization, furosemide

Decreased: Medications (thiazide diuretics, estrogens, oral contraceptives), hypothyroidism, renal failure, steatorrhea, rickets, osteomalacia

Catecholamines, Fractionated

Used to evaluate neuroendocrine tumors, including pheochromocytoma and neuroblastoma. Avoid caffeine and methyldopa (Aldomet) prior to test

Normal: Values are variable and depend on the assay method used. Norepinephrine 15–80 mg/24 h [SI: 89–473 nmol/24 h], epinephrine 0–20 mg/24 h [0–118 nmol/24 h], dopamine 65–400 mg/24 h [SI: 384–2364 nmol/24 h].

Increased: Pheochromocytoma, neuroblastoma, epinephrine administration, presence of drugs (methyldopa, tetracyclines cause false increases)

Cortisol, Free

Used to evaluate adrenal cortical hyperfunction, screening test of choice for Cushing's syndrome

Normal: 10–110 mg/24 h [SI: 30–300 nmol]

Increased: Cushing's syndrome (adrenal hyperfunction), stress during collection, oral contraceptives, pregnancy

Creatinine

• See pages 65 and 115

Cysteine

Used to detect cystinuria, homocystinuria, monitor response to therapy

Normal: 40–60 mg/g creatinine

Increased: Heterozygotes < 300 mg/g creatinine/day; homozygotes > 250 mg/g creatinine

5-HIAA (5-Hydroxyindoleacetic Acid)

5–HIAA is a serotonin metabolite useful in diagnosing carcinoid syndrome.

Normal: (2–8 mg [SI: 10.4–41.6] mmol/24–h urine collection)

Increased: Carcinoid tumors (except rectal), certain foods (banana, pineapple, tomato, walnuts, avocado), phenothiazine derivatives

Metanephrines

Detects metabolic products of epinephrine and norepinephrine, a primary screening test for pheochromocytoma

Normal: <1.3 mg/24 h (7.1 mmol/L) for adults, but variable in children

Increased: Pheochromocytoma, neuroblastoma (neural crest tumors), false-positive with drugs (phenobarbital, guanethidine, hydrocortisone, MAO inhibitors)

Protein

• See also Urine Protein Electrophoresis, pages 85 and 112.

Normal: <150 mg/24 h (<0.15 g/d)

Increased: Nephrotic syndrome usually associated with >4 g/24 h

17-Ketogenic Steroids (17-KGS, Corticosteroids)

Overall adrenal function test, largely replaced by serum or urine cortisol levels

Normal: Males 5–24 mg/24 h (17–83 mmol/24 h); females 4–15 mg/24 h (14–52 mmol/24 h)

Increased: Adrenal hyperplasia (Cushing's syndrome), adrenogenital syndrome

Decreased: Panhypopituitarism, Addison's disease, acute steroid withdrawal

17-Ketosteroids, Total (17-KS)

Measures DHEA, androstenedione (adrenal androgens); largely replaced by assay of individual elements

Normal: Adult males 8–20 mg/24 h (28–69 mmol/L); adult female 6–15 mg/dL (21–52 mmol/L). *Note:* Low values in prepubertal children

Increased: Adrenal cortex abnormalities (hyperplasia [Cushing's disease], adenoma, carcinoma, adrenogenital syndrome), severe stress, ACTH or pituitary tumor, testicular interstitial tumor and arrhenoblastoma (both produce testosterone)

Decreased: Panhypopituitarism, Addison's disease, castration in men

Vanillylmandelic Acid

VMA is the urinary product of both epinephrine and norepinephrine; good screening test for pheochromocytoma, also used to diagnose and follow up neuroblastoma and ganglioneuroma

Normal: <7–9 mg/24 h (35–45 mmol/L)

Increased: Pheochromocytoma, other neural crest tumors (ganglioneuroma, neuroblastoma), factitious (chocolate, coffee, tea, methyldopa)

OTHER URINE STUDIES

Drug Abuse Screen

• Normal = negative

  Tests urine for common drugs of abuse, often used for employment screening for critical jobs. Assay will vary by facility and may include tests for amphetamines, barbiturates, benzodiazepines, marijuana (cannabinoid metabolites), cocaine metabolites, opiates, phencyclidine.

Xylose Tolerance Test (D-Xylose Absorption Test)

• 5 g xylose in 5-h urine specimen after 25 g oral dose of xylose or 1.2 g after 5-g oral dose
• Collection: Patient is NPO after midnight except for water. • After voiding at 8 AM, 25 g of D-xylose (or 5 g if GI irritation is a concern) is dissolved in 250 mL water. • An additional 750 mL water is drunk and the urine collected for the next 5 h.

TABLE 6–1
Urinary Indices Useful in the Differential Diagnosis of Oliguria

Index	Prerenal	Renal (ATN)*
Urine osmolality	>500	<350
Urinary sodium	<20	>40
Urine/serum creatinine	>40	<20
Urine/serum osmolarity	>1.2	<1.2
Fractional excreted sodium†	<1	>1
Renal failure index (RFI)‡	<1	>1

*Acute tubular necrosis (intrinsic renal failure).

†Fractional excreted sodium = $\dfrac{\text{Urine / Serum sodium}}{\text{Urine / Serum creatinine}} \times 100$

‡Renal failure index = $\dfrac{\text{Urine sodium} \times \text{Serum creatinine}}{\text{Urine creatinine}}$

Used to assess proximal bowel function; differentiates between malabsorption due to pancreatic insufficiency or intestinal problems.

Decreased: Celiac disease (nontropical sprue, gluten-sensitive enteropathy), false de-creas0e with renal disease

URINARY INDICES IN RENAL FAILURE

Use Table 6–1 to help differentiate the causes (renal or prerenal) of oliguria. (See also Oliguria and Anuria, page 49.)

URINE OUTPUT

Although clinical situations vary greatly, the usual, minimal acceptable urine output for an adult is 0.5–1.0 mL/kg/h (daily volume normally 1000–1600 mL/d).

URINE PROTEIN ELECTROPHORESIS

See Protein Electrophoresis, Serum and Urine, page 85, and Figure 4–5, page 86.

CLINICAL MICROBIOLOGY

Staining Techniques
    Acid-Fast Stain
    Darkfield Examination
    Giemsa Stain
    Gonorrhea Smear
    Gram Stain
    Gram Stain Characteristics
      of Common Pathogens
    India Ink Preparation
    KOH Preparation
    Stool Leukocyte Stain
    Tzanck Smear
    Vaginal Wet Preparation
    Wayson Stain
Gonorrhea (GC) Cultures and Smear

Nasopharyngeal Cultures
Blood Cultures
Sputum Cultures
Stool Cultures
Throat Cultures
Urine Cultures
Viral Cultures and Serology
Scotch Tape Test
Molecular Microbiology
Susceptibility Testing (MIC, MBC,
    Schlichter Test)
Differential Diagnosis of Common
    Infections and Empiric Therapy
SBE Prophylaxis
Isolation Protocols

STAINING TECHNIQUES

Acid-Fast Stain (AFB Smear, Kinyoun Stain)

Clinical microbiology labs can also perform a "modified" acid-fast stain for organisms that are weakly acid-fast-staining (eg, *Nocardia* species).

Procedure

1. Spread the smear on a slide, allow it to air dry, and then gently heat fix it.
2. Stain the smear for 3–5 min with terpinol in carbol-fuchsin red solution.
3. Rinse the slide with tap water.
4. Decolorize with acid–alcohol solution for no longer than 30 s.
5. Rinse with tap water.
6. Counterstain with methylene blue for 1 min.
7. Rinse the slide with tap water and allow it to air dry.
8. Examine the smear with high dry and oil immersion lenses; search for the acid-fast bacilli that stain red to bright pink against the light blue background (*Mycobacterium tuberculosis* [TB], *M. scrofulaceum, M. avium-intracellulare,* others). These organisms have a beaded rod appearance under oil immersion.
9. These organisms must be cultured on specialized media. Rapid-growing AFB include *M. abscessus, M. chelonae, M. fortuitum* and can usually be cultured in fewer than 7 days. Most other AFB (*M. tuberculosis, M. avium* complex, *M. kansasii, M. marinum*) require at least 7–10 d to grow. *M. gordonae* is thought to be nonpathogenic.

Darkfield Examination

Darkfield examination is used to identify *Treponema pallidum,* the organism responsible for syphilis. Rectal and oral lesions cannot be examined by this technique due to the presence of nonpathogenic spirochetes.

Procedure

1. The chancre is cleansed with a saline-moistened swab and a slide is touched on the lesion and examined under darkfield illumination within 15 min of applying the specimen to the slide.
2. The organisms resemble tight corkscrews and are 1–1½ times the diameter of an RBC in length.

Giemsa Stain

Used to identify intracellular organisms such as chlamydiae, *Plasmodium* spp. (malaria), and other parasites.

Gonorrhea Smear (See the following section on Gonorrhea [GC] Cultures)
Gram Stain

The Gram stain is used to determine whether an organism can be decolorized with alcohol after being stained with crystal violet. This determination is based on the organism's cell wall characteristics. Gram staining is performed on bacteria from a variety of body fluids, including exudates, abscesses, sputum, and others as clinically indicated.

Procedure

1. Smear the specimen (sputum, peritoneal fluid, etc) on a glass slide in a fairly thin coat. If time permits, allow the specimen to air dry. The smear may also be fixed under very low heat (excessive heat can cause artifacts). If a Bunsen burner is not available, other possible methods for heating the sample include using a hot light bulb or setting an alcohol swab on fire. Heat the slide until it is warm, but not hot, when touched to the back of the hand.
2. Timing for the stain is not critical, but allow at least 10 s for each set of reagents.
3. Apply the **crystal violet (Gram stain)**, rinse the slide with tap water, apply iodine solution, and rinse with water.
4. Decolorize the slide carefully with the acetone–alcohol solution until the blue color is barely visible in the runoff. (Be careful; this is the step where most Gram stains are ruined.)
5. Counterstain with a few drops of safranin, rinse the slide with water, and blot it dry with lint-free bibulous or filter paper.
6. Use the high dry (100×) and oil immersion lenses on the microscope to examine the slide. If the Gram stain is satisfactory, any polys on the slide should be pink with light blue nuclei. On a Gram stain of **sputum,** an excessive number of epithelial cells (>25/hpf) means the sample contained more saliva than sputum. **Gram-positive organisms stain dark blue to purple; gram-negative ones stain red.**

Gram Stain Characteristics of Common Pathogens:

Initial lab reports identify the Gram stain characteristics of the organisms. Complete identification usually requires culturing the organism. The lab algorithm for gram-positive and

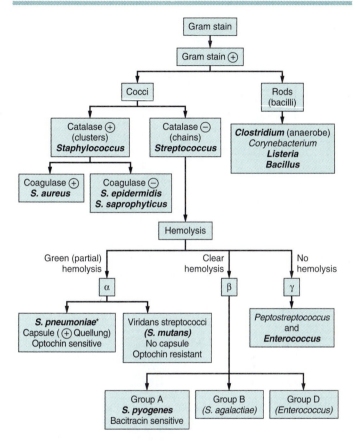

*Important pathogens are in **bold type**.
Note: Enterococcus is Group D but it is not β-hemolytic; it is α- or γ-hemolytic.

FIGURE 7–1   Lab algorithm for the identification of gram-positive organisms.
(Reprinted, with permission, from: Bhushan V [ed]: *First Aid for the USMLE, Step 1*,
Appleton & Lange, Norwalk, CT, 1999.)

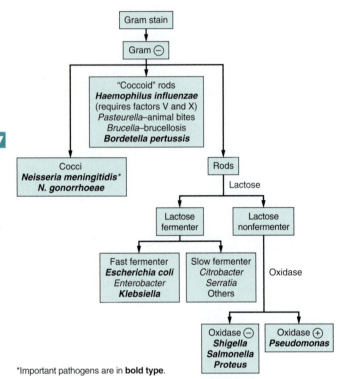

*Important pathogens are in **bold type**.

FIGURE 7–2 Lab algorithm for the identification of gram-negative organisms. (Reprinted, with permission, from: Bhushan V [ed]: *First Aid for the USMLE, Step 1,* Appleton & Lange, Norwalk, CT, 1999.)

TABLE 7-1
Gram Stain Characteristics and Key Features of Common Organisms*

Gram Staining Pattern and Organisms	Identifying Key Features
GRAM-POSITIVE COCCI	
Enterococcus spp. (*E. faecalis*) (*Note:* These are equivalent group D *Streptococcus*)	Pairs, chains; catalase-negative
Peptostreptococcus spp.	Anaerobic
Staphylococcus spp.	Clusters; catalase-positive
Staphylococcus aureus	Clusters; catalase-positive; coagulase-negative; beta-hemolytic; yellow pigment
Staphylococcus epidermidis	Clusters; catalase-positive; coagulase-positive; skin flora
Staphylococcus saprophyticus	Clusters; catalase-positive; coagulase-positive
Streptococcus spp.	Pairs, chains; catalase-negative
Streptococcus agalactiae (group B)	Pairs, chains; catalase-negative; vaginal flora
Streptococcus bovis (group D *Enterococcus*)	Pairs, chains; catalase-negative
Streptococcus faecalis (group D *Enterococcus*)	Pairs, chains; catalase-negative
Streptococcus pneumoniae (*Pneumococcus*, group B)	Pairs, lancet-shaped; alpha-hemolytic; Optochin-sensitive
Streptococcus pyogenes (group A)	Beta-hemolytic
Streptococcus viridans	Pairs, chains; catalase-negative; alpha-hemolytic, Optochin-resistant
GRAM-NEGATIVE COCCI	
Acinetobacter spp.	Filamentous, branching pattern
Moraxella (*Branhamella*) *catarrhalis*	Diplococci in pairs
Neisseria gonorrhoeae (gonococcus)	Diplococci in pairs, often intracellular; ferments glucose but not maltose
Neisseria meningitidis (meningococcus)	Diplococci in pairs; ferments glucose and maltose
Veillonella spp.	Anaerobic
GRAM-POSITIVE BACILLI	
Actinomyces	Branching, beaded, rods; anaerobic
Bacilli anthracis (anthrax)	Spore forming rod

(continued)

TABLE 7–1
(Continued)

Gram Staining Pattern and Organisms	Identifying Key Features
GRAM-POSITIVE BACILLI	
Clostridium spp. (*C. difficile, C. botulinum, C. tetani*)	Large, with spores; anaerobic
Corynebacterium spp. (*C. diphtheriae*)	Small, pleomorphic diphtheroid; skin flora
Eubacterium spp.	Anaerobic
Lactobacillus spp.	Common vaginal bacterium; anaerobic
Listeria monocytogenes	Beta-hemolytic
Mycobacterium spp. (limited staining)	Only rapidly growing species gram stain (*M. abscessus, M. chelonae, M. fortuitum*)
Nocardia	Beaded, branched rods; partially acid-fast-staining
Propionibacterium acne	Small, pleomorphic diphtheroid; anaerobic
GRAM-NEGATIVE BACILLI	
Acinetobacter spp.	Lactose-negative, oxidase-negative
Aeromonas hydrophilia	Lactose-negative (usually), oxidase-positive
Bacteroides fragilis	Anaerobic
Bordetella pertussis	Coccoid rod
Brucella (brucellosis)	Coccoid rod
Citrobacter spp.	Lactose-positive (usually)
Enterobacter spp.	Lactose-positive (usually)
Escherichia coli	Lactose-positive
Fusobacterium spp.	Long, pointed shape; anaerobic
Haemophilus ducreyi (chancroid)	Gram-negative bacilli
Haemophilus influenzae	Coccoid rod, requires chocolate agar to support growth
Klebsiella spp.	Lactose-positive
Legionella pneumophila	Stains poorly, use silver stain and special media
Morganella morganii	Lactose-negative, oxidase-negative
Proteus mirabilis	Lactose-negative, oxidase-negative, indole-negative
Proteus vulgaris	Lactose-negative, oxidase-negative, indole-positive

(continued)

**TABLE 7–1
(Continued)**

Gram Staining Pattern and Organisms	Identifying Key Features
GRAM-NEGATIVE BACILLI	
Providencia spp.	Lactose-negative, oxidase-negative
Pseudomonas aeruginosa	Lactose-negative, oxidase-positive blue-green pigment
Salmonella spp.	Lactose-negative, oxidase-negative
Serratia spp.	Lactose-negative, oxidase-negative
Serratia marcescens	Lactose-negative, oxidative-negative, red pigment
Shigella spp.	Lactose-negative, oxidase-negative
Stenotrophomonas (Xanthomonas) maltophilia	Lactose-negative, oxidase-negative
Vibrio cholerae (cholera)	Gram-negative bacilli
Yersinia enterocolitica	Gram-negative bacilli
Yersinia pestis (bubonic plague)	Gram-negative bacilli

*Organisms are aerobic unless otherwise specified.

gram-negative organisms is shown in Figures 7–1 and 7–2. Gram stain characteristics of clinically important bacteria are shown in Table 7–1.

India Ink Preparation

India ink is used primarily on CSF to identify fungal organisms (especially cryptococci).

KOH Preparation

KOH (potassium hydroxide) preps are used to diagnose fungal infections. Vaginal KOH preps are discussed in detail in Chapter 13, page 291.

Procedure

1. Apply the specimen (vaginal secretion, sputum, hair, skin scrapings) to a slide. Skin scrapings of a lesion are usually obtained by gentle scraping with a #15 scalpel blade (see page 242 for description).
2. Add 1–2 drops of 10% KOH solution and mix. Gentle heating (optional) may accelerate dissolution of the keratin. A fishy odor from a vaginal prep suggests the presence of *Gardnerella vaginalis* (see page 291)
3. Put a coverslip over the specimen, and examine the slide for the branching hyphae and blastospores that indicate the presence of a fungus. KOH should destroy most elements other than fungus. If dense keratin and debris are present, allow the slide to sit for several hours and then repeat the microscopic examination. Lowering the substage condenser provides better contrast between organisms and the background.

Stool Leukocyte Stain (Fecal Leukocytes, Löeffler Methylene Blue Stain)

Used to differentiate treatable diarrhea (ie, bacterial) from other causes. This method detects causes from Crohn's disease, ulcerative colitis, TB, and amebic infection as well, but it should be remembered that many causes of severe diarrhea are viral. The positive predictive value of the bacterial pathogen as a cause for the diarrhea is 70%.

Procedure

1. Mix a small amount of stool or mucus on a slide with 2 drops of Löeffler (methylene blue) stain. Mucus is preferred; if no mucus is present, use a small amount of stool from the outside of a formed stool.

2. Examine the smear after 2–3 min to allow the white cells to take up the stain; then place a coverslip. The presence of many leukocytes suggests a bacterial cause. Increased white cells (usually polys) are seen in *Shigella, Salmonella, Campylobacter, Clostridium difficile,* and enteropathogenic *Escherichia coli* infections, as well as ulcerative colitis and pseudo-membranous colitis-related diarrhea. White cells are absent or normal in cholera and in *Giardia* and viral (rotavirus, Norwalk virus, etc) infections.

Tzanck Smear

This technique (named after Arnault Tzanck) is used in the diagnosis of herpesvirus infections (ie, herpes zoster or simplex).

Procedure

1. Clean a vesicle (not a pustule or crusted lesion) with alcohol, allow it to air dry, and gently unroof it with a #15 scalpel blade. Scrape the base with the blade, and place the material on a glass slide.
2. Allow the sample to air dry, and stain with Wright's stain as used for peripheral blood. Giemsa stain can also be used, however, the sample must be fixed for 10 min with methyl alcohol before the Giemsa is applied.
3. Scan the slide under low power, and identify cellular areas. Then use high-power oil immersion to identify multinucleated giant cells (epithelial cells infected with herpes viruses). This strongly suggests viral infection; culture is necessary to identify the specific virus.

Vaginal Wet Preparation

• See Chapter 13, page 291

Wayson Stain

Wayson stain is a good quick scout stain that colors most bacteria.

Procedure

1. Spread the smear on a slide, and air or heat dry it.
2. Pour freshly filtered Wayson stain onto the slide, and allow it to stand for 10–20 s (timing is not critical).
3. Rinse the slide gently with tap water, and dry it with filter paper.
4. Use the high dry and oil immersion lenses to examine the slide.

GONORRHEA (GC) CULTURES AND SMEAR

Neisseria gonorrhea can be cultured from many different sites, including female genital tract (endocervix is the preferred site), male urethra, urine, anorectum, throat, and synovial fluid, and the specimen is plated on selective (**Thayer–Martin** or **Transgrow**) media. Due to the high incidence of coinfection with *Chlamydia* and *T. pallidum* (syphilis), *Chlamydia* cultures and syphilis serology should also be performed, especially in females with genital infections with GC. Anorectal stains may contain nonpathogenic *Neisseria* species; avoid fecal contact; apply swab to anal crypts. In males with a urethral discharge, insert a **calcium alginate swab (Calgiswab)** into the urethra to collect the specimen and then plate.

The GC smear (see Chapter 13, page 291) has a low sensitivity (<50% in female endocervical smear, but is fairly reliable (>95%) in males with urethral discharge. A rapid enzyme immunoassay (**gonococcal antigen assay [Gonozyme]**) is available to diagnose cervical or urethral GC (not throat or anus) infections in less than 1 h. DNA probe testing is becoming widespread for rapid diagnosis.

NASOPHARYNGEAL CULTURES

Ideally, the specimen for culture should be obtained from deep in the nasopharynx and not the anterior nares, and the swab should not touch the skin. Cultures of nasopharyngeal specimens are useful in identifying *Staphylococcus aureus* and *N. meningitidis* infections. Normal nasal flora include *Staphylococcus epidermidis* and *S. aureus, Streptococcus pneumoniae, Haemophilus influenzae,* and several others.

BLOOD CULTURES

Blood cultures are not usually indicated for the routine workup of fever. The best use is for

1. Fever of unknown origin, especially in adults with white blood counts of > 15,000/mm^3 and no localizing signs or symptoms to suggest the source.
2. Clinical situations in which the diagnosis is established by a positive blood culture (eg, acute and SBE).
3. Febrile elderly, neutropenic, or immunocompromised patients.

Chills and fever usually ensue from ½–2 h after sudden entry of bacteria into the circulation (bacteremia). If bacteremia is suspected, several sets of cultures are usually needed to improve the chances of culturing the offending organism. Ideally, more than one set of cultures should be done at least 1 h apart; drawing more than three sets of specimens a day does not usually increase the yield. Obtain the blood through venipuncture, and avoid sampling through venous lines. Each "set" of specimens for blood culture consists of both an aerobic and anaerobic culture bottle. If possible, culture the specimens before antibiotics are initiated; if the patient is already on antibiotics, use **ARD** culture bottles, which absorb the antibiotic that may otherwise destroy any bacteria. *Legionella, Mycobacterium, Bordetella,* and *Histoplasma* may require special blood collection devices.

Procedure

1. Review the section on the technique of venipuncture (Chapter 13 page 309). Apply a tourniquet above the chosen vein.

2. Paint the venipuncture site with a povidone–iodine solution. Repeat this procedure three times with a different pad. Then wipe the area around the vein with alcohol and allow the alcohol to dry.

3. Use an 18–22-gauge needle (or smaller if needed) and a 10–20-mL syringe. Enter the skin over the prepped vein, and aspirate a sufficient volume of blood (10–20 mL in adults,

1–5 mL in children); adequate volume will increase the detection rate. **Be careful not to touch the needle or the prepped skin site.** Draw about 10 mL of blood. Remove the tourniquet, and compress the venipuncture site and apply an adhesive bandage.

4. Discard the needle used in the puncture and replace it with a **new, sterile** 20–22-gauge needle. Place the blood in each of the bottles by allowing the vacuum to draw in the appropriate volume, usually specified on the collection device. Submit the samples to the lab promptly with the appropriate lab slips completed including current antibiotics being given.

Interpretation

Preliminary results are usually available in 12–48 h; cultures should not be formally reported as negative before 4 d. A single blood culture that is positive for one of the following organisms usually suggests contamination; however, on rare occasions these agents are the causative pathogen: *Staphylococcus epidermidis, Bacillus* sp., *Corynebacterium diphtheriae* (and other diphtheroids), *Streptococcus viridans.* Negative results do not rule out bacteremia, and false-positives can result for the contaminants noted. Gram-negative organisms, fungi, and anaerobes are considered to be pathogenic until proven otherwise.

SPUTUM CULTURES

Cultures of sputum remain controversial. Many clinicians do not even order them and treat only based on the Gram stain and clinical findings. One problem is that "sputum" samples often contain only saliva. If you do a Gram stain on the specimen and see only a few squamous cells, with many polys and histiocytes, the sample is good, and the culture will probably be reliable. Excessive numbers of squamous cells (see previous section on Gram stain) suggests that the sample is more saliva than sputum. An early morning sample is most likely to be from deep within the bronchial tree.

Steps to improve the quality of the sputum collection

1. Careful instructions to the patient.
2. If the patient cannot mobilize the secretions, P&PD along with nebulizer treatments may help.
3. Careful nasotracheal suctioning using a specimen trap.

In general most labs will not accept anaerobic sputum cultures (critical in the diagnosis of aspiration pneumonia and lung abscesses) unless obtained by **transtracheal aspirate** or **endobronchial endoscopic collection** and submitted in special anaerobic transport media. Viral, *Legionella, Mycoplasma,* and TB cultures require special culture materials available at most labs. **PCP** can be diagnosed by sputum culture only about 10% of the time; therefore open-lung biopsy, endobronchial lavage, or other invasive techniques must be used to demonstrate the organisms. Specialized staining techniques for identifying *Pneumocystis carinii* include the methenamine silver, Giemsa, and toluidine blue stains.

STOOL CULTURES

Stool cultures are most often done to diagnose the cause of diarrhea or to identify disease carriers. A fresh sample is essential to isolate the organisms. Most common pathogens (*Salmonella, Shigella,* enteropathogenic *E. coli,* etc) can be grown on standard media. *Yersinia* and *Campylobacter,* however, usually require a special culture medium, and a special lab request is usually necessary.

A quick bedside test for bacterial causes of diarrhea is to check the stool for white cells (fecal leukocyte smear) see page 128.

Clostridium difficile Assay

Clostridium difficile is usually best diagnosed by determining the presence of *C. difficile* enterotoxin on the stool and not by culture. A positive *C. difficile* assay is found in the following cases: >90% of pseudo-membranous colitis; 30–40% antibiotic associated colitis, and 6–10% cases of antibiotic-associated diarrhea.

Stool for Ova and Parasites

With toxic diarrhea, the possibility of parasitic disease must be considered and stool for **"ova and parasites"** should be ordered. Protozoa (ameba [*Entamoeba histolytica,* others], *Blastocystis, Giardia*) cannot be cultured and are identified by seeing mature, mobile organisms or cysts on microscopic examination of freshly passed feces. Immunosuppressed (eg,. HIV-positive) individuals may demonstrate *Cryptosporidium, Microsporidia,* and *Strongyloides.* The ova are most frequently identified in the stool of parasites such as nematodes (*Ascaris, Strongyloides*), cestodes (*Taenia, Hymenolepsis*), and trematodes (*Schistosoma*).

THROAT CULTURES

Used to differentiate viral from bacterial (usually group A beta-hemolytic streptococci, eg, *Streptococcus pyogenes*) pharyngitis.

Procedure

1. The best culture is obtained with the help of a tongue blade and a good light source.
2. **If epiglottitis (croup) is suspected (stridor, drooling), a culture should not be attempted.**
3. The goal is to use the culture swab and try not to touch the oral mucosa or tongue, but only the involved area. In the uncooperative patient, an arch-like swath touching both the tonsillar areas and posterior pharynx should be attempted.

   Many labs perform a specific **"strep screen"** to rapidly identify group A beta-hemolytic streptococci. Normal flora on routine culture can include alpha-hemolytic strep, non-hemolytic staph, saprophytic *Neisseria* species, *Haemophilus, Klebsiella, Candida,* and diphtheroids.

   Other pathogens can cause pharyngitis. If *Neisseria gonorrhoeae* is suspected, use the Thayer–Martin medium. Diphtheria (*C. diphtheriae*) with its characteristic pseudo-membrane, should be cultured on special media and the lab notified.

URINE CULTURES

As is true for sputum cultures, culturing for urinary tract pathogens is often controversial. Some clinicians base their decision to treat only when the culture is positive, whereas others rely on the presence of white blood cells or bacteria in the urinalysis, using cultures only for sensitivities in refractory infections. The introduction of urine dipsticks to detect leukocytes (by the detection of leukocyte esterase) aids in the decision making when cultures are not obtained or are confusing. Routine cultures fail to diagnose other urinary tract pathogens such as *N. gonorrhea* or *Chlamydia.*

A clean-catch urine (see Chapter 13, page 306) is about 85% accurate in women and uncircumcised males. In general, a positive culture is a colony count of >100,000 bacteria/mL of urine or a count from 10,000–100,000 bacteria/mL of urine in the presence of pyuria. If the culture is critical for diagnosis, obtain an in-and-out catheterized urine (page

308) or suprapubic aspiration in children (page 309). Any growth of bacteria on an in-and-out catheterized or suprapubic specimen is considered to represent a true infection.

If a urine specimen cannot be taken to the lab within 60 min, refrigerate it. The lab assumes that more than three organisms growing on a culture represents a contaminant and the specimen collection should be repeated. The exception occurs in patients with a chronic indwelling Foley catheter that may be colonized with multiple bacterial or fungal organisms; the lab should be told to "culture all organisms" in such cases.

VIRAL CULTURES AND SEROLOGY

The laboratory provides the proper collection container for the specific virus. Common pathogenic viruses cultured include **herpes simplex** (from genital vesicles, throat), **CMV** (from urine or throat), **varicella-zoster** (from skin vesicles in children with chickenpox and adults with shingles), and enterovirus (rectal swab, throat).

For serologic testing, obtain an **acute specimen (titer)** as early as possible in the course of the illness, and take a **convalescent specimen (titer)** 2–4 wk later. A fourfold or greater rise in the convalescent titer compared with the acute titer indicates an active infection (see Chapter 4 for selected viral antibody titers). With the development of PCR techniques, biopsies performed on older lesions may yield useful information when cultures might be negative.

SCOTCH TAPE TEST

Also known as a "pinworm preparation," this method is used to identify infestation with *Enterobius vermicularis*. A 3-in. piece of CLEAR Scotch tape is attached around a glass slide (sticky side out). The slide is applied to the perianal skin in four quadrants and examined under the microscope for pinworm eggs. The best sample is collected either in the early morning prior to bathing or several hours after retiring.

MOLECULAR MICROBIOLOGY

Molecular techniques can now identify many bacterial and viral organisms without culturing. Many tests rely on DNA probes to identify the pathogens. The following includes some microbes commonly identified from clinical specimens (ie, swab, serum, tissue). Availability varies with each clinical facility.

Common Microorganisms Identifiable by PCR/DNA Probe

- *Chlamydia trachomatis*
- *Borrelia burgdorferi* (Lyme disease)
- HIV
- *Mycoplasma pneumoniae*
- *Mycobacterium tuberculosis*
- *Neisseria gonorrhoeae*
- Hepatitis B
- HPV
- Many others under development

SUSCEPTIBILITY TESTING

To more effectively treat a specific infection by choosing the right antibiotic, many labs routinely provide the MIC or MBC. For more complex infections (endocarditis), Schlichter testing is sometimes used.

MIC (Minimum Inhibitory Concentration)

This is the lowest concentration of antibiotic that prevents an in vitro growth of bacteria. The organism is tested against a battery of antimicrobials in concentrations normally achieved in vivo and reported as

Susceptible (S):   The organism is inhibited by the agent in the usual dose and route, and the drug should be effective.

Intermediate (I):   Sometimes also reported as "indeterminate," this implies that high doses of the drug, such as those achieved with parenteral therapy (IM, IV), most likely inhibit the organism.

Resistant (R):   The organism is resistant to the usual levels achieved by the drug.

MBC (Minimum Bactericidal Concentration)

Similar to the MIC, but indicates the lowest antibiotic concentration that will kill 99.9% of the organisms. The MBC results in killing the organisms, and the MIC prevents growth but may not kill the organism.

Schlichter Test (Serum Bacteriocidal Level)

Used to determine the antibacterial level of the serum or CSF of patients who are receiving antibiotic therapy. The test uses eight serial dilutions of the patient's serum (1:1 through 1:128) to determine what dilution is bactericidal to the infecting organism. The test is usually coordinated by the departments of infectious disease and microbiology. One set of blood or CSF cultures must be negative for the infecting organism before the test is performed. Opinion varies greatly as to interpretation of the results. Optimal killing of the organism occurs at dilutions of blood (and CSF) ranging anywhere from a trough of 1:4 to a peak of 1:8. That is, a result such as "*S. aureus* bactericidal level = 1:8" means the infecting organism was killed at a serum dilution of 1:8. Some data suggest higher titers (1:32) are needed to treat bacterial endocarditis. For the test to be performed, the organisms responsible for the infection must be isolated from a patient specimen.

DIFFERENTIAL DIAGNOSIS OF COMMON INFECTIONS AND EMPIRIC THERAPY

The pathogens causing common infectious diseases are outlined in Table 7–2 along with some empiric therapeutic recommendations. The antimicrobial drug of choice for the treatment of infection is usually the most active drug against the pathogenic organism or the least toxic alternative among several effective agents. The choice of drugs is modified by the site of infection, clinical status (allergy, renal disease, pregnancy, etc), and susceptibility testing.

Tables 7–3 through 7–7 provide empiric treatment guidelines for some common infectious diseases, including bacterial, fungal, viral, HIV, parasitic, and tick-borne diseases.

TABLE 7-2
Organisms Responsible for Common Infectious Diseases with Recommended Empiric Therapy*

Site/Condition	Common Uncommon but Important	Common Empiric Therapy (Modify based on clinic factors such as Gram stain)
BONES AND JOINTS		
Osteomyelitis	*Staphylococcus aureus* Enterobacteriaceae If nail puncture: *Pseudomonas* spp.	Oxacillin, nafcillin
Joint, septic arthritis	*S. aureus* Group A strep Enterobacteriaceae Gonococci	Oxacillin; ceftriaxone if gonococci
Joint, prosthetic	*S. aureus, S. epididymis, Streptococcus* spp.	Vancomycin plus ciprofloxacin
BREAST		
Mastitis, postpartum	*S. aureus*	Cefazolin, nafcillin, oxacillin
BRONCHITIS	In adolescent/young patient: *Mycoplasma pneumoniae* Respiratory viruses In chronic adult infection: *Streptococcus pneumoniae* *Haemophilus influenzae* *M. catarrhalis* *Chlamydia pneumoniae*	Treatment controversial because most infections are viral; treat if febrile, or associated with sinusitis, positive sputum culture in patients with COPD or if duration >7 days; doxy-cycline, erythromycin, azithromycin, clarithromycin

(continued)

7

134

TABLE 7-2
(Continued)

Site/Condition	Common Uncommon but Important	Common Empiric Therapy (Modify based on clinic factors such as Gram stain)
CERVICITIS (nongonococcal)	*Chlamydia, M. hominis, Ureaplasma,* others	Azithromycin single dose, doxycycline (evaluate and treat partner)
CHANCHROID	*Haemophilus ducreyi*	Cefriaxone or azithromycin as single dose
CHLAMYDIA		
Urethritis, cervicitis, conjunctivitis, proctitis	*Chlamydia trachomatis*	Azithromycin, doxycycline (amoxicillin if pregnant)
Neonatal ophthalmia, pneumonia		Erythromycin
Lymphogranuloma venereum	*C. trachomatis* (specific serotypes, L1, L2, L3)	Doxycycline
DIVERTICULITIS (no perforation or peritonitis)	Enterobacteriaceae, enterococci, bacteroids	TMP-SMX, ciprofloxacin plus metronidazole
EAR		
Acute mastoiditis	*S. pneumoniae* Group A strep *S. aureus*	Amoxicillin, ampicillin/clavulanic acid, cefuroxime
Chronic mastoiditis	Polymicrobial: Anaerobes Enterobacteriaceae Rarely: *M. tuberculosis*	Ticarcillin/clavulanic acid, imipenem
Otitis externa (swimmer's ear)	*Pseudomonas* spp. Enterobacteriaceae	Topical agents such as Cortisporin otic, TobraDex

(continued)

7

135

TABLE 7-2
(Continued)

7

Site/Condition	Common Uncommon but Important	Common Empiric Therapy (Modify based on clinic factors such as Gram stain)
EAR		
Otitis externa (continued)	In diabetic or malignant otitis: Pseudomonas spp.	Malignant otitis externa: acutely aminoglycoside, plus ceftazidime, imipenem or piperacillin
Otitis media	S. pneumoniae, H. influenzae, M. catarrhalis, viral causes S. aureus, group A strep In nasal intubation: Enterobacteriaceae, Pseudomonas spp.	Amoxicillin, ampicillin/clavulanic acid, cefuroxime
EMPYEMA		
ENDOCARDITIS		
Native valve	S. pneumoniae, S. aureus S. viridans S. pneumoniae Enterococci S. bovis S. aureus	Cefotaxime, ceftriaxone Parenteral: penicillin or ampicillin plus oxacillin or nafcillin plus gentamicin; vancomycin plus gentamicin
IV drug user	Pseudomonas spp.	Nafcillin plus gentamicin
Prosthetic valve	If early (<6 mo after implant) S. epidermidis S. aureus Enterobacteriaceae	Vancomycin plus rifampin plus gentamicin

(continued)

**TABLE 7-2
(Continued)**

Site/Condition	Common Uncommon but Important	Common Empiric Therapy (Modify based on clinic factors such as Gram stain)
Prosthetic valve (continued)	If late (>6 mo after implant) S. viridans Enterococci S. epidermidis S. aureus	
EPIGLOTTITIS	H. influenzae S. pneumoniae S. aureus Group A strep	Chloramphenicol plus ceftriaxone, cefotaxime or ampicillin
GALL BLADDER Cholecystitis	Acute: E. Coli, Klebsiella, Enterococcus Chronic obstruction: anaerobes, coliforms, Clostridium	Ampicillin plus gentamicin w/wo metronidazole, imipenem
Cholangitis	E. coli, Klebsiella, Enterococcus	
GASTROENTERITIS Afebrile, no gross blood or no WBC in stool	Virus, mild bacterial infection	Supportive care only
Febrile, gross blood, and WBC in stool	Enteropathogenic E. coli Shigella Salmonella	Empiric treatment pending cultures: ciprofloxacin, norfloxacin

(continued)

TABLE 7-2
(Continued)

Site/Condition	Common Uncommon but Important	Common Empiric Therapy (Modify based on clinic factor such as Gram stain)
Febrile gastroenteritis (continued)	*Campylobacter* *Vibrio* *C. difficile* *L. monocytogenes*	
GRANULOMA INGUINALE	*Calymmatobacterium granulomatis*	Doxycycline, trimethoprim/sulfamethoxazole
GONORRHEA (urethra, cervix, rectal, pharyngeal)	*N. gonorrhea*	Cefixime, ciprofloxacin, ofloxacin, ceftriaxone all as single dose; (treat also for *Chlamydia*)
MENINGITIS (Empiric therapy before cultures)		
Neonate	Group B strep, *E. coli*, *Listeria monocytogenes*	Ampicillin plus cefotaxime
Infant 1–3 mo	*S. pneumoniae* *N. meningitidis*	
Child/adult, community acquired	*S. pneumoniae* *N. meningitidis*, *H. influenzae*	Vancomycin plus ceftriaxone
Postoperative or traumatic	*S. epidermitis*, *S. aureus*, *S. pneumoniae*, *Pseudomonas*	Vancomycin plus ceftazidime
Immunosuppressed (ie steroids)	Gram-negative bacilli, *L. monocytogenes*	Ampicillin plus ceftazidime
History of alcohol abuse	*S. pneumoniae* *N. meningitidis*, gram-negative bacilli	Ampicillin plus ceftriaxone or cefotaxime

(continued)

TABLE 7-2
(Continued)

Site/Condition	Common Uncommon but Important	Common Empiric Therapy (Modify based on clinic factors such as Gram stain)
Meningitis (continued)		
	Pseudomonas spp.	
	H. influenzae	
HIV infection	*Cryptococcus*	Amphotericin B (acutely), fluconazole
NOCARDIOSIS	*Nocardia asteroides*	Sulfisoxazole, TMP-SMX
PELVIC INFLAMMATORY DISEASE	Gonococci	Ofloxacin and metronidazole or ceftriaxone (single dose) plus doxycycline; parenteral cefotetan or cefoxitin plus doxycycline
	Enterobacteriaceae	
	Bacteroides spp.	
	Chlamydia	
	Enterococci	
	M. hominis	
PERITONITIS		
Primary (spontaneous)	*S. pneumoniae*	Cefotaxime or ceftriaxone
	Enterobacteriaceae	
Secondary to (bowel perforation, etc)	Enterobacteriaceae, *Bacteroides* spp.	Suspect small bowel: piperacillin, mezlocillin, meropenem, cefoxitin
	Enterococci	Suspect large bowel: clindamycin plus aminoglycoside
	Pseudomonas spp.	
Peritoneal dialysis-related	*S. epidermidis*	Based on culture
	S. aureus	
	Enterobacteriaceae	
	Candida	

(continued)

139

**TABLE 7–2
(Continued)**

Site/Condition	Common Uncommon but Important	Common Empiric Therapy (Modify based on clinic factors such as Gram stain)
PHARYNGITIS	Respiratory virus Group A strep Gonococci C. diphtheria Epstein–Barr virus (infectious monol); spirochetes, anaerobes	Exudative (group A strep): benzathine penicillin G, erythromycin, loracarbef, azithromycin
PNEUMONIA		
Neonate	Viral (CMV, herpes), bacterial (group B strep, L. monocytogenes, coliforms, S. aureus, Chlamydia)	Ampicillin or nafcillin plus gentamicin
Infant (1–24 mo)	Most viral such as RSV; S. pneumonia, Chlamydia, Mycoplasma	Cefuroxime; if critically ill, cefotaxime, ceftriaxone plus cloxacillin
Child (3 mo– 5 y)	As above	Erythromycin, clarithromycin; if critically ill, cefuroxime plus erythromycin
Child (5–18 y)	Mycoplasma, respiratory viruses, S. pneumoniae, C. pneumoniae	Clarithromycin, azithromycin; eryhthromycin
Adult community-acquired	M. pneumoniae, C. pneumoniae, S. pneumoniae Smokers: As above plus M. catarrhalis, H. influenzae	Clarithromycin, azithromycin If hospitalized, third-generation cephalosporin plus erythromycin or azithromycin

(continued)

TABLE 7-2
(Continued)

Site/Condition	Common Uncommon but Important	Common Empiric Therapy (Modify based on clinic factors such as Gram stain)
Adult, community-acquired aspiration	S. pneumoniae oral flora, including anaerobes (eg, Fusobacterium, Bacteroides sp.) Enterobacteriaceae	Clindamycin
Adult hospital-acquired or ventilator-associated	S. pneumonia, coliforms, Pseudomonas, Legionella	Imipenem, meropenem
HIV-associated	Pneumocystis Others as above TB, fungi	Pneumocystis: TMP–SMX;,may require steroids
SINUSITIS	S. pneumoniae H. influenzae M. catarrhalis Anaerobes In nosocomial, nasal intubations, etc: S. aureus Pseudomonas spp. Enterobacteriaceae	Acute: TMP-SMX ampicillin, amoxicillin/ clavulanic acid, ciprofloxacin, clarithromycin
SKIN/SOFT TISSUE Acne Acne rosacea Burns	Propionibacterium acne Possible skin mite S. aureus, Enterobacteriaceae,	Tetracycline, minocycline, topical clindamycin Topical: metronidazole, doxycycline Topical: silver sulfadiazine

7

(continued)

TABLE 7-2
(Continued)

Site/Condition	Common Uncommon but Important	Common Empiric Therapy (Modify based on clinic factors such as Gram stain)
Burns (continued)	*Pseudomonas, Proteus* Herpes simplex virus, *Providencia, Serratia, Candida*	Sepsis: Aztreonam or tobramycin plus cefoperazone, ceftazidime or piperacillin
Bite (human and animal)	Anaerobes *P. multiloculada*	Ampicillin/sulbactam IV or amoxicillin/clavulanic acid PO
Cellulitis	*Streptococcus* spp. (group. A. B. C, G) *S. aureus* Anaerobic	Diabetic: nafcillin, oxacillin with or without penicillin; if anaerobic, high-dose penicillin G, cefoxitin, cefotetan If acutely ill: imipenem, meropenem, ticarcillin/clavulanic acid
Decubitus	Group A strep (*S. pyogenes*) Anaerobes, *S. aureus,* Enterobacteria Polymicrobial anaerobic	
Erysipelas Impetigo	Group A strep (*S. pyogenes*) Group A strep *S. aureus*	Nafcillin, oxacillin, dicloxacillin, cefazolin Penicillin, erythromycin; oxacillin or nafcillin if *S. aureus*
Tinea capitis (scalp) "ringworm" Tinea corporis (body)	Fungus: *Trichophyton* spp., *Microsporum* spp. Fungus: *Trichophyton* spp., *Epidermophyton*	Terbinafine, itraconazole, fluconazole, Topical: ciclopirox, clotrimazole, econazole, ketoconazole, miconazole, terconazole, others
Tinea unguium	Various fungi	Itraconazole, fluconazole, terbinafine

(continued)

TABLE 7-2
(Continued)

Site/Condition	Common Uncommon but Important	Common Empiric Therapy [Modify based on clinic factors such as Gram stain]
SYPHILIS (less than 1 y duration)	*Treponema pallidum*	Benzathine penicillin G one dose; doxycycline, tetracycline, ceftriaxone
TUBERCULOSIS Pulmonary, HIV (–)	*Mycobacterium tuberculosis*	INH, rifampin ethambutol plus pyrazinamide at least 6 mo (+/– pyridoxine)
TB exposure, PPD (–)		Children <5 INH X3 mo (+/– pyridoxine), others observe
		INH 6–12 mo (+/– pyridoxine)
Prophylaxis in high-risk patients (diabetics, IV drug users, immuno-suppressed, etc) PPD + conversion		INH 6–12 mo (+/– pyridoxine)
URINARY TRACT INFECTIONS Cystitis	Enterobacteriaceae (*E. coli* most common) *S. saprophyticus* (young female) *Candida*	Quinolone, TMP–SMX
		Candida: fluconazole or amphotericin B bladder irrigation
Urethritis	Gonococci, *C. trachomatis*, Trichomonas	Ceftriaxone, cefixime, ciprofloxacin, ofloxacin (all one dose) plus

7

(continued)

TABLE 7-2
(Continued)

7

Site/Condition	Common Uncommon but Important	Common Empiric Therapy (Modify based on clinic factors such as Gram stain)
Urethritis (continued)	Herpesvirus Ureaplasma urealyticum	azithromycin (single dose) or doxycycline (treat partner)
Prostatitis, acute <35 y	C. trachomatis Gonococci Coliforms Cryptococcus (AIDS)	Ofloxacin
Prostatitis, acute >35 y	Coliforms	Quinolone, TMP–SMX; if acutely ill gentamicin/ampicillin IV
Prostatitis, chronic bacterial	Coliforms, enterococci, Pseudomonas	Long-term ciprofloxacin or ofloxacin
Pyelonephritis	Enterobacteriaceae (E. coli) Enterococci Pseudomonas spp.	If acutely ill, gentamicin/ampicillin IV; quinolone, TMP–SMX
ULCER DISEASE (duodenal or gastric, not NSAID related)	Helicobacter pylori	Omeprazole plus amoxicillin plus clarithromycin
VAGINA Candidiasis	C. albicans C. glabrata, C. tropicalis	Fluconazole, itraconazole

(continued)

TABLE 7-2
(Continued)

Site/Condition	Common Uncommon but Important	Common Empiric Therapy (Modify based on clinic factors such as Gram stain)
Trichomonas Vaginosis, bacterial	Trichomonas vaginalis Polymicrobial (Gardnerella vaginalis, Bacteroides, M. hominis	Metronidazole (treat partner) Metronidazole (PO or vaginal gel); clindamycin, PO or intravaginally

*All antimicrobial therapy should be based on complete clinical data, including results of Gram's stains and cultures. See also Tables 7–3 (Viral), 7–4 (HIV), 7–5 (Fungal), and 7–6 (Parasitic) 7–7 (Tick-Borne).
Note: These guidelines are based on agents commonly involved in adult infections. Actual microbial treatment should be guided by microbiologic studies interpreted in the clinical setting.
Abbreviations: AIDS = acquired immunodeficiency syndrome; COPD = chronic obstructive pulmonary disease; HIV = human immunodeficiency virus; INH = isoniazid; IV = intravenous; NSAID = nonsteroidal antiinflammatory drug; PO = by mouth; PPD = purified protein derivative; TB = tuberculosis; TMP–SMX = trimethoprim–sulfamethoxazole.

7

TABLE 7-3
Pathogens and Drugs of Choice for Treating Common Viral Infections*

Viral Infection	Drug of Choice	Adult Dosage
CMV		
Retinitis, colitis, esophagitis	Ganciclovir (Cytovene)†	5 mg/kg IV q12h × 14–21d, 5 mg/kg/d IV or 6 mg/kg IV 5×/wk or 1 g PO tid
	(Vitrasert) implants or Foscarnet (Foscavir)	4.5 mg intraocularly q 5–8 mo 60 mg/kg IV q8h or 90 mg/kg IV q1–2 h × 14–21 d followed by 90–120 mg/kg/d IV
	or Cidofovir (Vistide) or Fomivirsen (Vitravene)	5 mg/kg/wk IV × 2 wk, then 5 mg/kg IV q2 wk 330 μg intravitreally q2 wk × 2 then 1/mo
EBV		
Infectious mononucleosis	None	
HAV	None, but gamma globulin within 2 wk of exposure may limit infection	0.2 mL/kg IM × 1
HBV		
Chronic hepatitis	Lamivudine (Epivir HBV) Interferon alfa-2b (Intron A)	100 mg PO 1×/d × 1–3 y 5 million units/d or 10 million units 3×/wk SC or IM × 4 mo
HCV		
Chronic hepatitis	Interferon alfa-2b plus Ribavirin (Rebetron) Interferon alfa-2b (Intron A) Interferon alfa-2a (Roferon-A)	3 million units 3×/wk SC plus ribavirin 1000–1200 mg/d PO × 12 mo 3 million units SC or IM 3×/wk × 12–24 mo 3 million units SC or IM 3×/wk × 12–24 mo

(continued)

146

7

**TABLE 7-3
(Continued)**

Viral Infection	Drug of Choice	Adult Dosage
Chronic hepatitis (continued)	Interferon alfacon-1 (Infergen)	9 µg 3×/wk × 6 mo
HSV		
Orolabial herpes in the immunocompetent with multiple recurrences	Penciclovir (Denavir)	1% cream applied q2h while awake × 4 d
Genital herpes first episode	Acyclovir (Zovirax)	400 mg PO tid or 200 mg PO 5×/d × 7–10 d
	or Famciclovir (Famvir)	250 mg PO tid × 5–10 d
	or Valacyclovir (Valtrex)	1 g PO bid × 7–10 d
recurrence	Acyclovir (Zovirax)	400 mg PO tid × 5 d
	or Famciclovir (Famvir)	125 mg PO bid × 5 d 17
	or Valacyclovir (Valtrex)	500 mg PO bid × 5 d
chronic suppression	Acyclovir (Zovirax)	400 mg PO bid
	or Valacyclovir (Valtrex)	500–1000 mg PO 1×/d
	or Famciclovir (Famvir)	250 mg PO bid
Mucocutaneous in the immunocompromised	Acyclovir (Zovirax)	5 mg/kg IV q8h × 7–14 d
	or Acyclovir (Zovirax)	400 mg PO 5×/d × 7–14 d
Encephalitis	Acyclovir (Zovirax)	10–15 mg/kg IV q8h × 14–21 d
Neonatal	Acyclovir (Zovirax)	20 mg/kg IV q8h × 14–21 d
Acyclovir-resistant	Foscarnet (Foscavir)	40 mg/kg IV q8h × 14–21 d
Keratoconjunctivitis	Trifluridine (Viroptic)	1 drop 1% solution topically, q2h, up to 9 gtt/d × 10 d
HIV (See Table 7–4) INFLUENZA A AND B VIRUS	Zanamivir (Relenza)	10 mg bid × 5d by inhaler
	Oseltamivir (Tamiflu)	75 mg PO bid × 5 d

7

(continued)

TABLE 7-3
(Continued)

Viral Infection	Drug of Choice	Adult Dosage
INFLUENZA A VIRUS	Rimantadine (Flumadine)	200 mg PO 1×/d or 100 mg PO bid × 5 d
	Amantadine (Symmetrel)	100 mg PO bid × 5 d
MEASLES		
Children	None (immunize, See Table 22-9)	
Adults	None or ribavirin	20–35 mg/kg/d × 7 d
PAPILLOMA VIRUS (HPV)		
Anogenital warts	Podofilox or podophyllin	Topical application (see Chapter 22)
	Interferon alfa-2b (Intron A)	1 million units intralesional 3×/wk × 3 wk
	Imiquimod, 5% cream (Aldara)	Apply 3/wk hs, remove 6–10 h later up to 16 wk
RSV (bronchiolitis)	Ribavirin (Virazole)	Aerosol treatment 12–18 h/d × 3–7 d
VZV		
Exposure prophylaxis in the immunocompromised (HIV, steroids, etc)	VZIG, Varicella Zoster Immune Globulin	See package insert
Varicella (>12 y old)	Acyclovir (Zovirax)	20 mg/kg (800 mg max) PO qid × 5 d
	Valacyclovir (Valtrex)	1 g PO tid × 7 d
	or Famciclovir (Famvir)	500 mg PO tid × 7 d
Herpes zoster	or Acyclovir (Zovirax)	800 mg PO 5×/d × 7–10 d

(continued)

TABLE 7-3
(Continued)

Viral Infection	Drug of Choice	Adult Dosage
Varicella or zoster in the immunocompromised	Acyclovir (Zovirax)	10 mg/kg IV q8h × 7 d
Acyclovir-resistant	Foscarnet (Foscavir)	40 mg/kg IV q8h × 10 d

*Based on Guidelines from the CDC published in MMWR and the *Medical Letter* Vol. 41 December 3, 1999.

†The generic drug name appears in regular type; the trade name appears in parentheses afterward in *italics*.

Abbreviations: CMV = cytomegalovirus; EBV = Epstein-Barr virus; HAV = hepatitis A virus; HBV = hepatitis B virus; HCV = hepatitis C virus; HIV = human immunodeficiency virus; HPV = human papilloma virus; HSV = herpes simplex virus; RSV = respiratory syncytial virus; VZV = varicella zoster virus.

7

TABLE 7–4
Drugs of Choice for Treating HIV Infection in Adults

DRUGS OF CHOICE

2 nucleosides[1] + 1 protease inhibitor[2]
2 nucleosides[1] + 1 nonnucleoside[3]
2 nucleosides[1] + ritonavir[4] + another protease inhibitor[5]

ALTERNATIVES

1 protease inhibitor[2] + 1 nucleoside + 1 nonnucleoside[3]
2 protease inhibitors (each in low dose)[5] + 1 nucleoside +
    1 nonnucleoside[3]
abacavir + 2 other nucleosides[1]
2 protease inhibitors (each full dose)

1. One of the following: zidovudine + lamivudine; zidovudine + didanosine; stavudine + lamivudine; stavudine + didanosine; zidovudine + zalcitabine.
2. Nelfinavir, indinavir, saquinavir soft gel capsules, amprenavir or ritonavir. Ritonavir is used less frequently because of troublesome adverse effects. The Invirase formulation of saquinavir generally should not be used.
3. Efavirenz is often preferred. Nevirapine causes more adverse effects. Nevirapine and delavirdine require more doses, and have had shorter follow-up in reported studies. Combinations of Efavirenz and nevirapine with protease inhibitors require increasing the dosage of the protease inhibitor.
4. Ritonavir is usually given in dosage of 100–400 mg bid when used with another protease inhibitor.
5. Protease inhibitors that have been combined with ritonavir 100–400 mg bid include indinavir 400–800 mg bid, amprenavir 600–800 mg bid, saquinavir 400–600 mg bid and nelfinavir 500–750 mg bid.

Source: Reproduced, with permission, from *The Medical Letter* Vol 42, Issue 1089, January 10, 2000.

TABLE 7-5
Systemic Drugs for Treating Fungal Infections

Infection	Drug of Choice	Alternatives
ASPERGILLOSIS	Amphotericin B or itraconazole	Amphotericin B lipid complex, amphotericin cholesteryl complex liposomal amphotericin B
BLASTOMYCOSIS	Itraconazole or amphotericin B	Fluconazole
CANDIDIASIS		
Oral (thrush)	Fluconazole or itraconazole	Nystatin lozenge or swish and swallow
Stomatitis, eosphagitis, vaginitis in AIDS	Fluconazole or itraconazole	Parenteral or oral amphotericin B
Systemic	Amphotericin B or fluconazole	
Cystitis/vaginitis	See Table 7-2	
COCCIDIOIDOMYCOSIS		
Pulmonary (normal individual)	No drug usually recommended	
Pulmonary (high risk)	Itraconazole or fluconazole	Amphotericin B
CRYPTOCOCCOSIS		
In non-AIDS patient	Amphotericin B or fluconazole	Amphotericin B fluconazole
Meningitis (HIV/AIDS)	Amphotericin B plus 5-flucytosine; then long-term suppression with fluconazole	Amphotericin B lipid complex
HISTOPLASMOSIS		
Pulmonary, disseminated		
Normal individual	Moderate disease: itraconazole	Severe: amphotericin B
HIV/AIDS	Amphotericin B, followed by itraconazole suppression	Itraconazole

(continued)

7

151

TABLE 7–5
(Continued)

Infection	Drug of Choice	Alternatives
MUCORMYCOSIS	Amphotericin B	No dependable alternative
PARACOCCIDIOIDOMYCOSIS	Itraconazole	Amphotericin B
SPOROTRICHOSIS		
Cutaneous	Itraconazole	Potassium iodide 1–5 mL tid
Systemic	Itraconazole	Amphotericin B

Abbreviations: AIDS = acquired immunodeficiency syndrome; HIV = human immunodeficiency virus.

TABLE 7–6
Drugs for Treating Selected Parasitic Infections

Infection	Drug
Amebiasis (*Entamoeba histolytica*)	
Asymptomatic	Iodoquinol or paramomycin
Mild to moderate intestinal disease	Metronidazole or tinidazole
Severe intestinal disease, hepatic abscess	Metronidazole or tinidazole
Ascariasis (*Ascaris lumbricoides,* roundworm)	Albendazole, mebendazole or pyrantel pamoate
Cryptosporidiosis (*Cryptosporidium*)	Paromomycin
Cutaneous larva migrans (creeping eruption, dog and cat hookworm	Albendazole, thiabendazole or ivermectin
Cyclospora **infection**	Trimethoprim–sulfamethoxazole
Enterobius vermicularis (pinworm)	Pyrantel pamoate, mebendazole or albendazole
Filariasis (*Wuchereria bancrofti, Brugia malayi, Loa loa*)	Diethylcarbamazine
Giardiasis (*Giardia lamblia*)	Metronidazole
Hookworm infection (*Ancylostoma duodenale, Necator americanus*)	Albendazole, mebendazole, or pyrantel pamoate
Isosporiasis (*Isospora belli*)	Trimethoprim–sulfamethoxazole
Lice (*Pediculus humanus, P. capitis, Phthirus pubis*)	1% permethrin (topical) or 0.5% malathion
Malaria (*Plasmodium falciparum, P. ovale, P. vivax,* and *P. malariae*)	
Chloroquine-resistant *P. falciparum*	Quinine sulfate plus doxycycline, tetracycline, clindamycin or pyrimethamine–sulfadoxine (oral)
Chloroquine-resistant *P. vivax*	Quinine sulfate plus doxycycline, or pyrimethamine–sulfadoxine (oral)
All *Plasmodium* except chloroquine-resistant *P. falciparum*	Chloroquine phosphate (oral)
All *Plasmodium* (parenteral)	Quinine gluconate or quinine dihydrochloride
Prevention of relapses: *P. vivax,* and *P. ovale* only	Primaquine phosphate
Malaria, prevention	
Chloroquine-sensitive areas	Chloroquine phosphate
Chloroquine-resistant areas	Mefloquine or doxycycline
Mites, see Scabies	
Pinworm, see *Enterobius*	
Pneumocystis carinii **pneumonia**	Trimethoprim–sulfamethoxazole Alternative: pentamidine
Primary and secondary prophylaxis	Trimethoprim–sulfamethoxazole

7

(continued)

TABLE 7–6
(Continued)

Infection	Drug
Roundworm, see Ascariasis	
Scabies (*Sarcoptes scabiei*)	5% Permethrin topically Alternatives: ivermectin, 10% crotamiton
Strongyloidiasis (*Strongyloides stercoralis*)	Ivermectin
Tapeworm infection	
—Adult (intestinal stage)	
Diphyllobothrium latum (fish), *Taenia saginata* (beef), *Taenia solium* (pork), *Dipylidium caninum* (dog), *Hymenolepis nana* (dwarf tapeworm)	Praziquantel
—Larval (tissue stage)	
Echinococcus granulosus (hydatid cyst)	Albendazole
Cysticercus cellulosae (cysticercosis)	Albendazole or praziquantel
Toxoplasmosis (*Toxoplasma gondii*)	Pyrimethamine plus sulfadiazine
Trichinosis (*Trichinella spiralis*)	Steroids for severe symptoms plus mebendazole
Trichomoniasis (*Trichomonas vaginalis*)	Metronidazole or tinidazole
Hairworm infection (*Trichostrongylus colubriformis*)	Pyrantel pamoate
Trypanosomiasis (*Trypanosoma cruzi*, Chagas' disease)	Benznidazole
Trichuriasis (*Trichuris trichiuria*, whipworm)	Mebendazole or albendazole
Visceral larva migrans, toxocariasis (*Toxocara canis*)	Albendazole or mebendazole

Source: Based on data from *The Medical Letter* March 2000 www.medletter.com.

7

TABLE 7-7
Guide to Common Tick-borne Diseases

Disease	Causative Agent	Season	Vector Habits
Rocky Mountain spotted fever	*Rickettsia rickettsii* (bacterium)	Mostly spring, summer	*American Dog Tick* Found in high grass and low shrubs, fields *Lone Star Tick* Found in woodlands, forest edge, and old fields
Human granulocytic ehrlichiosis	*Ehrlichia* spp. (bacterium)	Under study	*Deer (black-legged)* Tick found in woodlands, old fields, landscaping with significant ground cover vegetation
Lyme disease	*Borrelia burgdorferi* (bacterium)	Mostly spring, but year-around	Same as for the deer tick
Babesiosis	*Babesia microti* (protozoan)	Mostly spring/summer	Same as for the deer tick

(continued)

TABLE 7–7
(Continued)

Classic Clinical Presentation	Incubation Period	Diagnosis	Treatment
Sudden moderate to high fever, severe headache, maculopapular rash (with planer/palmer presentation)	2–14 d	Clinical serology	Adults—doxycycline Children/pregnant women—chloramphenicol
Fever, headache, constitutional symptoms	1–30 d	Clinical serology	Adults—tetracyclines Children/pregnant women—consult specialist
EM rash, constitutional symptoms, arthritis, cardiovascular and nervous system involvement	3–30 d	Clinical serology, culture	Doxycycline, amoxicillin, cefuroxime for 14–21 d
Fever, hemolytic anemia, constitutional symptoms	1–52 wk	Thick and thin blood smears	Clindamycin/quinine

Abbreviation: EM = erythema multiforme.

Secretion/Discharge Precautions: (Handwashing and gloves with direct patient contact) Conjunctivitis, minor skin wounds, decubiti, colonization (but not infection that requires Wound and Skin Precautions) with MRSA, herpes, mucocutaneous candidiasis, ulcerative STDs, coccidioidomycosis, others

Pregnancy Precautions: (Handwashing) CMV, rubella, parvovirus

SBE PROPHYLAXIS

The following recommendations are based on guidelines published by the American Heart Association. (*JAMA* 1997;**277:**1794–1801). The guidelines now specify which patients are at high, moderate, or low risk of bacteremia and provide general guidelines for procedures that are more likely to be associated with bacterial endocarditis. SBE prophylaxis is recommended only for patients who are at high or moderate risk. See Tables 7–8 and 7–9 for regimens.

High-risk: Prosthetic cardiac valves, history of bacterial endocarditis, complex cyanotic congenital heart disease, surgically constructed systemic pulmonary shunts

Moderate-risk: Most other congenital cardiac malformations (other than those in the previous or following lists), acquired valvular disease (eg, rheumatic heart disease), hypertrophic cardiomyopathy, mitral valve prolapse with regurgitation or thickened leaflets

Low-risk: Isolated ASD secundum; repair of atrial/ventricular septal defect, or PDA; prior CABG; mitral valve prolapse without regurgitation; innocent heart murmurs; previous Kawasaki disease or rheumatic fever without valve dysfunction; pacemakers or implanted defibrillator

ISOLATION PROTOCOLS

To prevent the spread of infectious diseases from patient to patient, visitors, and hospital personnel, isolation procedures are recommended for various pathogens and clinical settings by various agencies such as the CDC in Atlanta, Georgia. Local hospital procedures may vary slightly from these recommendations.

Strict Isolation: (Single room, controlled airflow, handwashing, gown, gloves, mask) Varicella, herpes (localized, disseminated, neonatal), wound or burns infected with *S. aureus* or group A *Streptococcus, S. aureus* or group A *Streptococcus pneumoniae,* congenital rubella, rabies, smallpox, others

Contact Isolation: (Single room, controlled airflow, handwashing, gown, gloves, mask) All acute respiratory infections in infants and children (cough, cold, pneumonia, croup, pharyngitis, etc), extensive impetigo, gonococcal conjunctivitis in the newborn, others

Respiratory Isolation: (Single room, controlled airflow, handwashing, mask) TB (known or suspected), measles, mumps, rubella, pertussis, meningitis (suspected *N. meningitidis* or *H. influenzae* infection), pneumonia due to *H. influenzae,* epiglottitis, others

Wound and Skin Precautions: (Single room; handwashing; for direct contact with patient secretions: gown, gloves, mask) Major wound and skin infections, group A streptococcal endometritis, gas gangrene. Scabies and lice require only 24 h after effective therapy.

Enteric Precautions:(Single room; handwashing; for direct contact with patient secretions: gown, gloves) Known or suspected infectious gastroenteritis, including from rotavirus, enterovirus, *Salmonella, Shigella, E. coli, Giardia, and C. difficile* enterocolitis, acute hepatitis (all types)

Blood and Body Fluid Precautions:(Handwashing; for direct contact with patient secretions: gown, gloves) Known or suspected HIV infection, hepatitis (in acute and chronic carriers), syphilis, malaria, Lyme disease, all rickettsial infections, others

TABLE 7–8
SBE Prophylaxis for Oral, Respiratory or Esophageal Procedures*

Prophylaxis	Agent	Regimen[†]
Standard prophylaxis	Amoxicillin	Adults: 2.0 g; children: 50 mg/kg PO 1 h before procedure
Unable to take oral medications	Ampicillin	Adults: 2.0 g IM or IV; children: 50 mg/kg or IV 30 min before procedure
Allergic to penicillin	Clindamycin or	Adults: 600 mg; children: 20 mg/kg PO 1 h before procedure
	Cephalexin or cefadroxil	Adults: 2.0 g; children; 50 mg/kg PO 1 h before procedure
	Azithromycin or clarithromycin	Adults: 500 mg; children: 15 mg/kg PO 1 h before procedure
		Adults: 600 mg; children: 20 mg/kg IV 30 min before procedure
Penicillin allergic and unable to take oral medications	Clindamycin or cefazolin	Adults: 1.0 g; children: 25 mg/kg IM or IV 30 min before procedure

*See text page 157 for recommended risk groups.
[†]Total children's dose should not exceed adult dose.

TABLE 7–9
SBE Prophylaxis for GU/GI (Excluding Esophageal)
Procedures*

Patient	Agents	Regimen
High-risk	Ampicillin + gentamicin	Adults: ampicillin 2.0 g IM/IV + gentamicin 1.5 mg/kg (max 120 mg) within 30 min of procedure; 6 h later, ampicillin 1 g IM/IV or amoxicillin 1 g PO Children: ampicillin 50 mg/kg IM or IV (2.0 g max) + gentamicin 1.5 mg/kg within 30 min of procedure; 6 h later, ampicillin 25 mg/kg IM/IV or amoxicillin 25 mg/kg PO
High-risk allergic to ampicillin/ amoxicillin	Vancomycin + gentamicin	Adults: vancomycin 1.0 g IV over 1–2 h + gentamicin 1.5 mg/kg IV/IM (120 mg max); dose within 30 min of starting procedure Children: vancomycin 20 mg/kg IV over 1–2 h + gentamicin 1.5 mg/kg IV/IM; complete dose within 30 min of starting procedure
Moderate-risk	Amoxicillin or ampicillin	Adults: amoxicillin 2.0 g PO 1 h before procedure, or ampicillin 2.0 g IM/IV within 30 min of starting procedure Children: amoxicillin 50 mg/kg PO 1 h before procedure, or ampicillin 50 mg/kg IM/IV within 30 min of starting procedure
Moderate-risk allergic to ampicillin/ amoxicillin	Vancomycin	Adults: vancomycin 1.0 g IV over 1–2 h complete infusion within 30 min of starting procedure Children: vancomycin 20 mg/kg IV over 1–2 h; complete infusion within 30 min of starting procedure

*See text page 157 for recommended risk groups.
Total children's dose should not exceed adult dose.

BLOOD GASES AND ACID–BASE DISORDERS

Normal Blood Gas Values
Venous Blood Gases
Capillary Blood Gases
General Principles of Blood Gas
    Determinations
Acid–Base Disorders: Definition
Mixed Acid–Base Disorders
Interpretation of Blood Gases
Metabolic Acidosis: Diagnosis
    and Treatment

Metabolic Alkalosis: Diagnosis
    and Treatment
Respiratory Acidosis: Diagnosis
    and Treatment
Respiratory Alkalosis: Diagnosis
    and Treatment
Hypoxia
Sample Acid–Base Problems

NORMAL BLOOD GAS VALUES

The results of testing ABG are usually given as pH, pO_2, pCO_2, $[HCO_3^-]$, base excess/deficit (difference), and oxygen saturation. This test gives information on acid–base homeostasis (pH, pCO_2, $[HCO_3^-]$, and base difference) and on blood oxygenation (pO_2, O_2 saturation). Less frequently, venous blood gases and mixed venous blood gases are measured. Normal values for blood gas analysis are given in Table 8–1, page 162, and capillary blood gases are discussed in a following section. Note that the HCO_3^- from the blood gas is a calculated value and should not be used in the interpretation of the blood gas levels, instead the HCO_3^- from a chemistry panel should be used. The ABG and the chemistry panel $[HCO_3^-]$ should be obtained at the same time.

VENOUS BLOOD GASES

There is little difference between arterial and venous pH and bicarbonate (except in cases of CHF and shock); therefore, the venous blood gas level may occasionally be used to assess acid–base status. Venous oxygen levels, however, are significantly less than arterial levels (see Table 8–1).

CAPILLARY BLOOD GASES

A CBG is obtained from a highly vascularized capillary bed. (The heel is the most commonly used site.) The CBG is often used for pediatric patients because it is easier to obtain than the ABG and is less traumatic (no risk of arterial thrombosis, hemorrhage). The procedure is fully described in Chapter 13, page 274, under Heelstick.

When interpreting a CBG, apply the following rules:

- **pH:** Same as arterial or slightly lower (Normal = 7.35–7.40)
- **pCO₂:** Same as arterial or slightly higher (Normal = 40–45)
- **pO₂:** Lower than arterial (Normal = 45–60)
- **O₂ Saturation:** >70% is acceptable. Saturation is probably more useful than the pO_2 itself when interpreting a CBG.

TABLE 8–1
Normal Blood Gas Values

Measurement	Arterial Blood	Mixed Venous*	Venous
pH	7.40	7.36	7.36
(range)	(7.37–7.44)	(7.31–7.41)	(7.31–7.41)
pO$_2$ (mm Hg)	80–100	35–40	30–50
(decreases with age)			
pCO$_2$ (mm Hg)	36–44	41–51	40–52
O$_2$ saturation	>95	60–80	60–85
(decreases with age)			
HCO$_3^-$ (mEq/L)	22–26	22–26	22–28
[SI: mmol/L]			
Base difference	–2 to +2	–2 to +2	–2 to +2
(deficit/excess)			

*Obtained from the right atrium, usually through a pulmonary artery catheter.

GENERAL PRINCIPLES OF BLOOD GAS DETERMINATIONS

(Oxygen values are discussed on page 171.)

1. The blood gas machines in most labs actually measure the pH and the pCO$_2$ (as well as the pO$_2$). The [HCO$_3^-$] and the base difference are calculated values using the **Henderson–Hasselbalch equation:**

$$pH = pK_a + \frac{\log[HCO_3^-] \text{ in mEq} / L}{0.03 \times pCO_2 \text{ in mmHg}}$$

or the **Henderson equation:**

$$[H^+] \text{ in mEq} / L = \frac{24 \times pCO_2 \text{ in mmHg}}{[HCO_3^-] \text{ in mEq} / L}$$

2. For a rough estimate of [H$^+$], [H$^+$] = (7.80 – pH) × 100. This is accurate from a pH 7.25 – 7.48; 40 mEq/L = [H$^+$] at the normal pH of 7.40. Also pH is a log scale, and for every change of 0.3 in pH from 7.40 the [H$^+$] doubles or halves. For pH 7.10 the [H$^+$] = 2 × 40, or 80 nmol/L, and for pH 7.70 the [H$^+$] = ½ × 40, or 20 nmol/L.

3. The calculated [HCO$_3^-$] should be within 2 mEq/L of the bicarbonate concentration from a venous chemistry determination (eg, BMP) drawn at the same time. If not, an error has been made in the collection or the determination of the values, and the blood gas and serum bicarbonate should be recollected.

4. Two additional relationships that are derived from the Henderson–Hasselbalch equation should be committed to memory. These two rules are helpful in interpreting blood gas results, particularly in defining a simple versus a mixed blood gas disorder:

Rule I: A change in pCO_2 up or down 10 mm Hg is associated with an increase or decrease in pH of 0.08 units. As the pCO_2 decreases, the pH increases; as the pCO_2 increases, the pH decreases.

Rule II: A pH change of 0.15 is equivalent to a base change of 10 mEq/L. A decrease in base (ie, $[HCO_3^-]$) is termed a **base deficit,** and an increase in base is termed a **base excess.**

ACID–BASE DISORDERS: DEFINITION

1.   Acid–base disorders are very common clinical problems. **Acidemia** is a pH <7.37, and alkalemia is a pH >7.44. **Acidosis and alkalosis** are used to describe how the pH changes. The primary causes of acid–base disturbances are abnormalities in the respiratory system and in the metabolic or renal system. As from the Henderson–Hasselbalch equation, a respiratory disturbance leading to an abnormal pCO_2 alters the pH, and similarly a metabolic disturbance altering the $[HCO_3^-]$ changes the pH.
2.   Any primary disturbance in acid–base homeostasis invokes a **normal compensatory response.** A primary metabolic disorder leads to respiratory compensation, and a primary respiratory disorder leads to an acute metabolic response due to the buffering capacity of body fluids, *and* a more chronic compensation (1–2 days) due to alterations in renal function.
3.   The degree of compensation is well known and can be expressed in terms of the degree of the primary acid–base disturbance. Table 8–2, page 164, lists the major categories of primary acid–base disorders, the primary abnormality, the secondary compensatory response, and the expected degree of compensation in terms of the magnitude of the primary abnormality. These changes are defined graphically in Figure 8–1, page 165. The types of simple acid–base disorders are discussed in the following sections.

MIXED ACID–BASE DISORDERS

1.   Most acid–base disorders result from a single primary disturbance with the normal physiologic compensatory response and are called **simple acid–base disorders.** In certain cases, however, particularly in seriously ill patients, two or more different primary disorders may occur simultaneously, resulting in a **mixed acid–base disorder.** The net effect of mixed disorders may be additive (eg, metabolic acidosis and respiratory acidosis) and result in extreme alteration of pH; or they may be opposite (eg, metabolic acidosis and respiratory alkalosis) and nullify each other's effects on the pH.
2.   To determine a mixed acid–base disorder from a blood gas value, follow the six steps in the Interpretation of Blood Gases (in the following section). Alterations in either $[HCO_3^-]$ or pCO_2 that differ from expected compensation levels indicate a second process. Two of the examples given in the following section illustrate the strategies employed in identifying a mixed acid–base disorder.

INTERPRETATION OF BLOOD GASES

Use a uniform, stepwise approach to the interpretation of blood gases. (See also Figure 8–1.)

Step 1:   Determine if the numbers fit.

$$[H^+] = \frac{24 \times pCO_2}{[HCO_3^-]}$$

TABLE 8–2
Simple Acid-Base Disturbances

Acid–Base Disorder	Primary Abnormality	Expected Compensation	Expected Degree of Compensation
Metabolic acidosis	$\downarrow\downarrow\downarrow[HCO_3^-]$	$\downarrow\downarrow pCO_2$	$pCO_2 = (1.5 \times [HCO_3^-]) + 8$
Metabolic alkalosis	$\uparrow\uparrow\uparrow[HCO_3^-]$	$\uparrow\uparrow pCO_2$	$\uparrow$ in $pCO_2 = \Delta[HCO_3^-] \times 0.6$
Acute respiratory acidosis	$\uparrow\uparrow\uparrow pCO_2$	$\uparrow[HCO_3^-]$	$\uparrow$ in $[HCO_3^-] = \Delta pCO_2/10$
Chronic respiratory acidosis	$\uparrow\uparrow\uparrow pCO_2$	$\uparrow\uparrow[HCO_3^-]$	$\uparrow$ in $[HCO_3^-] = 4 \times \Delta pCO_2/10$
Acute respiratory alkalosis	$\downarrow\downarrow\downarrow pCO_2$	$\downarrow[HCO_3^-]$	$\downarrow$ in $[HCO_3^-] = 2 \times \Delta pCO_2/10$
Chronic respiratory alkalosis	$\downarrow\downarrow\downarrow pCO_2$	$\downarrow\downarrow[HCO_3^-]$	$\downarrow$ in $[HCO_3^-] = 5 \times \Delta pCO_2/10$

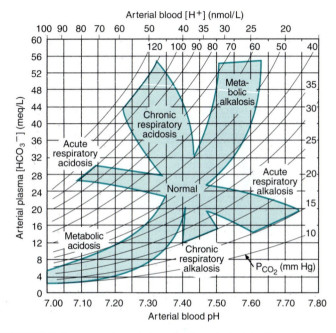

FIGURE 8–1 Nomogram for acid–base disorders. (Reprinted, with permission, from: Cogan MG: *Fluid and Electrolytes,* Appleton & Lange, Norwalk CT, 1991.)

The right side of the equation should be within about 10% of the left side. If the numbers do not fit, you need to obtain another ABG and chemistry panel for HCO_3^-.

Example. pH 7.25, pCO$_2$ 48, HCO_3^- 29 mmol/L

$$56 = 24 \times \frac{48}{29}$$

$$56 \neq 40$$

The blood gas is uninterpretable, and the ABG and HCO_3^- need to be recollected. The most common reason for the numbers not fitting is that the ABG and the chemistry panel [HCO_3^-] were obtained at different times.

Step 2: Next, determine if an acidemia (pH <7.37) or an alkalemia (pH >7.44) is present.

Step 3: Identify the primary disturbance as metabolic or respiratory. For example, if acidemia is present, is the pCO$_2$ >44 mm Hg (respiratory acidosis), or is the [HCO$_3^-$] <22 mmol/L (metabolic acidosis). In other words, identify which component, respiratory or metabolic, is altered in the same direction as the pH abnormality. If both components act in the same direction (eg, both respiratory [pCO$_2$ > 44 mm Hg] and metabolic [HCO$_3^-$ <22 mmol/L] acidosis are present), then this is a **mixed acid–base problem,** discussed later in this section. The primary disturbance will be the one that varies from normal the greatest, that is, with a [HCO$_3^-$] = 6 mmol/L and pCO$_2$ = 50 mm Hg, the primary disturbance would be a metabolic acidosis, the [HCO$_3^-$] is about one-quarter normal, whereas the increase in pCO$_2$ is only 25%.

Step 4: After identifying the primary disturbance, use the equations in Table 8–2, page 164, to calculate the expected compensatory response. If the difference between the actual value and the calculated value is significant, then a mixed acid–base disturbance is present.

Step 5: Calculate the anion gap. Anion gap = Na$^+$ – (Cl$^-$ + HCO$_3^-$). Normal anion gap is 8–12 mmol. If the anion gap is increased, proceed to step 6.

Step 6: If the anion gap is elevated, then compare the changes from normal between the anion gap and [HCO$_3^-$]. If the change in the anion gap is greater than the change in the [HCO$_3^-$] from normal, then a metabolic alkalosis is present in addition to a gap metabolic acidosis. If the change in the anion gap is less than the change in the [HCO$_3^-$] from normal, then a nongap metabolic acidosis is present in addition to a gap metabolic acidosis. See Examples 5, 6, and 7, page 174.

Finally, be sure the interpretation of the blood gas is consistent with the clinical setting.

METABOLIC ACIDOSIS: DIAGNOSIS AND TREATMENT

Metabolic acidosis represents an increase in acid in body fluids reflected by a decrease in [HCO$_3^-$] and a compensatory decrease in pCO$_2$.

Differential Diagnosis

The diagnosis of metabolic acidosis (Figure 8–2) can be classified as an anion gap or a nonanion gap acidosis. The **anion gap** (Normal range, 8–12 mmol/L) is calculated as:

$$\text{Anion gap} = [\text{Na}^+] - ([\text{Cl}^-] + [\text{HCO}_3^-])$$

Anion Gap Acidosis: Anion gap >12 mmol/L; caused by a decrease in [HCO$_3^-$] balanced by an increase in an unmeasured acid ion from either endogenous production or exogenous ingestion (**normochloremic acidosis**).

Nonanion Gap Acidosis: Anion gap = 8–12 mmol/L; caused by a decrease in [HCO$_3^-$] balanced by an increase in chloride (**hyperchloremic acidosis**). Renal tubular acidosis is a type of nongap acidosis that can be associated with a variety of pathologic conditions (Table 8–3 page 168). The anion gap is helpful in identifying metabolic gap acidosis, nongap acidosis, mixed metabolic gap and nongap acidosis. If an elevated anion gap is present, a closer look at the anion gap and the bicarbonate helps differentiate among (a) a pure metabolic gap acidosis, (b) a metabolic nongap acidosis, (c) mixed metabolic gap and nongap acidosis, and (d) a metabolic gap acidosis and metabolic alkalosis.

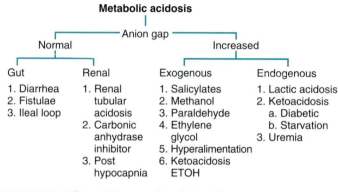

FIGURE 8–2   Differential diagnosis of metabolic acidosis.

Treatment of Metabolic Acidosis

1. Correct any underlying disorder (control diarrhea, etc).
2. Treatment with bicarbonate should be reserved for severe metabolic gap acidosis. If the pH <7.20, correct with sodium bicarbonate. The total replacement dose of $[HCO_3^-]$ can be calculated as follows:

$$[HCO_3^-] \text{ needed in mEq} = \frac{\text{Base deficit (mEq)} \times \text{Patient' s weight (kg)}}{4}$$

3. Replace with **one-half the total amount of bicarbonate over 8–12 h** and reevaluate. Be aware of sodium and volume overload during replacement. Normal or isotonic bicarbonate drip is made with 3 ampules $NaHCO_3$ (50 mmol $NaHCO_3$/ampule) in 1 L D_5W.

METABOLIC ALKALOSIS: DIAGNOSIS AND TREATMENT

Metabolic alkalosis represents an increase in $[HCO_3^-]$ with a compensatory rise in pCO_2.

Differential Diagnosis

In two basic categories of diseases the kidneys retain $[HCO_3^-]$ (Figure 8–3). They can be differentiated in terms of response to treatment with sodium chloride and also by the level of urinary $[Cl^-]$ as determined by ordering a "spot," or "random" urinalysis for chloride (U_{Cl}).

Chloride-Sensitive (Responsive) Metabolic Alkalosis: The initial problem is a sustained loss of chloride out of proportion to the loss of sodium (either by renal or GI

TABLE 8–3
Renal Tubular Acidosis: Diagnosis and Management

Clinical Condition	Renal Defect	GFR	Serum [HCO₃⁻] (meq/L)	Serum [K+] (mEq/L)	Minimal Urine pH	Associated Disease States	Treatment
Normal Proximal RTA (type II RTA)	None	N	24–28	3.5–5	4.8–5.2	None	N/A
	Proximal H⁺ secretion	N	15–18	↓	<5.5	Drugs, Fanconi's syndrome, various genetic disorders, dysproteinemic states, secondary hyperparathyroidism, toxins (heavy metals), tubulointerstitial diseases, nephrotic syndrome, paroxysmal nocturnal hemoglobinuria	NaHCO₃ or KHCO₃ (10–15 mEq/kg/d), thiazides
Classic distal RTA (type I RTA)	Distal H⁺ secretion	N	20–30	↓	>5.5	Various genetic disorders, autoimmune diseases, nephrocalcinosis, drugs, toxins, tubulointerstitial diseases, hepatic cirrhosis, empty sella syndrome	NaHCO₃ (1–3 meq/kg/d)
Buffer deficiency (type III RTA)	Distal NH₃ delivery	↓	15–18	N	<5.5	Chronic renal insufficiency, renal osteodystrophy, severe hypophosphatemia	NaHCO₃ (1–3 mEq/kg/d)
Generalized distal RTA (type IV RTA)	Distal Na+ reabsorption, K⁺ secretion, and H⁺ secretion	↓	24–28	↑	<5.5	Primary mineralocorticoid deficiency (eg, Addison's Disease), hyporeninemic hypoaldosteronism, diabetes mellitus, tubulointerstitial diseases, nephrosclerosis, drugs), salt-wasting mineralocorticoid-resistant hyperkalemia	Fludrocortisone (0.1–0.5 mg/d) dietary K⁺ restriction, NaHCO₃ (1–3 meq/kg/d) furosemide (40–160 mg/d)

8

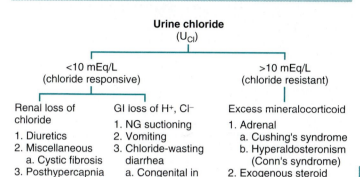

Urine chloride
(U_{Cl})

<10 mEq/L (chloride responsive)		>10 mEq/L (chloride resistant)

Renal loss of chloride
1. Diuretics
2. Miscellaneous
   a. Cystic fibrosis
3. Posthypercapnia

GI loss of H+, Cl−
1. NG suctioning
2. Vomiting
3. Chloride-wasting diarrhea
   a. Congenital in children
   b. Villous adenoma

Excess mineralocorticoid
1. Adrenal
   a. Cushing's syndrome
   b. Hyperaldosteronism (Conn's syndrome)
2. Exogenous steroid administration
3. Bartter's syndrome

FIGURE 8–3   Differential diagnosis of metabolic alkalosis.

losses). This chloride depletion results in renal sodium conservation leading to a corresponding reabsorption of [HCO_3^-] by the kidney. In this category of metabolic alkalosis, the urinary [Cl^-] is <10 mEq/L, and the disorders respond to treatment with intravenous NaCl.

Chloride-Insensitive (Resistant) Metabolic Alkalosis: The pathogenesis in this category is direct stimulation of the kidneys to retain bicarbonate irrespective of electrolyte intake and losses. The urinary [Cl^-] >10 mEq/L, and these disorders do not respond to NaCl administration.

Treatment of Metabolic Alkalosis

Correct the underlying disorder.
1. **Chloride-responsive**
   a. Replace volume with NaCl if depleted.
   b. Correct hypokalemia if present.
   c. NH_4Cl and HCl should be reserved for extreme cases.
2. **Chloride-resistant**
   a. Treat underlying problem, such as stopping exogenous steroids.

RESPIRATORY ACIDOSIS: DIAGNOSIS AND TREATMENT

Respiratory acidosis is a primary rise in pCO_2 with a compensatory rise in plasma [HCO_3^-]. Increased pCO_2 occurs in clinical situations in which decreased alveolar ventilation occurs.

Differential Diagnosis

1. **Neuromuscular Abnormalities with Ventilatory Failure**
   a. Muscular dystrophy, myasthenia gravis, Guillain–Barré syndrome, hypophosphatemia

2. **Central Nervous System**
   a. Drugs: Sedatives, analgesics, tranquilizers, ethanol
   b. CVA
   c. Central sleep apnea
   d. Spinal cord injury (cervical)
3. **Airway Obstruction**
   a. Chronic (COPD)
   b. Acute (asthma)
   c. Upper airway obstruction
   d. Obstructive sleep apnea
4. **Thoracic–Pulmonary Disorders**
   a. Bony thoracic cage: Flail chest, kyphoscoliosis
   b. Parenchymal lesions: Pneumothorax, severe pulmonary edema, severe pneumonia
   c. Large pleural effusions
   d. Scleroderma
   e. Marked obesity (Pickwickian syndrome)

Treatment of Respiratory Acidosis

Improve Ventilation: Intubate patient and place on ventilator, increase ventilator rate, reverse narcotic sedation with naloxone (Narcan), etc

RESPIRATORY ALKALOSIS: DIAGNOSIS AND TREATMENT

Respiratory alkalosis is a primary fall in pCO_2 with a compensatory decrease in plasma $[HCO_3^-]$. Respiratory alkalosis occurs with increased alveolar ventilation.

Differential Diagnosis

1. **Central stimulation**
   a. Anxiety, hyperventilation syndrome, pain
   b. Head trauma or CVA with central neurogenic hyperventilation
   c. Tumors
   d. Salicylate overdose
   e. Fever, early sepsis
2. **Peripheral stimulation**
   a. PE
   b. CHF (mild)
   c. Interstitial lung disease
   d. Pneumonia
   e. Altitude
   f. Hypoxemia: Any cause (See the section on Hypoxia, page 171.)
3. **Miscellaneous**
   a. Hepatic insufficiency
   b. Pregnancy
   c. Progesterone
   d. Hyperthyroidism
   e. Iatrogenic mechanical overventilation

Treatment of Respiratory Alkalosis

Correct the underlying disorder.

Hyperventilation Syndrome: Best treated by having the patient rebreathe into a paper bag to increase pCO_2, decrease ventilator rate, increase amount of dead space with ventilator, or treat underlying cause.

HYPOXIA

1. The second type of information gained from a blood gas level, in addition to acid–base results, pertains to the level of oxygenation. Usually, results are given as pO_2 and oxygen saturation (See Table 8–1 for normal values in page 162). These two parameters are related to each other.
2. Oxygen saturation at any given pO_2 is influenced by temperature, pH, and the level of 2,3-DPG as shown in Figure 8–4.

Differential Diagnosis

1. **V/Q abnormalities**
   a. COPD: Emphysema, chronic bronchitis
   b. Asthma
   c. Atelectasis
   d. Pneumonia
   e. PE
   f. ARDS
   g. Pneumothorax

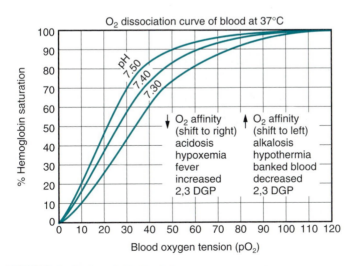

FIGURE 8–4   Oxyhemoglobin dissociation curve.

    h. Pneumoconiosis
    i. CF
    j. Obstructed airway
2. **Alveolar hypoventilation**
    a. Skeletal abnormalities
    b. Neuromuscular disorders
    c. Pickwickian syndrome
    d. Sleep apnea
3. **Decreased pulmonary diffusing capacity**
    a. Pneumoconiosis
    b. Pulmonary edema
    c. Drug-induced pulmonary fibrosis (Bleomycin)
    d. Collagen–vascular diseases
4. **Right-to-left shunt**
    a. Congenital heart disease: Tetralogy of Fallot, transposition, etc

8

SAMPLE ACID–BASE PROBLEMS

In each of the following examples, use the technique for blood gas interpretation on page 163 in this chapter to identify the acid–base disorder.

Example 1

A patient with COPD has a blood gas of pH 7.34, pCO$_2$ 55, and [HCO$_3^-$] of 29.

Step 1:

$$46 = 24 \times \frac{55}{29}$$

$$46 \approx 45$$

    The numbers fit because the difference between the calculated and observed is <10%.

Step 2:   pH < 7.37, the problem is an acidemia.

Step 3:   pCO$_2$ > 44 and [HCO$_3^-$] is **not** < 22, so it represents a respiratory acidosis.

Step 4:   Normal compensation for chronic (COPD) respiratory acidosis (from Table 8–2).

$$\Delta[HCO_3^-] = 4 \times \Delta\,(pCO_2\,/10) = 4 \times \frac{15}{10} = 6$$

    Expected [HCO$_3^-$] is 24 mEq/L + 6 = 30, which is reasonably close to the measured [HCO$_3^-$] of 29, therefore this is a simple respiratory acidosis. This patient has a chronic respiratory acidosis due to hypoventilation (simple acid–base disorder).

Example 2

Immediately after a cardiac arrest a patient has a pH 7.25, pCO$_2$ 28, and [HCO$_3^-$] 12.

Step 1:

$$56 = 24 \times \frac{28}{12}$$

$$56 = 56$$

    The numbers fit.

Step 2:   pH < 7.37, so the problem is an acidemia.

Step 3:   [HCO_3^-] is < 22 mEq/L and pCO_2 is **not** > 44, so this is a metabolic acidosis.

Step 4:   (See Table 8–2, page 164)

$$pCO_2 = (1.5 \times [HCO_3^-] + 8) = (1.5 \times 12) + 8 = 26$$

The expected pCO_2 of 26 mm Hg is very similar to the actual measured value of 28 mm HG, so this is a simple metabolic acidosis. This patient has a lactic acidosis following a cardiopulmonary arrest (simple acid–base disorder).

Example 3

A young man with a fever of 103.2°F and a fruity odor on his breath has a blood gas with pH = 7.36, pCO_2 = 9, and [HCO_3^-] = 5.

Step 1:

$$45 = \frac{24}{5} \times 9$$
$$43 \approx 45$$

The numbers fit.

Step 2:   The pH < 7.37 indicates an acidemia.

Step 3:   [HCO_3^-] < 22 and pCO_2 is **not** >44, thus a metabolic acidosis is present.

Step 4:   The expected compensation in pCO_2 can be calculated as follows (formula from Table 8–2):

$$pCO_2 = (1.5 \times [HCO_3^-]) + 8$$
$$= (1.5 \times 9) + 8$$
$$= 21.5$$

The expected pCO_2 is 15.5, but the actual result is 9 mm Hg, indicating a second process, which is a respiratory alkalosis. This patient had a metabolic acidosis due to diabetic ketoacidosis and a concomitant respiratory alkalosis due to early sepsis and fever (mixed acid–base disorder).

Example 4

A 30-y-old 30-wk pregnant female presents with nausea and vomiting. Blood gas reveals a pH 7.55, pCO_2 = 25 and [HCO_3^-] = 22.

Step 1:

$$28 = 24 \times \frac{25}{22}$$
$$28 \approx 27$$

The numbers fit.

Step 2:   pH < 7.44 indicates alkalemia.

Step 3: pCO_2 < 36 and the [HCO_3^-] is **not** >26, thus a respiratory alkalosis is present.

Step 4: The expected compensation for a chronic (pregnancy) respiratory alkalosis is calculated from Table 8–2, page 164:

$$\Delta[HCO_3^-] = 5 \times \Delta pCO_2 / 10$$
$$= 5 \times \frac{15}{10} = 7.5$$

The calculated $[HCO_3^-]$ is then $24 - 7.5$, or 16–17 mmol, but the actual bicarbonate level is 22, indicating a relative secondary metabolic alkalosis ($[HCO_3^-]$ is higher than expected).

This patient has a respiratory acidosis due to pregnancy and a relative secondary metabolic alkalosis due to vomiting.

Example 5

A 19-y-old diabetic has an anion gap of 29 and a $[HCO_3^-]$ of 6.

Step 1:

  29 mmol/L actual gap
−10 mmol/L normal gap
  19 mmol/L expected change in $[HCO_3^-]$

Step 2:

  24 mmol/L normal $[HCO_3^-]$
−19 mmol/L expected change in $[HCO_3^-]$
    5 mmol/L expected change in $[HCO_3^-]$

Actual bicarbonate is 6 mmol/L, which is very close to the expected of 5 mmol/L. Thus, a pure metabolic gap acidosis is present from DKA.

Example 6

A 21-y-old diabetic presents with nausea, vomiting, and abdominal pain. The anion gap was 23, and the $[HCO_3^-]$ was 18.

Step 1:

  23 mmol/L actual gap
−10 mmol/L normal gap
  13 mmol/L expected change in $[HCO_3^-]$ from normal

Step 2:

  24 mmol/L normal $[HCO_3^-]$
−13 mmol/L expected change in $[HCO_3^-]$
  11 mmol/L expected change in $[HCO_3^-]$

Actual bicarbonate is 18 mmol and not the 11 mmol/L expected from a pure metabolic gap acidosis. Because the actual bicarbonate was higher than expected, this must be a mixed metabolic gap acidosis and metabolic alkalosis. The patient has a metabolic gap acidosis from DKA and a metabolic alkalosis from the vomiting.

Example 7

A 55-y-old alcoholic with a 2-wk history of diarrhea. The anion gap was 17, and [HCO$_3^-$] was 10.

Step 1:

```
  17 mmol/L actual gap
−10 mmol/L normal gap
   7 mmol/L expected change in [HCO₃⁻] from normal
```

 17 mmol/L actual gap
−10 mmol/L normal gap
 7 mmol/L expected change in [HCO$_3^-$] from normal

Step 2:

 24 mmol/L normal [HCO$_3^-$]
−7 mmol/L expected change in [HCO$_3^-$]
 17 mmol/L expected change in [HCO$_3^-$]

Actual bicarbonate is 10 mmol/L and not the expected 17 mmol/L if there was a pure metabolic gap acidosis. Since the actual bicarbonate is lower than expected, there must be a mixed metabolic gap acidosis and metabolic nongap acidosis. The patient has a metabolic nongap acidosis from diarrhea and a metabolic gap acidosis from the alcoholic ketoacidosis.

8

9

FLUIDS AND ELECTROLYTES

Principles of Fluids and Electrolytes	Electrolyte Abnormalities: Diagnosis
Composition of Parenteral Fluids	and Treatment
Composition of Body Fluids	
Ordering IV Fluids	
Determining an IV Rate	

PRINCIPLES OF FLUIDS AND ELECTROLYTES

Fluid Compartments

9

- Example: 70-kg male

Total Body Water: 42,000 mL (60% of BW)

- Intracellular: 28,000 mL (40% of BW)
- Extracellular: 14,000 mL (20% of BW)
- Plasma: 3500 mL (5% of BW)
- Interstitial: 10,500 mL (15% of BW)

Total Blood Volume

Total blood volume = 5600 mL (8% of BW)

Red Blood Cell Mass

Male, 20–36 mL/kg (1.15–1.21 L/m^2); female, 19–31 mL/kg (0.95–1.0 L/m^2)

Water Balance

- 70-kg male

The minimum obligate water requirement to maintain homeostasis (assuming normal temperature and renal concentrating ability and minimal solute [urea, salt] excretion) is about 800 mL/d, which would yield 500 mL of urine.

"Normal" Intake: 2500 mL/d (about 35 mL/kg/d baseline)

- Oral liquids: 1500 mL
- Oral solids: 700 mL
- Metabolic (endogenous): 300 mL

"Normal" Output: 1400–2300 mL/d

- Urine: 800–1500 mL
- Stool: 250 mL

- Insensible loss: 600–900 mL (lungs and skin). (With fever, each degree above 98.6°F adds 2.5 mL/kg/d to insensible loss; insensible losses are decreased if a patient is on a ventilator; free water gain may occur from humidified ventilation.)

Baseline Fluid Requirement

Afebrile 70-kg Adult: 35 mL/kg/24 h

If not a 70-kg Adult: Calculate the water requirement according to the following **"kg Method"**:

- For the first 10 kg of body weight: 100 mL/kg/d plus
- For the second 10 kg of body weight: 50 mL/kg/d plus
- For the weight above 20 kg: 20 mL/kg/d

Electrolyte Requirements

- 70-kg adult, unless otherwise specified

Sodium (as NaCl):   80–120 mEq (mmol)/d (Pediatric patients, 3–4 mEq/kg/ 24 h [mmol/kg/24 h])

Chloride: 80–120 mEq (mmol)/d, as NaCl

Potassium: 50–100 mEq/d (mmol/d) (Pediatric patients, 2–3 mEq/kg/24 h [mmol/kg/24 h]). In the absence of hypokalemia and with normal renal function, most of this is excreted in the urine. Of the total amount of potassium, 98% is intracellular, and 2% is extracellular. Thus, assuming the serum potassium level is normal, about 4.5 mEq/L (mmol/L), the total extracellular pool of $K^+ = 4.5 \times 14$ L = 63 mEq (mmol). Potassium is easily interchanged between intracellular and extracellular stores under conditions such as acidosis. Potassium demands increase with diuresis and building of new body tissues (anabolic states).

Calcium: 1–3 gm/d, most of which is secreted by the GI tract. Routine administration is not needed in the absence of specific indications.

Magnesium: 20 mEq/d (mmol/d). Routine administration is not needed in the absence of specific indications, such as parenteral hyperalimentation, massive diuresis, ethanol abuse (frequently needed) or preeclampsia.

Glucose Requirements

100–200 g/d (65–75 g/d/m^2). During starvation, caloric needs are supplied by body fat and protein; the majority of protein comes from the skeletal muscles. Every gram of nitrogen in the urine represents 6.25 g of protein broken down. The **protein-sparing effect** is one of the goals of basic IV therapy. The administration of at least 100 g of glucose/d reduces protein loss by more than one-half. Virtually all IV fluid solutions supply glucose as dextrose (pure dextrorotatory glucose). Pediatric patients require about 100–200 mg/kg/h.

COMPOSITION OF PARENTERAL FLUIDS

Parenteral fluids are generally classified based on molecular weight and oncotic pressure. Colloids have a molecular weight of >8000 and have high oncotic pressure; crystalloids have a molecular weight of <8000 and have low oncotic pressure.

Colloids

- Albumin (see page 200)
- Blood products (RBCs, single-donor plasma, etc) (Chapter 10, page 197)
- Plasma protein fraction (Plasmanate) (See Chapter 22)
- Synthetic colloids (hetastarch [Hespan], dextran) (Chapter 22)

Crystalloids

Table 9–1 describes common crystalloid parenteral fluids.

COMPOSITION OF BODY FLUIDS

Table 9–2 gives the average daily production and the amount of some major electrolytes present in various body fluids.

ORDERING IV FLUIDS

One of the most difficult tasks to master is choosing appropriate IV therapy for a patient. The patient's underlying illness, vital signs, serum electrolytes, and a host of other variables all must be considered. The following are general guidelines for IV therapy. Specific requirements for each patient can vary tremendously from these guidelines.

Maintenance Fluids

These amounts provide the minimum requirements for routine daily needs:

1. **70-kg Male:** Five% dextrose in one-quarter concentration normal saline (D5¼NS) with 20 mEq KCl/L (20 mmol/L) at 125 mL/h. (This will deliver about 3 L of free water/day.)
2. **Other Adult Patients:** Also use D5¼ NS with 20 mEq KCl/L. Determine their 24-h water requirement by the "kg method" (page 178) and divide by 24 h to determine the hourly rate.
3. **Pediatric Patients:** Use the same solution, but determine the daily fluid requirements by either of the following methods:
   a. *kg Method:* (page 181)
   b. *Meter Squared Method:* Maintenance fluids are 1500 mL/m²/d. Divide by 24 to get the flow rate per hour. To calculate the surface area, use Table 9–3, page 181 "rule of sixes nomogram." Formal body surface area charts are in the Appendix.

Specific Replacement Fluids

These fluids are used to replace excessive, nonphysiologic losses.

Gastric Loss (Nasogastric Tube, Emesis): D_5½ NS with 20 mEq/L (mmol/L) potassium chloride (KCl)

Diarrhea: D_5LR with 15 mEq/L (mmol/L) KCl. Use body weight as a replacement guide (about 1 L for each 1 kg, or 2.2 lb, lost)

Bile Loss: D_5LR with 25 mEq/L (½ ampule) of sodium bicarbonate mL for mL

Pancreatic Loss: D_5LR with 50 mEq/liter (1 amp) HCO_3 mL for mL.

Burn Patients: Use the Parkland or "Rule of Nines" Formulas:

TABLE 9–1
Composition of Commonly Used Crystalloids

Fluid	Glucose (g/L)	Na$^+$	Cl$^-$	K$^+$	Ca^{2+}	HCO$_3^-$*	Mg^{2+}	HPO$_4^{-2}$	kcal/L
D_5W (5% dextrose in water)	50	—	—	—	—	—	—	—	170
D_{10}W (10% dextrose in water)	100	—	—	—	—	—	—	—	340
D_{20}W (20% dextrose in water)	200	—	—	—	—	—	—	—	680
D_{50}W (50% dextrose in water)	500	—	—	—	—	—	—	—	1700
½ NS (0.45% NaCl)	—	77	77	—	—	—	—	—	—
3% NS	—	513	513	—	—	—	—	—	—
NS (0.9% NaCl)	—	154	154	—	—	—	—	—	—
D_5¼NS	50	38	38	—	—	—	—	—	170
D_5¼NS (0.45% NaCl)	50	77	77	—	—	—	—	—	170
D_5½NS (0.9% NaCl)	50	154	154	—	—	—	—	—	170
D_5LR (5% dextrose in lactated Ringer's)	50	130	110	4	3	27	—	—	180
Lactated Ringer's	—	130	110	4	3	27	—	—	<10
Ionosol MB	50	25	22	20	—	23	3	3	170
Normosol M	50	40	40	13	—	16	3	—	170

*HCO$_3$ is administered in these solutions as lactate that is converted to bicarbonate.

TABLE 9–2
Composition and Daily Production of Body Fluids

Fluid	Na⁺	Cl⁻	K⁺	HCO₃⁻	Average Daily Production* (mL)
	Electrolytes (mEq/L)				

Fluid	Na^+	Cl^-	K^+	HCO_3^-	Average Daily Production* (mL)
Sweat	50	40	5	0	Varies
Saliva	60	15	26	50	1500
Gastric juice	60–100	100	10	0	1500–2500
Duodenum	130	90	5	0–10	300–2000
Bile	145	100	5	15	100–800
Pancreatic juice	140	75	5	115	100–800
Ileum	140	100	2–8	30	100–9000
Diarrhea	120	90	25	45	—

*In adults.

9

TABLE 9–3
"Rule of Sixes" Nomogram for Calculating Fluids in Children*

Weight (lb)	Body Surface Area (m²)
3	0.1
6	0.2
12	0.3
18	0.4
24	0.5
30	0.6
36	0.7
42	0.8
48	0.9
60†	1.0

*Over 100 lb, treat as an adult.
†After 60 lb, add 0.1 for each additional 10 lb.

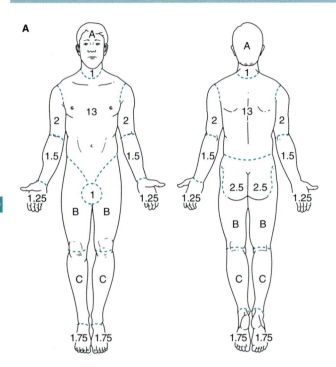

Relative Percentages of Areas Affected by Growth

Area	Age		
	10	15	Adult
A = half of head	5.5	4.5	3.5
B = half of one thigh	4.25	4.5	4.75
C = half of one leg	3	3.25	3.5

FIGURE 9–1 Tables for estimating the extent of burns in adults and children. In adults, a reasonable system for calculating the percentage of the body surface burned is the "rule of nines": Each arm equals 9%, the head equals 9%, the anterior and posterior each equal 18%, and the perineum equals 1%. (Reprinted, with permission, from: Way LW [ed]: *Current Surgical Diagnosis and Treatment,* 10th ed,. Appleton & Lange, Norwalk CT, 1994.)

B

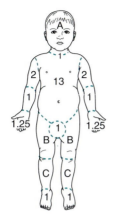
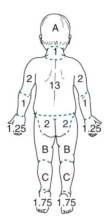

Relative Percentages of Areas Affected by Growth

Area	Age		
	0	1	5
A = half of head	9.5	8.5	6.5
B = half of one thigh	2.75	3.25	4
C = half of one leg	2.5	2.5	2.75

FIGURE 9-1 Continued.

Parkland Formula.

$$\text{Total fluid required during the first 24 h} = (\% \text{ body burn}) \times$$
$$(\text{body weight in kg}) \times 4 \text{ mL}$$

Replace with lactated Ringer's solution over 24 h. Use

- One-half the total over first 8 h (from time of burn)
- One-quarter of the total over second 8 h. One-quarter of the total over third 8 h
- *Rule of Nines.* Used for estimating percentage of body burned in adults. See Figure 9–1 for the exact calculation for the body burn in adults and children. This is also useful for determining ongoing fluid losses from a burn until it is healed or grafted. Fluid losses can be estimated as

$$\text{Loss in mL} = (25 \times \% \text{ Body burn}) \times \text{m}^2 \text{ Body surface area}$$

DETERMINING AN IV RATE

Most IV infusions are regulated by infusion pumps. If a mechanical infusion device is not available, use the following formulas to determine the infusion rate.

For a MAXI Drip Chamber: Use 10 drops/mL; thus

- 10 drops/min = 60 mL/h or
- 16 drops/min = 100 mL/h

For a MINI Drip Chamber: Use 60 drops/mL; thus

- 60 drops/min = 60 mL/h or
- 100 drops/min = 100 mL/h

ELECTROLYTE ABNORMALITIES: DIAGNOSIS AND TREATMENT

In all of the following situations, the primary goal should be to correct the underlying condition. Unless specified, all dosages are for adults. The complete differential diagnosis of laboratory findings can be found in Chapter 4.

Hypernatremia (Na$^+$ >144 mEq/L [mmol/L])

Mechanisms: Most frequently, a deficit of total body water.

- **Combined Sodium and Water Losses ("hypovolemic hypernatremia").** Water loss in excess of sodium loss results in low total body sodium. Due to renal (diuretics, osmotic diuresis due to glycosuria, mannitol, etc) or extrarenal (sweating, GI, respiratory) losses
- **Excess Water Loss ("isovolemic hypernatremia").** Total body sodium remains normal, but total body water is decreased. Caused by diabetes insipidus (central and nephrogenic), excess skin losses, respiratory loss, others.
- **Excess Sodium ("hypervolemic hypernatremia").** Total body sodium increased, caused by iatrogenic sodium administration (ie, hypertonic dialysis, sodium-containing medications) or adrenal hyperfunction (Cushing's syndrome, hyperaldosteronism).

Symptoms: Depend on how rapidly the sodium level has changed

- Confusion, lethargy, stupor, coma
- Muscle tremors, seizures

Signs: Hyperreflexia, mental status changes

Treatment: Check the serum sodium levels frequently while attempting to correct hypernatremia.

- **Hypovolemic Hypernatremia.** Determine if the patient volume is depleted by determining if orthostatic hypotension (see page 286) is present; if volume is depleted, rehydrate with NS until hemodynamically stable, then administer hypotonic saline (½ NS).
- **Euvolemic/Isovolemic.** (No orthostatic hypotension) calculate the volume of free water needed to correct the Na$^+$ to normal as follows:

$$\text{Body water deficit} = \text{Normal TBW} - \text{Current TBW}$$

where

$$\text{Normal TBW} = 0.6 \times \text{Body weight in kg}$$

and

$$\text{Current TBW} = \frac{\text{Normal serum sodium} \times \text{TBW}}{\text{Measured serum sodium}}$$

- Give free water as D_5W, one-half the volume in the first 24 h and the full volume in 48 h. (**Caution:** The rapid correction of the sodium level using free water (D_5W) can cause cerebral edema and seizures.)
- **Hypervolemic Hypernatremia.** Avoid medications that contain excessive sodium (carbenicillin, etc).Use furosemide along with D_5W.

Hyponatremia (Na$^+$ <136 mEq/L [mmol/L])

Mechanisms: Most often due to excess body water as opposed to decreased body sodium. To define the cause, determine serum osmolality.

- **Isotonic Hyponatremia.** Normal osmolality
- **Pseudo-Hyponatremia.** An artifact caused by hyperlipidemia or hyperproteinemia.
- **Hypertonic Hyponatremia.** High osmolality. Water shifts from intracellular to extracellular in response to high concentrations of such solutes as glucose or mannitol. The shift in water lowers the serum sodium; however, the total body sodium remains the same.
- **Hypotonic Hyponatremia.** Low osmolality. Further classified based on clinical assessment of extracellular volume status
- *Isovolemic.* No evidence of edema, normal BP. Caused by water intoxication (urinary osmolality <80 mOsm), SIADH, hypothyroidism, hypoadrenalism, thiazide diuretics, beer potomania
- *Hypovolemic.* Evidence of decreased skin turgor and an increase in heart rate and decrease in BP after going from lying to standing. Due to renal loss (urinary sodium >20 mEq/L) from diuretics, postobstructive diuresis, mineralocorticoid deficiency (Addison's disease, hypoaldosteronism) or extrarenal losses (urinary sodium <10 mEq/L) from sweating, vomiting, diarrhea, third spacing fluids (burns, pancreatitis, peritonitis, bowel obstruction, muscle trauma)
- *Hypervolemic.* Evidence of edema.(urinary sodium <10 mEq/L). Seen with CHF, nephrosis, renal failure, and liver disease
- **Excess Water Intake.** Primary (psychogenic water drinker) or secondary (large volume of sterile water used in procedures, eg, transurethral resection of the prostate or multiple tap water enemas)

Symptoms: Usually with Na$^+$ <125 mEq/L (mmol/L); severity of symptoms correlates with the rate of decrease in Na$^+$.

- Lethargy, confusion, coma
- Muscle twitches and irritability, seizures
- Nausea, vomiting

Signs: Hyporeflexia, mental status changes

Treatment: Based on determination of volume status. Evaluate volume status by physical examination HR and BP lying and standing after 1 min, skin turgor, edema and by determination of the plasma osmolality. Do not need to treat hyponatremia from pseudo-hyponatremia (increased protein or lipids) or hypertonic hyponatremia (hyperglycemia), treat underlying disorder (see above).

- **Life-Threatening.** (Seizures, coma) 3–5% NS can be given in the ICU setting. Attempt to raise the sodium to about 125 mEq/L with 3–5% NS.
- **Isovolemic Hyponatremia.** (SIADH)

Restrict fluids (1000–1500 mL/d).
Demeclocycline can be used in chronic SIADH.

- **Hypervolemic Hyponatremia**

Restrict sodium and fluids (1000–1500 mL/d).
Treat underlying disorder. CHF may respond to a combination of ACE inhibitor and furosemide.

- **Hypovolemic Hyponatremia**

Give D_5NS or NS.

Hyperkalemia

- (K^+ >5.2 mEq/L (mmol/L))

Mechanisms: Most often due to iatrogenic or inadequate renal excretion of potassium.

- **Pseudo-Hyperkalemia.** Due to leukocytosis, thrombocytosis, hemolysis, poor venipuncture technique (prolonged tourniquet time)
- **Inadequate Excretion.** Renal failure, volume depletion, medications that block potassium excretion (spironolactone, triamterene, others), hypoaldosteronism (including adrenal disorders and hyporeninemic states [such as Type IV renal tubular acidosis], NSAIDs, ACE inhibitors), long-standing use of heparin, digitalis toxicity, sickle cell disease, renal transplant
- **Redistribution.** Tissue damage, acidosis (a 0.1 decrease in pH increases serum K^+ approximately 0.5–1.0 mEq/L due to extracellular shift of K^+), beta-blockers, decreased insulin, succinylcholine
- **Excess Administration.** Potassium-containing salt substitutes, oral replacement, potassium in IV fluids

Symptoms: Weakness, flaccid paralysis, confusion.

Signs:

- Hyperactive deep tendon reflexes, decreased motor strength
- ECG changes, such as, peaked T waves, wide QRS, loss of P wave, sine wave, asystole
- K^+ = 7–8 mEq/L (mmol/L) yields ventricular fibrillation in 5% of cases
- K^+ = 10 mEq/L (mmol/L) yields ventricular fibrillation in 90% of cases

Treatment

- Monitor patient on ECG if symptomatic or if K^+ >6.5 mEq/L; discontinue all potassium intake, including IV fluids; order a repeat stat potassium to confirm.
- Pseudo-hyperkalemia should be ruled out. If doubt exists, obtain a plasma potassium in a heparinized tube; the plasma potassium will be normal if pseudo-hyperkalemia is present.
- **Rapid Correction.** These steps only protect the heart from potassium shifts, and total body potassium must be reduced by one of the treatments shown under Slow Correction.

Calcium chloride, 500 mg, slow IV push (only protects heart from effect of hyperkalemia)

Alkalinize with 50 mEq (1 ampule) sodium bicarbonate (causes intracellular potassium shift)

50 mL D50, IV push, with 10–15 units regular insulin, IV push (causes intracellular potassium shift)

- **Slow Correction**

Sodium polystyrene sulfonate (Kayexalate) 20–60 g given orally with 100–200 mL of sorbitol or 40 g Kayexalate with 40 g sorbitol in 100 mL water given as an enema. Repeat doses qid as needed.

Dialysis (hemodialysis or peritoneal)

- **Correct Underlying Cause.** Such as stopping potassium-sparing diuretics, ACE inhibitors, mineralocorticoid replacement for hypokalemia

Hypokalemia

- K^+ <3.6 mEq/L (mmol/L)

Mechanisms: Due to inadequate intake, loss, or intracellular shifts

- **Inadequate Intake.** Oral or IV
- **GI Tract Loss.** (Urinary chloride usually <10 mEq/d; "chloride-responsive alkalosis") vomiting, diarrhea, excess sweating, villous adenoma, fistula
- **Renal Loss.** Diuretics and other medications (amphotericin, high-dose penicillins, aminoglycosides, cisplatin), diuresis other than diuretics (osmotic, eg, hyperglycemia or ethanol-induced), vomiting (from metabolic alkalosis from volume depletion), renal tubular disease (renal tubular acidosis type II [distal], and [proximal]), Bartter's syndrome (due to increased renin and aldosterone levels), hypomagnesemia, natural licorice ingestion, mineralocorticoid excess (primary and secondary hyperaldosteronism, Cushing's syndrome, steroid use), and ureterosigmoidostomy
- **Redistribution (Intracellular Shifts).** Metabolic alkalosis (each 0.1 increase in pH lowers serum K^+ approximately 0.5–1.0 mEq/L, due to intracellular shift of K^+), insulin administration, beta-adrenergic agents, familial periodic paralysis, treatment of megaloblastic anemia

Symptoms

- Muscle weakness, cramps, tetany
- Polyuria, polydipsia

Signs

- Decreased motor strength, orthostatic hypotension, ileus
- ECG changes, such as flattening of T waves, "U" wave becomes obvious (U wave is the upward deflection after the T wave.)

Treatment: The therapy depends on the cause.

- A history of hypertension, GI symptoms, or use of certain medications may suggest the diagnosis.
- A 24-h urine for potassium may be helpful if the diagnosis is unclear. Levels <20 mEq/d suggest extrarenal/redistribution, >20 mEq/d suggest renal losses.

- A serum potassium level of 2 mEq/L (mmol/L) probably represents a deficit of at least 200 mEq (mmol) in a 70-kg adult; to change potassium from 3 mEq/L (mmol/L) to 4 mEq/L (mmol/L) takes about 100 mEq (mmol) of potassium in a 70-kg adult.
- Treat underlying cause.
- Hypokalemia potentiates the cardiac toxicity of digitalis. In the setting of digoxin use, hypokalemia should be aggressively treated.
- Treat hypomagnesemia if present. It will be difficult to correct hypokalemia in the presence of hypomagnesemia.
- **Rapid Correction.** Give KCl IV. Monitor heart with replacement >20 mEq/h. IV potassium can be painful and damaging to veins.

Patient <40 kg: 0.25 mEq/kg/h $\times$ 2 h
Patient >40 kg: 10–20 mEq/h $\times$ 2 h
Severe [<2 mEq/L (mmol/L)]: Maximum 40 mEq/h IV in adults
In all cases check a stat potassium following each 2–4 h of replacement.

- **Slow Correction.** Give KCl orally (see also Table 22–8, page 626) for potassium supplements).

Adult: 20–40 mEq two to three times a day (bid or tid)
Pediatric patients: 1–2 mEq/kg/d in divided doses

Hypercalcemia

- Ca^{2+} > 10.2 mg/dL (2.55 mmol/L)

Mechanisms

- **Parathyroid-Related.** Hyperparathyroidism with secondary bone resorption
- **Malignancy-Related.** Solid tumors with metastases (breast, ovary, lung, kidney), or paraneoplastic syndromes, (squamous cell, renal cell, transitional cell carcinomas, lymphomas, and myeloma)
- **Vitamin-D-Related.** Vitamin D intoxication, sarcoidosis, other granulomatous disease
- **High Bone Turnover.** Hyperthyroidism, Paget's disease, immobilization, vitamin A intoxication
- **Renal Failure.** Secondary hyperparathyroidism, aluminum intoxication
- **Other.** Thiazide diuretics, milk–alkali syndrome, exogenous intake

Symptoms

- Stones (renal colic) bones (osteitis fibrosa), moans (constipation), and groans (neuropsychiatric symptoms—confusion), as well as polyuria, polydipsia, fatigue, anorexia, nausea, vomiting

Signs

- Hypertension, hyporeflexia, mental status changes
- Shortening of the QT interval on the ECG.

Treatment: Usually emergency treatment if patient is symptomatic and Ca^{+2} >13 mEq/L (3.24 mmol/L)

- Use saline diuresis: D_5NS at 250–500 mL/h.

- Give furosemide (Lasix) 20–80 mg or more IV (saline and Lasix will treat most cases).
- Euvolemia or hypervolemia must be maintained. Hypovolemia results in calcium reabsorption.
- **Other Second-Line Therapies:**

Calcitonin 2–8 IU/kg IV or SQ q6–12h if diuresis has not worked after 2–3 h
Pamidronate 60 mg IV over 24 h (one dose only)
Gallium nitrate 200 mg/m^2 IV infusion over 24 h for 5 d
Plicamycin 25 μg/kg IV over 2–3 h (use as last resort—very potent)
Corticosteroids. Hydrocortisone 50–75 mg IV every 6 h.
Consider hemodialysis.

- **Chronic Therapy:**

Treat underlying condition, discontinue contributing medications (ie, thiazides).
Oral medications (prednisone 30 mg PO bid or phosphorus/potassium/sodium supplement [Neutra-Phos] 250–500 mg PO qid) can be effective in chronic therapy for such diseases as breast cancer or sarcoidosis.

Hypocalcemia

- Ca^{2+} < 8.4 mg/dL (2.1 mmol/L)

Mechanisms: Decreased albumin can result in decreased calcium (see discussion on page 61).

- **PTH.** Responsible for the immediate regulation of calcium levels
- **Critical Illness.** Sepsis and other ICU-related conditions can cause decreased calcium because of the fall in albumin often seen in critically ill patients, ionized calcium may be normal.
- **PTH Deficiency.** Acquired (surgical excision or injury, infiltrative diseases such as amyloidosis or hemachromatosis and irradiation) hereditary hypoparathyroidism (pseudo-hypoparathyroidism), hypomagnesemia
- **Vitamin D deficiency.** Chronic renal failure, liver disease, use of phenytoin or phenobarbital, malnutrition, malabsorption (chronic pancreatitis, postgastrectomy)
- **Other.** Hyperphosphatemia, acute pancreatitis, osteoblastic metastases, medullary carcinoma of the thyroid, massive transfusion

Symptoms

- Hypertension, peripheral and perioral paresthesia, abdominal pain and cramps, lethargy, irritability (in infants)

Signs

- Hyperactive DTRs, carpopedal spasm (Trousseau's sign, see page 27).

- Positive Chvostek's sign (facial nerve twitch, can be present in up to 25% of normal adults).
- Generalized seizures, tetany, laryngospasm
- Prolonged QT interval on ECG

Treatment

- **Acute Symptomatic**

100–200 mg of elemental calcium IV over 10 min in 50–100 mL of D_5W followed by an infusion containing 1–2 mg/kg/h over 6–12 h
10% calcium gluconate contains 93 mg of elemental calcium.
10% calcium chloride contains 272 mg of elemental calcium.
Check magnesium levels and replace if low.

- **Chronic**

For renal insufficiency, use vitamin D along with oral calcium supplements (see the following lists) and phosphate-binding antacids (Phospho gel, ALTernaGEL).

Calcium supplements

Calcium carbonate (Os-Cal) 650 mg PO qid (28% calcium)
Calcium citrate (Critical) 950-mg tablets (21% calcium)
Calcium gluconate 500- or 1000-mg tablets (9% calcium)
Calcium glubionate (Neo-Calglucon) syrup 115 mg/5 mL (6.4% calcium)
Calcium lactate 325- or 650-mg tablets (13% calcium)

Hypermagnesemia

- $Mg^{2+} > 2.1$ mEq/L (mmol/L)

Mechanisms

- **Excess Administration.** Treatment of preeclampsia with magnesium sulfate
- **Renal Insufficiency.** Exacerbated by ingestion of magnesium-containing antacids
- **Others.** Rhabdomyolysis, adrenal insufficiency

Symptoms and Signs

- 3–5 mEq/L(mmol/L): Nausea, vomiting, hypotension
- 7–10 mEq/L (mmol/L): Hyperreflexia, weakness, drowsiness
- >12 mEq/L (mmol/L): Coma, bradycardia, respiratory failure

Treatment: Clinical hypermagnesemia requiring therapy is infrequently encountered in
the patient with normal renal function.

- Calcium gluconate: 10 mL of 10% solution (93 mg elemental calcium) over 10–20
  min in 50–100 mL of D_5W given IV to reverse symptoms (useful in patients being
  treated for eclampsia).
- Stop magnesium-containing medications (hypermagnesemia is most often encountered in patients in renal failure on magnesium-containing antacids).
- Insulin and glucose as for hyperkalemia (page 186). Furosemide and saline diuresis
- Dialysis

Hypomagnesemia

- $Mg^{2+} < 1.5$ mEq/L (mmol/L)

Mechanisms

- **Decreased Intake or Absorption.** Malabsorption, chronic GI losses, deficient intake (alcoholics), TPN without adequate supplementation
- **Increased Loss.** Diuretics, other medications (gentamicin, cisplatin, amphotericin B, others), RTA, diabetes mellitus (especially DKA), alcoholism, hyperaldosteronism, excessive lactation
- **Other.** Acute pancreatitis, hypoalbuminemia, vitamin D therapy.

Symptoms

- Weakness, muscle twitches, asterixis
- Vertigo
- Symptoms of hypocalcemia (hypomagnesemia may cause hypocalcemia and hypokalemia)

Signs

- Tachycardia, tremor, hyperactive reflexes, tetany, seizures
- ECG may show prolongation of the PR, QT, and QRS intervals as well as ventricular ectopy, sinus tachycardia

Treatment

- **Severe: Tetany or Seizures**

Monitor patient with ECG in ICU setting.

2 g magnesium sulfate in D_5W infused over 10–20 min. Follow with magnesium sulfate: 1 g/h for 3–4 h follow DTR and levels. Repeat replacement if necessary.

These patients are often hypokalemic and hypophosphatemic as well and should be supplemented.

Hypocalcemia may also result from hypomagnesemia.

- **Moderate**

Mg^{2+} <1.0 mg/dL but asymptomatic

Magnesium sulfate: 1 g/h for 3–4 h, follow TR and levels and repeat replacement if necessary.

- **Mild**

Magnesium oxide: 1 g/d PO (available over the counter in 140-mg capsules, and in 400- and 420-mg tablets). May cause diarrhea.

Hyperphosphatemia

- PO_4^{-3} > 4.5 mg/dL (1.45 mmol/L)

Mechanisms

- **Increased Intake/Absorption.** Iatrogenic, abuse of laxatives or enemas containing phosphorus, vitamin D, granulomatous disease
- **Decreased Excretion** (Most Common Cause). Renal failure, hypoparathyroidism, adrenal insufficiency, hyperthyroidism, acromegaly, sickle cell anemia
- **Redistribution/Cellular Release.** Rhabdomyolysis, acidosis, chemotherapy-induced tumor lysis, hemolysis, plasma cell dyscrasias

Symptoms and Signs: Mostly related to tetany as a result of hypocalcemia (see page 189) caused by the hyperphosphatemia or metastatic calcification (deposition of calcium phosphate in various soft tissues)

Treatment

- Low-phosphate diet
- Phosphate binders like aluminum hydroxide gel (Amphojel) or aluminum carbonate gel (Basaljel) orally
- Acute, severe cases: Acetazolamide 15 mg/kg q4h or insulin and glucose infusion, dialysis as last resort

Hypophosphatemia

- PO_4^{-3} < 2.5 mg/dL (0.8 mmol/L)

Mechanisms

- **Decreased Dietary Intake.** Starvation, alcoholism, iatrogenic (hyperalimentation without adequate supplementation), malabsorption, vitamin D deficiency, phosphate-binding antacids (ie, ALTernaGEL)
- **Redistribution.** Conditions associated with respiratory or metabolic alkalosis (alcohol withdrawal, salicylate poisoning, etc), endocrine (insulin, catecholamine, etc), anabolic steroids, hyper- or hypothermia, leukemias and lymphomas, hypercalcemia, hypomagnesemia
- **Renal Losses.** RTA, diuretic phase of ATN, hyperparathyroidism, hyperthyroidism, hypokalemia, diuretics, hypomagnesemia, alcohol abuse, diabetes mellitus (poorly controlled)
- **Other.** Refeeding in the setting of severe protein-calorie malnutrition, severe burns, treatment of DKA

Symptoms and Signs: < 1 mg/dL (0.32 mmol/L): Weakness, muscle pain and tenderness, paresthesia, cardiac and respiratory failure, CNS dysfunction (confusion and seizures). rhabdomyolysis, hemolysis, impaired leukocyte and platelet function

Treatment: IV therapy is reserved for severe potentially life-threatening hypophosphatemia (<1.0–1.5 mg/dL) because too rapid correction can lead to severe hypocalcemia. With mild to moderate hypophosphatemia (1.5–2.5 mg/dL), oral replacement is preferred.

- **Severe.** (<1.0–1.5 mg/dL)

Potassium or sodium phosphate. 2 mg/kg (0.08 mM/kg) given IV over 6 h. (**Caution:** Rapid replacement can lead to hypocalcemic tetany.)

- **Mild to Moderate.** (levels > 1.5 mg/dL)

Sodium–potassium phosphate (Neutra-Phos) or potassium phosphate (K-Phos): 1–2 tablets (250–500 mg PO_4 or 8 mM/tablet) PO bid or tid
Sodium phosphate (Fleet's Phospho-soda). 5 mL PO, bid or tid (128 mg PO_4 or 4 mM/mL)

BLOOD COMPONENT THERAPY

Blood Banking Procedures
Routine Blood Donation
Autologous Blood Donation
Donor-Directed Blood Products
Irradiated Blood Components
Apheresis
Preoperative Blood Set-Up
Emergency Transfusions

Blood Groups
Basic Principles of Blood Component
Therapy
Blood Bank Products
Transfusion Procedures
Transfusion Reactions
Transfusion-Associated Infectious
Disease Risks

BLOOD BANKING PROCEDURES

T&S or T&H: The blood bank types the patient's blood (ABO and Rh) and screens for antibodies. If a rare antibody is found, the physician will usually be notified, and if it is likely that blood will be needed, the type and screen order may be changed to a type and cross. This usually takes less than 1 h.

T&C: The blood bank types and screens the patient's blood as described in the previous section and matches specific donor units for the patient. The cross-match involves testing the recipient's serum against the donor blood cells.

STAT Requests: The bank sets up blood immediately and usually holds it for 12 h. For routine requests, the blood is set up at a date and time that you specify and usually held for 36 h.

ROUTINE BLOOD DONATION

Voluntary blood donation is the mainstay of the blood system in the United States. Donors must usually be >18 y old, in good health, afebrile. and weigh >110 lb. Donors are usually limited to 1 unit every 8 wk and 6 donations/y. Patients with a history of hepatitis, HB_sAg positivity, insulin-dependent diabetes, IV drug abuse, heart disease, anemia, and homosexual activity are excluded from routine blood donation. Patients are counseled about high-risk behaviors that may risk others if they have transmissible diseases and donate blood. Donor blood is tested for ABO, Rh, antibody screen, HB_sAg, antihepatitis B core antigen, hepatitis C antibody, anti-HIV-1 and 2, and anti-HTLV-1 and 2.

AUTOLOGOUS BLOOD DONATION

Preadmission autologous blood banking (predeposit phlebotomy) is popular for some patients anticipating elective surgery in which blood may be needed. General guidelines for autologous banking include good overall health status, a hematocrit greater than 34%, and arm veins that can accommodate a 16-gauge needle. Patients can usually donate up to 1 unit every 3–7 days, until 3–7 days prior to surgery (individual blood banks have their own specifications), depending on the needs of the planned surgery. Iron supplements (eg, ferrous gluconate 325 mg PO tid) are usually given prior to and several months after the donation. The use of erythropoietin is being investigated in this preoperative setting. Units of whole blood can be held for up to 35 days.

DONOR-DIRECTED BLOOD PRODUCTS

This method of donation involves a relative or friend donating blood for a specific patient. This technique cannot be used in the emergency setting because it takes up to 48 h to process the blood for use.

   This system has some drawbacks: Relatives may be unduly pressured to give blood, risk factors that would normally exclude the use of the blood (hepatitis or HIV positivity) become problematic, and ultimately the routine donation of blood for emergency transfusion may be adversely affected. These units are usually stored as packed red cells and released into the general transfusion pool 8 h after surgery unless otherwise requested.

IRRADIATED BLOOD COMPONENTS

Transfusion-associated GVHD, a frequently fatal condition, can be minimized through the highly selected irradiation of blood components. Patients who are at risk for GVHD include recipients of donor-directed units or HLA-matched platelets, fetal intrauterine transfusions, and selected immunocompromised and bone marrow recipients.

APHERESIS

Apheresis procedures are used to collect single-donor platelets (**plateletpheresis**) or white blood cells (**leukapheresis**); the remaining components are returned to the donor. **Therapeutic apheresis** is the separation and removal of a particular component to achieve a therapeutic effect (eg, **erythrocytapheresis** to treat polycythemia).

PREOPERATIVE BLOOD SET-UP

Most institutions have established parameters (MSBOS) for setting up blood before procedures. Some typical guidelines are given in Table 10–1 for the number of units of packed red cells or if only a T&S is requested.

EMERGENCY TRANSFUSIONS

Non-cross-matched blood is rarely transfused because most blood banks can do a complete cross-match within 1 h. In cases of massive, exsanguinating hemorrhage, type-specific blood (ABO- and Rh-matched only), usually available in 10 min, can be used. If even this delay is too long, type O, Rh-negative, packed red blood cells can be used as a last resort. When possible, it is generally preferable to support blood pressure with colloid or crystalloid until properly cross-matched blood is available.

BLOOD GROUPS

Table 10–2 gives information on the major blood groups and their relative occurrences. O– is the **"universal donor"** and AB+ is the **"universal recipient."**

TABLE 10–1
Guidelines for Blood Required for Surgical Procedures

Procedure	Number of Units Needed
Amputation (lower extremity)	2
Cardiac procedure (CABG, valve)	4
Cholecystectomy (open and laparoscopic)	T&S
Colon resection	2
Colostomy	T&S
Cystectomy, radical with diversion	4
Esophageal resection	2
Exploratory laparotomy	2
Gastrectomy	2
Gastrostomy	T&S
Hemorrhoidectomy	T&S
Hernia	T&S
Hysterectomy	2
Liver resection	6
Live transplant	6
Mastectomy	T&S
Nephrectomy	2
Pancreatectomy	4
Parathyroidectomy	T&S
Pulmonary resection	2
Radical neck dissection	2
Radical prostatectomy	3 — 4
Renal transplant	2
Small bowel resection	2
Splenectomy	2
Thyroidectomy	T&S
Tracheostomy	2
Total hip replacement	2
TURP	2
VASCULAR PROCEDURES	
Abdominal aortic aneurysm	6
Aortofemoral bypass	4
Aortoiliac bypass	4
Carotid endarterectomy	T&S
Femoral popliteal bypass	4
Iliofemoral bypass	4
Portacaval shunt	6
Splenorenal shunt	6
Vein stripping	T&S

Abbreviations: CABG = coronary artery bypass graft; T&S = type and screen; TURP = transurethral resection of the prostate.

TABLE 10–2
Blood Groups and Guidelines for Transfusion

Type (ABO/Rh)	Occurrences	Can Usually Receive* Blood From
O+	1 in 3	O (+/–)
O–	1 in 15	O (–)
A+	1 in 3	A (+/–) or O (+/–)
A–	1 in 16	A (–) or O (–)
B+	1 in 12	B (+/–) or O (+/–)
B–	1 in 67	B (–) or O (–)
AB+	1 in 29	AB, A, B, or O (all + or –)
AB–	1 in 167	AB, A, B, or O (all –)

*First choice is always the identical blood type, other acceptable combinations are shown. An attempt is also made to match Rh status of donor and recipient; Rh negative can usually be given to an RH+ recipient safely

10

BASIC PRINCIPLES OF BLOOD COMPONENT THERAPY

Table 10–3 provides some common indications and uses for transfusion products. The following are the basic transfusion principles for adults.

Red Cell Transfusions

Acute Blood Loss: Normal, healthy individuals can usually tolerate up to 30% blood loss without need for transfusion; patients may manifest tachycardia, mild hypotension without evidence of hypovolemic shock. Replace loss with volume (IV fluids, etc) replacement.

- Hgb >10 g/dL, rarely needs transfusion.
- Hgb 6–10 g/dL, transfuse based on clinical symptoms, unless patient has severe medical problems (ie, CAD, respiratory conditions).
- Hgb <6 g/dL usually requires transfusion.

"Allowable Blood Loss":   Often used to guide acute transfusion in the operating room setting. Losses less than allowable are usually managed with IV fluid replacement.

$$\text{Weight in kg} \times 0.08 = \text{Total blood volume}$$

$$\text{Total volume} \times 0.3 = \text{Allowable blood loss (assumes normal hemoglobin)}$$

Example: A 70-kg adult

$$\text{Estimated allowable blood loss} = 70 \times 0.08 = 5600 \text{ mL} \times 0.3 = 1680 \text{ mL}$$

Chronic Anemia: Common in certain chronic conditions such as renal failure, rarely managed with blood transfusion; typically managed with pharmacologic therapy (eg, erythropoietin). However, transfusion is generally indicated if Hgb < 6 g/dL or in the face of symptoms due to low hemoglobin.

TABLE 10-3
Blood Bank Products

Product	Description	Common Indications
Whole blood (see also page 196)	No elements removed 1 unit = 450 mL ± 45 mL (HCT ≈ 40%) Contains RBC, WBC, plasma and platelets (WBC & platelets may be nonfunctional) Deficient in factors V & VII	Not for routine use Acute, massive bleeding Open heart surgery Neonatal total exchange
Packed Red Cells (PRBC) (see also page 196)	Most plasma, WBC, platelets removed; unit = 250–300 mL. (HCT ≈ 75%) 1 unit should raise HCT 3%	Replacement in chronic and acute blood loss, GI bleeding, trauma
Universal Pedi-Packs	250–300 mL divided into 3 bags Contains red cells, some white cells, some plasma and platelets	Transfusion of infants
Leukocyte-Poor (Leukocyte-reduced) Red Cells	Most WBC removed by filtration to make it less antigenic <5 × 10⁶ WBC, few platelets, minimal plasma 1 unit = 200–250 mL	Potential renal transplant patients Previous febrile transfusion reactions Patients requiring multiple transfusions (leukemia, etc.)
Washed RBCs	Like leukocyte-poor red cells, but WBC almost completely removed <5 × 10⁸ WBC, no plasma 1 unit = 300 mL	As for leukocyte-poor red cells, but very expensive and much more purified

(continued)

10

TABLE 10-3
(Continued)

Product	Description	Common Indications
Granulocytes (pheresis)	1 unit ≈220 mL Some RBC, >1 × 10¹⁰ PMN/unit, Lymphocytes, platelets	See page 194
Platelets (see also page 201)	1 "pack" should raise count by 5000–8000 "6-pack" means a pool of platelets from 6 units of blood	Decreased production or destruction (ie, aplastic anemia, acute leukemia, postchemo, etc) Counts <5000–10,000 (risk of spontaneous hemorrhage) must transfuse Counts 10,000–30,000 if risk of bleeding (headache, GI losses, contiguous petechiae) or active bleeding Counts <50,000 if life-threatening bleed Prophylactic transfusion >20,000 for minor surgery or >50,000 for major surgery Usually not indicated in ITP or TTP unless life-threatening bleeding or preoperatively
	1 pack = about 50 mL >5 × 10¹⁰ platelets unit, contains RBC, WBC	See Platelets, may be HLA matched
Platelets, pheresis	>3 × 10¹⁰ platelets/unit 1 unit = 300 mL	
Platelets, leukocyte-reduced	As above, but <5 × 10⁶ WBC/unit	See Platelets, may decrease febrile reactions and CMV transmission, alloimmunization to HLA antigens
Cryoprecipitated Antihemophilic Factor ("Cryo")	Contains factor VIII, factor XIII, von Willebrand's factor, and fibrinogen 1 unit = 10 mL	Hemophilia A (factor VII deficiency), when safer factor VIII concentrate not available; von Willebrand's disease, fibrinogen deficiency, fibrin surgical glue

(continued)

**TABLE 10-3
(Continued)**

Product	Description	Common Indications
Fresh-Frozen Plasma (FFP)	Contains factors II, VII, IX, X, XI, XII, XIII and heat-labile V and VII About 1 h to thaw 150–250 ml (400–600 ml if single-donor pheresis)	Emergency reversal of Coumadin Massive transfusion (>5 L in adults) Hypoglobulinemia (IV immune globulin preferred) Suspected or documented coagulopathy (congenital or acquired) with active bleeding or before surgery Clotting factor replacement when concentrate unavailable Not recommended for volume replacement If PT <22 s or PTT <70 s, 1 unit is usually sufficient
Single Donor Plasma	Like FFP, but lacks factors V and VIII About 1 h to thaw; 150–200 ml	No longer routinely used for plasma replacement Stable clotting factor replacement Coumadin reversal, hemophilia B (Christmas disease)
Rho Gam (Rho D immune globulin)	Antibody against Rh factor (volume = 1 ml)	Rh-mother with Rh+ baby, within 72 h of delivery, to prevent hemolytic disease of newborn; autoimmune thrombocytopenia

(continued)

10

TABLE 10-3
(Continued)

Product	Description	Common Indications
ALL OF THE AFOREMENTIONED ITEMS USUALLY REQUIRE A "CLOT TUBE" TO BE SENT FOR TYPING. THE FOLLOWING PRODUCTS ARE USUALLY DISPENSED BY MOST HOSPITAL PHARMACIES AND ARE USUALLY ORDERED AS A MEDICATION.		
Factor VII (purified antihemophilic factor)	From pooled plasma, pure Factor VIII Increased hepatitis risk	Routine for hemophilia A (factor VII deficiency)
Factor IX concentrate (prothrombin complex)	Increased hepatitis risk Factors II, VII, IX, and X Equivalent to 2 units of plasma	Active bleeding in Christmas disease (Hemophilia B or factor IX deficiency)
Immune serum globulin	Precipitate from plasma "gamma globulin"	Immune globulin deficiency Disease prophylaxis (hepatitis A, measles, etc.)
5% Albumin or 5% plasma protein fraction	Precipitate from plasma (see Drugs, Chapter 22)	Plasma volume expanders in acute blood loss
25% Albumin	Precipitate from plasma	Hypoalbuminemia, volume expander, burns Draws extravascular fluid into circulation

Abbreviations: RBC = red blood cells; WBC = white blood cells; HCT = hematocrit; GI = gastrointestinal; ITP = idiopathic thrombocytopenic purpura; TTP = thrombotic thrombocytopenic purpura; HLA = histocompatibility locus antigen; PT = prothrombin time; PTT = partial thromboplastin time.

RBC Transfusion Formula: As a guide, one unit of packed RBCs raises the HCT by 3% (Hgb 1 g/dL) in the average adult. To roughly determine the volume of whole blood or packed red cells needed to raise a hematocrit to a known amount, use the following formula:

$$\text{Volume of cells} = \frac{\text{Total blood volume of patient} \times (\text{Desired HCT} - \text{Actual HCT})}{\text{HCT of transfusion product}}$$

where total blood volume is 70 mL/kg in adults, 80 mL/kg in children; the HCT of packed cells is approximately 70, and that of whole blood is approximately 40.

White Cell Transfusions

- The use of white cell transfusions is rarely indicated today due to the use of genetically engineered myeloid growth factors such as GM-CSF (see Chapter 22)
- Indicated for patients being treated for overwhelming sepsis and severe neutropenia (<500 PMN/μL)

Platelet Transfusions

For indications, see Table 10–3

Platelet Transfusion Formula: Platelets are often transfused at a dose of 1 unit/10 kg of body weight. After administration of 1 unit of multiple-donor platelets, the count should rise 5000–8000/mm^3 within 1 h of transfusion and 4500 mm^3 within 24 h. Normally, stored platelets that are transfused survive in vivo 6–8 d after infusion. Clinical factors (DIC, alloimmunization) can significantly shorten these intervals. To standardize the corrected platelet count to an individual patient, use the CCI. Measure the platelet count immediately before and 1 h after the platelet infusion. If the correction is less than expected, do a workup to determine the possible cause (antibodies, splenomegaly, etc). Many institutions are now using platelet pheresis units. One platelet pheresis unit has enough platelets to raise the count by 6000–8000/mm^3. Using a single unit has the advantage of exposing the patient to only one donor versus possibly six to eight. This limits HLA exposures and reduces the risks of infection transmission.

$$\text{CCI} = \frac{\text{Posttransfusion platelet count} - \text{Pretransfusion count} \times \text{Body surface area (m}^2)}{\text{Platelets given} \times 10^{11}}$$

BLOOD BANK PRODUCTS

Table 10–3 describes products used in blood component therapy and gives recommendations for use of these products.

TRANSFUSION PROCEDURES

1. Draw a clot tube (red top), and sign the lab slips to verify that the sample came from the correct patient. The patient should be identified by referring to the ID bracelet and asking the patient, if able, to state his or her name. Place the patient's name, hospital number, date, and your signature on the tube label. **Prestamped labels are not accepted by most blood banks.**
2. Obtain the patient's informed consent by discussing the reasons for the transfusion and the potential risks and benefits from it. Follow hospital procedure regarding the need

for the patient to sign a specific consent form. At most hospitals, chart documentation is usually all that is necessary.

3. When the blood products become available, ensure good venous access for the transfusion (18-gauge needle or larger is preferred in an adult).

4. Verify the information on the request slip and blood bag with another person, such as a nurse, and with the patient's ID bracelet. Many hospitals have defined protocols for this procedure; check your institutional guidelines.

5. Mix blood products to be transfused with isotonic (0.9%) NS only. Using hypotonic products such as D_5W may result in hemolysis of the blood in the tubing. Lactated Ringer's should NOT be used because the calcium could chelate the anticoagulant citrate.

6. Red cells are infused through a special filter. Specific leukocyte reduction filters are available and may be used in very specific circumstances (febrile transfusion reactions, to reduce potential CMV transmission, to reduce risk of alloimmunization to WBC antigens).

7. When transfusing large volumes of packed red cells (>10 units), monitor coagulation, Mg^{2+}, Ca^{2+}, and lactate levels. It is usually necessary to also transfuse platelets and FFP. Also, a calcium replacement is sometimes needed because the preservative used in the blood is a calcium binder and hypocalcemia can result after large amounts of blood are transfused. Also, for massive transfusions (usually >50 mL/min in adults and 15 mL/min in children), the blood should be warmed to prevent hypothermia and cardiac arrhythmias.

TRANSFUSION REACTIONS

Several types of transfusion reactions are possible:

1. **Acute intravascular hemolysis.** Over 85% of adverse hemolytic reactions involving the transfusion of RBCs result from clerical error.. Usually caused by ABO incompatible transfusion. Can result in renal failure (<1/250,000 units transfused).

2. **Nonhemolytic febrile reaction.** Usually mild, fever, chills, rigors, mild dyspnea. Due to a reaction to donor white cells (HLA) and more common in patients who have had multiple transfusions or delivered several children. ($\cong$2–3:100 units transfused)

3. **Mild allergic reaction.** Urticaria or pruritus can be caused by sensitization to plasma proteins in transfusion product. ($\cong$1/100 units transfused)

4. **Anaphylactic reaction.** Acute hypotension, hives, abdominal pain and respiratory distress; seen mostly in IgA-deficient recipients. (<1/1000 units transfused)

5. **Sepsis.** Usually caused by transfusion of a bacterially infected transfusion product, with platelets becoming an increasing risk. *E. coli, Pseudomonas, Serratia, Salmonella,* and *Yersinia* some of the more commonly implicated bacteria. (<1/500,000 RBC units transfused, 1/12,000 platelet units transfused)

6. **Acute lung injury.** Fever, chills, and life-threatening respiratory failure; probably induced by antibodies from donor against recipient white cells. (<1/5000 units transfused)

7. **Volume overload.** Usually due to excess volume infusion; can exacerbate CHF.

Detection of a Transfusion Reaction

1. Spin an HCT to look for a pink plasma layer (indicates hemolysis).

2. Order serum for free hemoglobin and serum haptoglobin assays (haptoglobin decreases with a reaction) and urine for hemosiderin levels. Obtain a stat CBC to determine the presence of schistocytes, which can be present with a reaction.

3. If you suspect acute hemolysis, request a DIC screen (PT, PTT, fibrinogen, and fibrin degradation products).

Treatment of Transfusion Reactions

1. Stop the blood product immediately, and notify the blood bank.
2. Keep the IV line open with NS, and monitor the patient's vital signs and urine output carefully.
3. Save the blood bag, and have the lab verify the type and cross-match. Verify that the proper patient received the proper transfusion. Redraw blood samples for the blood bank.
4. Make specific recommendations, using the following guidelines; modifications should be based on clinical judgment.

- **Nonhemolytic febrile reaction:** Antipyretics can be used and the transfusion continued with monitoring. Use leukocyte-washed transfusion products in future.
- **Mild allergic reaction:** Administer Benadryl (25–50 mg IM/PO/IV). Resume the transfusion carefully only if the patient improves promptly.
- **Anaphylactic reaction.** Terminate transfusion, monitor closely, give antihistamines (Benadryl 25–50 mg IM/PO/IV), corticosteroids (Solu-Medrol 125 mg IV, 2 mg/kg Peds IV), epinephrine (1:1000 0.3–0.5 mL SQ adults, 0.1 mL/kg Peds), and pressors as needed. Premedicate (antihistamines, steroids) for future transfusions; use only leukocyte-washed red cells.
- **Acute lung injury.** Give ventilatory support as needed; use only leukocyte-washed red cells for future transfusions.
- **Sepsis:** Culture the transfusion product and specimens from the patient; treat sepsis empirically by monitoring and administering pressors and antibiotics (third/fourth-generation cephalosporin or piperacillin/tazobactam along with an aminoglycoside) until cultures returns.
- **Volume overload.** Employ a slow rate of infusion with selective use of diuretics.
- **Acute intravascular hemolysis.** Prevent acute renal failure. Place a Foley catheter, monitor the urine output closely, and maintain a brisk diuresis with plain D_5W, mannitol (1–2 g/kg IV), furosemide (20–40 mg IV), and/or dopamine (2–10 μg/kg/min IV) as needed. Consider alkalinization of the urine with bicarbonate (see Chapter 22). Beware of DIC. A renal and hematology consult are usually indicated with a severe hemolytic reaction. Support pressure as needed (fluids, vasopressors such as dopamine).

TRANSFUSION-ASSOCIATED INFECTIOUS DISEASE RISKS

Hepatitis

Incidence of posttransfusion hepatitis for Hep B is 1:63,000 units transfused and for Hep C is 1:103,000 units transfused. Anicteric hepatitis is much more common than hepatitis with jaundice. Screening of donors for HB_sAg and hepatitis C has greatly reduced these forms of hepatitis. Historically, the greatest risk is with pooled factor products (concentrates of Factor VIII). Use of albumin and globulins involves no risk of hepatitis.

HIV

Incidence is <1:600,000 units transfused. Antibody testing is routinely performed on the donor's blood. A positive antibody test means that the donor may be infected with the HIV virus; a confirmatory Western blot is necessary. Do a follow-up test on any donor found to be HIV-positive because false-positives can occur. With screening, AIDS transmission has decreased. Because there is a delay of 22 d between HIV exposure and the development of the HIV antibody, a potential risk of HIV transmission exists even with blood from a donor who is HIV-negative. Newer molecular detection methods should decrease this to approximately 11 d.

CMV

Incidence in donors is very high (approaches 100% in many series), but clinically represents a major risk mostly for immunocompromised recipients and neonates. Leukocyte filters can reduce the risk of transmission if procedures are strictly followed.

HTLV-I, II

Very rare (<<1/641,000 units transfused). Use of leukocyte filters can decrease risk of transmission of HTLV.

Bacteria and Parasites

Sepsis due to bacteria is discussed on page 414. Parasites are very rarely transmitted, but careful donor screening is necessary, especially in endemic regions (eg, Chagas' disease in Central America).

10

DIETS AND CLINICAL NUTRITION

Hospital Diets
Nutritional Assessment
Nutritional Requirements
Determining the Route of Nutritional
    Support

Principles of Enteral Tube Feeding
Postoperative Nutritional Support
Infant Formulas and Feeding

HOSPITAL DIETS

The most commonly ordered standard hospital diets and their indications are listed in Table 11–1, page 206. The vast majority of patients admitted to the hospital can be given one of these hospital diets without any specific supplementation or modification. Most hospitals have diet manuals available for reference, and registered dietitians are usually on staff for nutritional consultation. A physician order for diet instruction by a clinical dietitian is recommended for all patients being discharged with a therapeutic or modified diet.

NUTRITIONAL ASSESSMENT

Nutritional screening should be incorporated into the history and physical evaluation of all patients. Identifying patients at nutrition risk is crucial because malnutrition is prevalent among hospitalized patients and has been associated with adverse clinical outcomes. Situations that predispose a patient to malnutrition include recent and continuing nausea, vomiting, diarrhea, inability to feed oneself, inadequate food intake (cancer-related, others), decreased nutrient absorption or utilization, and increased nutrient losses and nutritional requirements. If needed, detailed nutritional assessment may be needed for some patients and is discussed in the following section.

Although many patients are admitted to the hospital in a nutritionally depleted state, some patients become malnourished during their hospital stay. According to guidelines from the American Society for Parenteral and Enteral Nutrition, "patients should be considered malnourished or at risk of developing malnutrition if they have inadequate nutrient intake for 7 days or more or if they have a weight loss of 10% or more of their preillness body weight."

Formal evaluation is often necessary to identify patients at nutritional risk and to provide a baseline to assess whether therapeutic goals are being achieved with specialized nutritional support. The patient's history is useful in evaluating weight loss; dietary intolerance, including that for glucose or lactose; and disease states that may influence nutritional tolerance. Anthropometric evaluations include comparisons of actual body weight to ideal and usual body weight. Other anthropometric measurements, such as MAMC and TCF, have much

TABLE 11–1
Hospital Diets

Diet	Guidelines	Indications
House/regular	Adequate in all essential nutrients All foods are permitted Can be modified according to patient's food preferences	No diet restrictions or modifications
Mechanical soft	Includes soft-textured or ground foods that are easily masticated and swallowed	Decreased ability to chew or swallow Presence of oral mucositis or esophagitis May be appropriate for some patients with dysphagia
Pureed	Includes liquids as well as strained and pureed foods	Inability to chew or swallow solid foods Presence of oral mucositis or esophagitis May be appropriate for some patients with dysphagia
Full liquid	Includes foods that are liquid at body temperature Includes milk/milk products Can provide approximately: 2500–3000 mL fluid 1500–2000 Cal 60–80 g high-quality protein <10 g dietary fiber 60–80 g fat per day	May be appropriate for patients with severely impaired chewing ability Not appropriate for a lactase-deficient patient unless commercially available lactase enzyme tablets are provided
Clear liquid	Includes foods that are liquid at body temperature Foods are very low in fiber lactose-free virtually fat-free Can provide approximately: 2000 mL fluid 400–600 Cal	Ordered as initial diet in the transition from NPO to solids Used for bowel preparation before certain medical or surgical procedures For management of acute medical conditions warranting minimized biliary contraction or pancreatic exocrine secretion

(continued)

11

TABLE 11-1
(Continued)

Diet	Guidelines		Indications
Clear liquid (continued)	<7 g low-quality protein <1 g dietary fiber <1 g fat/day This diet is inadequate in all nutrients and should not be used >3 d without supplementation		
Low-fiber	Foods that are low in indigestible carbohydrates Decreases stool volume, transit time, and frequency		Management of acute radiation enteritis and inflammatory bowel disease when narrowing or stenosis of the gut lumen is present
Carbohydrate controlled diet (ADA)	Calorie level should be adequate to maintain or achieve desirable body weight Total carbohydrates are limited to 50–60% of total calories Ideally fat should be limited to ≈30% of total calories		Diabetes mellitus
Acute renal failure	Protein (g/kg DBW) Calories Sodium (g/day) Potassium (g/day) Fluid (mL/day)	0.6 35–50 1–3 Variable Urine output + 500	For patients in renal failure who are not undergoing dialysis
Renal failure/Hemodialysis	Protein (g/kg DBW) Calories (per kilogram DBW) Sodium (g/d) Potassium (g/d) Fluid (mL/d)	1.0–1.2 30–35 1–2 1.5–3 Urine output + 500	For patients in renal failure on hemodialysis

(continued)

TABLE 11–1
(Continued)

Diet	Guidelines		Indications
Peritoneal dialysis	Protein (g/kg DBW) Calories (per kilogram DBW) Sodium (g/d) Potassium (g/d) Fluid (mL/d)	1.2–1.6 25–35 3–4 3–4 Urine output + 500	For patients in renal failure on peritoneal dialysis
Liver failure	In the absence of encephalopathy do not restrict protein In the presence of encephalopathy initially restricted protein to 40–60 g/d then liberalize in increments of 10 g/d as tolerated Sodium and fluid restriction should be specified based on severity of ascites and edema		Management of chronic liver disorders
Low lactose/ lactose-free	Limits or restricts mild products Commercially available lactase enzyme tablets are available on the market		Lactase deficiency
Low-fat	<50 g total fat per day		Pancreatitis Fat malabsorption Hypercholesterolemia
Fat/cholesterol restricted	Total fat >30% total calories Saturated fat limited to 10% of calories <300 mg cholesterol <50% calories from complex carbohydrates		
Low-sodium	Sodium allowance should be as liberal as possible to maximize nutritional intake yet control symptoms "No-added salt" is 4 g/d; no added salt or highly salted food; 2 g/d avoids processed foods (ie, meats) <1 g/d is unpalatable and thus compromises adequate intake		Indicated for patients with hypertension, ascites, and edema associated with the underlying disease

11

208

interobserver variability and are generally not useful unless performed by an experienced evaluator. Absolute lymphocyte count is sometimes used as a marker of visceral proteins and immunocompetence. Visceral protein markers, such as prealbumin and transferrin, may be helpful in evaluating nutritional insult as well as catabolic stress. Although the most commonly quoted laboratory parameter of nutritional status is albumin, the albumin concentration often reflects hydration status and metabolic response to injury (ie, the acute phase response) more than the nutritional state of the patient, especially in patients with intravascular volume deficits. Due to its long half-life, albumin may be normal in the malnourished patient. Prealbumin is superior as an indicator of malnutrition only because of its shorter half-life. Use of these serum proteins as indicators of malnutrition is subject to the same limitation, however, because they are all affected by catabolic stress. Table 11–2, page 210, lists the parameters for identifying potentially malnourished patients; however, no single criterion should be used to assess a patient's nutritional status. Patients can generally be classified as mildly, moderately, or severely nutritionally depleted based on these parameters.

NUTRITIONAL REQUIREMENTS

Determining the patient's nutritional requirements is one of the first steps in prescribing a modified diet order or supplementation for a patient. The following list provides guidelines for estimating nutritional needs. Monitoring the patient's progress and adjusting nutritional goals on the basis of clinical judgment is important for ensuring that the patient's specific needs are being met. Caloric needs can be determined by one of two means: the Harris–Benedict BEE and the "rule of thumb" method.

Caloric Needs

A patient's caloric needs can be calculated by the following methods:

Harris–Benedict BEE

For men:

$$BEE = 66.47 + 13.75 \, (w) + 5.00 \, (h) - 6.76 \, (a)$$

For women:

$$BEE = 655.10 + 9.56 \, (w) + 1.85 \, (h) - 4.689 \, (a)$$

where w = weight in kilograms; h = height in centimeters; and a = age in years.

After the BEE has been determined from the Harris–Benedict equation, the patient's total daily maintenance energy requirements are estimated by multiplying the BEE by an activity factor and a stress factor.

$$\text{Total energy requirements} = \text{BEE} \times \text{Activity factor} \times \text{Stress factor}$$

Use the following correction factors:

Activity Level	Correction Factor
Bedridden	1.2
Ambulatory	1.3

Level of Physiologic Stress	Correction Factor
Minor operation	1.2
Skeletal trauma	1.35
Major sepsis	1.60
Severe burn	2.10

TABLE 11-2
Parameters Used to Identify the Malnourished Patient

Parameters	Measurement/Interpretation	Usefulness/Limitations
ANTHROPOMETRIC MEASUREMENT		
Actual body weight (ABW) compared with ideal body weight (IBW)	"Rule-of-thumb" method to determine IBW	
	Step 1	
	For men: IBW (lb) = 106 lb for 5 ft of height, plus 6 lb for each inch of height over 5 ft	
	For women: IBW (lb) = 100 lb for first 5 ft of height plus an additional 5 lb for each inch over 5 ft	
	Step 2	
	$\%\ IBW = \dfrac{ABW}{IBW} \times 100$	
	% of IBW	
	90–110 Normal nutritional status	
	80–90 Mild malnutrition	
	70–80 Moderate malnutrition	
	<70 Severe malnutrition	
Actual body weight compared with usual body weight (UBW)	$\%\ UBW = \dfrac{ABW}{UBW} \times 100$	
	% of UBW	
	85–95% Mild malnutrition	
	75–84% Moderate malnutrition	
	<75% Severe malnutrition	

(continued)

TABLE 11-2
(Continued)

Parameters	Measurement/Interpretation	Usefulness/Limitations
BIOCHEMICAL PARAMETERS		
Serum albumin	3.5–5.2 g/dL Normal 2.8–3.4 g/dL Mild depletion 2.1–2.7 g/dL Moderate depletion <2 g/dL Severe depletion	Routinely available Valuable prognostic indicator: depressed levels predict increased mortality and morbidity Inexpensive Large body stores and relatively long half-life (approximately 20 d) limit usefulness in evaluating short-term changes in nutritional status
Transferrin (TFN)	200–300 mg/dL Normal 150–200 mg/dL Mild visceral depletion 100–150 mg/dL Moderate depletion <100 mg/dL Severe depletion TFN can be calculated from the total iron-binding capacity (TIBC) as follows: $TFN = (0.8 \times TIBC) - 43$	Frequently available Depressed levels predict increased mortality and morbidity Smaller body pool and shorter half-life (8–10 days) than serum albumin If TFN is calculated from TIBC, levels will be increased with the presence of iron deficiency or chronic blood loss Levels are increased during pregnancy Levels are decreased if iron stores are increased as a result of hemosiderosis, hemochromatosis, thalassemia

(continued)

11

TABLE 11-2
(Continued)

11

Parameters	Measurement/Interpretation		Usefulness/Limitations
Prealbumin	16-30 mg/dL	Normal	Half-life is 2 d. Thus is more sensitive indicator of acute change in nutritional status than is albumin or TFN
	10-15 mg/dL	Mild depletion	
	5-10 mg/dL	Moderate depletion	
	<5 mg/dL	Severe depletion	Not routinely available Levels are quickly depleted after trauma or acute infection. Also decreased in response to cirrhosis, hepatitis, and dialysis, and therefore, should be interpreted with caution
Absolute lymphocyte count (calculated as WBC × % lymphocytes)	1400-2000	Mild depletion	May not be valid in cancer patients. Not used by some nutritionists
	900-1400	Moderate depletion	
	<900	Severe depletion	

"Rule of Thumb" Method

- Maintenance of the patient's nutritional status without significant metabolic stress requires 25–30 Cal/kg body weight/d.
- Maintenance needs for the hypermetabolic, severely stressed patient or for supporting weight gain in the underweight patient without significant metabolic stress requires 35–40 Cal/kg body weight/d.
- Greater than 40 Cal/kg body weight/d may be needed to meet the needs of severely burned patients.

Protein Needs

Maintenance requirements for nonstressed patients are 0.8 g of protein per kilogram of body weight. Repletion requirements of the nutritionally compromised patient are 1.2–2.5 g of protein per kilogram of body weight.

DETERMINING THE ROUTE OF NUTRITIONAL SUPPORT

Once nutritional support is indicated, the route for administration is chosen. Enteral supplementation by mouth or tube and parenteral nutrition are the main routes for providing nutritional support.

Enteral Supplementation and Tube Feeding

Enteral nutrition encompasses both supplementation by mouth and feeding by tube into the GI tract. If the patient's oral intake is inadequate, every effort should be made to increase intake by providing nutrient-dense foods, frequent feedings, or oral supplements. If such attempts are unsuccessful, tube feeding may be indicated. In addition, patients who have a functioning GI tract but for whom oral nutrition intake is contraindicated should be considered for tube feedings.

If the GI tract is functioning and can be used safely, tube feedings should be ordered instead of parenteral nutrition when nutrition support is necessary because it

- Is more easily absorbed physiologically
- Is associated with fewer complications than TPN
- Maintains the gut barrier to infection
- Maintains the integrity of the GI tract
- Is more cost-effective than TPN
- Contraindications to tube feeding can be found in Table 11–3.

Parenteral Nutrition

Parenteral nutrition usually offers no advantage to the patient with a functioning GI tract. Because it does not achieve greater anabolism nor provide greater control over a patient's nutritional regimen, parenteral nutrition is indicated only when the enteral route is not usable; therefore, the following rule applies: If the gut works, use it.

Some patients, because of their disease states, cannot be fed enterally and require parenteral feedings. Enteral nutrition is to be avoided in the situations noted in Table 11–3. TPN is typically used in these patients and is discussed in detail in Chapter 12.

Although parenteral nutrition can be given either via central veins (TPN) or by peripheral veins (PPN), the tonicity of the fluid required to administer all nutritional requirements

TABLE 11–3
Contraindications to Tube Feeding

Complete bowel obstruction
GI bleeding
High-output (>500 mL/d) enterocutaneous fistula or fistula not located in the
    proximal or distal GI tract
Hypovolemic or septic shock
Ileus
Inability to obtain safe enteral tube feeding access
Poor prognosis not warranting invasive nutritional support
Severe acute pancreatitis
Severe intractable diarrhea
Severe intractable nausea and vomiting
Severe malabsorption
Anticipated duration of tube feeding therapy <5 d

intravenously requires central administration, and thus PPN may be used as a supplement, but is not adequate to provide all nutritional requirements.

PRINCIPLES OF ENTERAL TUBE FEEDING

The factors involved in choosing the route for enteral nutrition include the projected duration of feeding by this method, GI tract pathophysiology, and the risk for aspiration. Nasally placed tubes are the most frequently used. Patient comfort is maximized by using a small-bore flexible tube. When enteral feedings are started, it is often important to assess gastric residual volumes. The small-bore tubes do not allow for aspiration of residual volumes, however, which may be significant if gastric emptying is questionable. Thus, larger bore tubes are often used to start, and, once feeding tolerance is ensured, the tube is changed to a small-bore tube, which can be left in place comfortably for prolonged periods. Feeding directly into the stomach (as opposed to the bowel) is often preferable because the stomach is the best line of defense against hyperosmolarity. Patients at risk for aspiration require longer tubes into the jejunum or duodenum. Types of feeding tubes and placement procedures are discussed in detail in Chapter 13, page 272.

When long-term feeding is anticipated, a tube enterostomy is usually required. **PEG tubes** can usually be placed without general anesthesia. Patients with tumors, GI obstruction, adhesions, or abnormal anatomy, however, may require open surgical placement. A jejunal feeding tube may be threaded through a PEG for small-bowel feeding. The placement of a needle catheter or Witzel's jejunostomy during surgery generally allows for earlier postoperative feeding with an elemental formulation than waiting for the return of gastric emptying and colonic function.

Enteral Products

A variety of enteral products and tube feedings are available (see Table 11–4, page 215, for some examples). Check the enteral formulary for the specific products available in your facility.

TABLE 11-4
Composition of Some Commonly Available Enteral Formulas

Product	kcal/ mL	Protein (g)	Fat (g)	Carbohydrates (g)	Na$^+$ (mEq)	K$^+$ (mEq)	mOsm/ kg
Meal replacements							
Compleat B	Require normal proteolytic and lipolytic function. Contain lactose.						
	1.00	4.00	4.00	12.0	5.20	3.40	390
Lactose-free	Provides proximal absorption. Requires normal proteolytic and lipolytic function. Low residue.						
Ensure	1.06	3.70	3.70	14.5	3.60	4.0	450
Ensure Plus	1.50	5.50	5.30	19.7	4.90	5.90	600
Isocal	1.06	3.70	3.80	14.4	2.40	2.60	300
Magnacal	2.0	3.5	4.0	12.5	2.20	1.60	590
Osmolite	1.06	3.70	3.80	14.4	2.40	2.60	300
Sustacal	1.00	6.10	2.30	13.8	4.10	5.40	620–700
Travasorb MCT	1.00	4.90	3.30	12.2	1.50	4.50	312
Elemental formulas	Provide rapid proximal absorption. Indicated for pancreatic-biliary dysfunction, selective malabsorption, fistulas, and short bowel syndrome (SBS). Low residue. Nutrients predigested.						
Peptamen	1.0	4.0	3.9	12.7	2.20	3.21	270
Reabilan	1.0	3.15	4.30	13.2	3.05	3.20	350
Reabilan HN	1.33	4.36	4.30	11.9	3.26	3.18	490
Vital HN	1.00	4.20	1.00	18.8	2.70	3.40	450
Vivonex TEN	1.00	3.82	0.28	20.5	2.00	2.00	630
Vivonex	1.00	2.04	0.15	22.6	2.00	3.00	550

(continued)

11

TABLE 11-4
(Continued)

Product	kcal/ mL	Protein (g)	Fat (g)	Carbohydrates (g)	Na⁺ (mEq)	K⁺ (mEq)	mOsm/ kg
Special metabolic	May require vitamin-mineral supplement if used as principal source of nutrition.						
Amin-Aid	2.00	1.90	4.70	37.3	>1	>1	850
Glucerna	1.0	4.18	5.57	9.37	4.03	4.0	375
Pulmocare	1.5	4.17	6.14	7.04	3.80	2.95	490
Hepatic Aid II	1.17	4.30	3.60	16.8	>1	>1	560
Travasorb Hepatic	1.10	2.90	1.40	20.9	1.9	2.9	690
Travasorb Renal	1.35	2.30	1.80	27.1	>1	>1	590
Fiber-containing	Nutritionally complete tube feeding that may help maintain normal bowel function and useful in patients who demonstrate intolerance to low-residue feedings.						
Enrich	1.1	3.62	3.39	14.3 (1.3 g fiber)	3.35	3.94	480
Jevity	1.06	4.20	3.48	14.4 (1.36 g fiber)	3.81	3.77	310

Note: Formulation of products at the time of publication. Actual components may vary slightly.

Component (per 100 kcal)

11

To simplify selection, the nutritional components and osmolality of the enteral product are listed and help classify the formulations. The protein component can be supplied as intact proteins, partially digested hydrolyzed proteins, or crystalline amino acids. Each gram of protein provides 4 Cal. The carbohydrate source may be intact complex starches, glucose polymers, or simpler disaccharides such as sucrose. Carbohydrates provide 4 Cal/g. Fat in enteral products is usually supplied as long-chain fatty acids. Some enteral products, however, contain MCTs, which are transported directly in the portal circulation rather than via chyle production. Because MCT oil does not contain essential fatty acids, it cannot be used as the sole fat source. Long-chain fatty acids provide 9 Cal/g, and MCT oil provides 8 Cal/g.

The osmolality of an enteral product is determined primarily by the concentration of carbohydrates, electrolytes, amino acids, or small peptides. The clinical importance of osmolality is often debated. Hyperosmolal formulations, with osmolalities exceeding 450 mOsm/L, may contribute to diarrhea by acting in a manner similar to osmotic cathartics. Hyperosmolal feedings are well tolerated when delivered into the stomach (as opposed to the small bowel) because gastric secretions dilute the feeding before it leaves the pylorus to traverse the small bowel. Thus, feedings administered directly to the small bowel (eg, via feeding jejunostomy) should not exceed 450 mOsm/L.

Oral supplements differ from other enteral feedings in that they are designed to be more palatable so as to improve compliance. Although most enteral products do not contain lactose (Ensure, Osmolite, others), several oral supplements, commonly referred to as "meal replacements" (such as Compleat B) contain lactose and are therefore not appropriate for patients with lactase deficiency and are not normally used for tube feedings.

Based on osmolality and macronutrient content, enteral products can be classified into several categories. Low-osmolality formulas are isotonic and contain intact macronutrients. They usually provide 1 Cal/mL and require approximately 2 L to provide the RDA for vitamins. These products are appropriate for the general patient population and include products such as Ensure.

High-density formulas may provide up to 2 Cal/mL. These concentrated solutions are hyperosmolar and also contain intact nutrients. The RDA for vitamins can be met with volumes of 1500 mL or less. These products are used for volume-restricted patients. Examples are Nutren 2.0 and Ensure Plus HN.

Chemically defined or elemental formulas provide the macronutrients in the predigested state. These formulations are usually hyperosmolar and have poor palatability. Patients with compromised nutrient absorption abilities or GI function may benefit from elemental type products. Vivonex and Peptamen are two such products.

Disease-specific (special metabolic) enteral formulas have been developed for various disease states. Products for pulmonary patients, such as Pulmocare, contain a higher percentage of calories from fat to decrease the carbon dioxide load from the metabolism of excess glucose. Patients with hepatic insufficiency may benefit from formulations (eg, Hepatic-Aid II) containing a higher concentration of the branched-chain amino acids and a lower concentration of aromatic amino acids in an attempt to correct their altered serum amino acid profile. Formulas containing only essential amino acids have been marketed for the patient in renal failure (Amin-Aid). A low-carbohydrate, high-fat product for persons with diabetes (Glucerna) is available that also contains fiber to help regulate glucose control. Other fiber-containing enteral feedings are available to help regulate bowel function (Enrich, Jevity). The clinical utility of many of the specialty products remains controversial.

Initiating Tube Feedings

Guidelines for ordering enteral feedings are outlined in Table 11–5, page 218. In summary, when using enteral feedings:

TABLE 11–5
Routine Orders for Enteral Nutrition Administered by Tube Feeding

1. Confirm tube placement. (Usually by x-ray)
2. Elevate head of bed to 30–45 degrees
3. Check gastric residuals in patients receiving gastric feedings. Hold feedings if >1.5–2x infusion rate. Significant residuals should be reinstilled and rechecked in 1 h. If continues to be elevated, hold tube feeding and begin NG suction.
4. Check patient weight 3x/wk.
5. Record strict I&O
6. Request routine laboratory studies

1. Determine nutritional needs.
2. Assess GI tract function and appropriateness of enteral feedings.
3. Determine fluid requirements and volume tolerance based on overall status and concurrent disease states.
4. Select an appropriate enteral feeding product and method of administration.
5. Verify that the regimen selected satisfies micronutrient requirements.
6. Monitor and assess nutritional status to evaluate the need for changes in the selected regimen.

The tube feeding can be given into the stomach (bolus, intermittent gravity drip, or continuous) or into the small intestine by continuous infusion (Table 11–6, page 219). Enteral nutrition is best tolerated when instilled into the stomach because this method produces fewer problems with osmolarity or feeding volumes. The stomach serves as a barrier to hyperosmolarity, thus the use of isotonic feedings is mandated only when instilling nutrients directly into the small intestine. The use of gastric feedings is thus preferable and should be used whenever appropriate. Patients at risk for aspiration or with impaired gastric emptying may need to be fed past the pylorus into the jejunum or the duodenum. Feedings via a jejunostomy placed at the time of surgery can often be initiated on the first postoperative day, obviating the need for parenteral nutrition.

Although enteral nutrition is generally safer than parenteral nutrition, aspiration can be a significant morbid event in the care of these patients. Appropriate monitoring for residual volumes in addition to keeping the head of the bed elevated can help prevent this complication. A "significant residual" may be defined as 1½ times the instillation rate. This can be treated in a number of ways. Any transient postoperative ileus can best be treated by waiting for the ileus to resolve. Metoclopramide or erythromycin may be useful pharmacologic therapy for postop ileus (Chapter 22). Patients who have been tolerating feedings and develop intolerance should be carefully assessed for the cause. Feeding intolerance is characterized by vomiting, abdominal distention, diarrhea, or high gastric residual volumes.

Complications of Enteral Nutrition

Diarrhea: Diarrhea occurs in about 10–60% of patients receiving enteral feedings. The physician must be certain to evaluate the patient for other causes of diarrhea. Formula-related causes include contamination, excessively cold temperature, lactose intolerance, osmolality, and an incorrect method or route of delivery. Eliminate potential causes before using antidiarrheal medications.

TABLE 11-6
Tube Feeding Delivery Methods

Delivery Site/ Indication	Delivery Method	Notes	Suggested Feeding Progression
INTRAGASTRIC Appropriate for alert patients with intact gag and cough reflexes and for those with normal gastric emptying	Bolus	Rapid infusion of formula into the stomach by syringe or other feeding reservoir; generally 240–480 mL of formula is given every 3–6 h Feedings are usually given over a period of 5–15 min Associated symptoms of GI distress, such as bloating, nausea, and distention	Typical starter regimen: 60–120 mL of full-strength formula is generally provided Typical feeding progression: Volume of formula provided at each feeding may be increased in 60–120 mL increments every 12 h or as tolerated
INTRAGASTRIC	Intermittent gravity drip	Generally 240–480 mL of formula is allowed to drip from a feeding container through tubing over a 30–60 min period four to eight times per day Rate of formula administration is controlled with a clamp in the tubing May reduce the incidence of GI complications associated with bolus delivery Highly viscous formulas, such as those that contain 2 Cal/mL, may not flow through the tubing	Typical starter regimen: 60–120 mL of full-strength formula is generally provided Typical feeding progression: Volume of formula provided at each feeding may be increased to 60–120 mL increments every 12 h or as tolerated

(continued)

11

219

TABLE 11–6
(Continued)

Delivery Site/ Indication	Delivery Method	Notes	Suggested Feeding Progression
		More expensive than bolus method because feeding containers are necessary Not recommended for critically ill patients	
INTRAGASTRIC	Continuous	Preferred method to administer formula if gastric feeding is necessary for a critically ill patient because it reduces risk of aspiration Use of a feeding pump to deliver precise volumes of formula at a constant rate Goal feeding rates are typically between 80 and 125 mL/h, depending on the individual's nutritional requirements Volume- and rate-controlled delivery minimizes gastric emptying and reduces the incidence of osmotic diarrhea secondary to dumping syndrome	Typical starter regimen: Full-strength formula is generally initiated at a rate of 40 or 50 mL/h Typical feeding progression: Feeding rate is generally increased in increments of 10–15 mL/h every 12 h or as tolerated until the goal feeding rate is achieved

(continued)

TABLE 11-6
(Continued)

Delivery Site/ Indication	Delivery Method	Notes	Suggested Feeding Progression
		In the hospital setting, the formula is usually provided over a 24-h period; home patients may cycle feedings over an 8–14-h period	
		May be necessary to deliver formulas with high viscosity	
		Necessity of feeding pump in addition to feeding bag and tubing increases cost	
		Restricts ambulation in patients who are not critically ill	
INTRAINTESTINAL Appropriate for patients who are at high risk for aspiration, including those who cannot keep the proper position during feeding (head of bed 30 degrees upright)	Continuous	Feeding pump required because excessively rapid formula delivery, as would occur with bolus or gravity drip administration, would probably result in dumping syndrome; allows tube feeding formula to be delivered in a more physiologic manner	Typical starter regimen: Full-strength formula is generally initiated at a rate of 40–50 mL/h; markedly hypertonic formulas (>600 mOsm/L) occasionally may be diluted to half-strength if dumping syndrome is present or if a prolonged period without enteral nutrition has elapsed
		Goal rates are usually	Typical feeding progression: Feeding rate is generally increased in increments of

(continued)

11

TABLE 11-6
(Continued)

Delivery Site/ Indication	Delivery Method	Notes	Suggested Feeding Progression
and those without an intact gag reflex Required feeding route when proximal (ie, oral, esophageal, or gastric) GI obstruction or impairment is present Preferred delivery site for critically ill patients		80–125 mL/h, depending on the patient's nutritional needs Usually 24-h infusions are given in the hospital, but cyclic infusions are an option for the ambulatory or home patient Associated with high cost because of necessity of feeding containers and infusion pump Continuous infusions may restrict patient ambulation	10–12 mL/h every 12 h or as tolerated until the goal feeding rate is achieved; if hypertonic formula was initially diluted, the patient can be switched to full-strength formula after the goal feeding rate is achieved

11

- Check medication profile for possible drug-induced cause.
- Rule out *Clostridium difficile* colitis in patients receiving antibiotics (see Chapter 7).
- Attempt to decrease the feeding rate or try an alternative regimen such as bolus feeding.
- Change the formulation, for example, limit lactose or reduce the osmolality.
- Use pharmacologic therapy only after eliminating treatable causes (eg, give *Lactobacillus* powder [one packet tid to replenish gut flora]; most effective in patients on antibiotics) or antidiarrheal medications (loperamide [Lomotil], calcium carbonate).

Constipation: Although less common than diarrhea, constipation can occur in the enterally fed patient. Check to ensure that adequate fluid volume is being given. Patients with additional requirements may benefit from water boluses or dilution of the enteral formulation. Fiber can be added to help regulate bowel function.

Aspiration: Aspiration is a serious complication of enteral feedings and is more likely to occur in the patient with diminished mental status. The best approach is prevention. Elevate the head of the bed and carefully monitor residual fluid volume. Further evaluate any patient who may have aspirated or who is assessed as being at increased risk for aspiration prior to instituting enteral feedings. Such patients may not be candidates for gastric feedings, and small-bowel feedings may be necessary.

Drug Interactions: The vitamin K content of various enteral products varies from 22 to 156 mg/1000 Cal. This can significantly affect the anticoagulation profile of a patient receiving warfarin therapy. Tetracycline products should not be administered 1 h before or 2 h after enteral feedings to avoid the inhibition of absorption. Similarly, enteral feedings should be stopped 2 h before and after the administration of phenytoin.

POSTOPERATIVE NUTRITIONAL SUPPORT

Most patients can be started on oral feedings postoperatively, the question is when to begin them. Begin feedings once the bowel recovers motility. Motility is delayed in patients undergoing laparotomy, whereas feedings begin fairly quickly for patients who undergo surgery on other parts of the body, once they recover consciousness sufficiently to protect their airway. Remember that the gut recovers motility as follows: The small intestine never loses motility (peristalsis is observed in the OR), the stomach regains motility about 24 h postoperatively, and the colon is the last to recover at 72–96 h postoperatively. Thus, by the time a patient reports flatus, one can assume that the entire gut has regained motility. Feedings then begin, depending on the exact operation performed and the resulting gastrointestinal anatomy. Patients who are to begin oral feedings are usually started on clear liquids (see Table 11–1). As long as the patient is willing to eat regular food, there is no reason not to progress to a regular diet rapidly (after one meal of clear liquids), and there is **no need** to step through a progression from clear liquids to full liquids to a regular diet.

INFANT FORMULAS AND FEEDING

Bottle feeding is often chosen by the mother and, in general, commercially available formulas are recommended over homemade formulas because of their ease of preparation and their standardization of nutrients. Occasionally, special formulas are medically indicated and can only be supplied by commercially available formulas. Commonly used formulas are outlined in Table 11–7.

TABLE 11–7
Commonly Used Infant Formulas

Formula	Indications*
Human milk	
Donor	Preterm infant <1200 g
Maternal	All infants
Breast milk fortifiers	
Standard formulas	
Isoosmolar	
Enfamil 20	Full-term infants: as supplement to breast milk
Similac 20	Preterm infants >1800–2000 g
SMA 20	
Higher Osmolality	
Enfamil 24	Term infants: for infants on fluid restriction or
Similac 24 & 27	who cannot handle required volumes of 20-Cal
SMA† 24 & 27	formula to grow
Low Osmolality	
Similac 13	Preterm and term infants: for conservative initial feeding in infants who have not been fed orally for several days or weeks. Not for long-term use.
Soy formulas	
ProSobee (lactose- and sucrose-free)	Term infants: milk sensitivity, galactosemia, carbo-hydrate intolerance. Do not use in preterm in-fants. Phytates can bind calcium and cause rickets
Isomil (lactose-free)	
Nursoy (lactose-free)	
Protein hydrosylate formulas	
Nutramigen	Term infants: Gut sensitivity to proteins, multiple food allergies, persistent diarrhea, galac-tosemia.
Pregestimil	Preterm and term infants: disaccharidase defi-ciency, diarrhea, GI defects, cystic fibrosis, food allergy, celiac disease, transition from TPN to oral feeding
Alimentum	Term infants: protein sensitivity, pancreatic insuf-ficiency, diarrhea, allergies, colic, carbohydrate and fat malabsorption
Special formulas	
Portagen	Preterm and term infants: pancreatic or bile acid insufficiency, intestinal resection
Similac PM 60/40	Preterm and term infants: problem feeders on standard formula; infants with renal, cardio-vascular, digestive diseases that require de-creased protein and mineral levels, breast-feeding supplement, initial feeding

(continued)

**TABLE 11–7
(Continued)**

Formula	Indications*
Premature formulas	
Low osmolality	
Similac Special Care 20 Enfamil Premature 20 Preemie SMA 20	Premature infants (<1800–2000 g) who are growing rapidly. These formulas promote growth at intrauterine rates. Vitamin and mineral concentrations are higher to meet the needs of growth. Usually started on 20 Cal/oz and advanced to 24 Cal/oz as tolerated.
Isoosmolar	
Similac Special Care 24 Enfamil Special Care 24 Preemie SMA 24	Same as for low-osmolality premature formulas

*Multivitamin supplementation such as Polyvisol (Mead Johnson) ½ mL/d may be needed for commercial formulas if baby is taking <2 oz/d.
†SMA has decreased sodium content and can be used in patients with congestive heart failure, bronchopulmonary dysplasia, and cardiac disease. Modified and produced with permission from Gomella, TL (ed) Neonatology, 4th ed. Norwalk, CT, Appleton & Lange, 1999

11

Principles of Infant Feeding

Criteria for Initiating Infant Feeding: Most normal full-term infants are fed within the first 4 h after birth. The following criteria should usually be met before initiating infant feedings.

- The infant should have no history of excessive oral secretions, vomiting, or bile-stained gastric aspirate.
- An examination should have been performed with particular attention to the abdomen. The examination should be normal with normal bowel sounds and a nondistended, soft abdomen.
- The infant should be clinically stable.
- At least 6 h should pass before recently extubated infants are fed. The infant should be tolerating extubation well and have little respiratory distress.
- The respiratory rate should be <60 breaths/min for oral feeding and <80 breaths/min for gavage (tube) feeding. Tachypnea increases the risk of aspiration.

Prematurity: Considerable controversy remains concerning the timing of initial enteral feeding for the preterm infant. For the stable larger (>1500 g) premature infant, the first feeding may be given within the first 24 h of life. Early feeding may allow the release of enteric hormones that exert a trophic effect on the intestinal tract. On the other hand, apprehension about necrotizing enterocolitis (mostly in very low birth weight infants) in the following circumstances often precludes the initiation of enteral feeding: perinatal asphyxia, mechanical ventilation, presence of umbilical vessel catheters, patent ductus arteriosus, indomethacin treatment, sepsis, and frequent episodes of apnea and bradycardia.

No established policies are available, and delay and duration of delay in establishing feeding with those conditions varies for every institution. In general, enteral feeding is started in the first 3 d of life, with the objective of reaching full enteral feeding by 2–3 wk of life. Parenteral nutrition including amino acids and lipids should be started at the same time to provide for adequate caloric intake.

Choice of Formula: (See Table 11–7, page 224.) Human breast milk is recommended for feeding infants whenever possible. Breast-feeding has many advantages: It is ideal for virtually all infants, produces fewer infantile allergies, is immunoprotective to the infant due to the presence of immunoglobulins, is convenient and economical, and offers several theoretical psychologic benefits to both the mother and child. Occasionally, an infant cannot be breast-fed due to extreme prematurity or other problems such as a cleft palate.

If commercial infant formula is chosen, no special considerations are needed for normal full-term newborns. Selection of the best formula for preterm infants may require more care. The majority of infant formulas are isoosmolar (Similac 20, Enfamil 20, and SMA 20 with and without iron). These formulas are used most often for healthy infants. Formulas for premature infants, containing 24 Cal/oz (Similac 24, Enfamil 24, "preemie" SMA 24), are also isoosmolar and are indicated for rapidly growing premature infants. Many other "specialty" formulas are available for such conditions as milk and protein sensitivity, among others. Many pediatricians recommend vitamin supplements with some formulas if the infant is taking <32 oz/day. An iron-containing formula is generally recommended.

Feeding Guidelines

1. **Initial feeding.** For the initial feeding for all infants, use sterile water or 5% dextrose in water (D_5W) if the infant is not being breast-fed. Ten % dextrose in water ($D_{10}W$) should not be used because it is a hypertonic solution.

2. **Subsequent feedings.** There is controversy over whether infant formulas should be diluted for the next several feedings if the infant tolerates the initial one. Some clinicians advocate diluting formulas with sterile water and advance as tolerated (eg, ¼ strength, increase to ½ and then ¾ strength). Others feel this is unnecessary and that full-strength formula can be used if infants tolerate the initial feeding without difficulty. Breast milk is never diluted.

Oral Rehydration Solutions: Infants with mild or moderate dehydration, often due to diarrhea or vomiting, may benefit from oral rehydration formulas. These solutions typically include glucose, sodium, potassium, and bicarbonate or citrate. Common formulations include **Pedialyte, Lytren, Infalyte, Resol** and **Hydrolyte.**

12

TOTAL PARENTERAL NUTRITION

Common Indications
Nutritional Principles
Nitrogen Balance
TPN Solutions
Peripheral Parenteral Nutrition
TPN Additives

Fat Emulsions
Starting TPN
Assessing TPN Therapy
Stopping TPN
Disease-Specific TPN Formulations
Common TPN Complications

COMMON INDICATIONS

Total parenteral nutrition, also called "hyperalimentation," is the provision of all essential nutrients—protein, carbohydrates, lipids, vitamins, electrolytes, and trace elements—by the intravenous route. Nutrients may be supplied by either a peripheral or central vein. To provide a patient's entire nutritional requirement by vein, however, a central venous line must be used because of the tonicity of the fluid required. Peripheral veins simply cannot tolerate these hypertonic fluids, and thus peripheral IV alimentation can be used only as a supplement. Parenteral nutrition bypasses the GI tract and should be reserved for patients who are unable to receive nutritional support enterally. The principle of "if the gut works use it" is sound practice. How to determine the route of nutritional support is discussed on page 213. The following indications are appropriate for TPN initiation:

- Preoperatively, in the malnourished patient. There is no benefit for patients who are not malnourished.
- Postoperatively, for patients with a slow return of GI function or in patients with complications that limit or prohibit the use of the GI tract. The interval between surgery and initiation of nutritional support to prevent complications is not definitively known. However, many practitioners wait 7–10 d after surgery, anticipating the return of bowel function. If this does not occur, nutritional support is begun.
- Patients with Crohn's disease, ulcerative colitis, pancreatitis, fistulas, and short-bowel syndrome.
- Patients who are malnourished secondary to a disease or injury that results in inadequate oral intake. This may include patients with organ failure, severe metabolic stress, malignancies, burns, or trauma.

NUTRITIONAL PRINCIPLES

Nutritional assessment to determine the need for TPN requires a history (which includes weight changes over the previous 6 mo), physical, and laboratory evaluation. Indicators of long-term nutritional depletion include serum albumin and prealbumin levels, anthropometrics, and total lymphocyte count. Nutritional assessment is presented in detail in Chapter 11, page 206.

To establish the appropriate caloric amount for TPN therapy, estimate the patient's daily nonprotein calories and nitrogen requirements. The best method for calculating the BEE requirements for nonprotein calories is the Harris–Benedict equation (Chapter 11, page 209). The weight used in this equation determines the amount of calories needed to maintain that weight; therefore, if the patient is morbidly obese, the ideal weight should be established as a goal.

Calculation of Caloric Requirements in Stressed Patients

The BEE obtained from the Harris–Benedict equation reflects the number of calories from carbohydrate and fat that should be provided to maintain the patient's weight under non-stressed conditions. Stress, in nutritional terms, is correlated with the amount of catecholamines and cortisol released endogenously. These biochemical mediators promote protein breakdown, which is necessary to provide glucose for the brain and red blood cells.

- Mild stress: Supply total calories at approximately $1.2–1.4 \times$ BEE.
- Moderate stress: $1.5–1.75 \times$ BEE.
- Severe stress: $1.75–2.0 \times$ BEE.
- Ideally, 25–35 Cal/kg/d should be the dosing range. Bear in mind the patient's safety may be of concern should these values exceed a daily intake greater than 3000 Cal. In the event this occurs, dose conservatively until nitrogen balance data confirms the need for more aggressive caloric replacement.

12   Nutritional Component Considerations

The fundamental principle of TPN is the administration of sufficient protein to avoid catabolism of endogenous protein (muscle). Carbohydrates must be given to supply necessary calories (at a ratio of 150 Cal/g of nitrogen) to support these anabolic processes. Fat is given as a source of essential fatty acids. The basis for using TPN explains the necessity for protein, carbohydrate, and fat administration. In addition, TPN includes all necessary fluids, electrolytes, vitamins, and trace elements required to support life.

Studies have shown that doses between 4–7 mg/kg/min of carbohydrate (generally, do not exceed 5 mg/kg/min) provide optimal protein sparing with minimal liver toxicity. Assessment of the carbohydrate intake is important in order to limit complications from TPN.

Lipid calories should not exceed 3 g/kg/d due to increased complications. Additionally, no more than 50% of total daily calories should be administered as fat.

The best method for establishing a protein need for a given patient is the 24-h urine sample testing for **UUN levels.** This value reflects the amount of protein catabolism occurring daily. Urinary losses of 8–12 g/d are consistent with a mild stress condition, 14–18 g/d moderate stress, and greater than 20 g/d with severe stress.

Protein dosing should be modified based on the 24-h UUN and daily nitrogen balance. Initially, however, if the patient is considered mildly stressed, 0.8–1.2 g/kg/d is appropriate. In cases of moderate and severe stress (burned and head injured patients) 1.3–1.75 g/kg/d and 2–2.5 g/kg/d may be required, respectively. (*Note:* Generally, do not exceed 2.0 g/kg/d.) Several studies suggest that doses of protein in this range exceed the patients utilization capacity and may increase BUN. Adequate renal function must be present to provide such high protein loads. Patients with renal failure who are not receiving dialysis may be dosed at the minimum daily allowance, 0.6 g/kg/d, until a decision for dialysis is made. Once the patient is receiving dialysis, normal dosing may be instituted.

NITROGEN BALANCE

The best method for determining the adequacy of nutritional support is the calculation of nitrogen balance. A **positive nitrogen balance** implies that the amount of protein being administered is sufficient to cover the losses of endogenous protein that occur secondary to catabolism. This is the best therapeutic goal for TPN because it is impossible to determine whether the prescribed protein is preventing muscle breakdown or not. Once positive nitrogen balance has been achieved, however, protein replacement has been optimized. In critical care patients, nitrogen losses may be very high, and an attempt should be made to at least achieve nitrogen equilibrium. This may be impossible in the acute phase of injury, in severe trauma, or in burn cases. Thus, minimizing protein loss (–2 to –4 g/d) may be the goal during this period.

A **negative nitrogen balance** is indicative of insufficient protein replacement for the degree of skeletal muscle loss. Under most circumstances, an attempt to achieve positive nitrogen balance should be made. Patients with renal dysfunction or those who are severely stressed may not be able to achieve a positive balance due to safety concerns. The efficacy of protein doses exceeding 2.5 g/kg/d has not been established. Investigational agents (growth hormone, IGF-1) and specialized formulas (branched-chain amino acids, essential amino acids, glutamine) are being studied in these populations to assess their potential in improving nitrogen retention under these circumstances. The following are key concepts in determining nitrogen balance:

- Nitrogen balance = Nitrogen input – Nitrogen output.
- 1 g of nitrogen = 6.25 g of protein.
- Nitrogen input = (Protein in grams/6.25 g nitrogen).
- Nitrogen output = 24-h UUN + 4 g/d (nonurine loss).
- The conditions and disease states that increase the amount of nonurine losses for nitrogen include high-output fistulas and massive diarrhea. Fecal nitrogen measurements can be obtained but are difficult for nursing staff to perform.

Sample Determination of Nitrogen Balance

A patient is receiving 2 L TPN/24 h with 27.5 g crystalline amino acid (protein) solution per liter.

1. 27.5 g protein/L × 2 L = 55 g protein/24 h.
2. Recall that 1 g of nitrogen = 6.25 g of protein.
3. Nitrogen input = 55 g protein/6.25 g protein per gram N = 8.8 g.
4. Patient voided 22.5 dL urine/ 24 h with UUN 66 mg/dL.
5. Nitrogen lost in urine = 22.5 dL × 66 mg/dL = 1485 mg, or about 1.5 g.
6. Add 4.0 g for nonurine nitrogen loss.
7. Nitrogen output = 1.5 g + 4.0 = 5.5 g.
8. Nitrogen balance = Input – output = 8.8 – 5.5 = +3.3 g nitrogen.

TPN SOLUTIONS

Different strength CAA solutions are available (Table 12–1) to which the pharmacy can add varying concentrations of dextrose, electrolytes, vitamins, and trace elements. Most hospitals supply a "house," or standard, formula for patients with normal renal and hepatic function. Changes in the standard formulas can be made when necessary while a TPN solution is being infused based on measured laboratory parameters. Administration of TPN is never an emergency and in most cases can be provided within 24 h of prescribing. If a formula change is necessary based on a change in patient status, discontinue the TPN and replace it with $D_{10}W$ at the same rate until a new bag of TPN can be provided.

TABLE 12–1
Typical TPN Solutions for Adults

Component	Solution 1	Solution 2
CAA	4.25% (42.5 g/L)	4.25% (42.5 g/L)
Dextrose	25% (250 g/L, 850 Cal/L)	12.5% (125 g/L, 425 Cal/L)
Na	50 mEq/L	50 mEq/L
K	50 mEq/L	50 mEq/L
Ca	6 mEq/L	6 mEq/L
Mg	6 mEq/L	6 mEq/L
PO$_4$	15 mMol/L	15 mMol/L
Cl	45 mEq/L	45 mEq/L

Abbreviation: CAA = crystalline amino acids.

Amino acid formulas are supplied as CAA or SAA in concentrations ranging from 3.5–15%. These are diluted by the pharmacy to varying concentrations to provide for the necessary protein dose (2.75%, 4.25%, etc). The final concentrations of dextrose vary, but are usually either 12.5% or 25%. Examples of typical TPN solutions for adults are provided in Table 12–1.

The maximum rate of infusion of solution 1 from Table 12–1 should be 100–125 mL/h to avoid excessive glucose administration (remember to consider the patient's weight and the dosing guidelines of 4–7 mg/kg/min). Fat emulsions should be given with solution 1 to provide essential fatty acids (10%, 500 mL 3×/wk) or as an additional calorie source. Solution 2 is designed to be given at a maximum rate of 125 mL/h, but this only provides 1275 Cal from dextrose and must be supplemented with a fat emulsion (10% 500 mL = 550 Cal, 20% 500 mL = 1000 Cal).

Many hospitals have adopted a "three-in-one" solution for the standard house formula. This involves the administration of protein, carbohydrate, and fat from the same TPN bag over a 24-h period; in other words, the fat is not administered peripherally through a separate site. Caution should be used when altering the standard formula in this situation because the fat emulsion may be less stable to additives and makes incompatibilities less visible. For example, the solution will be milky in color, and a calcium–phosphate problem, normally easily seen, would not be apparent. Additions to these formulations should be done in conjunction with a pharmacist to ensure that precautions are taken for appropriate additive concentrations.

Remember, the solutions described in Table 12–1 contain full concentrations of electrolytes and are for patients with normal renal function. For patients with renal impairment, the concentrations of potassium, magnesium, phosphorus, and protein should be reduced (see page 235).

PERIPHERAL PARENTERAL NUTRITION

If a deep line is contraindicated or impossible, a peripheral TPN solution (<7% dextrose with 2.75% SAA, electrolytes, and vitamins) can be given. The majority of nonprotein calories must be given as an IV fat emulsion. In this case, caloric goals will not be met. A positive nitrogen balance will not be achieved in most patients receiving parenteral nutrition by this route. This is usually used only as a supplement to enteric feedings.

TPN ADDITIVES

Vitamins are a necessary component to TPN solutions. A product conforming to recommendations of the American Medical Association Nutrition Advisory Group is usually used, such as multivitamin infusion-12 (MVI-12). The contents of 2 vials is added to 1 L of TPN solution daily (Table 12–2).

In addition to MVI-12, 5–10 mg of vitamin K (phytonadione) must be given IM weekly. Vitamin K may also be added to the TPN and given as a 1-mg IV dose daily.

Several manufacturers sell a trace element supplement that conforms to the AMA group's guidelines. Each milliliter contains 1.0 mg zinc, 0.4 mg copper, 4.0 mg chromium, and 0.1 mg manganese. Suggested doses for trace elements are listed in Table 12–3, page 232.

Trace element deficiencies are rare in hospitalized patients receiving short-term TPN supplements. Supplementation should be routine, however, to ensure trace element availability for cell restoration. In patients receiving long-term support or home TPN, additional trace element supplementation may be necessary.

Iron can be given as an injectable iron–dextran complex (Dexferrum, InFeD). Note, however, that owing to the inconvenience of its administration, many clinicians avoid injectable iron–dextran. A complete medical and hematologic work-up is often indicated before instituting parenteral iron replacement. Prior to receiving the first dose, a test IV dose of 0.5 mL is recommended. Anaphylaxis is rare, but a period of 1h should elapse before the therapeutic dose of iron is administered. Use the following equation to determine the dose of iron:

$$\text{Total replacement dose (mL)} = 0.0476 \times \text{Weight (kg)} \times$$
$$[\text{Desired hemoglobin (g/dL)} - \text{Measured hemoglobin (g/dL)}]$$
$$+ \text{1 mL/5 kg weight (max 14 mL)}$$

12

Maximum Daily Dose: Adults >50 kg: 100 mg iron; Peds <5 kg: 25 mg iron, 5–10 kg: 50 mg iron, 0–50 kg: 100 mg iron

The iron–dextran is supplied in an injectable form of 50 mg (Fe)/mL. The calculated dose should be added to TPN at 2 mL/L until the entire dose has been given.

TABLE 12–2
Typical Vitamins Provided in 1 L of TPN by Adding 2 Vials of Standard MVI–12

Ascorbic acid	100 mg	Pyridoxine (B$_6$)	4 mg
Vitamin A	3300 IU	Dexpanthenol	15 mg
Vitamin D	200 IU	Vitamin E (α tocopherol)	10 IU
Biotin	60 µg	Thiamine (B$_1$)	3 mg
Folic acid	400 µg	Riboflavin (B$_2$)	3.6 mg
Vitamin B$_{12}$	5 µg	Niacin	40 mg

Abbreviation: MVI–12 = multivitamin infusion–12.

TABLE 12–3
Suggested Trace Element Dosing

Trace Element	Parenteral Dose per Day
Zinc	2.5–4.0 mg*
Copper	0.5–1.5 mg
Selenium	20–40mg
Chromium	10–15mg
Manganese	0.15–0.8 mg

*May be higher, up to 15 mg/d, in severe stress or in patients with high-output fistulas.

Insulin, when required, can be given subcutaneously as regular insulin using a sliding scale, as shown in Table 12–4. **But the preferred method is to add the insulin directly to the TPN solution.** This allows a constant infusion of insulin along with the infusion of dextrose, which avoids the peaks and valleys in blood glucose that occur when the sliding scale is used. The usual starting dose per liter of TPN is 10 units of regular insulin. Doses from 10 to 90 units/L may often be required. Insulin drips are not advised because TPN can be temporarily or permanently discontinued, which would then stop the insulin. Other additives include H_2 antagonists and heparin.

12

FAT EMULSIONS

Lipid emulsions were initially used only to provide essential fatty acids (linoleic acid, and linolenic acid in children). This could be done with minimal supplementation; as little as 4% of total calories per day would prevent the syndrome of EFAD. Most clinicians prescribe 500 mL of 10% lipid emulsion three times weekly to prevent this syndrome. The signs and symptoms of this deficiency include scaling skin rash, alopecia, and wound healing failure.

TABLE 12–4
Sliding Scale for Insulin Orders

Urine Glucose*	Regular Insulin Dose (Units, given SQ)
0–1+	0
2+	5
3+	10
4+	15
Any acetone: call house officer	

*Should be checked every 6 h as part of standing TPN orders.

Linoleic acid is a precursor to arachidonic acid, which is essential for prostaglandin and leukotriene synthesis. Once data became available establishing the problems associated with overfeeding of carbohydrate calories, the use of lipid for caloric supplementation became more recognized.

Commercially available intravenous fat emulsions are derived from soybean oil, with one product (**Liposyn II**) combining both soybean and safflower oil. The 10% products provide 1.1 Cal/mL, and the 20% products provide 2.0 Cal/mL. Pediatricians often prefer the Liposyn II product because of its higher percentage of linolenic acid.

Because the particle size of these emulsions closely approximates naturally occurring chylomicrons, parenteral infusion is possible. In addition, the emulsions are cleared from the bloodstream in a manner and rate similar to that for chylomicrons.

Before beginning the IV fat emulsion, the serum triglyceride level should be checked to ensure that hypertriglyceridemia is not present. Provided that the serum triglyceride level is below 400 mg/dL, the fat emulsion can be given over a 6–12-h period. The longer infusion rate is preferred. The first bottle should be given slowly (1 mL/min for 15 min to check for hypersensitivity reaction). Adverse reactions can include dyspnea, fever, chills, chest tightness, wheezing, headaches, and nausea.

Currently, the only absolute contraindication to the use of IV fat emulsion is type IV hypertriglyceridemia, although isolated cases of nontype IV intolerance to the solution have been reported. To monitor for the clearing of the fat from the bloodstream, a trough serum triglyceride level should be tested 8–12 h following the daily infusion of the fat emulsion. Because fat emulsions are primarily composed of triglycerides (essentially cholesterol free), if the blood is mistakenly drawn while the fat is being infused or shortly thereafter, the serum triglyceride level will be markedly elevated. Other possible contraindications include lipoid nephrosis, severe hepatic failure, and allergy to eggs (egg phosphatides are used as the emulsifying agent).

Fat emulsions can be administered through peripheral veins, although the vein may be damaged and cease to be functional in 2–3 days. For this reason, it is usually recommended that the fat emulsion be infused into the central line under strict aseptic technique via a sterile Y-connector. As mentioned earlier, some institutions combine the lipid with the TPN formula in one bag for 24-h administration. This limits the clinicians ability to validate fat clearance from the blood and makes baseline triglyceride data extremely important.

STARTING TPN

In general, TPN should not be started until a patient has a stable fluid and electrolyte profile. It is usually unwise to begin TPN in a patient who requires large amounts of fluid, may need resuscitation for trauma, or is septic. Once a patient's fluid and electrolyte requirements are reasonably stable, TPN can be started safely. The initiation of TPN is never an emergency.

Placement of a deep line must be done aseptically, as outlined in Chapter 13, page 253. Infection (bacteremia, fungemia) arising from the catheter or the catheter–skin interface is the most common complication of TPN. Many hospitals now have standardized order forms for starting patients on TPN.

1. **Baseline laboratory tests:**
   a. CBC with differential and platelets
   b. PT and PTT
   c. SMA-7 and SMA-12; in particular check phosphate, glucose, and routine electrolytes (Na, K, Cl)
   d. Urinalysis
   e. Baseline weight

2. **Order the type of TPN** desired along with the additives and supplements. Medications are generally not added to TPN solutions except insulin and H_2 receptor blockers. A 0.22-μm filter should be used with aqueous TPN (no fat). A 1.2-μm filter should be used with three-in-one TPN.
3. **Nursing orders:**
    a. Check urine for sugar and acetone every 6-8 h, house officer should be called if sugar is >2+ or acetone is present.
    b. Take vital signs every shift.
    c. Change tubing and deep-line dress every other day (or per hospital procedure).
    d. Weigh patient every other day.
    e. Monitor daily fluid balance
4. **Laboratory monitoring:**
    a. SMA-7 daily until patient is stable, then every other day.
    b. CBC with differential, platelets, PT/PTT, twice weekly.
    c. SMA-12 twice weekly (especially liver function tests).
    d. Triglyceride trough level (obtained at least 6 h after infusion has stopped, preferably prior to hanging next bottle of fat) once or twice weekly.
    e. 24-h urine for nitrogen balance determinations and creatinine clearance once or twice weekly.
5. **Begin the solution at 25–50 mL/h** when using a 25% or 50–75 mL/h when using a 12.5% dextrose solution. Increase by 25 mL/h every 24 h, providing the urine sugar levels are negative. Advance to the maximum rate based on the calculated daily caloric need (page 209). **Begin the IV fat emulsion the next day,** provided that the serum triglyceride levels are less than 400 mg/dL. Remember that glucose intolerance is the major adverse effect seen during the initial infusion period. Urine sugar and acetone levels should be less than 2+, and serum glucose values less than 180–200 mg/dL. If the sugar level rises above these levels, insulin must be given to achieve the desired level of caloric intake. If glucose intolerance develops when using a 25% dextrose solution, consider decreasing the amount of calories from dextrose and increasing the calories from fat. (Be sure to check that overfeeding is not occurring, ie, >4–7 mg/kg/min, in this case reduce the dose of carbohydrate prior to the addition of insulin). Glucose intolerance arising once the patient has been stabilized may signify sepsis.

ASSESSING TPN THERAPY

Nitrogen balance is a good measure of the success of the TPN regimen because the goal is protein-sparing (see page 229). Serum albumin will not change appreciably during TPN therapy lasting less than 3 wk. This is due to albumin's long half-life of 22–24 d. In stressed patients, albumin often falls due to reduced production because the body shifts to increased production of acute-phase reactant proteins.

STOPPING TPN

TPN can usually be stopped when necessary. Although widely practiced, there is rarely a need for a formal weaning schedule. If there are concerns about hypoglycemia, then a 10% dextrose solution can be administered after cessation of the TPN.

DISEASE-SPECIFIC TPN FORMULATIONS

Cardiac Failure: In patients with CHF, reduce water from 1 to 0.5 mL/Cal or 500 mL insensible loss plus measured water losses. This limits overloading with water from TPN. Other considerations include providing energy needs at the BEE + 30% for initiation of TPN calories, limiting protein initially to 0.8–1 g/kg and reducing sodium to 0.5–1.5 g/d.

Diabetes: Consider increasing the percentage of calories provided from fat. Ideally, blood sugar should be well controlled or at least not >200 when initiating TPN. Remember that no more than 50% of total intake should be from fat and not more than 3 g/kg/d. Fat provides 9 Cal/g. Commercial lipid emulsions provide 1.1 or 2 Cal/mL. Insulin should be added to the solution initially at 5–10 units/bag in patients requiring >20 units of insulin daily.

Geriatrics: Patients older than 75 years have a documented need for fewer calories. Use caution in monitoring total fluids to prevent overload.

Inflammatory Bowel Disease: TPN can be initiated in these patients at approximately 1.5 × RME at 30 Cal/kg of ideal body weight. Protein needs vary from 1 to 2 g/kg of ideal body weight daily. Dose the protein based on a 24-h UUN. *Note:* Patients with fistulas lose nitrogen via this route and need additional protein. Zinc losses may be greater in this group of IBD patients also.

Liver Disease: Specialized formulas of amino acids that contain primarily branched-chain amino acids (leucine, isoleucine, and valine) are available for use in cases of liver disease. Theoretically, these products may improve arousal from hepatic encephalopathy by competing with the aromatic amino acids that are precursors for some centrally active amines. There is no definitive evidence that branched-chain formulas improve patient outcome. The specialized formulas should only be used in cases of severe hepatic disease accompanied by encephalopathy. In other clinical conditions of liver disease, standard formulas should be used. Lipid emulsions are not recommended in cases of severe hepatic failure when hypertriglyceridemia is present.

Pancreatic Disease: Total energy needs may be high in this disease (35 Cal/kg). Protein should be initiated at 1.5 g/kg/d. Intravenous fat may be administered in these cases because it is metabolized by peripheral tissue lipases. A reasonable nonprotein system would be 70% carbohydrate and 30% fat.

Pulmonary Disease: Carbohydrate metabolism produces higher amounts of CO_2 than does fat metabolism. Consequently, the patient with CO_2 retention problems often is stressed if overfed with carbohydrates. Increasing the percentage of daily nonprotein calories provided by fat (not >60%) may decrease the CO_2 load and assist with ventilator weaning. Higher fat percentages influence oxygen diffusion capacity and are not beneficial, especially in cases of mild pulmonary compromise. Phosphate depletion is a second clinically relevant concern in this population due to the depression of the hypoxic ventilatory drive. Once patients are started on TPN, PO_4^{-2} often decreases due to the incorporation into ATP. Adequate supplementation and monitoring is very important in this group of patients.

Renal Failure: Several considerations become important in this disease. If a patient is not receiving dialysis or is not a dialysis candidate, protein must be restricted to 0.6–0.8 g/kg/d, and total energy needs must be limited to approximately 30 Cal/kg/d. Weight should be ideal or admission weight, so as to control for the influence of water retention. Specialized amino acid formulas have been developed for this group of patients. These products provide higher concentrations of essential amino acids than the standard amino acid products. Theoretically, the nitrogen waste products are recycled to make the nonessential amino acids, thereby reducing the BUN content. Risks exist, however, for elevations in ammonia when arginine is not also supplemented. Consequently, manufacturers have modified the original formulas to include several nonessential amino acids. Due to these changes, the renal products provide a very similar amino acid profile to those of the SAA solutions at very low concentrations (2.5%). The cost differential can be significant. It is therefore recommended that patients with renal dysfunction receive SAA formulas at a reduced concentration to provide the minimum daily allowance of protein. TPN should not be supplemented with potassium or magnesium, and sodium should be reduced to 40–180 mEq/d once the GFR is <10 mL/min.

Patients receiving hemodialysis or peritoneal dialysis may be fed protein similarly to patients without renal disease. Doses of 1–1.2 g/kg/d may be used. Nitrogen balance calculations are not useful in this population due to the problem of renal clearance of urea waste inherent to kidney disease.

Sepsis or Trauma: Sepsis and trauma causes hypermetabolism and requires greater numbers of calories from nonprotein (30–35 Cal/kg) and protein (2–2.5 g/kg/d) sources. Estimates of RME should be increased by 50% initially, and some cases may support up to 100%. Note that feeding >3000 Cal/d is not recommended. Specialized amino acid formulas are also available for this group of patients. Again, these formulas include higher concentrations of the branched-chain amino acids. The reason for their inclusion in this population is to provide substrate directly to the skeletal muscle undergoing catabolism to provide gluconeogenic precursors. Although these formulas have been shown to normalize the amino acid profile and in some cases improve nitrogen balance, no studies have demonstrated an improved patient outcome. The additional cost of these formulas is a deterrent to their routine use in these populations until further data are available. Additional zinc supplementation is often recommended in this group of patients. Studies have shown losses to be increased in stress; therefore, daily supplementation of up to 15 mg of zinc may be appropriate.

COMMON TPN COMPLICATIONS

Hyperosmolar Nonketotic Coma: Usually found in improperly monitored patients with impaired insulin responses. Caused by excessive glucose levels, usually corrected by administration of insulin and rehydration. Sustained hyperglycemia (>220 mg/dL) depresses monocyte activity and could compromise the immune defenses.

Infection (Sepsis): The care of the deep-line site and tubing must be meticulous. Suspect sepsis if a previously stable patient becomes glucose-intolerant. If the patient becomes septic, the deep line should be considered a possible source. If no other source of infection can be identified, the deep line must be removed or changed and the tip sent for routine culture and sensitivity. *Candida albicans* is the most frequently encountered pathogen on the catheter, followed by *Staphylococcus aureus, Staphylococcus epidermidis* and gram-negative rods.

Hypophosphatemia: Severe hypophosphatemia can occur in patients started on TPN after severe weight loss and those with conditions such as anorexia nervosa (refeeding syndrome). This may also result from increased metabolic processes requiring phosphate and can significantly hamper weaning from the ventilator.

Elevated Liver Function Tests: The usual cause is excessive glucose infusion. When the primary metabolic pathway for glucose becomes saturated, excess glucose is converted to intracellular triglycerides in the liver. This is especially seen when rates exceed 4–7 mg/kg/min. A reduction in carbohydrate calories, supplementing with fat, is recommended.

Cholestasis: This often occurs secondary to overfeeding of fat calories (>3 g/kg/d or >60% of total nonprotein calories).

Hyperkalemia: This is the most common electrolyte disturbance seen with TPN. Most TPN formulations contain potassium 40–50 mEq/L and are intended for patients with normal renal function. Excess potassium over and above that required for maintenance and urine losses (usually 3–5 mEq/g nitrogen) is included. Potassium must be closely followed in the elderly and those with impaired renal function. Additionally, many drugs contribute to potassium balance problems. These include some antibiotics that are potassium salts (eg, penicillins); oral phosphate supplements (Neutra-Phos); ACE inhibitors, which reduce potassium excretion (Captopril, Enalapril); and potassium-sparing diuretics (triamterene, spironolactone).

Metabolic Alkalosis: Modern SAAs are present as the acetate salt (80–100 mEq/L), which is converted to bicarbonate in vivo. In postoperative patients with nasogastric tubes, the loss of chloride, together with the high infusion of the acetate, can lead to a metabolic alkalosis. The increased use of histamine blockers and antacids in intensive care patients has also contributed to a higher incidence of this problem. Treating this condition requires increasing the chloride level in the solution and reducing the acetate.

Hyponatremia: Serum sodium levels of 127–135 mEq/L are commonly seen in patients on TPN. The cause is controversial but is probably due to mild SIADH; therefore the problem is probably an excess of water and not deficiency of sodium. It is usually asymptomatic and does not require a change in formula unless the sodium drops below 125 mEq/L.

Hypermagnesemia: This is usually seen in patients with renal failure. Antacid therapy may also contribute to this condition. If potassium is reduced in the TPN, magnesium should also be reduced.

12

13

BEDSIDE PROCEDURES

Procedure Basics
Amniotic Fluid Fern Test
Arterial Line Placement
Arterial Puncture
Arthrocentesis (Diagnostic and
    Therapeutic)
Bone Marrow Aspiration and Biopsy
Central Venous Catheterization
Chest Tube Placement
Cricothyrotomy (Needle and Surgical)
Culdocentesis
Doppler Pressures
Electrocardiogram
Endotracheal Intubation
Fever Work-up
Gastrointestinal Intubation
Heelstick
Internal Fetal Scalp Monitoring
Injection Techniques

Intrauterine Pressure Monitoring
IV Techniques
Lumbar Puncture
Orthostatic Blood Pressure
    Measurement
Pelvic Examination
Pericardiocentesis
Peripherally Inserted Central Catheter
    (PICC Line)
Peritoneal Lavage
Peritoneal (Abdominal) Paracentesis
Pulmonary Artery Catheterization
Pulsus Paradoxus Measurement
Sigmoidoscopy (Rigid)
Skin Biopsy
Skin Testing
Thoracentesis
Urinary Tract Procedures
Venipuncture

13

PROCEDURE BASICS

Universal Precautions

Universal precautions should be used whenever an invasive procedure exposes the operator to potentially infectious body fluids. Not all patients infected with transmissible pathogens can be identified at the time of hospital admission or even later in their course. Because pathogens transmitted by bloody and body fluids pose a hazard to personnel caring for such patients, particularly during invasive procedures, certain precautions are now *required* for *routine* care of **all** patients whether or not they have been placed on isolation precautions of any type. For these reasons, the CDC calls these Universal Precautions.

1. Wash hands before and after **all** patient contact.
2. Wash hands before and after **all** invasive procedures.
3. Wear gloves in **every** instance in which contact with blood is certain or likely. For example, wear gloves for all venipunctures, for all IV starts, for IV manipulation, and for wound care.
4. Wear gloves once and discard. Do not wear the same pair to perform tasks on two different patients or two different tasks at different sites on the same patient.
5. Wear gloves in **every** instance in which contact with any body fluid is likely, including urine, feces, wound secretions, respiratory tract care, thoracentesis, paracentesis, etc.

6. Wear gown when splatter of blood or of body fluids on clothing seems likely.
7. Additional barrier precautions may be necessary for certain invasive procedures when significant splatter or aerosol generation seems likely. This does not occur during most routine patient care activities. It may occur in certain instances in the operating room, emergency room, the ICUs, during invasive procedures, and during cardiopulmonary resuscitation. Always wear masks when goggles are worn and vice versa.

Informed Consent

Patients should be counseled before any procedure concerning the reason for it and the potential risks and benefits from it. Explaining the various steps often can make the patient more cooperative and the procedure easier on both parties. In general, procedures such as bladder catheterization, NG intubation, or venipuncture do not require a written informed consent beyond normal hospital sign in protocols. More invasive procedures, such as thoracentesis or lumbar puncture, for example, require written consent and must be obtained by a licensed physician.

Basic Equipment

Table 13–1 lists useful collections of instruments and supplies, often packaged together, that aid in the completion of the procedures outlined in this chapter. Local anesthesia is discussed in Chapter 17.

The size of various catheters, tubes and needles is often designated by **French unit (1 french = ⅓ mm in diameter)** or by "gauge." Reference listings for these designations can be found in Figure 13–1A. Designations of surgical scalpels, used in the performance of many basic bedside procedures and in the operating room are shown in Figure 13–1B.

TABLE 13–1
13
Instruments and Supplies Used in the Completion of Common Bedside Procedures

---

MINOR PROCEDURE TRAY

Sterile gloves
Sterlile towels/drapes
4×4 gauze sponges
Povidone–iodine (Betadine) prep solution
Syringes: 5-, 10-, 20-mL
Needles: 18-, 20-, 22-, 25-gauge
1% Lidocaine (with or without epinephrine)
Adhesive tape

INSTRUMENT TRAY

Scissors
Needle holder
Hemostat
Scalpel and blade (No. 10 for adult, No. 15 for children or delicate work)
Suture of choice (2-0 or 3-0 silk or nylon on cutting needle; cutting needle best for suturing to skin)

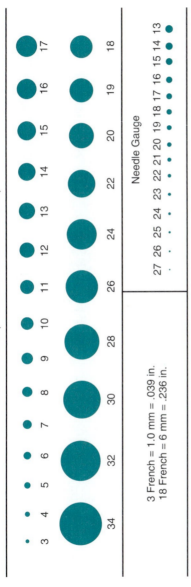

FIGURE 13-1A: French catheter guide and needle gauge reference. (Courtesy Cook Urological.)

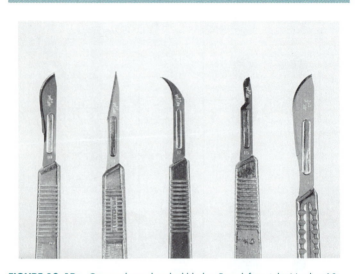

FIGURE 13–1B: Commonly used scalpel blades. From left to right: Number 10, 11, 12, 15, and 20. The No. 10 is the standard surgical blade; No. 11 is useful for press cuts into abscesses; No. 12 is used to open tubular structures; No. 15 is widely used for bedside procedures and for more delicate work; the No. 20 blade is used when large incisions are called for.

13

AMNIOTIC FLUID FERN TEST

Indication

- Assessment of rupture of membranes

Materials

- Sterile speculum and swab
- Glass slide and microscope
- Nitrazine paper (optional)

Procedure

1. After placing a sterile speculum in the vagina, a sample of fluid which has "pooled" in the vault is swabbed onto a glass slide and allowed to air dry.
2. Amniotic fluid produces a microscopic arborization or "fern" pattern, which may be visualized with 10× magnification. False-positive results may occur if cervical mucus is collected; however, the ferning pattern of mucus is coarser. This test is unaffected by meconium, vaginal pH, and blood-to-amniotic-fluid ratios ≤ 1:10. Samples heavily contaminated with blood may not fern.

3. An additional test used to detect ruptured membranes entails the use of nitrazine paper, which has a pH turning point of 6.0. Normal vaginal pH in the pregnant woman ranges from 4.5 to 6.0; the pH of amniotic fluid is 7.0–7.5. A positive nitrazine test is manifested by a color change in the paper from yellow to blue. False-positive results are more common with the nitrazine paper test because blood, meconium, semen, alkalotic urine, cervical mucus, and vaginal infections can all raise the pH.

Complication

- Bacteria may be introduced if sterile technique is not used.

ARTERIAL LINE PLACEMENT
Indications

- Continuous blood pressure readings are needed (for patients on pressors, with unstable pressures, etc).
- Frequent arterial blood gases are needed.

Contraindications

- Arterial insufficiency with poor collateral circulation (See Allen test, page 246)
- Thrombolytic therapy or coagulopathy (relative)

Materials

- Minor procedure and instrument tray (page 240)
- Heparin flush solution (1:1000 dilution)
- Arterial line set-up per local ICU routine (transducer, tubing and pressure bag with preheparinized saline, monitor)
- Arterial line catheter kit **or** 20-gauge catheter over needle, 1½–2 in. (Angiocath) with 0.025-in. guidewire (optional)

13

Procedure

(See Fig. 13–2)

1. The radial artery is most frequently used and that approach is described here. Other sites, in decreasing order of preference, are the ulnar, dorsalis pedis, femoral, brachial, and axillary arteries. Never puncture the radial and ulnar arteries in the same hand because this may compromise blood supply to the hand and fingers.
2. Verify the patency of the collateral circulation between the radial and ulnar arteries using the Allen test (page 246) or Doppler ultrasound probe. Have the ICU staff prepare the flush bag, tubing, and transducer, paying particular attention to removing the air bubbles.
3. Place the extremity on an armboard with a roll of gauze behind the wrist to hyperextend the joint. Prep with povidone–iodine, and drape with sterile towels. Wear gloves and a mask.
4. Carefully palpate the artery, and choose the puncture site where it appears most superficial. Raise a very small skin wheal at the puncture site with 1% lidocaine using a 25-gauge needle.
5. a. **Standard technique:** See Figure 13–2. While palpating the path of the artery with the left hand, advance the 20-gauge (preferably 2 in. long) catheter-over-needle assembly into the artery at a 30-degree angle to the skin. Once a "flash" of blood is

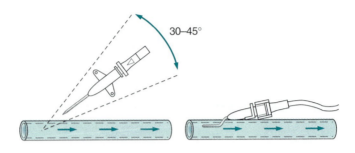

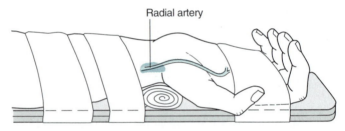

FIGURE 13–2 Technique for arterial line placement. (Reprinted, with permission, from: Gomella TL [ed]: *Neonatology: Basic Management, On-Call Problems, Diseases, Drugs,* 4th ed. Appleton & Lange, Norwalk CT, 1998.)

seen in the hub, advance the entire unit 1–2 mm, so that the needle and catheter are in the artery. If blood flow in the hub stops, carefully pull the entire unit back until flow is reestablished. Once the catheter is in the artery, hold the needle steady, and advance the catheter over the needle into the artery. The catheter should slide smoothly into the artery. Withdraw the needle completely and check for arterial blood flow from the catheter. A catheter that does not spurt blood is not in position. Briefly occlude the artery with manual pressure while the pressure tubing is being connected. *Note:* The pressure tubing system must be preflushed to clear all air bubbles prior to connection.

b. **Alternative procedure** ("through-and-through" technique): Use the same approach to the artery as in part a, however, purposely puncture the artery through the anterior and the posterior walls. This method is probably most useful in children and infants. Once a flash of blood is seen in the hub, advance the entire unit together until blood no longer fills the hub. (This can be done in a single motion.) S-l-o-w-l-y withdraw the entire unit until blood starts to fill the hub, then advance the catheter as the needle is withdrawn. Connect the tubing.

   c. **Prepackaged kit technique:** Kits, sometimes referred to as "quick catheters" are available with a needle and guidewire that allow the Seldinger technique to be used. Place the entry needle at a 30-degree angle to the skin site and insert until a flash of blood rises in the catheter. The catheter does not need to be advanced, but advance both the guidewire portion (orange handle in some kits) and the catheter into the vessel. Remove the wire and connect it to the pressure tubing.

6. If placement is not successful, apply pressure to the site for 5 min and reattempt one or two more times. If still not successful, move to another site.

7. Suture in place with 3-0 silk, and apply a sterile dressing. Splint the dorsum of the wrist to limit mobility and provide catheter stability.

8. If larger vessels such as the femoral artery are used, the clinician can employ the **Seldinger technique** for femoral artery cannulation: locate the vessel lumen with a small-gauge, thin-walled needle; pass a 0.035 floppy-tipped J("J" describes the configuration of the end of the floppy wire) guidewire into the lumen; and use the guidewire to pass a larger catheter into the vessel. Use a 16-gauge catheter assembly at least 6 in. long for the femoral artery.

9. Replace arterial lines using a different site every 4–7 d to decrease risk of infection.

10. Any amount of heparin can make the results of coagulation studies (PTT) inaccurate. If the blood is drawn from the arterial line and unexpectedly high results are obtained, always repeat the test and consider using standard venipuncture technique (see page 309). Despite the removal of the first 5–10 mL from the line, some of the heparinized flush solution can still get into the lab sample tube, yielding unreliable results.

11. Always compare the arterial line pressure with a standard cuff pressure. An occasional difference is normal (10–20 mm Hg) and should be incorporated when following the blood pressure.

Complications

Thrombosis, hematoma, arterial embolism, arterial spasm, arterial insufficiency with tissue loss, infection, hemorrhage, pseudo-aneurysm formation

ARTERIAL PUNCTURE

Indications

- Blood gas determinations and when arterial blood is needed for chemistry determinations (eg, ammonia levels)

Materials

- Blood gas-sampling kit
or
- 3–5-mL syringe
- 23–25-gauge for radial; 20–22 acceptable for femoral artery
- Heparin (1000 U/mL), 1 mL
- Alcohol or povidone–iodine swabs
- Cup of ice

Procedure

1. Use a "heparinized" syringe for blood gas and a "nonheparinized" syringe for chemistry determinations. If a blood gas kit is not available, a 3–5-mL syringe can be heparinized by drawing up 1 mL of 1:1000 solution of heparin through a small-gauge

needle (23–25-gauge) into the syringe, pulling the plunger all the way back. The heparin is then expelled, leaving only a small amount, which coats the syringe.

2. In order of preference, the arteries are radial, femoral, and brachial. If using the radial artery, perform an **Allen test** prior to puncture of the artery to verify the patency of the ulnar artery. You do not want to damage the radial artery if there is no flow in the ulnar artery. To perform the Allen test, have the patient make a tight fist. Occlude both the radial and ulnar arteries at the wrist and have the patient open the hand. While maintaining pressure on the radial artery, release the ulnar artery. If the ulnar artery is patent, the hand should flush red within 6 s. A radial puncture can then be safely performed. If the color return is delayed on part of the hand or remains pale, do **not** perform the puncture because the collateral flow is inadequate. Choose an alternative site.

3. If using the femoral artery, use the mnemonic **NAVEL** to aid in locating the important structures in the groin. Palpate the femoral artery just below the inguinal ligament. From lateral to medial the structures are **N**erve, **A**rtery, **V**ein, **E**mpty space, **L**ymphatic.

4. Palpate the chosen artery carefully. You may wish to inject 1 lidocaine subcutaneously for anesthesia (use a small needle such as a 25–27-gauge), but this often turns a "one-stick procedure" into a "two-stick" one. Palpate the artery proximally and distally with two fingers, or trap the artery between two fingers placed on either side of the vessel. Hyperextension of the joint often brings the radial and brachial arteries closer to the surface.

5. Prep the area with either a povidone–iodine solution or alcohol swab.

6. Hold the syringe like a pencil with the needle bevel up, and enter the skin at a 60–90-degree angle. Often you can feel the arterial pulsations as you approach the artery.

7. Maintaining a slight negative pressure on the syringe, obtain blood on the downstroke or on slow withdrawal (after both sides of the artery have been punctured). Aspirate very slowly. A good arterial sample, because of the pressure in the vessel, should require only minimal back pressure. If a glass syringe or special blood-gas syringe is used, the barrel usually fills spontaneously and it is not necessary to pull on the plunger.

8. If the vessel is not encountered, withdraw the needle without coming out of the skin, and redirect it to the pulsation.

9. After obtaining the sample, withdraw the needle quickly and apply **firm** pressure at the site for **at least 5 min** or longer if the patient is receiving anticoagulants. Apply pressure even if a sample was not obtained in order to prevent a compartment syndrome from extravasated blood.

10. If the sample is for a blood-gas determination, expel any air from the syringe, mix the contents thoroughly by twirling the syringe between your fingers, remove and dispose of the needle, and make the syringe airtight with a cap. Place the syringe in an ice bath if more than a few minutes will elapse before the sample is processed. Note the inspired oxygen concentration and time of day on the lab slip.

ARTHROCENTESIS (DIAGNOSTIC AND THERAPEUTIC)

Indications

- **Diagnostic.** Arthrocentesis is helpful in the diagnosis of new-onset arthritis; to rule out infection in acute or chronic, unremitting joint effusion.
- **Therapeutic.** To instill steroids and maintain drainage of septic arthritis; relief of tense hemarthrosis or effusion

Contraindications

Cellulitis at injection site. Relative contraindication is a bleeding disorder; use caution if coagulopathy or thrombocytopenia is present or if the patient is receiving anticoagulants.

Materials

- Minor procedure tray (page 240) (18- or 20-gauge needle (smaller for finger or toe)
- Ethyl chloride spray can be substituted for lidocaine.
- Two heparinized tubes for cell count and crystal examination
- Discuss with your microbiology lab their preference for transporting fluid for bacterial, fungal, AFB culture, and Gram's stain. A Thayer–Martin plate is needed if *Neisseria gonorrhoeae* (GC) is suspected.
- A small syringe containing a long-acting corticosteroid such as Depo-Medrol or triamcinolone is optional for therapeutic arthrocentesis.

Procedures, General

1. Obtain the patient's consent after describing the procedure and complications.
2. Determine the optimal site for aspiration, identify landmarks, and mark site with indentation or sterile marking pen. Avoid injection of tendons.
3. When aspiration is to be followed by corticosteroid injection, maintaining a sterile field with sterile implements minimizes the risk of infection.
4. Clean the area with povidone–iodine, dry and wipe over the aspiration site with alcohol. Povidone–iodine can render cultures negative. Let the alcohol dry before beginning procedure.
5. Anesthetize the area with lidocaine using a 25-gauge needle, taking care not to inject into the joint space. Lidocaine is bactericidal. Avoid preparations containing epinephrine, especially in a small digit. Alternatively, spray the area with ethyl chloride ("freeze spray") just prior to needle aspiration.
6. Insert the aspirating needle, applying a small amount of vacuum to the syringe. When the capsule is entered, fluid usually flows easily. Remove as much fluid as possible, repositioning the syringe if necessary.
7. If corticosteroid is to be injected, remove the aspirating syringe from the needle, which is still in the joint space. It is helpful to ensure that the syringe can easily be removed from the needle before step 6. Attach the syringe containing corticosteroid, pull back on the plunger to ensure you are not in a vein, and inject contents. Never inject steroids when there is any possibility of an infected joint. Remove the needle, and apply pressure to the area (leakage of subcutaneous steroids can lead to localized atrophy of the skin. Generally, the equivalent of 40 mg of methylprednisolone is injected into large joints such as the knee and 20 mg into medium-size joints such as the ankle or wrist. Warn the patient that a postinjection "flare" characterized by pain several hours after the injection can be treated with ice and NSAIDs.
8. Note the volume aspirated from the joint. As an example, the knee typically contains 3.5 mL of synovial fluid; in inflammatory, septic, or hemorrhagic arthritis, the volume can be much higher. A quick bedside test for viscosity is to allow a drop of fluid to fall from the tip of the needle. Normal synovial fluid is highly viscous and forms a several-inch long string; decreased viscosity is seen in infection. A mucin clot test (normally forms in < 1 min; a delayed result suggests inflammation) was once a standard test for RA, but is not now routinely performed.
9. Joint fluid is usually sent for:

   - Cell count and differential (purple or green top tube)
   - Microscopic crystal exam using polarized light microscopy (purple or green top tube); **normally** no debris, crystals, or bacteria are seen; urate crystals are present with gout; calcium pyrophosphate in pseudo-gout.
   - Glucose (red top tube) See Table 13–2.

- Gram's stain, and cultures for bacteria, fungi, and AFB as indicated (check with your lab or deliver immediately in a sterile tube with no additives.)
- Cytology if a malignant effusion is suspected clinically.

Arthrocentesis of the Knee

1. Fully extended the knee with the patient supine. Wait until the patient has a relaxed quadriceps muscle because its contraction plants the patella against the femur, making aspiration painful.
2. Insert the needle posterior to the *medial* portion of the patella into the patellar-femoral groove. Direct the advancing needle slightly posteriorly and inferiorly (Fig. 13–3)

Arthrocentesis of the Wrist

1. The easiest site for aspiration is between the navicular bone and radius on the dorsal wrist. Locate the distal radius between the tendons of the extensor pollicis longus and the extensor carpi radialis longus to the second finger. This site is just ulnar to the anatomic snuff box. Direct the needle perpendicular to the mark (Fig. 13–4).

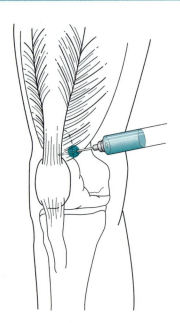

FIGURE 13–3 Arthrocentesis of the knee. (Reprinted, with permission, from: Haist SA et al [eds]: *Internal Medicine on Call,* 3rd ed. McGraw-Hill, New York, 2001.)

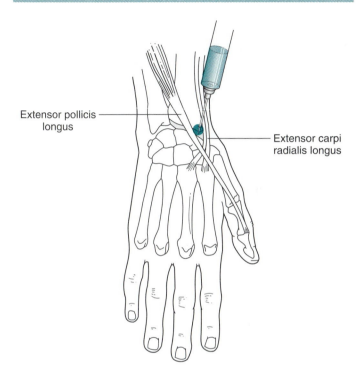

Extensor pollicis
longus

Extensor carpi
radialis longus

13

FIGURE 13–4   Arthrocentesis of the wrist. (Reprinted, with permission, from: Haist
SA et al [eds]: *Internal Medicine on Call,* 3rd ed. McGraw-Hill, New York, 2001.)

Arthrocentesis of the Ankle

1.   The most accessible site is between the tibia and the talus. Position the angle of the foot
     to leg at 90 degrees. Make a mark lateral and anterior to the medial malleolus and me-
     dial and posterior to the tibialis anterior tendon. Direct the advancing needle posteriorly
     toward the heel.
2.   The **subtalar ankle joint** does not communicate with the ankle joint and is difficult to
     aspirate even by an expert. Be aware that "ankle pain" may originate in the subtalar
     joint rather than in the ankle (Fig. 13–5).

Synovial Fluid Interpretation

Normal synovial fluid values and values in disease states are found in Table 13–2.

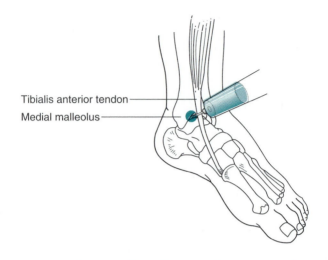

FIGURE 13–5   Arthrocentesis of the ankle. (Reprinted, with permission, from: Haist SA et al [eds]: *Internal Medicine on Call,* 3rd ed. McGraw-Hill, New York, 2001.)

Noninflammatory Arthritis: Osteoarthritis, traumatic, aseptic necrosis, osteochondritis desiccans

Inflammatory Arthritis: Gout (usually associated with elevated serum uric acid), pseudo-gout, RA, rheumatic fever, collagen–vascular disease

Septic Arthritis: Pyogenic bacterial (*S. aureus* GC and *S. epidermidis* most common), TB

Hemorrhagic: Hemophilia or other bleeding diathesis, trauma, with or without fracture

Complications

Infection, bleeding, pain. Postinjection flare of joint pain and swelling can occur after steroid injection and persist for up to 24 h. This complication is felt to be a crystal-induced synovitis due to the crystalline suspension used in long-acting steroids.

BONE MARROW ASPIRATION AND BIOPSY

Indications

- Evaluation of unexplained anemia, thrombocytopenia, leukopenia
- Evaluation of unexplained leukocytosis, thrombocytosis, search for malignancy primary to the marrow (leukemia, myeloma) or metastatic to the marrow (small-cell lung cancer, breast cancer)

TABLE 13–2
Synovial Fluid Analysis and Categories for Differential Diagnosis*

Parameter	Normal	Noninflammatory	Inflammatory	Septic	Hemorrhagic
Viscosity	High	High	Decreased	Decreased	Variable
Clarity	Transparent	Transparent	Translucent-opaque	Opaque	Cloudy
Color	Clear	Yellow	Yellow to opalescent	Yellow to green[†]	Pink to red
WBC (per µL)	<200	<3000	3000–50,000	>50,000[†]	Usually <2000
Polymorphonuclear leukocytes (%)	<25%	<25%	50% or more	75% or more	30%
Culture	Negative	Negative	Negative	Usually positive	Negative
Glucose (mg/dL)	Approx. serum	Approx. serum	>25, but <serum	<25, ≤serum	>25

*See page 249 for additional information.
[†]May be lower if antibiotics initiated.
Abbreviation: WBC = white blood cells.

13

- Evaluation of iron stores; evaluation of possible disseminated infection (tuberculosis, fungal disease)
- Bone marrow donor harvesting (aspiration)

Contraindications

- Infection, osteomyelitis near the puncture site
- Relative contraindications include severe coagulopathy or thrombocytopenia (may be corrected by platelet transfusion); prior radiation to the region

Materials

Commercial kits are usually available that contain all the materials necessary. A technician from the hematology lab or BMT facility is necessary to ensure delivery and processing of specimens.

Procedure

1. Explain the procedure to the patient and/or the legally responsible surrogate in detail, and obtain informed consent.
2. Usually local anesthesia is all that is required; however, in extremely anxious patients, premedication with an anxiolytic or sedative such as diazepam (Valium) or midazolam (Versed) or an analgesic is reasonable.
3. Bone marrow can be obtained from numerous sites, the most common being the sternum, the anterior iliac crest, and the posterior iliac crest. The posterior iliac crest is the safest and usually the site of choice and is described here. Position the patient on either the abdomen or on the side opposite the side from which the biopsy specimen is to be taken.
4. Identify the posterior iliac crest by palpation and mark the desired biopsy site with indelible ink.
5. Use sterile gloves and follow strict aseptic technique for the remainder of the procedure.
6. Prep the biopsy site with sterile povidone–iodine solution and allow the skin to dry. Then wipe the site free of the povidone–iodine with sterile alcohol. Use surgical drapes to cover the surrounding areas.
7. With a 26-gauge needle, administer 1% lidocaine solution intradermally to raise a skin wheal. Then, with the 22-gauge needle, infiltrate the subcutaneous and deeper tissues with lidocaine until the periosteum is reached. At this point, advance the needle just through the periosteum and infiltrate lidocaine subperiosteally. Infiltrate an area approximately 2 cm in diameter, using repeated periosteal punctures.
8. Once you obtain local anesthesia, use a No. 11 scalpel blade to make 2–3-mm skin incision over the biopsy site.
9. Insert the bone marrow biopsy needle through the skin incision and then advance with a rotating motion and gentle pressure until the periosteum is reached. Once it is firmly seated on the periosteum, advance the needle through the outer table of bone into the marrow cavity with the same rotating motion and gentle pressure. Generally, a slight change in the resistance to needle advancement signals entry into the marrow cavity. At this point, advance the needle 2–3 mm.
10. Remove the stylet from the biopsy needle and attach a 10-mL syringe to the hub of the biopsy needle. Withdraw the plunger on the syringe briskly, and aspirate 1–2 mL of marrow into the syringe. This may cause severe, instantaneous pain, but slow withdrawal of the plunger or collection of more than 1–2 mL of marrow with each aspiration results in excessive contamination of the specimen with peripheral blood.

13

11. The marrow aspiration specimen can be used to prepare coverslips for viewing under the microscope or sent for special studies such as cytogenetics and cell markers or for culture. Repeat aspirations may be required to obtain enough marrow to perform all of the studies needed. Also note that certain studies may require heparin or EDTA for collection. Contact the appropriate lab prior to the procedure to ensure that specimens are collected in the appropriate solution.

12. If a biopsy is to be obtained, replace the stylet and withdraw the needle. Then reinsert the needle at a slightly different angle and location, still within the area of periosteum previously anesthetized. Once the marrow cavity has been reentered, again remove the stylet and advance the needle d 5–10 mm, using the same rotating motion with gentle pressure. Withdraw the needle several millimeters (but not outside of the marrow cavity) and redirect it at a slightly different angle and then advance again. Repeat this step several times. This should result in 2–3 cm of core material entering the needle. Rotate the needle rapidly on its long axis in a clockwise and then a counterclockwise manner. This severs the biopsy specimen from the marrow cavity. Withdraw the needle completely without replacing the stylet. Some operators prefer to hold their thumb over the open end of the needle to create a negative pressure in the needle as it is withdrawn. This may help prevent loss of the core biopsy specimen.

13. Remove the core biopsy by inserting a probe (provided with the biopsy needle) into the distal end of the needle and gently pushing the specimen the full length of the needle and **out the hub end.** This is important because attempting to push the specimen out the distal end may damage the specimen. Most biopsy needles are tapered at the distal end, presumably allowing the specimen to expand once in the needle and preventing it from being lost when the needle is withdrawn from the patient.

14. The core biopsy specimen is usually collected in formalin solution. Again, plans for special studies should be made prior to the procedure so that any special handling of the biopsy can be done.

15. Observe the biopsy site for excess bleeding and apply local pressure for several minutes. Clean the area thoroughly with alcohol and apply an adhesive bandage or gauze patch. Instruct the patient to assume a supine position and place a pressure pack between the bed or table and the biopsy site to apply pressure for 10–15 min. This is not an absolute requirement in patients without an underlying coagulopathy or thrombocytopenia, but still serves to decrease local hematoma formation. Patients with an underlying bleeding tendency should maintain pressure for 20–25 min. A patient who is stable at this point may resume normal activities.

Complications

Local bleeding and hematoma, retroperitoneal hematoma, pain, bone fracture, infection

CENTRAL VENOUS CATHETERIZATION
Indications

- Administration of fluids and medications, especially when no peripheral access is available
- Administration of hyperalimentation solutions or other hypertonic fluids (eg, amphotericin B) that damage peripheral veins
- Measurement of CVP (See Chapter 20, page 397)
- Acute dialysis or plasmapheresis (Shiley catheter)
- Insertion of a pulmonary artery catheter or transvenous pacemaker

Contraindications

- Coagulopathy dictates the use of the femoral or median basilic vein approach to avoid bleeding complications.

Background

A central venous catheter (also known as a **"deep line"**) is a catheter introduced into the superior vena cava, inferior vena cava, or one of their main branches. Generally, two techniques are used to place central venous lines. One of these **(Seldinger technique)** involves puncturing the vein with a relatively small needle through which a thin guidewire is placed in the vein. After the needle has been withdrawn, the intravascular appliance or a sheath through which a smaller catheter will be placed is introduced into the vein over the guidewire. The other technique involves puncturing the vein with a larger bore needle through which the intravascular catheter will fit. The ensuing discussion focuses on the **Seldinger technique** and placement of either a triple-lumen catheter or a sheath through which a smaller catheter (eg, a pulmonary artery catheter) will eventually be placed. The internal jugular and subclavian approaches are commonly used, but the femoral approach, although infrequently utilized, offers several advantages (see following discussion). Another technique, the PICC line is designed for more long-term outpatient administration of medications and is described on page 292.

Materials

Commercially available disposable trays provide all the necessary needles, wires, sheaths, dilators, suture materials, and anesthetics. If needles, guidewires, and sheaths are collected from different places, it is very important to make sure that the needle will accept the guidewire, that the sheath and dilator will pass over the guidewire, and that the appliance to be passed through the sheath will indeed fit the inside lumen of the sheath. Supplies should include the following items:

- Minor procedure and instrument tray (page 240); 1% lidocaine (mixed 1:1 with sodium bicarbonate 1 mEq/L removes the sting)
- Guidewire (usually 0.035 floppy-tipped J wire)
- Vessel dilator
- Intravascular appliance (triple-lumen catheter or a sheath through which a pulmonary artery catheter could be placed)
- Heparinized flush solution 1 mL of 1:100 U heparin in 10 mL of NS (to be used to fill all lumens prior to placement to prevent clotting of the catheter during placement)
- Mask, sterile gown, highly recommended

Subclavian Approach (Left or Right)

The left subclavian approach affords a gentle, sweeping curve to the apex of the right ventricle and is the preferred entry site for placement of a temporary transvenous pacemaker without fluoroscopic assistance. Hemodynamic measurements are often easier to record from the left subclavian approach. From the left subclavian vein approach, the catheters do not have to negotiate an acute angle, as is commonly the case at the junction of the right subclavian with the right brachiocephalic vein en route to the superior vena cava. This is also a common site for kinking of the deep line. It also has the lowest risk of infection of various central line sites. However, remember that the thoracic duct is on the left side, and the dome of the pleura rises higher on the left.

1. Use sterile technique (povidone–iodine prep, gloves, mask, and a sterile field) whenever possible.
2. Place the patient flat or head down in the Trendelenburg position with the head in the center or turned to the opposite side (the "ideal" position is somewhat controversial, and left up to operator preference). It may be helpful to place a towel roll along the patient's spine.
3. Use a 25-gauge needle to make a small skin wheal 2 cm below the midclavicle with 1% lidocaine (mixed 1:1 with sodium bicarbonate 1 mEq/L to help remove the sting). At this point, a larger needle (eg, 22-gauge) can be used to anesthetize the deeper tissues as well as locate the vein.
4. Attach a large-bore, deep-line needle (a 14-gauge needle with a 16-gauge catheter at least 8–12 in. long) to a 10–20-mL syringe and introduce it into the site of the skin wheal.
5. Advance the needle under the clavicle, aiming for a location halfway between the suprasternal notch and the base of the thyroid cartilage. The vein is encountered under the clavicle, just medial to the lateral border of the clavicular head of the sternocleidomastoid muscle. In most patients this is roughly two finger-breadths lateral to the sternal notch. Apply gentle pressure on the needle at the skin entrance site to assist in lowering the needle under the clavicle (Fig. 13–7).
6. Apply back pressure as the needle is advanced deep to the clavicle, but above the first rib, and watch for a "flash" of blood.
7. Free return of blood indicates entry into the subclavian vein. Remember that occasionally the vein is punctured through *both* walls, and a flash of blood may not appear as the needle is advanced. Therefore, if a free return of blood does not occur on needle advancement, withdraw the needle slowly with intermittent pressure. A free return of blood heralds the entry of the end of the needle into the lumen. Bright red blood that forcibly enters the syringe indicates that the subclavian artery has been entered. If the arterial entry occurs, remove the needle. In the majority of patients, the surrounding tissue will tamponade any bleeding from the arterial puncture. Because the artery is under the clavicle, holding pressure has little effect on bleeding.
8. a. If you are using an Intracath, remove the syringe, place a finger over the needle hub, and advance the catheter an appropriate distance through the needle. Then withdraw the needle to just outside the skin and snap the protective cap over the tip of the needle.
   b. If you are using the Seldinger wire technique, advance the wire through the needle and then withdraw the needle. The pulse or ECG should be monitored during wire passage because the wire can induce ventricular arrhythmias. Arrhythmias usually resolve by calmly pulling the wire out several centimeters. Nick the skin with a No. 11 blade, and advance the dilator approximately 5 cm; remove the dilator and advance catheter in over the guidewire (use the brown port on the triple-lumen catheter). While advancing either the dilator or the catheter over the wire, periodically ensure that the wire moves freely in and out. When placing a Cordis, advance the catheter and dilator over the guidewire as one unit (see Chapter 20 Pulmonary Artery Catheter Insertion, page 402, for more details). If the wire does not move freely, it usually is kinked, and the catheter or dilator should be removed and repositioned. Maintain a firm grip on the guidewire at all times. Remove the wire and attach the IV tubing. Note that the wire used to insert a single-lumen catheter is

13

shorter than the wire supplied with the triple-lumen catheter. This is most critical when exchanging a triple-lumen for a single-lumen catheter; use the longer triple-lumen wire and insert the wire into the brown port. Place Shiley catheters using the Seldinger wire technique.

9. Attach the catheter to the appropriate IV solution, and place the IV bottle below the level of the deep-line site to ensure a good backflow of blood into the tubing. If no backflow occurs, the catheter may be kinked or not in the proper position.

10. Securely suture the assembly in place with 2-0 or 3-0 silk. Apply an occlusive dressing with povidone–iodine ointment.

11. Obtain a chest x-ray film immediately to verify placement of the catheter tip and to rule out pneumothorax. Ideally, the catheter tip lies in the superior vena cava at its junction with the right atrium, at about the fifth thoracic vertebra. Malpositioned catheters that go into the neck veins may be used only for saline infusion and not for monitoring or TPN infusion.

12. Catheters that cannot be manipulated at the bedside into the chest can usually be positioned properly in the interventional radiology suite with the aid of fluoroscopy.

Right Internal Jugular Vein Approach

Three different sites are described and used in accessing the right internal jugular vein: anterior (medial to the sternocleidomastoid muscle belly), middle (between the two heads of the sternocleidomastoid muscle belly), and posterior (lateral to the sternocleidomastoid muscle belly). The middle approach is most commonly used and has the advantage of using well-defined landmarks. The major disadvantage of the internal jugular site is the patient discomfort it causes. The site is difficult to dress and is uncomfortable for patients, particularly when turning the head.

Procedure

13

1. Sterilize the site with povidone–iodine, and drape area with sterile towels.
2. Administer local anesthesia with lidocaine in the area to be explored.
3. Place the patient in the **Trendelenburg** (head down) position.
4. Use a small-bore, thin-walled needle (21-gauge) with syringe attached to locate the internal jugular vein. It may be helpful to have a small amount of anesthetic in the syringe to inject during exploration for the vein if the patient notes some discomfort. Some prefer to leave this needle and syringe in the vein and place the large-bore needle directly over the smaller needle, into the vein. This is commonly called the "seeker needle" technique.
5. The internal diameter of the needle used to locate the internal jugular vein should be large enough to accommodate the passage of the guidewire.
6. Percutaneous entry should be made at the apex of the triangle formed by the two heads of the sternocleidomastoid muscle and the clavicle. (See Fig. 13–6.)
7. Direct the needle slightly lateral toward the ipsilateral nipple and enter at a 45-degree angle to the skin.
8. Often a notch can be palpated on the posterior surface of the clavicle. This actually can help locate the vein in the lateral/medial plane because the vein lies deep to this shallow notch.
9. Successful puncture of the vein is accomplished usually at an unnerving depth of needle insertion and is heralded by sudden aspiration of nonpulsatile venous blood. Bedside localizing Doppler ultrasound units are available in most operating rooms or intensive care units. They can aid in localization of the internal jugular vein if the standard techniques fail.

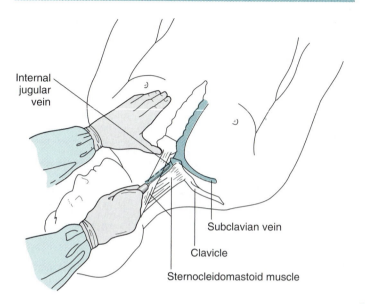

Internal jugular vein

Subclavian vein

Clavicle

Sternocleidomastoid muscle

FIGURE 13–6   Technique for the catheterization of the internal jugular vein.

13

10. Inadvertent puncture of the carotid artery is common if the needle is inserted medial to where it should be on the middle approach and is common with the anterior approach. With arterial puncture, the syringe fills without negative pressure because of arterial pressure, and bright red blood pulsates from the needle after the syringe is removed. In this case remove the needle and apply manual pressure for 10–15 min to ensure adequate hemostasis.
11. Follow steps 8–12 as for subclavian line (page 255). On chest x-ray, the catheter tip should lie in the superior vena cava in the vicinity of the right atrium, at about the fifth thoracic vertebra.

Complications

Overall this is a safe procedure when the small-bore needle is first used to identify the vein.

- Pneumothorax can be detected when a sudden gush of air is aspirated instead of blood. A postprocedure chest x-ray should always be done to rule out pneumothorax and check for line placement. A pneumothorax requires chest tube placement in virtually all cases, especially when the patient is being supported on a ventilator. The left-sided approach is associated with higher risk for pneumothorax because of the higher dome of the left pleura compared with the right.
- Perforation of endotracheal tube cuffs

- Hemothorax from vascular injury or hydrothorax from administration of IV fluids into the pleural space
- Catheter tip embolus: **Never** withdraw the catheter through the needle. It can shear off the tip.
- **Air embolus:** Make sure that the open end of a deep line is **always** covered with a finger. As little as 50–100 mL of air in a vein can be fatal. **If you suspect that air embolization has occurred, place the patient's head down and turn on left side to keep the air in the right atrium.** Obtain a **STAT** portable chest film to see if air is present in the heart.

Left Internal Jugular Vein Approach

The left internal jugular vein is not commonly used for central line placement. Better options exist and should be exhausted before resorting to this approach. The procedure is similar to right internal jugular vein approach. In addition to the usual procedural complications common to central lines, this approach has some unique complications, including inadvertent left brachiocephalic vein and superior vena cava puncture with intravascular wires, catheters, and sheaths and laceration of the thoracic duct resulting in chylothorax.

External Jugular Vein Approach

This is a safe approach to central venous catheterization but a very technically demanding procedure due to the difficulty in threading the catheter into the central venous system. This is also an uncomfortable insertion site for the patient because the dressing and IV tubing is on the neck. If the central venous system cannot be entered, this is also a site of last resort for placing a standard IV catheter ("peripheral") for the administration of routine nonsclerosing IV fluids. The external jugular vein is usually visible with the patient in the 30° Trendelenburg position. The vein, located in the subcutaneous tissues, crosses the sternocleidomastoid muscle arising from just behind the angle of the jaw inferiorly where it drains into the subclavian vein just lateral to the inferior aspect of the sternocleidomastoid muscle.

13

Procedure

1. Place the patient in the Trendelenburg position with the head turned away from the side of insertion. Prep and drape the neck from the ear to the subclavicular area.
2. Having the patient perform the Valsalva maneuver or gently occluding the vein near its insertion into the subclavian vein will help engorge the vein.
3. At the approximate midportion of the vein, make a skin wheal with a 25-gauge needle and lidocaine solution. Use a 21-gauge needle to anesthetize the deeper subcutaneous tissue and to locate the vein.
4. Remove the syringe from the needle and insert a floppy-tipped J wire into the needle. Use the guidewire with gentle pressure to negotiate the turns into the intrathoracic portion of the venous system. If there is difficulty passing the wire, have the patient turn the head slightly to help direct the wire. **Never forcibly push the wire.** As a last resort, fluroscopy can be used to direct the wire into the superior vena cava.
5. Once a sufficient length of guidewire is passed, the locating needle can be removed.
6. An incision in the skin may have to be made to accommodate the catheter. The catheter is then slid over the guidewire and the guidewire is removed. Aspirate blood from the end of the catheter to confirm that it is in the venous system.
7. Follow steps 8–12 as for placement via the subclavian vein (page 255).

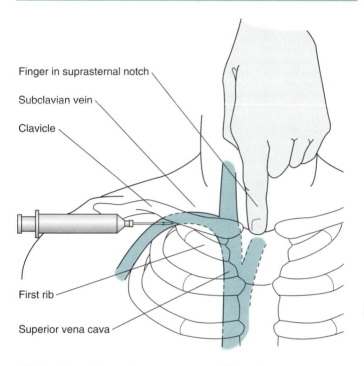

Finger in suprasternal notch

Subclavian vein

Clavicle

First rib

Superior vena cava

FIGURE 13–7   Technique for the catheterization of the subclavian vein.

Complications

See Right Internal Jugular Vein Approach, page 257.

Femoral Vein Approach

The femoral vein approach has several advantages. The procedure is safe, in that arterial and venous sites are more easily compressible, and it is impossible to cause pneumothorax from this site. Placement can be accomplished without interrupting cardiopulmonary resuscitation. This site can be used to place a variety of intravascular appliances, including temporary pacemakers, pulmonary artery catheters (expertise with fluoroscopy may be needed), and triple-lumen catheters. The major disadvantages are the high risk of sepsis, the immobilization it causes, and the occasional need for fluoroscopy to ensure proper placement of pulmonary artery catheters or transvenous pacemakers.

Procedure

1. Place the patient in the supine position.
2. Use sterile preparation and appropriate draping. Administer local anesthesia in the area to be explored.
3. Palpate the femoral artery. Use the "NAVEL" technique to locate the vein (see page 246).
4. Guard the artery with the fingers of one hand.
5. Explore for the vein just medial to the operator's fingers with a needle and syringe.
6. It may be helpful to have a small amount of anesthetic in the syringe to inject with exploration.
7. Direct the needle cephalad at about a 30-degree angle and insert below the femoral crease.
8. Puncture is heralded by the return of venous, nonpulsatile blood on application of negative pressure to the syringe.
9. Advance the guidewire through the needle.
10. The guidewire should pass with ease into the vein to a depth at which the distal tip of the guidewire is always under the operator's control even when the sheath/dilator or catheter is placed over the guidewire.
11. Remove the needle once the guidewire has advanced into the femoral vein.
12. If the catheter is a French 6 or larger, a skin incision with a scalpel blade and the use of a vessel dilator are generally needed. The catheter can then be advanced along with the guidewire in unison into the femoral vein. Be sure always to control the distal end of the guidewire.
13. Follow steps 13 through 18 for the right internal jugular vein approach.

13

Complications

- The femoral deep line has the highest incidence of contamination and sepsis. If an occlusive dressing can remain in place and remain free from contamination, this is a safe option.
- DVT has occurred from femoral vein catheterization. The risk for DVT increases if the catheter remains in place for prolonged periods.
- Uncontrolled retroperitoneal bleeding can occur if the iliac/common femoral artery is inadvertently punctured above the inguinal ligament.

Removal of a Central Venous Catheter

1. Turn off the IV flow.
2. Cut the retention sutures, and gently withdraw the catheter. Visually inspect the catheter to ensure it is intact.
3. Apply pressure for at least 2–3 min, and apply a sterile dressing.

CHEST TUBE PLACEMENT (CLOSED THORACOSTOMY, TUBE THORACOSTOMY)
Indications

- Pneumothorax (simple or tension)

- Hemothorax, hydrothorax, chylothorax, or empyema evacuation
- Pleurodesis for chronic recurring pneumothorax or effusion that is refractory to standard management (eg, malignant effusion)

Materials

- Chest tube (20–36 French for adults, 12–4 French for children)
- Water-seal drainage system (Pleurovac, etc) with connecting tubing to wall suction
- Minor procedure tray and instrument tray (see page 240)
- Silk or nylon suture (0 to 2-0)
- Petrolatum gauze (Vaseline) (optional)
- 4×4 gauze dressing and cloth tape

Background

A chest tube is usually placed to treat an ongoing intrathoracic process that cannot be managed by simple thoracentesis (see page 304). The traditional methods of chest tube placement are described. Percutaneous tube thoracostomy kits are also available based on the Seldinger technique. It can be used in dealing with small pneumothoraces when there is no risk of ongoing air leak, but it should not be used with more significant conditions (empyema, major pneumothorax >20%, tension pneumothorax, chronic effusions)

Procedure

If a patient manifests signs of a tension pneumothorax (acute shortness of breath, hypotension, distended neck veins, tachypnea, tracheal deviation) before a chest tube is placed, urgent treatment is needed. Insert a 14-gauge needle into the chest in the second intercostal space in the midclavicular line to rapidly decompress the tension pneumothorax and proceed with chest tube insertion.

13

1. Prior to placing the tube, review the chest x-ray unless an emergency does not allow enough time. For a pneumothorax, choose a high anterior site, such as the second or third intercostal space, midclavicular line, or subaxillary position (more cosmetic). Place a low lateral chest tube in the fifth or sixth intercostal space in the midaxillary line and direct posteriorly for fluid removal. (In most patients this location corresponds to the inframammary crease.) For a traumatic pneumothorax, use a low lateral tube because this condition usually is associated with bleeding. Rarely, a loculated apical pneumothorax or effusion may require placement of an anterior tube in the second intercostal space at the midclavicular line.
2. Choose the appropriate chest tube. Use a 24–28 French tube for pneumothorax and 36 French for fluid removal. A "**thoracic catheter**" has multiple holes and works best for nearly all purposes. The vast majority of tubes can be inserted painlessly with generous use of local anesthetics. If the procedure is elective, the patient is extremely anxious, and the patient's respiratory status is not compromised, sedation **occasionally** may be helpful.
3. Prep the area with povidone–iodine solution and drape it with sterile towels. Use 1idocaine (with or without epinephrine) to anesthetize the skin, intercostal muscle, and periosteum of the rib; start at the center of the rib and gently work over the top. Remember, the neurovascular bundle runs under the rib (Fig. 13–8). The needle then can be gently "popped" through the pleura and the aspiration of air or fluid confirms the correct location for the chest tube.

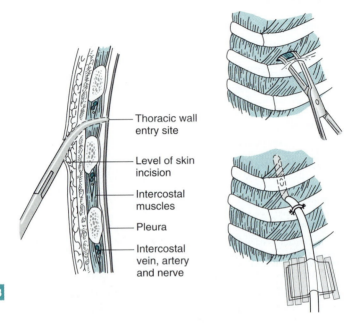

Thoracic wall entry site

Level of skin incision

Intercostal muscles

Pleura

Intercostal vein, artery and nerve

13

FIGURE 13–8   Chest tube technique demonstrating the procedure for creating a subcutaneous tunnel. *Note:* The skin incision is lower than the thoracic wall entry site. (Reprinted, with permission, from: Gomella TL [ed]: *Neonatology: Basic Management, On-Call Problems, Diseases, Drugs,* 4th ed. Appleton & Lange, Norwalk CT, 1998.)

4. Make a 2–3-cm transverse incision over the center of the rib with a No. 15 or 11 scalpel blade. Use a blunt-tipped clamp to dissect over the top of the rib and create a subcutaneous tunnel (see Fig. 13–8).

5. Puncture the parietal pleura with the hemostat, and spread the opening. **BE CAREFUL NOT TO INJURE THE LUNG PARENCHYMA WITH THE HEMOSTAT TIPS.** Insert a gloved finger into the pleural cavity to gently clear any clots or adhesions and to make certain the lung is not accidentally punctured by the tube.

6. Carefully insert the tube into the desired position with a hemostat or gloved finger as a guide. Make sure all the holes in the tube are in the chest cavity. Attach the end of the tube to a water-seal or Pleur-Evac suction system. Some chest tubes are provided with sharp trocars that are used to pierce the chest wall and place the chest tube simultane-

ously with minimal amounts of dissection. These instruments are extremely dangerous and are usually placed in the anterior high position (ie, second, third, or fourth ICS).

7. Suture the tube in place. Place a heavy silk (0 or 2-0) suture through the incision next to the tube. Tie the incision together, then tie the ends around the chest tube. Make sure to wrap around the tube several times. Alternatively, a purse string suture (or "U stitch") can be placed around the insertion site. Make sure all of the suction holes are in the chest cavity before the tube is secured.

8. Cover the insertion site with plain gauze. Make the dressing as airtight as possible with tape, and secure all connections in the tubing to prevent accidental loss of the water seal. Some physicians still wrap the insertion site with petroleum (Vaseline or Xeroform) gauze; however, these materials are not foolproof: they are not water-soluble (therefore, they act as foreign bodies), inhibit wound healing, and do not actually provide a true seal.

9. Start suction (usually –20 cm in adults, –16 cm in children) and take a portable chest x-ray immediately to check the placement of the tube and to evaluate for residual pneumothorax or fluid.

10. **To remove a chest tube,** make sure the pneumothorax or hemothorax is cleared. Check for an air leak by having the patient cough; observe the water-seal system for bubbling that indicates either a system (tubing) leak or persistent pleural air leak.

11. Take the tube off suction **but not off water seal,** and cut the retention suture. Have the patient inspire deeply and perform the Valsalva maneuver while you apply pressure with petrolatum gauze or with a sufficient amount of antibiotic ointment on 4 × 4 gauze with additional 4 × 4 gauze squares. Pull the tube rapidly while the patient performs the Valsalva maneuver and make an airtight seal with tape. Check an "upright" exhalation chest x-ray film for pneumothorax.

Complications

Infection, bleeding, lung damage, subcutaneous emphysema, persistent pneumothorax/hemothorax, poor tube placement, cardiac arrhythmia

13

CRICOTHYROTOMY (NEEDLE AND SURGICAL)
Background

Cricothyrotomy is a true emergency procedure that should be performed when obtaining an airway using endotracheal or orotracheal intubation is impossible.

Indications

- When immediate mechanical ventilation is indicated, but an endotracheal or orotracheal tube cannot be placed (eg, severe maxillofacial trauma, excessive oropharyngeal hemorrhage)

Contraindications

- Surgical cricothyrotomy is contraindicated in children < 12 y; use needle approach.

Basic Materials

- Oxygen connecting tubing, high-flow oxygen source (tank or wall)
- Bag ventilator

Needle Cricothyrotomy

- 12–14-gauge catheter over needle (Angiocath or other),
- 6–12-mL syringe
- 3-mm pediatric endotracheal tube adapter

Surgical Cricothyrotomy (minimum requirements)

- Minor procedure and instrument tray (page 240) plus tracheal spreader if available
- No. 5–7 tracheostomy tube (6–8 French endotracheal tube can be substituted)
- Tracheostomy tube adapter to connect to bag-mask ventilator

Procedures

Needle Cricothyrotomy

1. With the patient supine, place a roll behind the shoulders to gently hyperextend the neck.
2. Palpate the cricothyroid membrane, which resembles a notch located between the caudal end of the thyroid cartilage and the cricoid cartilage. Prep the area with povidone–iodine solution. Local anesthesia can be used if the patient is awake.
3. Mount the syringe on the 12- or 14-gauge catheter-over-needle assembly, and advance through the cricothyroid membrane at a 45-degree angle, applying back pressure on the syringe until air is aspirated.
4. Advance the catheter, and remove the needle. Attach the hub to a 3-mm endotracheal tube adapter that is connected to the oxygen tubing. Allow the oxygen to flow at 15 L/min for 1–2 s on, then 4 s off by the use of a Y-connector or a hole in the side of the tubing to turn the flow on and off.
5. The needle technique is only useful for about 45 min because the exhalation of CO_2 is suboptimal.

13

Surgical Cricothyrotomy

1. Follow steps 1 and 2 as for needle cricothyrotomy.
2. Make a 3–4-cm vertical skin incision through the cervical fascia and strap muscles in the midline over the cricothyroid membrane. Expose the cricothyroid membrane, and make a horizontal incision. Insert the knife handle, and rotate it 90 degrees to open the hole in the membrane. Alternatively, a hemostat or tracheal spreader can be used to dilate the opening.
3. Insert a small (5–7-mm) tracheostomy tube, inflate the balloon (if present), and secure in position with the attached cotton tapes.
4. Attach to oxygen source and ventilate. Listen to the chest for symmetrical breath sounds.
5. A surgical cricothyrotomy should be replaced with a formal tracheostomy after the patient has been stabilized and generally within 24–36 h.

Complications

- Bleeding, esophageal perforation, subcutaneous emphysema, pneumomediastinum, and pneumothorax, CO_2 retention (especially with the needle procedure)

CULDOCENTESIS

Indications

- Diagnostic technique for problems of acute abdominal pain in the female

- Evaluation of female patient with signs of hypovolemia and possible intraabdominal bleeding
- Evaluation of ascites, especially in possible cases of gynecologic malignancy

Materials

- Speculum
- Antiseptic swabs
- Povidone–iodine or chlorhexidine
- 1% lidocaine
- 18–21-gauge spinal needle
- 2 (10 mL) syringes and tenaculum

Procedure

1. Culdocentesis should be preceded with a careful pelvic exam to document uterine position and rule out pelvic mass at risk of perforation by the culdocentesis.
2. After obtaining the patient's informed consent, the vagina is prepped with antiseptic, such as iodine or chlorhexidine.
3. Inject 1% lidocaine submucosally in the posterior cervical fornix prior to tenaculum application.
4. Traction is improved by application of the tenaculum to the posterior cervical lip.
5. Apply an 18–21-gauge spinal needle to a 10-mL syringe, filled with 1 mL of air.
6. As you move the needle forward through the posterior cervical fornix, apply light pressure to the syringe until the air passes. Maintain traction on the tenaculum as you advance the spinal needle to maximize the surface area of the cul de sac for needle entry.
7. After intraabdominal entry, ask the patient to elevate herself on elbows to permit gravity drainage into the area of needle entry. Apply negative pressure to the syringe. Slow rotation of the needle followed by slow removal may enable a pocket of fluid to be found and aspirated.
8. If first culdocentesis attempt is not successful, the procedure can be repeated with a different angle of approach.
9. Although perforation of viscus is a possibility, the complication rate has been very low. Fresh blood that clots rapidly is probably secondary to traumatic tap, and the procedure can be repeated.
10. If blood is aspirated, it should be spun for hematocrit and placed into an empty glass test tube to demonstrate the presence or absence of a clot. Failure of blood to clot suggests old hemorrhage.
11. If pus is aspirated, send specimens for GC, aerobic, anaerobic, *Chlamydia, Mycoplasma,* and *Ureaplasma* cultures.
12. If a malignancy is suspected, send fluid for cytologic evaluation.

Complications

Infection, hemorrhage, air embolus, perforated viscus

DOPPLER PRESSURES

Indications

- Evaluation of peripheral vascular disease (ankle-brachial or ankle-arm index)
- Routine blood pressure measurement in infants or critically ill adults

Materials

- Doppler flow monitor
- Conductive gel (lubricant jelly can also be used)
- Blood pressure cuff

Procedure (Ankle-Brachial or Ankle-Arm Index)

1. Determine the blood pressure in each arm.
2. Measure the pressures in the popliteal arteries by placing a BP cuff on the thigh. The pressures in the dorsalis pedis arteries (on the top of the foot) and the posterior tibial arteries (behind the medial malleolus) are determined with a BP cuff on the calf.
3. Apply conductive jelly and place the Doppler probe over the artery. Inflate the BP cuff until the pulsatile flow is no longer heard. Deflate the cuff until the flow returns. This is the systolic, or Doppler, pressure. *Note:* The Doppler cannot routinely determine the diastolic pressure, and a palpable pulse need not be present to use the Doppler.
4. The **A/B or AAI index** is often computed from Doppler pressure. It is equal to the pressure in the ankle (usually the posterior tibial) divided by the systolic pressure in the arm. An A/B index of >0.9 is usually normal, and an index of <0.5 is usually associated with significant peripheral vascular disease.

ELECTROCARDIOGRAM

Basic ECG interpretation can be found in Chapter 19, page 367.

Indications

- Useful in the evaluation of chest pain and other cardiac conditions

Materials

13

- ECG machine with paper and lead electrodes
- Adhesive electrode pads

Procedure

1. Most hospitals have converted to fully automated ECG machines. It is important to become acquainted with your particular machine prior to using it. The following is a general outline.
2. Start with the patient in a comfortable, recumbent position. Explain the procedure to dispel any myths. Instruct the patient to lie as still as possible to cut down on artifacts in the tracing.
3. Plug in the ECG machine and turn it on.
4. Attach the electrodes as outlined here:
   a. **Patient Cables.** The standard ECG machine has five lead wires, one for each limb and one for the chest leads. Newer machines have six precordial electrodes, which are all placed in the proper positions prior to performing the procedure. These may be color-coded in the following fashion:
      - RA: White—right arm
      - LA: Black—left arm
      - RL: Green—right leg
      - LL: Red—left leg
      - C: Brown—chest

b. **Limb Electrodes.** The limb electrodes are flat, rectangular plates held in place by rubber or Velcro straps that encircle the limb; newer machines may use self-adhering electrode pads. Place each electrode on the limb indicated, wrist or ankle, usually on the ventral surface. In case of amputation or a cast, the lead may be placed on the shoulder or groin with almost no effect on the tracing.

c. **Chest (Precordial) Electrodes.** The chest electrode is brown and designated by the letter "C." It is attached to a suction cup that is attached in sequence to each of the positions on the precordium (see the following description). Newer machines allow all leads to be placed prior to running the ECG with all pads applied at the same time. This makes locating the proper positions much quicker and easier (Fig. 13–9). Precordial leads are placed as follows:

- V_1 = fourth intercostal space just to the **right** of the sternal border
- V_2 = fourth intercostal space just to the **left** of the sternal border
- V_3 = midway between leads V_2 and V_4
- V_4 = midclavicular line, above the fifth interspace

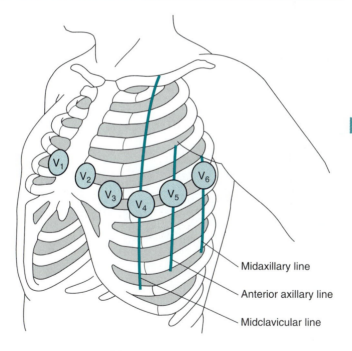

Midaxillary line

Anterior axillary line

Midclavicular line

FIGURE 13–9 Location of the precordial chest leads used in obtaining a routine ECG.

- V_5 = anterior axillary line at the same level as V_4
- V_6 = midaxillary line at the same level as leads V_4 and V_5

4. Once the machine is warmed up and the electrodes are positioned or ready for position-ing, make sure that the paper speed is set at 25 mm/s. When everything is ready, follow the directions for your particular machine to obtain the ECG tracing. It should include 12 different leads, that is, I, II, III, AVR, AVL, and V_{1-6}.

5. Label the tracing with the patient's name, date, time, and any other useful information, such as medications, and your name. A routine 12-lead ECG should take 4–8 min.

Helpful Hints

1. The second rib inserts at the sternal angle, and therefore the second intercostal space is directly inferior to the sternal angle. Feel down two more intercostal spaces and you have the fourth intercostal space to position V_1 and V_2.

2. When you start seeing a solid blue or red line at the top or bottom of the strip, you are about to run out of paper. **Always** leave enough paper for the next user.

3. Learn the color scheme for the leads; it could be very useful in an emergency. Some memory aids include
   a. Red and green go to the legs: "Christmas on the bottom" or "When driving your car you use your left leg to brake (red light) and your right leg to go (green light)."
   b. Black (left) and white (right) go to the arms: "Remember white is right and black is left."
   c. Brown is for the chest.

ENDOTRACHEAL INTUBATION
Indications

- Airway management during cardiopulmonary resuscitation
- Any indication for using mechanical ventilation (respiratory failure, coma, general anesthesia, etc)

Contraindications

- Massive maxillofacial trauma (relative)
- Fractured larynx
- Suspected cervical spinal cord injury (relative)

Materials

- Endotracheal tube of appropriate size (Table 13–3)
- Laryngoscope handle and blade (straight [Miller] or curved [MAC]; size No. 3 for adults, No. 1–1.5 for small children)
- 10-mL syringe, adhesive tape, benzoin
- Suction equipment (Yankauer suction)
- Malleable stylet (optional)
- Oropharyngeal airway

Technique

1. Orotracheal intubation is most commonly used and is described here. Orotracheal intu-bation should be done only with great care in cases of suspected cervical spine injuries. In such cases nasotracheal intubation is preferred.

TABLE 13–3
Recommended Endotracheal Tube Sizes

Patient	Internal Diameter (mm)	
Premature infant	2.5–3.0	(uncuffed)
Newborn infant	3.5	(uncuffed)
3–12 mo	4.0	(uncuffed)
1–8 y	4.0–6.0	(uncuffed)*
8–16 y	6.0–7.0	(cuffed)
Adult	7.0–9.0	(cuffed)

*Rough estimate is to measure the little finger.

2. Any patient who is hypoxic or apneic must be ventilated prior to attempting endotracheal intubation (bag mask or mouth to mask). Remember to avoid prolonged periods of no ventilation if the intubation is difficult. A rule of thumb is to hold your breath while attempting intubation. When you need to take a breath, so must the patient, and you should resume ventilation, and reattempt intubation in a minute or so.

3. Extend the laryngoscope blade to 90 degrees to verify the light is working, and check the balloon on the tube (if present) for leaks.

4. Place the patient's head in the "sniffing position" (neck extended anteriorly and the head extended posteriorly). Use suction to clear the upper airway if needed.

5. Hold the laryngoscope in the left hand, hold the mouth open with the right hand, and use the blade to push the tongue to patient's left while keeping it anterior to the blade. Advance the blade carefully toward the midline until the epiglottis is visualized. Use suction if needed.

6. If the **straight laryngoscope blade** is used, pass it under the epiglottis and **lift** upward to visualize the vocal cords (Fig. 13–10). If the **curved blade** is used, place it anterior to the epiglottis (into the vallecula) and gently lift anteriorly. In either case, do **not** use the handle to pry the epiglottis open, but rather gently lift to expose the vocal cords.

7. While maintaining visualization of the cords, grasp the tube in your right hand and pass it through the cords. With more difficult intubations, the malleable stylet can be used to direct the tube.

8. In patients who may have eaten recently, gentle pressure placed over the cricoid cartilage by an assistant helps to occlude the esophagus and prevent aspiration during intubation. "Cricoid pressure" can also help visualize the vocal cords in patients whose larynx is situated more anteriorly than usual.

9. When using a cuffed tube (adult and older children), gently inflate air with a 10-mL syringe until the seal is adequate (about 5 mL). Ventilate the patient while auscultating and visualizing both sides of the chest to verify positioning. If the left side does not seem to be ventilating, it may signify that the tube has been advanced down the right mainstem bronchus. Withdraw the tube 1–2 cm, and recheck the breath sounds. Also auscultate over the stomach to ensure the tube is not mistakenly placed in the esophagus. Confirm positioning with a chest x-ray. The tip of the endotracheal tube should be a few centimeters above the carina.

13

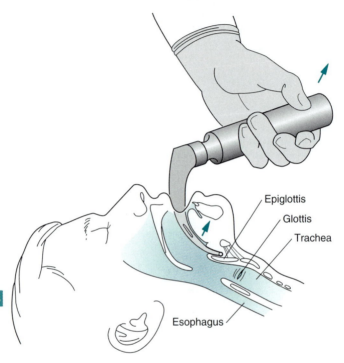

FIGURE 13–10   Endotracheal intubation using a curved laryngoscope blade.

10. Tape the tube in position, and insert an oropharyngeal airway to prevent the patient from biting the tube. Consider an orogastric tube to prevent regurgitation.

Complications

- Bleeding, oral or pharyngeal trauma, improper tube positioning (esophageal intubation, right mainstem bronchus), aspiration, tube obstruction or kinking

FEVER WORK-UP

Although not a "procedure" in the true sense of the word, a fever work-up involves judicious use of invasive procedures. The true definition of a *fever* can vary from service to service. General guidelines to follow are a temperature of >100.4°F orally on a medical or surgical service, or a temperature greater than or equal to 101°F rectally or 100°F orally in an infant or immunocompromised patient.

When evaluating a patient for a fever, consider if the temperature is oral, rectal, tympanic, or axillary (rectal and tympanic temperatures are about 1° higher and axillary temperatures are about 1° lower than oral); has the patient drunk any hot or cold liquids or smoked around the time of the determination; and is the patient on any antipyretics. Differential diagnosis of fever and fever of unknown origin are discussed in Chapter 3.

General Fever Work-Up

1. Quickly review the chart and medication record if the patient is not familiar to you.
2. Question and examine the patient to locate any obvious sources of fever.
   a. **Ears, nose, and throat:** Especially in children
   b. **Neck:** Tenderness or stiffness present
   c. **Nodes:** Adenopathy
   d. **Lungs:** Rales (crackles), rhonchi (wheezes), decreased breath sounds, or dullness to percussion. Can the patient generate an effective cough?
   e. **Heart:** Heart murmur, which may suggest SBE
   f. **Abdomen:** Presence or absence of bowel sounds, guarding, rigidity, tenderness, bladder fullness, or costovertebral angle tenderness
   g. **Genitourinary:** When a Foley catheter is in place; appearance of the urine, grossly and microscopically
   h. **Rectal Exam:** Tenderness or fluctuance to suggest an abscess, or acute prostatitis
   i. **Pelvic Exam:** Especially in the postpartum patient
   j. **Wounds:** Erythema, tenderness, swelling, or drainage from surgical sites
   k. **Extremities:** Signs of inflammation at IV sites. Look for thigh or calf tenderness and swelling.
   l. **Miscellaneous:** Consider the possibility of a drug fever (eosinophil count on the CBC may be elevated) or NG tube fever. Do all this before you begin to investigate the less common or less obvious causes of a fever
3. **Laboratory Studies**
   a. **Basic:** CBC with differential, urinalysis, cultures as indicated: urine, blood, sputum, wound, spinal fluid (**especially** in children less than 4–6 mo old)
   b. **Other:** Studies based on your evaluation:
      (i) **Radiographic:** Chest or abdominal films, CT or ultrasound exams
      (ii) **Invasive:** LP, thoracentesis, paracentesis are more aggressive procedures that may be indicated.

Miscellaneous Fever Facts

1. **Causes of Fever in the Postop Patient:** Think of the "Six W's":
   a. **Wind:** Atelectasis secondary to intubation and anesthesia is the most common cause of a fever immediately after surgery. To treat, have the patient up and ambulating, getting incentive spirometry, P&PD, etc.
   b. **Water:** UTI; may be secondary to a bladder catheter
   c. **Wound:** Infection
   d. **Walking:** Phlebitis, DVT
   e. **Wonder drugs:** Drug fever (common causes are listed on page 46).
   f. **Woman:** Endometritis, or mastitis. (These are common only in postpartum patients.)
2. **Elevated White Cell Counts:** Commonly elevated secondary to catecholamine discharge after a stress such as surgery or childbirth

3. **Temperatures of 103–105°F:** In adults, think of lung or kidney infections, or bacteremia.
4. **Lethargy, Combativeness, Inappropriate Behavior:** Strongly consider doing an LP to rule out meningitis.
5. **Elderly Patients:** Can be extremely ill without many of the typical manifestations; they may be hypothermic or deny any tenderness. You must be very aggressive to identify the cause.
6. **Infants and Children:** Have normally elevated baseline temperatures (up to 3 mo 99.4°F, 1 y 99.7°F, 3 y 99.0°F)

GASTROINTESTINAL INTUBATION

Indications

- GI decompression: ileus, obstruction, pancreatitis, postoperatively
- Lavage of the stomach with GI bleeding or drug overdose
- Prevention of aspiration in an obtunded patient
- Feeding a patient who is unable to swallow

Materials

- Gastrointestinal tube of choice (see following list)
- Lubricant jelly
- Catheter tip syringe
- Glass of water with a straw, stethoscope

Types of Gastrointestinal Tubes

1. **Nasogastric Tubes**
    a. **Levin:** A tube with a single lumen, a perforated tip, and side holes for the aspiration of gastric contents. Connect it to an intermittent suction device to prevent the stomach lining from obstructing the lumen. Sometimes it is necessary to cut off the tip to allow for the aspiration of larger pills or tablets. The size varies from 10 to 18 French (1 French unit = ⅓ mm in diameter, see page 241).
    b. **Salem-sump:** A double-lumen tube, with the smaller tube acting as an air intake vent so that continuous suction can be applied. This is the best tube for irrigation and lavage because it will not collapse on itself. If a Salem-sump tube stops working even after it is repositioned, often a "shot" of air from a catheter-tipped syringe in the air vent will clear the tube. Both the Salem-sump and Levin tubes have radiopaque markings.
2. **Intestinal Decompression Tubes** ("long intestinal tubes")
    a. **Cantor tube:** A long single-lumen tube with a rubber balloon at the tip. The balloon is partially filled with mercury (5–7 mL using a tangentially directed 21-gauge needle, then the air is aspirated), which allows it to gravitate into the small bowel with the aid of peristalsis. Used for decompression when the bowel is obstructed distally.
    b. **Miller–Abbott tube:** A long double-lumen tube with a rubber balloon at the tip. One lumen is used for aspiration; the other connects to the balloon. After the tube is in the stomach, inflate the balloon with 5–10 mL of air, inject 2–3 mL of mercury into the balloon, and then aspirate the air. Functioning and indications are essentially the same as for the Cantor tube. **Do not** tape these intestinal tubes to the patient's nose or the tube will not descend. The progress of the tube can be followed on x-ray.

13

3. **Feeding Tubes**

Virtually any NG tube can be used as a feeding tube, but it is preferable to place a specially designed nasoduodenal feeding tube. These are of smaller diameter (usually 8 French) and are more pliable and comfortable for the patient. Weighted tips tend to travel into the duodenum, which helps prevent regurgitation and aspiration. Most are supplied with stylets that facilitate positioning, especially if fluoroscopic guidance is needed. Always verify the position of the feeding tube with an x-ray prior to starting tube feeding. Commonly used tubes include the mercury-weighted varieties (**Keogh tube, Duo-Tube, Dobbhoff, Entriflex**), the tungsten-weighted (**Vivonex tube**), and the unweighted pediatric feeding tubes.

4. **Miscellaneous**

a. **Sengstaken–Blakemore tube:** A triple-lumen tube used exclusively for the control of bleeding esophageal varices by tamponade. One lumen is for gastric aspiration, one is for the gastric balloon, and the third is for the esophageal balloon. Other types of tubes used to control esophageal bleeding include the **Linton** and **Minnesota** tubes.

b. **Ewald tube:** An orogastric tube used almost exclusively for gastric evacuation of blood or drug overdose. The tube is usually double lumen and large diameter (18–36 French).

c. **Dennis, Baker, Leonard tubes:** These are used for intraoperative decompression of the bowel and are manually passed into the bowel at the time of laparotomy.

Procedure (For Nasogastric and Feeding Tubes)

1. Inform the patient of the nature of the procedure and encourage cooperation if the patient is able. Choose the nasal passage that appears most open. Have the patient sitting up if able.

2. Lubricate the distal 3–4 in. of the tube with a water-soluble jelly (K-Y Jelly or viscous lidocaine), and insert the tube gently along the floor of the nasal passageway. Maintain gentle pressure that will allow the tube to pass into the nasopharynx.

3. When the patient can feel the tube in the back of the throat, ask patient to swallow small amounts of water through a straw as you advance the tube 2–3 in. at a time.

4. To be sure that the tube is in the stomach, aspirate gastric contents or blow air into the tube with a catheter-tipped syringe and listen over the stomach with your stethoscope for a "pop" or "gurgle." The position of feeding tubes **must** be verified by a chest x-ray prior to institution of feedings to prevent accidental bronchial instillation.

5. NG tubes are usually attached either to low wall suction (Salem-sump type tubes with a vent) or to intermittent suction (Levin type tubes). The latter allows the tube to fall away from the gastric wall between suction cycles.

6. Feeding and pediatric feeding tubes in adults are more difficult to insert because they are more flexible. Many are provided with stylets that make their passage easier. Feeding tubes are best placed into the duodenum or jejunum in order to decrease the risk of aspiration. Administering 10 mg of metoclopramide (Reglan) IV 10 min before insertion of the tube assists in placing the tube into the duodenum. Once the feeding tube is in the stomach, the bell of the stethoscope can be placed on the right side of the patient's midabdomen. As the tube is advanced, air can be injected to confirm progression of the tube to the right, toward the duodenum. If the sound of the air becomes fainter, the tube is probably curling in the stomach. Pass the tube until a slight resistance is felt, heralding the presence of the tip of the tube at the pylorus. Holding constant pressure and slowly injecting water through the tube is often rewarded with a "give," which signifies passage through the pylorus. The tube often can be advanced far into the

13

duodenum with this method. The duodenum usually provides constant resistance which will give with slow injection of water. Placing the patient in the right lateral decubitus position may help the tube enter the duodenum. Always confirm the location of the tube with an abdominal x-ray.

7. Tape the tube securely in place but do not allow it to apply pressure to the ala of the nose. (*Note:* Intestinal decompression tubes should not be taped because they are allowed to pass through the intestine). Patients have been disfigured because of ischemic necrosis of the nose caused by a poorly positioned NG tube.

Complications

*   Inadvertent passage into the trachea may provoke coughing or gagging in the patient.
*   Aspiration
*   If the patient is unable to cooperate, the tube often becomes coiled in the oral cavity.
*   The tube is irritating and may cause a small amount of bleeding in the mucosa of the nose, pharynx, or stomach. The drying and irritation can be lessened by throat lozenges or antiseptic spray.
*   Intracranial passage in patient with a basilar skull fracture
*   Esophageal perforation
*   Esophageal reflux caused by the tube-induced incompetence of the distal esophageal sphincter
*   Sinusitis can result from the tube, causing edema of the nasal passages that blocks drainage from the nasal sinuses.

HEELSTICK
Indication

*   Frequently used to collect blood samples from infants

Materials

*   Alcohol swabs
*   Lancet
*   Capillary or caraway collection tubes
*   Clay tube sealer

Technique

1. Although called a "heelstick," any highly vascularized capillary bed can be used (finger, ear lobe, or great toe). The heel can be warmed for 5–10 min by wrapping it in a warm washcloth.
2. Wipe the area with an alcohol swab. Use Figure 13–11 to choose the site for the puncture on the foot. Use of these sites helps decrease the incidence of osteomyelitis.
3. Use a 4-mm lancet, and make a quick, deep puncture so that blood flows freely. Automated safety lancets (eg, BD Genie lancet for fingersticks and the BD Quick Heel Lancer for heelsticks) are also available. Wipe off the first drop of blood. Gently squeeze the heel and touch a collection tube to the drop of blood. The tube should fill by capillary action. Seal the end of the tube in clay.
4. Most labs can usually make laboratory determinations on small samples from the pediatric age group. A **Caraway tube** can hold 0.3 mL of blood. One to three caraway tubes can be used for most routine tests. For a capillary blood gas, the blood is usually transferred to a 1-mL heparinized syringe and placed on ice.
5. Wrap the foot with 4×4 gauze squares or apply an adhesive bandage.

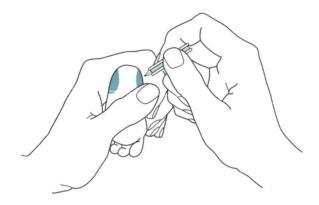

FIGURE 13–11   Demonstration of the preferred sites and technique of performing a heelstick in an infant. (Reprinted, with permission, from: Gomella TL [ed]: *Neonatology: Basic Management, On-Call Problems, Diseases, Drugs,* 4th ed. Appleton & Lange, Norwalk CT, 1998.)

INTERNAL FETAL SCALP MONITORING

Indication

- To accurately assess FHR patterns during labor to screen for possible fetal distress

Contraindications

- Presence of placenta previa
- When it is otherwise impossible to identify the portion of the fetal body where application is contemplated

Materials

- Fetal scalp monitoring electrode
- Sterile vaginal lubricant or povidone–iodine spray
- Spiral electrode
- Leg plate/fetal monitor

Technique

1. Position the patient in the dorsal lithotomy position (knees flexed and abducted), and perform an aseptic perineal prep with sterile vaginal lubricant or povidone–iodine spray.
2. Perform a manual vaginal exam, and clearly identify the fetal presenting part. The membranes **must** be ruptured prior to attachment of the spiral electrode.

3. Remove the spiral electrode from the sterile package and place the guide tube firmly against the fetal presenting part. Electrode should not be applied to fetal face, fontanels, or genitalia.
4. Advance the drive tube and electrode until the electrode contacts the presenting part. Maintaining pressure on the guide tube and drive tube, rotate the drive tube clockwise until mild resistance is met (usually one turn).
5. Press together the arms on the drive tube grip, which releases the locking device. Carefully slide the drive and guide tubes off the electrode wires while holding the locking device open.
6. Attach the spiral electrode wires to the color-coded leg plate, which is then connected to the electronic fetal monitor.

Complications

- Fetal or maternal hemorrhage, fetal infection (usually scalp abscess at the site of insertion)

Interpretation

Normal FHR is 120–160 bpm. **Accelerations** are increases in the FHR, and although they can be associated with fetal distress (usually in association with late decelerations), they are almost always a sign of fetal well-being. **Decelerations** are transient falls in FHR related to a uterine contraction and are of three types:

1. **Early Decelerations:** Seen in normal labor, slowing of the FHR clearly associated with the onset of the contraction and the FHR promptly returns to normal after the contraction is over. Usually caused by head compression, and occasionally by cord compression.
2. **Late Deceleration:** Slowing of the FHR that occurs after the uterine contraction starts and the rate does not return to normal until well after the contraction is over. This type of pattern is often associated with uteroplacental insufficiency (fetal acidosis or hypoxia).
3. **Variable Decelerations:** Irregular pattern of decelerations unassociated with contractions caused by cord compression. If bradycardia persists, evaluate with scalp pH.

Other patterns seen include **beat-to-beat variability** (small fluctuations in FHR 5–15 BPM over the baseline FHR usually associated with fetal well-being); **tachycardia** (often an early sign of fetal distress, seen with febrile illnesses, hypoxia, fetal thyrotoxicosis); and **bradycardia** (associated with maternal and fetal hypoxia, fetal heart lesions including heart block). **Sinusoidal** pattern can be drug-induced and is seen occasionally with severe fetal anemia.

INJECTION TECHNIQUES

Indications

- **Intradermal:** Most commonly used for skin testing
- **Subcutaneous:** Useful for low-volume medications such as insulin, heparin and some vaccines
- **Intramuscular:** Administration of parenteral medications that cannot be absorbed from the subcutaneous layer or of high volume (up to 10 mL)

Contraindications

- Allergy to any components of the injectate
- Active infection or dermatitis at the injection site
- Intramuscular injections are generally contraindicated with coagulopathy

Procedures

Intradermal (see Skin Testing, page 303)

Subcutaneous

1. Deposit the drug within the fat but above the muscle. With careful placement nerve injury is rarely a danger.
2. Choose a site free of scarring or active infection. Injection sites include the outer surface of the upper arm, anterior surface of the thigh, and lower abdominal wall. With repeated injections (diabetics, etc) sites should be rotated.
3. 25–27-gauge ¾–1-in. needles are most commonly used; volume of medication must not exceed 5 mL. Draw up the medication, making certain to expel any air bubbles.
4. Clean site with an alcohol swab. Bunch up the skin between the thumb and forefinger so that the subcutaneous tissue is off the underlying muscle.
5. Warn the patient that there will be "pinch" or "sting," and insert the needle firmly and rapidly at a 45-degree angle until a sudden release signifies penetration of the dermis.
6. Release the skin, and aspirate to make certain a blood vessel has not been entered and inject slowly.
7. Withdraw the needle and apply gentle pressure. A dressing is not usually necessary. Apply pressure longer if there is bleeding from the site.

Intramuscular

1. Common sites include the deltoid, gluteus, and the vastus lateralis.
   - **Deltoid Muscle:** The safe zone includes only the main body of the deltoid muscle lying lateral and a few centimeters beneath the acromion. Low risk of radial nerve injury unless the needle strays into the middle or lower third of the arm.
   - **Gluteus Muscles:** This is the preferred site in children > 2 y and in adults. Draw an imaginary line from the femoral head to the posterior superior iliac spine. This site (upper outer quadrant of the buttocks) is safe for injections because it is away from the sciatic nerve and superior gluteal artery.
   - **Vastus Lateralis Muscle** (anterior thigh): A very safe site in all patients and the site of choice in infants. The only disadvantage of this site is that the firm fascia lata overlying the muscle can make needle insertion somewhat more painful.
2. A 22-gauge, 1½-in. needle is acceptable for most intramuscular injections. Remove air bubbles from the syringe and needle. Wipe the skin with alcohol.
3. Gently stretch the skin to one side and warn the patient of a sting. Penetrate the skin at a 90-degree angle, and advance approximately 1 in. into the muscle. (Obese patients may require deeper penetration with a longer needle).
4. Aspirate to make sure that you have not entered a vessel. Administer the medication. Gently massage the site with alcohol swab or gauze to promote absorption.

Complications

- Nerve and arterial injury
- Abscesses (sterile or septic). Use good technique and rotate injection sites.
- Bleeding can usually be controlled with pressure.

INTRAUTERINE PRESSURE MONITORING
Indication

- To accurately assess uterine contraction during labor

Contraindication

- Presence of placenta previa

Materials

- Pressure catheter and introducer
- Transducer connected to fetal monitor
- Sterile gloves, vaginal lubricant, povidone–iodine spray
- 10-mL syringe, 30 mL sterile water

Procedure

1. Prime the transducer with sterile water.
2. Position the patient in the dorsal lithotomy position (knees flexed and abducted), and perform an aseptic perineal prep with sterile vaginal lubricant or povidone–iodine spray.
3. Perform a manual vaginal exam, and clearly identify the fetal presenting part. The membranes must be ruptured prior to insertion of catheter.
4. Remove the catheter from the sterile package, and place the guide tube through fingers around the presenting part into the uterine cavity.
5. Prime the catheter with sterile water and thread through the guide tube.
6. Attach the distal catheter to transducer and zero to air.

Complications

Infection, placental perforation if low lying

IV TECHNIQUES

Indication

13

- To establish an intravenous access for the administration of fluids, blood, or medications
- (Other techniques include Central Venous Catheters, page 253 and PICC lines (page 292)

Materials

- IV fluid
- Connecting tubing
- Tourniquet
- Alcohol swab
- Intravenous cannulas (a catheter over a needle [eg, Angiocath, Insyte] or a butterfly needle)
- Antiseptic ointment, dressing, and tape

Technique

1. It helps to rip the tape into strips, attach the IV tubing to the solution, and flush the air out of the tubing before you begin. Using a catheter–needle assembly (Angiocath, etc) often helps to "break the seal" between the needle and catheter prior to the time that the catheter is in the vein so that dislodging the catheter is less likely.
2. The upper, nondominant extremity is the site of choice for an IV, unless the patient is being considered for placement of permanent hemodialysis access. In this instance, the

upper nondominant extremity should be "saved" as the access site for hemodialysis. Choose a distal vein (dorsum of the hand) so that if the vein is lost, you can reposition the IV more proximally. Figure 13–12 demonstrates some common upper extremity

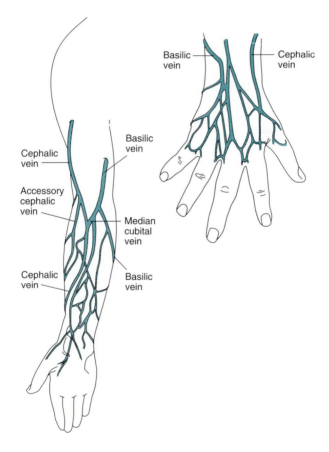

FIGURE 13–12 Principle veins of the arm used to place IV access and in venipuncture, the pattern can be highly variable. (Reprinted, with permission, from: Stillman RM [ed]: *Surgery, Diagnosis, and Therapy,* Appleton & Lange, Norwalk, CT, 1989.)

veins; however, avoid veins that cross a joint space. Also avoid the leg because the incidence of thrombophlebitis is high with IVs placed there.

3. Apply a tourniquet above the proposed IV site. Use the techniques described in the section on venipuncture to help expose the vein (page 309). Carefully clean the site with an alcohol or povidone–iodine swab. If a large-bore IV is to be used (16 or 14), local anesthesia (1idocaine injected with a 25-gauge needle) is helpful.

4. Stabilize the vein distally with the thumb of your free hand. Using the catheter-over-needle assembly (Intracath or Angiocath), either enter the vein directly or enter the skin alongside the vein first and then stick the vein along the side at about a 20-degree angle. Direct entry and side entry IV techniques are illustrated in Figures 13–13 and 13–14. Once the vein is punctured, blood should appear in the "flash chamber" of a catheter-over-needle assembly. Advance a few more millimeters to be sure that **both** the needle **and** the tip of the catheter have entered the vein. Carefully withdraw the needle as you advance the catheter into the vein (see Fig. 13–13). **Never withdraw the catheter over the needle because this procedure can shear off the plastic tip and cause a catheter embolus.** Remove the tourniquet, and connect the IV line to the catheter. Blood loss can be minimized by compressing the vein with the thumb just proximal to the catheter.

5. With the IV fluid running, observe the site for signs of induration or swelling that indicate improper placement or damage to the vein. See Chapter 9 for choosing IV fluids and how to determine infusion rates.

6. Tape the IV securely in place, apply a drop of povidone–iodine or antibiotic ointment and sterile dressing. Ideally, the dressing should be changed every 24–48 h to help reduce infections. Arm boards are also useful to help maintain an IV site.

7. **"Butterfly"** or **"scalp vein"** needle can sometimes be used (see Fig. 13–14). This is a small metal needle with plastic "wings" on the side. It is very useful in infants, who often have poor peripheral veins but prominent scalp veins, children, and in adults who have small, fragile veins.

8. Troubleshooting difficult IV placement

    • If the veins are deep and difficult to locate, a small 3–5-mL syringe can be mounted on the catheter assembly. Proper positioning inside the vein is determined by aspiration of blood. If blood specimens are needed on a patient who also needs an IV, this technique can be used to start the IV and to collect samples at the same time.

    • **Whaid's maneuver** can be attempted (*J Emerg Nurs,* 1993;**19:**186). Spend about 1 min using both hands to "milk" blood from the arm toward the forearm. While holding the arm compressed with both hands, place a tourniquet above the elbow. Milk the blood from the fingers to the forearm for 3–5 min. When a vein becomes prominent, wrap your hand around the patient's wrist and place the IV.

    • If no extremity vein can be found, try the external jugular. Placing the patient in the head down position can help distend the vein.

    • If all these fail, the next alternative is a central venous line insertion.

LUMBAR PUNCTURE

Indications

    • **Diagnostic purposes:** Analysis of CSF for conditions such as meningitis, encephalitis, Guillain-Barré syndrome, staging work-up for lymphoma, others

    • Measurement of CSF pressure or its changes with various maneuvers (Valsalva, etc)

    • **Injection of various agents:** Contrast media for myelography, antitumor drugs, analgesics, antibiotics

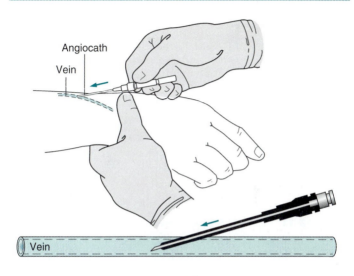

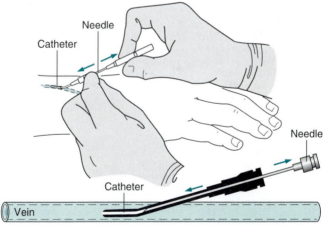

FIGURE 13–13   To insert a catheter-over-needle assembly into a vein, stabilize the skin and vein with gentle traction. Enter the vein and advance the catheter while removing the needle.

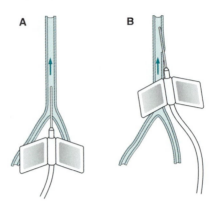

FIGURE 13–14 Example of a "butterfly" needle assembly and the two different techniques of entering a vein for intravenous access: A direct puncture; and B side entry. (Reprinted, with permission, from: Gomella TL [ed]: *Neonatology: Basic Management, On-Call Problems, Diseases, Drugs,* 4th ed. Appleton & Lange, Norwalk CT, 1998.)

Contraindications

- Increased intracranial pressure (papilledema, mass lesion)
- Infection near the puncture site
- Planned myelography or pneumoencephalography
- Coagulation disorders

Materials

- A sterile, disposable LP kit

or

- Minor procedure tray (see page 240)
- Spinal needles (21-gauge for adults, 22-gauge for children)

Background

The objective of an LP is to obtain a sample of CSF from the subarachnoid space. Specifically, during an LP the fluid is obtained from the **lumbar cistern,** the volume of CSF located between the termination of the spinal cord (the conus medullaris) and the termination of the dura mater at the coccygeal ligament. The cistern is surrounded by the subarachnoid membrane and the overlying dura. Located within the cistern are the filum terminale and the nerve roots of the cauda equina. When an LP is done, the main body of the spinal cord is avoided and the nerve roots of the cauda are simply pushed out of the way by the needle.

The termination of the spinal cord in the adult is usually between L1 and L2, and in the pediatric patient between L2 and L3. The safest site for an LP is the interspace between L4 and L5. An imaginary line drawn between the iliac crests (the supracristal plane) intersects the spine at either the L4 spinous process or the L4–L5 interspace.

A spinal needle introduced between the spinous processes of L4 and L5 penetrates the layers in the following order: skin, supraspinous ligament, interspinous ligament, ligamentum flava, epidural space (contains loose areolar tissue, fat, and blood vessels), dura, "potential space," subarachnoid membrane, subarachnoid space (lumbar cistern) (Fig. 13–15).

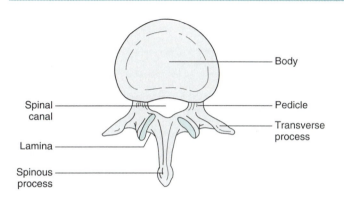

Body

Spinal canal

Pedicle

Transverse process

Lamina

Spinous process

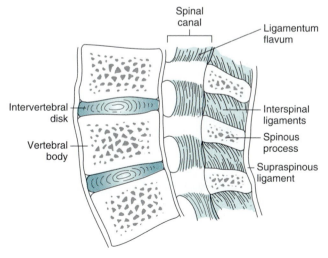

Spinal canal

Ligamentum flavum

Intervertebral disk

Interspinal ligaments

Spinous process

Vertebral body

Supraspinous ligament

FIGURE 13–15 Basic anatomy for a lumbar puncture.

Technique

1. Examine the fundus for evidence of papilledema, and review the CT or MRF of the head if available. Discuss the relative safety and lack of discomfort to the patient to dispel any myths. Some clinicians prefer to call the procedure a "subarachnoid analysis" rather than a spinal tap. As long as the procedure and the risks are outlined, most patients will agree to the procedure. Have the patient sign an informed consent form.

2. Place the patient in the lateral decubitus position close to the edge of the bed or table. The patient (held by an assistant, if possible) should be positioned with knees pulled up toward stomach and head flexed onto chest (Fig. 13–16). This position enhances flexion of the vertebral spine and widens the interspaces between the spinous processes. Place a pillow beneath the patient's side to prevent sagging and ensure alignment of the spinal column. In an obese patient or a patient with arthritis or scoliosis, the sitting position, leaning forward, may be preferred.

3. Palpate the supracristal plane (see under Background) and carefully determine the location of the L4–L5 interspace.

4. Open the kit, put on sterile gloves, and prep the area with povidone–iodine solution in a circular fashion and covering several interspaces. Next, drape the patient.

5. With a 25-gauge needle and 1idocaine, raise a skin wheal over the L4–L5 interspace. Anesthetize the deeper structures with a 22-gauge needle.

6. Examine the spinal needle with a stylet for defects and then insert it into the skin wheal and into the spinous ligament. Hold the needle between your index and middle fingers, with your thumb holding the stylet in place. Direct the needle cephalad at a 30–45-degree angle, in the midline and parallel to the bed (see Fig. 13–16).

7. Advance through the major structures and pop into the subarachnoid space through the dura. An experienced operator can feel these layers, but an inexperienced one may need to periodically remove the stylet to look for return of fluid. It is important to always replace the stylet prior to advancing the spinal needle. The needle may be withdrawn, however, with the stylet removed. This technique may be useful if the needle has passed through the back wall of the canal. Direct the bevel of the needle parallel to the long axis of the body so that the dural fibers are separated rather than sheared. This method helps cut down on "spinal headaches."

8. If no fluid returns, it is sometimes helpful to rotate the needle slightly. If still no fluid appears, and you think that you are within the subarachnoid space, inject 1 mL of air because it is not uncommon for a piece of tissue to clog the needle. **Never** inject saline or distilled water. If no air returns and if spinal fluid cannot be aspirated, the bevel of the needle probably lies in the epidural space; advance it with the stylet in place.

9. When fluid returns, attach a manometer and stopcock and measure the pressure. Normal opening pressure is 70–180 mm water in the lateral decubitus. Increased pressure may be due to a tense patient, CHF, ascites, subarachnoid hemorrhage, infection, or a space-occupying lesion. Decreased pressure may be due to needle position or obstructed flow (you may need to leave the needle in for a myelogram because if it is moved, the subarachnoid space may be lost).

10. Collect 0.5–2.0-mL samples in serial, labeled containers. Send them to the lab in this order:

    - **First tube for bacteriology:** Gram's stain, routine C&S, AFB, and fungal cultures and stains
    - **Second tube for glucose and protein:** If a work-up for MS, order electrophoresis to detect oligoclonal banding and assay for myelin basic protein characteristic of MS
    - **Third tube for cell count:** CBC with differential

13

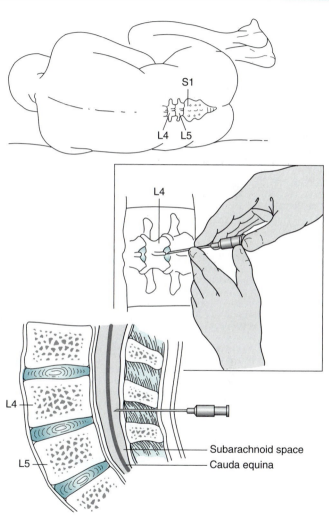

FIGURE 13–16 When performing a lumbar puncture, place the patient in the lateral decubitus position, and locate the L4–L5 interspace. Control the spinal needle with two hands, and enter the subarachnoid space.

- **Fourth tube for special studies as clinically indicated:**

VDRL neurosyphilis

CIEP (counterimmunoelectrophoresis) for bacterial antigens such as *H. influenzae, S. Pneumoniae, N. meningitidis*)

PCR assay for tuberculous meningitis or herpes simplex encephalitis (allows rapid diagnosis)

If *Cryptococcus neoformans* is suspected (most common cause of meningitis in AIDS patients) India ink preparation and cryptococcal antigen (latex agglutination test)

Note: Some clinicians prefer to send the first and last tubes for CBC because this procedure permits a better differentiation between a **subarachnoid hemorrhage** and a **traumatic tap.** In a traumatic tap, the number of RBCs in the first tube should be much higher than in the last tube. In a subarachnoid hemorrhage, the cell counts should be equal, and **xanthochromia** of the fluid should be present, indicating the presence of old blood.

11. Withdraw the needle and place a dry, sterile dressing over the site.
12. Instruct the patient to remain recumbent for 6–12 h, and encourage an increased fluid intake to help prevent "spinal headaches."
13. Interpret the results based on Table 13–4.

Complications

- **Spinal headache:** The most common complication (about 20%), this appears within the first 24 h after the puncture. It goes away when the patient is lying down and is aggravated when the patient sits up. It is usually characterized by a severe throbbing pain in the occipital region and can last a week. It is thought to be caused by intracranial traction caused by the acute volume depletion of CSF and by persistent leakage from the puncture site. To help prevent spinal headaches, keep the patient recumbent for 6–12 h, encourage the intake of fluids, use the smallest needle possible, and keep the bevel of the needle parallel to the long axis of the body to help prevent a persistent CSF leak.
- **Trauma to nerve roots or to the conus medullaris:** Much less frequent (some anatomic variation does exist, but it is very rare for the cord to end below L3). If the patient suddenly complains of paresthesia (numbness or shooting pains in the legs), stop the procedure.
- **Herniation of either the cerebellum or the medulla:** Occurs rarely, during or after a spinal tap, usually in a patient with increased intracranial pressure. This complication can often be reversed medically if it is recognized early.
- **Meningitis.**
- **Bleeding** in the subarachnoid/subdural space can occur with resulting paralysis especially if the patient is receiving anticoagulants or has severe liver disease with a coagulopathy.

ORTHOSTATIC BLOOD PRESSURE MEASUREMENT
Indication

- Assessment of volume depletion

Materials

- Blood pressure cuff and stethoscope

TABLE 13-4
Differential Diagnosis of Cerebrospinal Fluid

Condition	Color	Opening Pressure (mm H$_2$O)	Protein (mg/ 100 mL)	Glucose (mg/ 100 mL)	Cells (#/mm^3)
NORMAL					
Adult	Clear	70–180	15–45	45–80	0–5 lymphocytes
Newborn	Clear	70–180	20–120	2/3 serum	40–60 lymphocytes
INFECTIOUS					
Viral infection ("aseptic meningitis")	Clear or opalescent	Normal or slightly increased	Normal or slightly increased	Normal	10–500 lymphocytes PMNs
Bacterial infection	Opalescent yellow, may clot	Increased	Increased, 50–10,000	Increased, usually <20	25–10,000 PMNs
Granulomatous infection (TB, fungal)	Clear or opalescent	Often increased	Increased, but usually <500	Decreased, usually <20–40	10–500 lymphocytes
NEUROLOGIC					
Guillain–Barré Syndrome	Clear or Cloudy	Normal	Markedly increased	Normal	Normal or increased lymphocytes

13

(continued)

287

TABLE 13-4 (Continued)

Condition	Color	Opening Pressure (mm H_2O)	Protein (mg/100 mL)	Glucose (mg/100 mL)	Cells (#/mm³)
Multiple sclerosis	Clear	Normal	Normal or increased	Normal	0–20 lymphocytes
Pseudotumor cerebri	Clear	Increased	Normal	Normal	Normal
MISCELLANEOUS					
Neoplasm	Clear or xanthochromic	Increased	Normal or increased	Normal or decreased	Normal or increased lymphocytes
Traumatic tap	Bloody, no xanthochromia	Normal	Normal	Sl increased	RBC = peripheral blood; Less RBC in tube 4 than in tube 1
Subarachnoid hemorrhage	Bloody or xanthochromic after 2–8 h	Usually increased	Increased	Normal	WBC/RBC ratio same as blood

Abbreviations: WBC = white blood cell; RBC = red blood cell; PMNs = polymorphonuclear neutrophils.

13

288

Procedure

1. Changes in blood pressure and pulse when a patient moves from supine to the upright position are very sensitive guides for detecting early volume depletion. Even before a person becomes overtly tachycardic or hypotensive because of volume loss, the demonstration of orthostatic hypotension aids in the diagnosis.
2. Have the patient assume a supine position for 5–10 min. Determine the BP and pulse.
3. Then have the patient stand up. If the patient is unable to stand, have the patient sit at the bedside with legs dangling.
4. After about 1 min, determine the BP and pulse again.
5. A drop in systolic BP greater than 10 mm Hg or an increase in pulse rate greater than 20 (16 if elderly) suggests **volume depletion.** A change in heart rate is more sensitive and occurs with a lesser degree of volume depletion. Other causes include peripheral vascular disease, surgical sympathectomy, diabetes, and medications (prazosin, hydralazine, or reserpine).

PELVIC EXAMINATION
Indications

- Part of a complete physical examination in the female
- Used to assist in the diagnosis of diseases and conditions of the female genital tract

Materials

- Gloves
- Vaginal speculum and lubricant
- Slides, fixative (Pap aerosol spray, etc), cotton swabs, endocervical brush and cervical spatula prepared for a Pap smear
- **Materials for other diagnostic tests:** Culture media to test for gonorrhea, *Chlamydia,* herpes; sterile cotton swabs, plain glass slides, KOH, and normal saline solutions, as needed

Procedure

1. The pelvic exam should be carried out in a comfortable fashion for both the patient and physician. A female assistant **must** be present for the procedure. The patient should be draped appropriately with her feet placed in the stirrups on the examining table. Prepare a low stool, a good light source, and all needed supplies before the exam begins. In unusual situations examinations are conducted on a stretcher or bed; raise the patients buttocks on one or two pillows to elevate the perineum off the mattress.
2. Inform the patient of each move in advance. Glove hands before proceeding.
3. **General inspection:**
   a. Observe the skin of the perineum for swelling, ulcers, condylomata (venereal warts), or color changes.
   b. Separate the labia to examine the clitoris and vestibule. Multiple clear vesicles on an erythematous base on the labia suggest herpes.
   c. Observe the urethral meatus for developmental abnormalities, discharge, neoplasm, and abscess of Bartholin's gland at the 4 or 8 o'clock positions.
   d. Inspect the vaginal orifice for discharge, or protrusion of the walls (cystocele, rectocele, urethral prolapse).
   e. Note the condition of the hymen.

4. **Speculum examination:**
   a. Use a speculum moistened with warm water **not** with lubricant (lubricant will interfere with Pap tests and slide studies). Check the temperature on the patient's leg to see if the speculum is comfortable.
   b. Because the anterior wall of the vagina is close to the urethra and bladder, do not exert pressure in this area. Pressure should be placed on the posterior surface of the vagina. With the speculum directed at a 45-degree angle to the floor, spread the labia and insert the speculum fully, pressing posteriorly. The cervix should pop into view with some manipulation as the speculum is opened.
   c. Inspect the cervix and vagina for color, lacerations, growths, nabothian cysts, and evidence of atrophy.
   d. Inspect the cervical os for size, shape, color, discharge.
   e. Inspect the vagina for secretions and obtain specimens for a Pap smear, other smear, or culture (see tests for vaginal infections and Pap smear in item 7).
   f. Inspect the vaginal wall; rotate the speculum as you draw it out to see the entire canal.

5. **Bimanual examination:**
   a. For this part, stand up. It is best to use whichever hand is comfortable to do the internal vaginal exam. Remove the glove from the hand that will examine the abdomen.
   b. Place lubricant on the first and second gloved fingers, and then, keeping pressure on the posterior fornix, introduce them into the vagina.
   c. Palpate the tissue at 5 and 7 o'clock between the first and second fingers and the thumb to rule out any abnormality of Bartholin's gland. Likewise, palpate the urethra and paraurethral (Skene's) gland.
   d. Place the examining fingers on the posterior wall of the vagina to further open the introitus. Ask the patient to bear down. Look for evidence of prolapse, rectocele, or cystocele.
   e. Palpate the cervix. Note the size, shape, consistency, and motility, and test for tenderness (the so-called **chandelier sign** or marked cervical tenderness, which is positive in PID).
   f. With your fingers in the vagina posterior to the cervix and your hand on the abdomen placed just above the symphysis, force the corpus of the uterus between the two examining hands. Note size, shape, consistency, position, and motility.
   g. Move the fingers in the vagina to one or the other fornix, and place the hand on the abdomen in a more lateral position to bring the adnexal areas under examination. Palpate the ovaries, if possible, for any masses, consistency, and motility. Unless the fallopian tubes are diseased, they usually are not palpable.

6. **Rectovaginal examination:**
   a. Insert your index finger into the vagina, and place the well-lubricated middle finger in the rectum.
   b. Palpate the posterior surface of the uterus and the broad ligament for nodularity, tenderness, or other masses. Examine the uterosacral and rectovaginal septum. Nodularity here may represent endometriosis.
   c. It may also be helpful to do a test for occult blood if a stool specimen is available.

7. **Papanicolaou (Pap) smear:**
   The Pap smear is helpful in the early detection of cervical intraepithelial neoplasia and carcinoma. Endometrial carcinoma is occasionally identified on routine Pap smears. It is recommended that low-risk patients have routine Pap smears done every 2–3 y, but only after three annual Pap smears are negative. High-risk patients such as those exposed to in utero DES, patients with HPV infections, history of cervical dysplasia or cervical intraep-

13

ithelial neoplasia, more than two sexual partners in the patient's lifetime, and intercourse prior to age 20 should obtain an annual Pap smear.

    a. With the unlubricated speculum in place, use a wooden cervical spatula to obtain a scraping from the squamocolumnar junction. Rotate the spatula 360 degrees around the external os. Smear on a frosted slide that has the patient's name written on it in pencil. Fix the slide either in a bottle of fixative or with commercially available spray fixative. The slide must be fixed within 10 s or a drying artifact may occur.

    b. Next, obtain a specimen from the endocervical canal using a cotton swab or commercial available endocervical brush and prepare the slide as described in part a.

    c. Using a wooden spatula, an additional specimen should be obtained from the posterior/lateral vaginal pool of fluid and smeared on a slide.

    d. Complete the appropriate lab slips. Forewarn the patient that she may experience some spotty vaginal bleeding following the Pap smear.

8. **Tests for cervical/vaginal infections:**

    a. **GC culture:** Use a sterile cotton swab to obtain a specimen from the endocervical canal and plate it out on **Thayer–Martin** medium.

    b. **Vaginal saline (wet) prep:** Helpful in the diagnosis of *Trichomonas vaginalis* or *Gardnerella vaginalis*. A thin, foamy, white, pruritic discharge is associated with a **Trichomonas** infection. Mix a drop of discharge with a drop of NS on a glass slide and cover the drop with a coverslip. It is important to observe the slide while it is still warm to see the flagellated, motile trichomonads. If a patient has a thin, watery, gray, malodorous discharge, an infection with *Gardnerella vaginalis* may be present. Bacterial vaginosis is most often caused by *G. vaginalis* and can be diagnosed by the presence of "clue cells," which represent polymorphonuclear white cells dotted with the *G. vaginalis* bacteria, a vaginal pH of > 4.5 and a fishy amine odor with addition of KOH to the secretions. Alternatively, these can be seen by using a hanging drop of saline and a concave slide. *Lactobacillus* is normally the predominant bacteria in the vagina in the absence of specific infection and the normal pH is usually < 4.5.

    c. **Potassium hydroxide prep:** If a thick, white, curdy discharge is present, the patient may have a *Candida albicans* (monilial) yeast infection. Prepare a slide with one drop of discharge and one drop of aqueous 10% KOH solution. The KOH dissolves the epithelial cells and debris and facilitates viewing of the hyphae and mycelia of the fungus that causes the infection.

    d. **Gram's stain:** Material can easily be stained in the usual fashion (Chapter 7, page 122). Gram-negative intracellular diplococci (so-called GNIDs) are pathognomonic of *Neisseria gonorrhoeae.* The most commonly found bacteria in Gram's stains are large gram-positive rods (lactobacilli), which are normal vaginal flora.

    e. **Herpes cultures:** A routine Pap smear of the cervix or a Pap smear of the herpetic lesion (multiple, clear vesicles on a painful, erythematous base) may demonstrate herpes inclusion bodies. A herpes culture may be done by taking a viral culture swab of the suspicious lesion or of the endocervix.

    f. *Chlamydia* cultures: Special swabs can be obtained from the microbiology lab for *Chlamydia* cultures.

PERICARDIOCENTESIS

Indications

- Emergency treatment of cardiac tamponade
- Diagnose the cause of pericardial effusion

Contraindications

- Minimal pericardial effusion (< 200 mL)
- After CABG due to risk of injury to grafts
- Uncorrected coagulopathy

Materials

- Electrocardiogram machine
- Prepackaged pericardiocentesis kit **or** Procedure and instrument tray (page 240) with pericardiocentesis needle or 16–18-gauge needle 10 cm long

Background

Cardiac tamponade results in decreased cardiac output, increased right atrial filling pressures, and a pronounced pulsus paradoxus.

Procedure

1. If time permits, use sterile prep and draping with gown, mask, and gloves.
2. Draining the pericardium can be approached either through the left para xiphoid or the left parasternal fourth intercostal space. The para xiphoid is safer, more commonly used, and described here (Fig. 13–17).
3. Anesthetize the insertion site with lidocaine. Connect the needle with an alligator clip to lead V on the ECG machine. Attach the limb leads, and monitor the machine.
4. Insert the pericardiocentesis needle just to the left of the xiphoid and directed upward 45 degrees toward the left shoulder.
5. Aspirate while advancing the needle until the pericardium is punctured and the effusion is tapped. If the ventricular wall is felt, withdraw the needle slightly. Additionally, if the needle contacts the myocardium, pronounced ST segment elevation will be noted on the ECG.
6. If performed for cardiac tamponade, removal of as little as 50 mL of fluid dramatically improves blood pressure and decreases right atrial pressure.
7. Blood from a bloody pericardial effusion is usually defibrinated and will not clot, whereas blood from the ventricle will clot.
8. Send fluid for hematocrit, cell count, or cytology if indicated. Serous fluid is consistent with CHF, bacterial infection, TB, hypoalbuminemia, or viral pericarditis. Bloody fluid (HCT >10%) may result from trauma; be iatrogenic; or due to MI, uremia, coagulopathy, or malignancy (lymphoma, leukemia, breast, lung most common)
9. If continuous drainage is necessary, use a guidewire to place a 16-gauge intravenous catheter.

Complications

Arrhythmia, ventricular puncture, lung injury

PERIPHERALLY INSERTED CENTRAL CATHETER (PICC LINE)
Indications

- Home infusion of hypertonic or irrigating solutions and drugs
- Long-term infusion of medications (antibiotics, chemotherapeutics)
- TPN
- Repetitive venous blood sampling

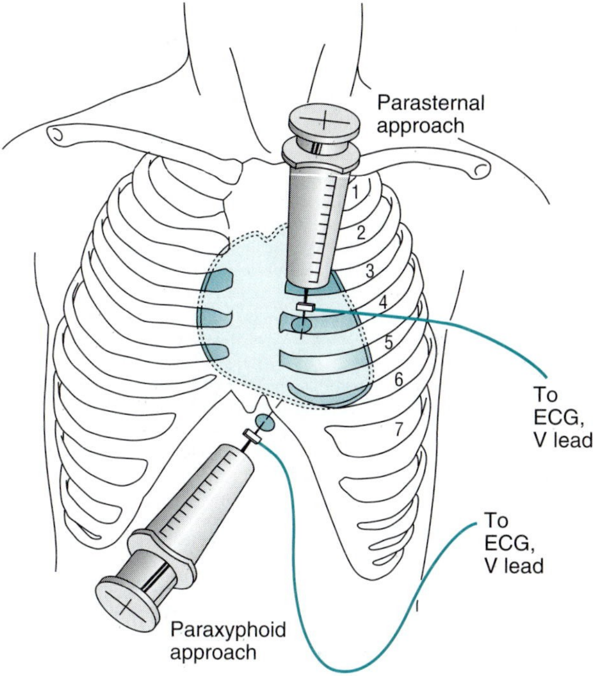

FIGURE 13–17 Techniques for pericardiocentesis. The paraxiphoid approach is the most popular. (Reprinted, with permission, from: Stillman RM [ed]: *Surgery, Diagnosis, and Therapy,* Appleton & Lange, Norwalk CT, 1989.)

Contraindications

- Infection over placement site
- Failure to identify veins in an arm with a tourniquet in place

Materials

- PICC catheter kit (contains most items necessary including the silastic long arm line)
- Tourniquet, sterile gloves, mask, sterile gown, heparin flush, 10-mL syringes

Background

Installation of a PICC allows for central venous access through a peripheral vein. Typically, a long-arm catheter is placed into the basilic or cephalic vein (See Fig. 13–12) and is threaded into the subclavian vein/superior vena cava. PICCs are useful for long-term home infusion therapies. The design of PICC catheters can vary, and the operator should be familiar with the features of the device (attached hub or detachable hub designs).

Procedure

1. Explain the procedure to the patient and then obtain informed consent. Position the patient in a sitting or reclining position with the elbow extended and the arm in a dependent position. The arm should be externally rotated.
2. Using a measuring tape, determine the length of the catheter required. Measure from the extremity vein insertion site to the subclavian vein.
3. Wear mask, gown, protective eyewear, and sterile gloves. Prep and drape the skin in the standard fashion. Set up an adjacent sterile working area.
4. Anesthetize the skin at the proposed area of insertion. Apply a tourniquet above the proposed IV site.
5. Trim the catheter to the appropriate length. Most PICC lines have an attached hub, and the distal end of the catheter is cut to the proper length. Flush with heparinized saline.
6. Insert the catheter and introducer needle (usually 14-gauge) into the chosen arm vein as detailed in the section on IV techniques (page 279). Once the catheter is in the vein, remove the introducer needle.
7. Place the PICC line in the catheter and advance (use a forceps if provided by the manufacturer of the kit to advance the PICC line). Remove the tourniquet and gradually advance the catheter the requisite length. Remove the inner stiffening wire slowly once the catheter has been adequately advanced.
8. Peel away the introducer catheter. Attach the Luer-lock, and flush the catheter again with heparin solution. Attempt to also aspirate blood to verify patency.
9. Attach the provided securing wings, and suture in place. Apply a sterile dressing over the insertion site.
10. Confirm placement in the central circulation with a chest x-ray. Always document the type of PICC, the length inserted, and the site of its radiologically confirmed placement.
11. If vein cannulation is difficult, a surgical cutdown may be necessary to cannulate the vein. If the catheter will not advance, fluoroscopy may be helpful.
12. Instruct the patient on the maintenance of the PICC. The PICC should be flushed with heparinized saline after each use. Dressing changes should be performed at least every 7 d under sterile conditions. Patient must be instructed to evaluate the PICC site for signs and symptoms of infection. Patient must also be instructed to come to the emergency room for evaluation of any fevers.
13. For venous samples, a specimen of at least the catheter volume (1–3 mL) must first be withdrawn and then discarded. The PICC must always be flushed with heparinized saline after each blood draw.

PICC Removal

Position the patient's arm at a 90-degree angle to his body. Remove the dressing and gently pull the PICC out. Apply pressure to site for 2–3 min. Always measure the length of the catheter and check prior documentation to ensure that the PICC line has been removed in its entirety. If a piece of a catheter is left behind, an emergency interventional radiology consult is in order.

Complications

Site bleeding, clotted catheter, subclavian thrombosis, infection, broken catheter (leakage or embolization), arrhythmia (catheter inserted too far)

PERITONEAL LAVAGE

Indications

- **Diagnostic peritoneal lavage (DPL)** is used in the evaluation of intraabdominal trauma (bleeding, perforation) (*Note:* Spiral CT of the abdomen has largely replaced this as an initial screening for intraabdominal trauma in the emergency setting.)
- Acute peritoneal dialysis and the treatment of severe pancreatitis

Contraindications

- None are absolute. Relative contraindications include multiple abdominal procedures, pregnancy, known retroperitoneal injury (high false-positive rates) cirrhosis, morbid obesity and any coagulopathy.

Materials

- Prepackaged diagnostic peritoneal lavage or peritoneal dialysis tray

Procedure

1. A Foley catheter and a nasogastric or oro gastric tube **must** be in place. Prep the abdomen from above the umbilicus to the pubis.
2. The site of choice is in the midline 1–2 cm below the umbilicus. Avoid the site of old surgical scars (danger of adherent bowel). If a subumbilical scar or pelvic fracture is present, a supraumbilical approach is recommended.
3. Infiltrate the skin with 1idocaine with epinephrine. Incise the skin in the midline vertically, and expose the fascia.
4. Either pick up the fascia and incise it, or puncture it with the trocar and peritoneal catheter. Caution is needed to avoid puncturing any organs. Use one hand to hold the catheter near the skin and to control the insertion while using the other hand to apply pressure to the end of the catheter. After entering the peritoneal cavity, remove the trocar and direct the catheter inferiorly into the pelvis.
5. During a diagnostic lavage, gross blood indicates a positive tap. If no blood is encountered, instill 10 mL/kg (about 1 L in adults) of lactated Ringer's solution or NS into the abdominal cavity.
6. Gently agitate the abdomen to distribute the fluid and after 5 min, drain off as much fluid as possible into a bag on the floor. (Minimum fluid for a valid analysis is 200 mL in an adult.) If the drainage is slow, try instilling additional fluid, carefully repositioning the catheter.
7. Send the fluid for analysis (amylase, bile, bacteria, hematocrit, cell count). See Table 13–5 for interpretation.
8. Remove the catheter and suture the skin. If the catheter is inserted for pancreatitis or peritoneal dialysis, suture it in place.

13

TABLE 13–5
Criteria for Evaluation of Peritoneal Lavage Fluid

Positive	>20 mL gross blood on free aspiration (10 mL in children)
	≥100,000 RBC/mL
	≥500 WBC/mL (if obtained >3 h after the injury)
	≥175 units amylase/dL
	Bacteria on Gram's stain
	Bile (by inspection or chemical determination of bilirubin content)
	Food particles (microscopic analysis of strained or spun specimen)
Intermediate	Pink fluid on free aspiration
	50,000–100,000 RBC/mL in blunt trauma
	100–500 WBC/mL
	75–175 units amylase/dL
Negative	Clear aspirate
	≤ 100 WBC/mL
	≤75 units amylase/dL

Source: Reprinted, with permission, from: Way L (ed): *Current Surgical Diagnosis and Treatment,* 10e. Appleton and Lange, Norwalk CT. 1994.
Abbreviations: RBC = red blood cells; WBC = white blood cells.

13

9. A negative DPL does not rule out retroperitoneal trauma. A false-positive DPL can be caused by a pelvic fracture or bleeding induced by the procedure (eg, laceration of an omental vessel).

Complications

Infection/peritonitis or superficial wound infection, bleeding, perforated viscus (bladder, bowel)

PERITONEAL (ABDOMINAL) PARACENTESIS
Indications

- To determine the cause of ascites
- To determine if intraabdominal bleeding is present or if a viscus has ruptured (Diagnostic peritoneal lavage is considered a more accurate test. See preceding procedure.)
- Therapeutic removal of fluid when distention is pronounced or respiratory distress is associated with it (acute treatment only)

Contraindications

- Abnormal coagulation factors
- Bowel obstruction, pregnancy

- Uncertainty if distention is due to peritoneal fluid or to a cystic structure (ultrasound can usually differentiate)

Materials

- Minor procedure tray (see page 240)
- Catheter-over-needle assembly (Angiocath, Insyte 18–20-gauge with a 1½-in. needle)
- 20–60-mL syringe
- Sterile specimen containers

Procedure

Peritoneal paracentesis is surgical puncture of the peritoneal cavity for the aspiration of fluid. Ascites is indicated by abdominal distention, shifting dullness, and a palpable fluid wave.

1. Explain the procedure and have the patient sign an informed consent form. Have the patient empty the bladder, or place a Foley catheter if voiding is impossible or if significant mental status changes are present.
2. The entry site is usually the midline 3–4 cm below the umbilicus. Avoid old surgical scars because the bowel may be adhering to the abdominal wall. Alternatively, the entry site can be in the left or right lower quadrant midway between the umbilicus and the anterior superior iliac spine or in the patient's flank, depending on the percussion of the fluid wave (Fig. 13–18).
3. Prep and drape the patient appropriately. Raise a skin wheal with the lidocaine over the proposed entry site.
4. With the catheter mounted on the syringe, go through the anesthetized area carefully at an oblique angle while gently aspirating. You will meet some resistance as you enter the fascia. When you get free return of fluid, leave the catheter in place, remove the needle, and begin to aspirate. Sometimes it is necessary to reposition the catheter because of abutting bowel.
5. Aspirate the amount of fluid needed for tests (20–30 mL). If the tap is therapeutic, 10–15 L can be safely removed. This large volume must be removed relatively slowly.
6. Quickly remove the needle, apply a sterile 4 × 4 gauze square, and apply pressure with tape.
7. Depending on the clinical picture of the patient, send samples for total protein, specific gravity, LDH, amylase, cytology, culture, stains, or CBC.

Complications

Peritonitis, perforated viscus, hemorrhage, precipitation of hepatic coma if patient has severe liver disease, oliguria, hypotension

Diagnosis of Ascitic Fluid

A complete listing is found in Chapter 3, page 43. **Transudative ascites** is found with cirrhosis, nephrosis, and CHF. **Exudative ascites** is found with tumors, peritonitis (TB, perforated viscus), hypoalbuminemia. See Table 13–6 to interpret the results of fluid analysis.

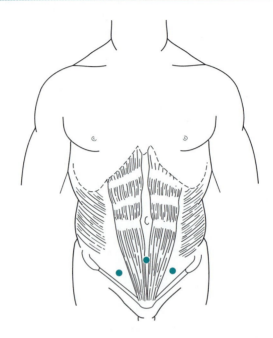

FIGURE 13–18 Preferred sites for abdominal (peritoneal) paracentesis. Be sure to avoid old surgical scars. (Reprinted, with permission, from: Krupp MA [ed]: *The Physician's Handbook,* 21st ed. Lange Medical Publications, Los Altos CA, 1985.)

PULMONARY ARTERY CATHETERIZATION

(See Chapter 20, page 399)

PULSUS PARADOXUS MEASUREMENT

(See also Chapter 20, page 393)

Indication

- Used in the evaluation of cardiac tamponade and other diseases

Materials

- Blood pressure cuff and stethoscope

TABLE 13–6
Differential Diagnosis of Ascitic of Pleural Fluid

Lab Value	Transudate	Exudate
Appearance	Clear yellow	Clear or turbid
Specific gravity	<1.016	>1.016
Absolute protein	<3 g/100 mL	>3 g/100 mL
Protein (ascitic or pleural to serum ratio)	<0.5	>0.5
LDH (ascitic or pleural to serum ratio)	<0.6	>0.6
Absolute LDH	<200 IU	>200 IU
Glucose (serum to ascitic or pleural ratio)	<1	>1
Fibrinogen (clot)	No	Yes
WBC (ascitic)	<500/mm^3	>1000/mm^3
WBC (pleural)	Very low	>2500/mm^3
Differential (pleural)		PMNs early, monocytes later
RBC (ascitic)		>100 RBC/mm^3

OTHER SELECTED TESTS

Cytology: Bizarre cells with large nuclei may represent reactive mesothelial cells and not a malignancy. Malignant cells suggest a tumor.
pH (pleural): Generally >7.3. If between 7.2 and 7.3, suspect TB or malignancy or both. If <7.2, suspect empyema.
Glucose (pleural): Normal pleural fluid glucose is ⅔ serum glucose. Pleural fluid glucose is much lower than serum glucose in effusions due to rheumatoid arthritis (0–16 mg/100 mL); low <40 mg/100 mL in empyema.
Triglycerides and positive Sudan stain (pleural fluid): Chylothorax.
Food fibers (ascitic): Perforated viscus.

Abbreviations: LDH = lactate dehydrogenase; WBC = white blood cells; RBC = red blood cells; PMNs = polymorphonuclear neutrophils; TB = tuberculosis.

Background

Pulsus paradoxus is an exaggeration of the normal inspiratory drop in arterial pressure. Inspiration decreases intrathoracic pressure. The result is increased right atrial and right ventricular filling with an increase in right ventricular output. Because the pulmonary vascular bed also distends, these changes lead to a delay in left ventricular filling and subsequently a decreased left ventricular output. This drop in systolic blood pressure is usually <10 mm Hg.

In the case of cardiac compression (eg, acute asthma or pericardial tamponade), the right side of the heart fills more with inspiration and decreases the left ventricular volume to even greater degree as a result of compression of the pericardial sac. This exaggerated decrease in left ventricular output drops the systolic pressure >10 mm Hg. See Figure 20–1 (page 394) for a graphic representation of a paradoxical pulse.

Procedure

1. A simple, **qualitative method** involves palpating the radial pulse, which "disappears" on normal inspiration.
2. A more precise **quantitative method** requiring that the patient take a breath, let it out, and hold it. Determine the systolic BP.
3. Ask the patient to breathe again. Once the patient is breathing normally, drop the pressure in the cuff **slowly** until you hear the pulse during inspiration.
4. The difference in systolic pressure should be <10 mm Hg. If not, a so-called paradox exists.
5. Differential diagnosis includes pericardial effusion, cardiac tamponade, pericarditis, COPD, bronchial asthma, restrictive cardiomyopathies, hemorrhagic shock

SIGMOIDOSCOPY (RIGID)
Indications

- Diagnosis and treatment of lower gastrointestinal problems
- Part of the standard work-up of blood in the stool

Materials

- Examination gloves, lubricant, tissues
- Occult blood stool test kit (Hemoccult paper and developer)
- Sigmoidoscope with obturator and light source
- Insufflation bag
- Long (rectal) swabs and suction catheter
- Proctologic examination table (helpful but not essential)

Procedure

1. Several techniques can be used to examine the distal large bowel. These include rigid **sigmoidoscopy** (endoscopic examination of the last 25 cm of the GI tract), **flexible sigmoidoscopy** (examination up to 40 cm from the end of the GI tract), **proctoscopy** (roughly synonymous to sigmoidoscopy, but technically means examination of the last 12 cm), and **anoscopy** (examination of the anus and most distal rectum).
2. Enemas and cathartics are not routinely given before sigmoidoscopy, although some people prefer to give a mild prep such as a Fleet's enema just before the exam. Explain the procedure, and have the patient sign a consent form.
3. Sigmoidoscopy can be performed with the patient in bed lying on side in the knee–chest position, but the best results are obtained with the patient in the "jackknife" position on the procto table. Do not position the patient until all materials are at hand and you are ready to start.
4. Converse with the patient to create distraction and to relieve apprehension. Announce each maneuver in advance. Glove before proceeding.
5. Observe the anal region for skin tags, hemorrhoids, fissures, and so on. Do a careful rectal exam with a gloved finger and plenty of lubricant, and check for fecal occult blood (**Hemoccult test**) on the stool recovered on the glove.

13

6. Lubricate the sigmoidoscope well with water-soluble jelly, and insert it with the obturator in place. Aim toward the patient's umbilicus initially. Advance 2–3 cm past the internal sphincter, and remove the obturator.

7. Always advance under direct vision and make sure that the lumen is always visible (Fig. 13–19). **Insufflation** (introducing air) may be used to help visualize the lumen, but remember this may be painful. It is necessary to follow the curve of the sigmoid toward the sacrum by directing the scope more posteriorly toward the back. A change from a smooth mucosa to concentric rings signifies entry into the sigmoid colon. The scope should reach 15 cm with ease. Use suction and the rectal swabs as needed to clear the way.

8. At this point, the sigmoid curves to the patient's left. Warn the patient that he or she may feel a cramping sensation. If you ever have difficulty negotiating a curve, do not force the scope.

9. After advancing as far as possible, slowly remove the scope; use a small rotary motion to view all surfaces. Observation here is critical. Remember to release the air from the colon before withdrawing the scope.

10. Inform the patient that he or she may experience mild cramping after the procedure.

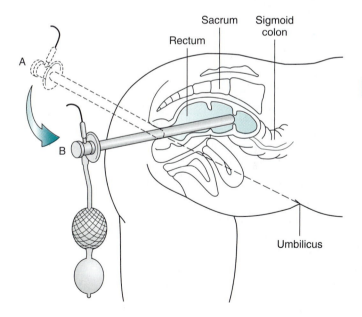

FIGURE 13–19   The sigmoidoscope is advanced under direct vision as shown.

Complications

- Bleeding, bowel perforation (rare)

SKIN BIOPSY

Indications

- Any skin lesion or eruption for which the diagnosis is unclear
- Any refractory skin condition

Contraindications

- Any skin lesion that is suspected to be a malignancy (eg, melanoma) should be referred to a plastic surgeon or dermatologist for excisional biopsy rather than a punch biopsy.

Materials

- 2-, 3-, 4-, or 5-mm skin punch
- Minor procedure tray (page 240)
- Curved iris scissors and fine-toothed forceps (Ordinary forceps may distort a small biopsy specimen and should not be used.)
- Specimen bottle containing 10% formalin
- Suturing materials (3-0 or 4-0 nylon)

Procedure

1. If more than one lesion is present, choose one that is well developed and representative of the dermatosis. For patients with vesiculobullous disease, an early edematous lesion should be chosen rather than a vesicle. Avoid lesions that are excoriated or infected.
2. Mark the area to be biopsied with a skin-marking pen. Inject the lidocaine to form a skin wheal over the site of the biopsy.
3. After putting on sterile gloves and preparing a sterile field, take the punch biopsy specimen. First, immobilize the skin with the fingers of one hand, applying pressure perpendicular to the skin wrinkle lines with the skin punch. Core out a cylinder of skin by twirling the punch between the fingers of the other hand. As the punch enters into the subcutaneous fat, resistance will lessen. At this point, the punch should be removed. The core of tissue usually pops up slightly and can be cut at the level of the subcutaneous fat with curved iris scissors without using forceps. If a tissue core does not pop up, it may be elevated by use of a hypodermic needle or fine-toothed forceps. Be sure to include a portion of the subcutaneous fat in the specimen.
4. Place the specimen in the specimen container.
5. Hemostasis can be achieved by pressure with the gauze pad.
6. Defects from 1.5 and 2-mm punches usually do not require suturing and heal with very minimal scarring. Punch defects that are 2–4 mm can generally be closed with a single suture.
7. A dry dressing should be applied and removed the following day.
8. Sutures can be removed as early as 3 d from the face and 7–10 d from other areas.

Complications

Infection (unusual); hemorrhage (usually controlled by simple application of pressure); keloid formation, especially in a patient with a prior history of keloid formation

SKIN TESTING

Indications

- Screening for current or past infectious agent (TB, coccidioidomycosis, etc)
- Screening for immune competency (so-called anergy screen) in debilitated patients

Materials

- Appropriate antigen (usually 0.1 mL)(eg, 5 TU PPD)
- A small, short needle (25-, 26-, or 27-gauge)
- 1-mL syringe
- Alcohol swab

Procedure

1. Skin tests for **delayed type hypersensitivity (type IV, tuberculin)** are the most commonly administered and interpreted. Delayed hypersensitivity (so called because a lag time of 12–36 h is required for a reaction) is caused by the activation of sensitized lymphocytes after contact with an antigen. The inflammatory reaction results from direct cytotoxicity and the release of lymphokines. Allergy tests (immediate wheal and flare) are rarely performed by the student or house officer.
2. The most commonly used site is the flexor surface of the forearm, approximately 4 in. below the elbow crease.
3. Prep the area with alcohol. With the bevel of the 27-gauge needle up, introduce the needle into the upper layers of skin, but **not** into the subcutis. Inject 0.1 mL of antigen such as the PPD. The goal is to inject the antigen intradermally. If done properly, you will raise a discrete white bleb, approximately 10 mm in diameter (known as the **Mantoux test**). The bleb should disappear soon, and no dressing is needed. If a bleb is not raised, move to another area and repeat the injection.
4. Mark the test site with a pen, and if multiple tests are being administered, identify each one. Also, document the site in the patient's chart.
5. To interpret the skin test, examine the injection site at 48–72 h. If nonreactive, check again at 72 h. **Measure the area of induration (the firm raised area), not the erythematous area.** Use a ballpoint pen held at approximately a 30-degree angle and bring it lightly toward the raised area. Where the pen touches is the area of induration. Measure two diameters and take the average.
6. It is important to check the PPD and other tests at intervals. If the patient develops a severe reaction to the skin test, apply hydrocortisone cream to prevent skin sloughing.

13

Specific Skin Tests

TST (Tuberculin Skin Testing): Routine TST in low-risk individuals is not currently recommended. High-risk individuals should undergo periodic TST (CXR findings suspicious for TB, recent contact of known or suspected TB cases, [includes health care workers], high-risk immigrants [Asia, Africa, Middle East, Latin America] , medically underserved (IV drug abusers, alcoholics, homeless), chronically institutionalized, HIV-infected or immunosuppression)

The **Mantoux test** is the standard technique for TST and relies on the intradermal injection of **PPD**. The **tine test** for TB is no longer recommended by the CDC. The PPD comes in three tuberculin unit "strengths": 1 TU ("first"), 5 TU ("intermediate"), and 250 TU ("second"). 1 TU is used if the patient is expected to be hypersensitive (history of a positive skin test); 5 TU is the standard initial screening test. A patient who has a negative response to a 5-TU test dose may react to the 250-TU solution. A patient who does not respond to the 250-TU is considered nonreactive to PPD. A patient may not react if he or she has not been exposed to the antigen or if the patient is anergic and unable to respond to any antigen challenge. A positive TST indicates the presence of *M. tuberculosis* infection, either active or past (dormant) and an intact cell-mediated immunity.

Interpretation of a positive PPD test is based on the clinical scenario. **Patients who have been previously immunized with percutaneous BCG may give a false-positive PPD, usually 10 mm or less.**

- 0–5 mm induration: Negative response
- ≥5 mm: Considered positive in contacts of known TB cases, CXR findings consistent with TB infection, HIV infection or in patients who are immunosuppressed, occasionally in non-TB mycobacterial infection due to cross reactivity
- ≥10 mm induration: Considered positive in patients with chronic diseases (diabetics, alcoholics, IV drug abusers, other chronic diseases), homeless, immigrants from known TB regions, children <4 y
- >15 mm induration: Positive in individuals who are healthy and otherwise do not meet the preceding risk categories

Anergy Screen (Anergy Battery): An anergy screen is based on the assumption that a patient has been exposed in the past to certain common antigens and a healthy patient is able to mount a reaction to them. To perform the screen, antigens such as mumps, or *Candida.* These are generally applied and read just like the PPD test (a reaction of >5 mm induration is considered a positive test and indicates intact cellular immunity). Anergy screens are sometimes used to evaluate a patient's immunological status and in the following specific situations: If you suspect a patient is PPD-positive, and the patient does not react to the test, do an anergy screen along with the PPD test to see if the patient has **any** cellular immune response.

13

THORACENTESIS
Indications

- Determining the cause of a pleural effusion
- Therapeutically removing pleural fluid in the event of respiratory distress
- Aspirating small pneumothoraces where the risk of recurrence is small (ie, postoperative without lung injury)
- Instilling sclerosing compounds (eg, tetracycline) to obliterate the pleural space

Contraindications

- None are absolute (pneumothorax, hemothorax, or any major respiratory impairment on the contralateral side, or coagulopathy)

Materials

- Prepackaged thoracentesis kit with either needle or catheter (preferred)
or
- Minor procedure tray (page 240)
- 20–60 mL syringe, 20- or 22-gauge needle 1½-in. needle, three-way stopcock
- Specimen containers

Procedure

Thoracentesis is the surgical puncture of the chest wall to aspirate fluid or air from the pleural cavity. The area of pleural effusion is dull to percussion with decreased whisper or breath sounds. Pleural fluid causes blunting of the costophrenic angles on chest x-ray. Blunting usually indicates that at least 300 mL of fluid is present. If you suspect that less than 300 mL of fluid is present or you suspect that the fluid is loculated (trapped and not free-flowing), a lateral decubitus film is helpful. Loculated effusions do not layer out. Thoracentesis can be done safely on fluid visualized on lateral decubitus film if at least 10 mm of fluid is measurable on the decubitus x-ray. Ultrasound may also be used to localize a small or loculated effusion.

1.   Explain the procedure, and have the patient sign an informed consent form. Have the patient sit up comfortably, preferably leaning forward slightly on a bedside tray table. Ask the patient to practice increasing intrathoracic pressure using the Valsalva maneuver or by humming.
2.   The usual site for thoracentesis is the posterior lateral aspect of the back over the diaphragm but under the fluid level. Confirm the site by counting the ribs based on the x-ray and percussing out the fluid level. Avoid going below the eighth intercostal space because the risk of peritoneal perforation is great.
3.   Use sterile technique, including gloves, povidone–iodine prep, and drapes. Thoracentesis kits come with an adherent drape with a hole in it.
4.   Make a skin wheal over the proposed site with a 25-gauge needle and 1idocaine. Change to a 22-gauge, 1½-in. needle and infiltrate up and over the rib (Fig. 13–20); try

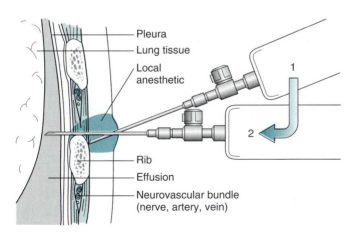

FIGURE 13–20   When performing a thoracentesis, the needle is passed over the top of the rib to avoid the neurovascular bundle.

to anesthetize the deeper structures and the pleura. During this time, you should be aspirating back for pleural fluid. Once fluid returns, note the depth of the needle and mark it with a hemostat. This gives you an approximate depth. Remove the needle.

5. Use a hemostat to measure the 14–18-gauge thoracentesis needle to the same depth as the first needle. Penetrate through the anesthetized area with the thoracentesis needle. **Make sure that you "march" over the top of the rib** to avoid the neurovascular bundle that runs below the rib (see Fig. 13–20). With the three-way stopcock attached, advance the thoracentesis catheter through the needle, withdraw the needle from the chest, and place the protective needle cover over the end of the needle to prevent injury to the catheter. Next, aspirate the amount of pleural fluid needed. Turn the stopcock, and evacuate the fluid through the tubing. **Never remove more than 1000–1500 mL per tap!** This may result in hypotension or the development of pulmonary edema due to reexpansion of compressed alveoli.

6. Have the patient hum or do the Valsalva maneuver as you withdraw the catheter. This maneuver increases intrathoracic pressure and decreases the chances of a pneumothorax. Bandage the site.

7. Obtain a chest x-ray to evaluate the fluid level and to rule out a pneumothorax. An expiratory film may be best because it helps reveal a small pneumothorax.

8. Distribute specimens in containers, label slips, and send them to the lab. Always order pH, specific gravity, protein, LDH, cell count and differential, glucose, Gram's stain and cultures, acid-fast cultures and smears, and fungal cultures and smears. Optional lab studies are cytology if you suspect a malignancy, amylase if you suspect an effusion secondary to pancreatitis (usually on the left) or esophageal perforation, and a Sudan stain and triglycerides (>110 mg/dL) if a chylothorax is suspected.

Complications

- Pneumothorax, hemothorax, infection, pulmonary laceration, hypotension, hypoxia due to ventilation–perfusion mismatch in the newly aerated lung segment

13

Differential Diagnosis of Pleural Fluid

For a more complete differential, see Chapter 3. **Transudate** is usually associated with nephrosis, CHF, cirrhosis; an **exudate** is associated with infection (pneumonia, TB), malignancy, empyema, peritoneal dialysis, pancreatitis, chylothorax. See Table 13–6, page 299, for the differential diagnosis.

URINARY TRACT PROCEDURES
Bladder Catheterization

Indications

- Relieving urinary retention
- Collecting an uncontaminated urine specimen for diagnostic purposes
- Monitoring urinary output in critically ill patients
- Performing bladder tests (cystogram, cystometrogram)

Contraindications

- Urethral disruption, often associated with pelvic fracture
- Acute prostatitis (relative contraindication)

Materials

- Prepackaged bladder catheter tray (may or may not include a Foley catheter)
- Catheter of choice (see Fig. 13–21):

Foley: Balloon at the tip to keep it in the bladder. Use a 16–18 French for adults (the higher the number, the larger the diameter). Irrigation catheters ("three-way Foley") should be larger (20–22 French).

Coudé (pronounced "COO-DAY"): An elbow-tipped catheter useful in males with prostatic hypertrophy (the catheter is passed with the tip pointing to 12 o'clock).

Red rubber catheter (Robinson): Plain rubber or latex catheter without a balloon, usually used for "in-and-out catheterization" in which urine is removed but the catheter is not left indwelling.

Procedure

1. Each insertion of a catheter implants bacteria into the bladder, so strict aseptic technique is mandatory.
2. Have the patient lie supine in a well-lighted area; females with knees flexed wide and heels together to get adequate exposure of the meatus.
3. Get all the materials ready before you attempt to insert the catheter. Open the kit, and put on the gloves. Open the prep solution, and soak the cotton balls. Apply the sterile drapes.

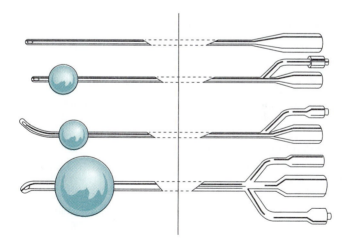

FIGURE 13–21 Types of bladder catheters include (from the top) the straight "Robinson" catheter [or red rubber catheter], Foley catheter with standard 5-mL balloon, the Coudé catheter, and "three-way" irrigating catheter with 30-mL balloon. Catheters have been shortened for illustrative purposes.

4. Inflate and deflate the balloon of the Foley catheter to ensure its proper function. Coat the end of the catheter with lubricant jelly.

5. In females, use one gloved hand to prep the urethral meatus in a pubis-toward-anus direction; hold the labia apart with the other gloved hand. With uncircumcised males, retract the foreskin to prep the glans; use a gloved hand to hold the penis still.

6. The hand used to hold the penis or labia should not touch the catheter to insert it; a disposable forceps in the kit can be used to insert it. Or the forceps can be used to prep, then the gloved hand can insert the catheter.

7. In the male, **stretch** the penis upward perpendicular to the body to eliminate any internal folds in the urethra that might lead to a false passage. Use **steady, gentle** pressure to advance the catheter. The bulbous urethra is the most likely part to tear. Any significant resistance encountered may represent a stricture and requires urological consultation. In males with BPH, a Coudé tip catheter may facilitate passage. Some tricks used to get a catheter to pass in a male are to make sure that the penis is well stretched and to instill 30–50 mL of sterile water-based surgical lubricant (K-Y jelly) into the urethra with a catheter-tipped syringe prior to passage of the catheter. Viscous lidocaine jelly for urologic use can help lubricate and relieve the discomfort of difficult catheter placement. Allow at least 5 min after instillation of the lidocaine jelly for the anesthetic effect to take place.

8. In both males and females, insert the catheter to the hilt of the drainage end. Compress the penis toward the pubis. These maneuvers ensure that the balloon inflates in the bladder and not in the urethra. Inflate the balloon with 5–10 mL of sterile water or, occasionally, air. After inflation, pull the catheter back so that the balloon comes to rest on the bladder neck. There should be good urine return when the catheter is in place. If a large amount of lubricant jelly was placed into the urethra, the catheter may need to be flushed with sterile saline to clear the excess lubricant. A catheter that will not irrigate is **in the urethra, not the bladder.**

9. Any male who is uncircumcised should have the foreskin repositioned to prevent massive edema of the glans after the catheter is inserted.

10. Catheters in females can be taped to the leg. In males, the catheter should be taped to the abdominal wall to decrease stress on the posterior urethra and help prevent stricture formation. The catheter is usually attached to a gravity drainage bag or some device for measuring the amount of urine. Many new kits come with the catheter already secured to the drainage bag. These systems are considered "closed" and should not be opened if at all possible.

"In-and-Out" Catheterized Urine

1. If urine is needed for analysis or for culture and sensitivity, especially in a female patient, a so-called in-and-out cath can be done. This is also useful for measuring residual urine in males or females. The incidence of inducing infection with this procedure is about 3%.

2. The procedure is identical to that described for bladder catheterization. The main difference is that a red rubber catheter (no balloon) is often used and is removed immediately after the specimen is collected.

Clean-Catch Urine Specimen

1. A clean-catch urine is useful for routine urinalysis, is usually good for culturing urine from males, but is only fair for culturing urine from females because of the potential for contamination.

2. For males:
    a. Expose the glans, clean with a povidone–iodine solution and dry it with a sterile pad.
    b. Collect a midstream urine in a sterile container after the initial flow has escaped.
3. **For females:**
    a. Separate the labia widely to expose the urethral meatus; keep the labia spread throughout the procedure.
    b. Cleanse the urethral meatus with povidone–iodine solution from front to back, and rinse with sterile water.
    c. Catch the midstream portion of the urine in a sterile container.

Percutaneous Suprapubic Bladder Aspiration
Indications

(Used most frequently in young children)

- When urine cannot be obtained by a less invasive method
- In the presence of urethral abnormalities
- In the presence of a refractory UTI

Contraindications

- If the child has voided within the last hour, or if the bladder cannot be percussed

Procedure

1. This procedure is almost exclusively limited to the very young pediatric patient (usually <6 months).
2. Immobilize the child. Do not attempt this procedure if the child has voided within the last hour.
3. Palpate the bladder above the pubic symphysis (the bladder sticks high above the pubis in a young child when it is full). Some suggest occluding the urethra by holding the penis in a male and by inserting a finger in the rectum to exert pressure in the female. Percuss out the limits of the bladder.
4. Obtain a 20-mL syringe with a 23- or 25-gauge, 1½-in. needle. Prep with povidone–iodine and alcohol 0.5–1.5 cm above the pubis. Anesthesia is not routinely used.
5. Insert the needle perpendicular to the skin in the midline; maintain negative pressure on the downstroke and on withdrawal until urine is obtained (Fig.13–22).
6. If no urine is obtained, wait at least 1 h before reattempting the procedure.

VENIPUNCTURE
Materials

- A tourniquet (a 1½-in. Penrose drain or glove is acceptable)
- Alcohol prep sponge
- Proper specimen tubes for desired studies (red top, purple top, etc.) (Table 13–7)
- Appropriate-sized syringe for volume of blood needed (5 mL, 10 mL, etc), or a Vacutainer tube and appropriate needle and Vacutainer holder
- A 20–22-gauge needle (Larger needles are uncomfortable, and smaller ones can cause hemolysis or clotting; the higher the gauge number, the smaller the needle.)

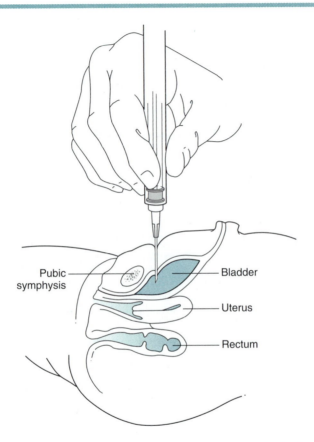

FIGURE 13–22 The technique and anatomic structures in suprapubic bladder aspiration. (Reprinted, with permission, from: Gomella TL [ed]: *Neonatology: Basic Management, On-Call Problems, Diseases, Drugs,* 4th ed. Appleton & Lange, Norwalk CT, 1998.)

Procedure

Venipuncture (**phlebotomy**) is the puncture of a vein to obtain a sample of venous blood for analysis. Blood cultures, IV techniques, and arterial punctures are discussed in other sections of the chapter.

TABLE 13-7
Tube Guide for Venipuncture Using the Vacutainer System*

Vacutainer Tubes	Vacutainer Hemogard Closure	Additive	Number or Inversions at Blood Collection (Invert gently, do not shake)	Laboratory Use
Black/red marbled ("Tiger Top")	Gold	Clot activator and gel for serum separation	5	SST brand tube for serum demonstrations in chemistry. Tube inversions ensure mixing of clot activator with blood and clotting within 30 min
Green/red marbled	Light green	Lithium heparin and gel for plasma separation	8	PST brand tube for plasma determinations in chemistry. Tube inversions prevent clotting
Red	Red	None	0	For serum determinations in chemistry, serology, and blood banking.
Yellow/black marbled	Orange	Thrombin	8	For stat serum determinations in chemistry. Tube inversions prevent clotting, usually in less than 5 min
Royal blue	Royal blue	Sodium heparin Na EDTA None	8 8 0	For trace element, toxicology, and nutrient determinations. Special stopper formulation offers the lowest verified levels of trace elements available. (See package insert)
Green	Green	Sodium heparin Lithium heparin Ammonium heparin	8 8 8	For plasma determinations in chemistry. Tube inversions prevent clotting

(continued)

13

TABLE 13-7
(Continued)

13

Vacutainer Tubes	Vacutainer Hemogard Closure	Additive	Number or Inversions at Blood Collection (Invert gently, do not shake)	Laboratory Use
Gray	Gray	Potassium oxalate/ Sodium fluoride Sodium fluoride Lithium iodoacetate	8 8 8 8	For glucose determinations. Tube inversions ensure proper mixing of additive and blood. Oxalate and heparin, anticoagulants, will give samples that are serum
Brown	Brown	Sodium heparin	8	For lead determinations. This tube is certified to contain less than .01 µ/mL (ppm) lead. Tube inversions prevent clotting
Yellow	Yellow	Sodium polyanetholesulfonate (SPS)	8	For blood culture specimen collections in microbiology. Tube inversions prevent clotting.
Lavender	Lavender	Liquid EDTA Freeze-dried Na EDTA	8 8	For whole blood hematology determinations. Tube inversions prevent clotting
Light blue	Light blue	0.105 M sodium citrate (3.2%) 0.129 M sodium citrate (3.8%)	8 8	For coagulation determinations on plasma specimens. Tube inversions prevent clotting. *Note:* Certain tests require chilled specimens. Follow recommended procedures for collection and transport of specimen

*Based on products from Becton-Dickinson.
Abbreviation: EDTA = ethylene diamine tetraacetic acid.

1. Collect the necessary materials before you begin.

2. The most commonly used sites for routine venipuncture are the veins of the antecubital fossa (see Fig. 13–12, page 279). Other sites that can be used include the dorsum of the hand, the forearm, the saphenous vein near the medial malleolus, or the external jugular vein. If all the routine peripheral sites are unacceptable, the femoral vein can be used. **Never draw a blood sample proximal to an IV site. The high concentration of IV fluid in the veins** at this location may make the laboratory studies invalid.

3. Apply the tourniquet at least 2–3 in. above the venipuncture site. Have the patient make a fist to help engorge the vein. If veins are difficult to locate, some helpful techniques include slapping the vein to cause reflex dilation, hanging the extremity in a dependent position, wrapping the extremity in a warm soak, substituting a blood pressure cuff for the standard tourniquet, or applying nitroglycerin paste below and over the area may help dilate the veins.

4. Swab the site with the alcohol prep pad, and allow the alcohol to evaporate.

5. Use the syringe and needle with the bevel up and puncture the skin alongside the vein. After the needle is through the skin, use the thumb of your free hand to stabilize the vein and prevent it from rolling.

6. Enter the vein on the side at about a 30-degree angle while applying gentle back pressure on the syringe. Withdraw the sample slowly to prevent the vein from collapsing. An alternative acceptable technique is to enter both the skin and vein in one stick, however this maneuver requires practice because the vein is often stuck through and through.

7. The **Vacutainer system** is a very useful means of collecting blood, especially if several different sample tubes need to be filled. Mount a 20–22-gauge Vacutainer needle on the Vacutainer cup. Enter the vein as directed previously. Advance the collection tube onto the needle inside the Vacutainer. The vacuum inside the tube automatically collects the sample. If you hold the Vacutainer steady, several tubes can be collected in this fashion.

8. After the blood is collected (by whatever method), remove the tourniquet, withdraw the needle, and apply firm pressure with the alcohol swab or sterile gauze for 2–3 min. Elevation of the extremity is helpful. Current evidence indicates that bending the arm actually increases the size of the venipuncture site and should be discouraged.

9. If a needle and syringe are used, distribute the samples to the blood tubes. The best technique is to insert the needle into the tube and allow the vacuum to draw in the appropriate volume of blood for a given tube (this is most critical for coagulation studies). Distribute the blood to the coagulation and CBC tubes first because clotting of the blood in the syringe can invalidate the results. Mix the tubes thoroughly. Blood drawn for typing and cross-matching usually has special labels that require signature of the person that obtained the sample.

10. If no peripheral veins can be located, puncture of the **femoral vein** can be attempted. Locate the femoral artery. The mnemonic of lateral to medial structures in the groin is **NAVEL: N**erve, **A**rtery, **V**ein, **E**mpty space, **L**ymphatic. The femoral vein should be just medial to the femoral artery. After prepping the skin, insert the needle perpendicular to the skin, and gently aspirate. The vein should be about 1–1½ in. below the skin. Apply firm pressure after the collection of the sample because hematomas are frequent complications of femoral venipunctures. Should you accidentally enter the femoral artery, it is acceptable to collect the sample. Apply pressure for a longer period if the artery is entered.

11. In children and the elderly with fragile veins, a butterfly (21–25-gauge) can be used to obtain a sample (see Fig. 13–12).

12. When completed with the venipuncture needle, follow the CDC recommendations and **DO NOT reshield the needle** with the protective cap. Whenever possible, dispose of the needle immediately into the sharps collection container located on each hospital unit where blood is routinely drawn. Newer "safe needles" (Safety-Lok, ProGuard, Puncture-Guard, etc) are designed to attach to the Vacutainer system and have mechanisms to help protect the tip and hopefully diminish the incidence of accidental needlesticks.

PAIN MANAGEMENT

Terminology
Classification of Pain
Adverse Physiologic Effects of Pain
Principles of Pain Control

Evaluation of Patient with Pain
Pain Measurement
Practical Pain Management
Patient-Controlled Analgesia

"Men do not fear death, they fear the pain of dying."

TERMINOLOGY

Pain is the most common symptom that brings patients to see a physician, and it is frequently the first alert of an ongoing pathologic process. The International Association for the Study of Pain defines pain as: An "unpleasant sensory and emotional experience associated with actual or potential tissue damage." Acute pain is common postoperatively and in acute injury. Chronic pain can be associated with conditions such as cancer and arthritis.

Oligoanalgesia is the failure to recognize or properly treat pain. This may result because the physician makes a judgment without asking the patient if she or he hurts or discredits the patient's response and bases the determination of pain severity on the physician's own subjective past pain experience. Accordingly, the gold standard for determining if a patient is in pain is to ask the patient if he or she hurts and then to attempt to objectively verify the report with monitors, touch, or direct vision.

Nociception is derived from the Latin word *noci,* meaning "harm or injury." It refers to the detection, transduction, and transmission of noxious stimuli. Stimuli generated from thermal, mechanical, or chemical tissue damage may activate nociceptors, which are free nerve endings. (All nociception produces pain but not all pain results from nociception.)

CLASSIFICATION OF PAIN

Pain can be broadly divided into acute and chronic pain.

Acute Pain

Acute pain is caused by noxious stimulation due to injury or disease process or abnormal function of muscle or viscera. It is a manifestation of autonomic, psychologic, and behavior responses, which can be self-limited and resolve with treatment (eg, after trauma, after surgery, MI, pancreatitis, or renal calculi). Acute pain is further classified as

- **Superficial.** Nociception from skin, subcutaneous tissue, or mucous membrane. Localized, sharp, pricking, throbbing, or burning
- **Deep somatic.** From muscle, tendon, joints, bones. Less localized, dull aching in character

- **Visceral.** From internal organ or coverings (parietal pleura, pericardium, or peritoneum). Can be localized or referred. May accompany sympathetic or parasympathetic manifestations as changes in BP or heart rate, nausea and vomiting

Chronic Pain

The determination of whether pain is chronic should not be based on its duration, but rather on the substantial damage it causes to an individual in terms of functional loss, psychologic distress (sleep and affective disturbances), and social and vocational dysfunction. This pain usually results from peripheral nociception of the peripheral or central nervous system, and it usually lacks neuroendocrine stress response: musculoskeletal disorders, chronic visceral disorders, lesions of peripheral nerves, nerve root, dorsal root ganglia (causalgia, phantom limb pain, postherpetic neuralgia), stroke, spinal cord injury, MS, or cancer.

ADVERSE PHYSIOLOGIC EFFECTS OF PAIN

This is usually associated with acute pain and is proportional to pain intensity. (Table 14–1)

PRINCIPLES OF PAIN CONTROL

- Proper patient evaluation, including pain measurement
- Good physician–patient relationship built on trust
- Consideration of both psychologic and emotional aspects
- Acknowledgment that treatment depends on patient's compliance, understanding, and cooperation
- Possible combination therapy
- Explanation of side effects (if unavoidable) and how to treat them
- Proper follow-up

EVALUATION OF PATIENT WITH PAIN

1. Ask the patient if she or he is in pain? Bear in mind that you must trust and believe what the patient says.
2. Obtain a detailed history of this pain:

   - Character of the pain (dull, colicky, sharp)
   - Duration of pain

3. Is the pain referred to other sites of the body (eg, ureteral calculi may be referred to the ipsilateral testicle)?
4. What relieves the pain: Rest, position?
5. What makes it worse: Movement, positions, activities?
6. Are there any accompanying symptoms: Nausea, vomiting, headache?

   - Perform a physical examination and request imaging studies if an organic cause is suspected.
   - Chronic pain frequently affects daily activity and social interaction so psychosocial evaluation may be indicated.

PAIN MEASUREMENT

The most commonly used two methods of pain measurement are Visual Analogue Scale (VAS) and McGill Pain Questionnaire (MPQ).

TABLE 14-1
Adverse Physiologic Sequelae of Pain

Organ System	Adverse Effect
RESPIRATORY	
Increased skeletal muscle tension	Hypoxia, hypercapnia
Decreased total lung compliance	Ventilation–perfusion abnormality, atelectasis, pneumonitis
ENDOCRINE	
Increased adrenocorticotropic hormone	Protein catabolism, lipolysis, hyperglycemia
Decreased insulin, decreased testosterone	Decreased protein anabolism
Increased aldosterone, increased antidiuretic hormone	Salt and water retention, congestive heart failure
Increased catecholamines	Vasoconstriction
Increased angiotensin II	Increased myocardial contractility
CARDIOVASCULAR	
Increased myocardial work	Dysrhythmias, angina
IMMUNOLOGIC	
Lymphopenia, depression of reticuloendothelial system, leukocytosis	Decreased immune function
Reduced killer T-cell cytotoxicity	

(continued)

14

TABLE 14-1
(Continued)

Organ System	Adverse Effect
COAGULATION EFFECTS	
Increased platelet adhesiveness, diminished fibrinolysis	Increased incidence of thromboembolic phenomena
Activation of coagulation cascade	
GASTROINTESTINAL	
Increased sphincter tone	Ileus
Decreased smooth muscle tone	
GENITOURINARY	
Increased sphincter tone	Urinary retention
Decreased smooth muscle tone	

14

Visual Analogue Scale

The **VAS** is a 10-cm horizontal line with the words *NO PAIN* at one end and *WORST PAIN IMAGINABLE* at the other end. The patient is asked to put a mark on this line at the point that identifies the intensity but not quality of his or her pain. This has been called the "fifth vital sign" and is commonly used in the hospital setting to guide pain management.

0   1   2   3   4   5   6   7   8   9   10
No pain   Worst possible pain

McGill Pain Questionnaire

The **MPQ** (Melzack R: The McGill Pain Questionnaire: Major properties and scoring methods. *Pain* 1975;**1**:277–299.) is a checklist of words describing symptoms. Scores are then analyzed in various dimensions (sensory and affective) to identify the quality of pain. This tool is usually used in the detailed management of pain syndromes.

Psychologic Evaluation: A psychologic evaluation is indicated if medical examination fails to reveal any apparent cause for the patient's pain. The Minnesota Multiple Personality Inventory (Hathaway SR and McKinley JC: *MMPI.* University of Minnesota Press, Minneapolis, 1989.) and Beck Depression Inventory (Beck AT, Steer RA: Internal consistencies of the original and revised Beck Depression Inventory. *J Clin Psychol* 1984;**40**(**6**): 1365–1367.) are two commonly used tools for evaluating chronic pain and depression. These questionnaires should not only determine the patient's psychologic status but also evaluate his or her behavior and response to pain and its management.

Electromyography and Nerve Conduction Testing: This method differentiates between neurogenic and myogenic causes and confirms diagnoses of nerve entrapment, neural trauma, and polyneuropathies.

Thermography: Normally, heat from body surfaces is emitted in the form of infrared energy; this emission is symmetrical in homologous areas. Neurogenic pathophysiologic changes result in asymmetry. This infrared energy can be measured and displayed; hyperemission indicates an acute stage and hypoemission a chronic stage.

Diagnostic and Therapeutic Neural Blockade: Neural blockade with local anesthetics can be used to diagnose and manage both acute and chronic pain.

PRACTICAL PAIN MANAGEMENT

The goal of pain management is to provide the patient adequate relief with minimum side effects (eg, drowsiness). Always begin therapy with the lowest dose of any medication that provides relief. Oral, rectal, or transdermal routes are preferred over parental therapy.

Pain management can be generally divided into

- Pharmacologic
- Nonpharmacologic
- Combinations according to the patient response and compliance

Pharmacologic

The World Health Organization has made specific recommendations concerning pain management. These principles apply primarily to cancer pain but can be used in any clinical setting. Start at step 1 and advance to the next level based on patient response.

Step 1: Nonopioid agents (NSAIDs, acetaminophen, etc)
Step 2: Weak opioids (codeine, oxycodone)
Step 3: Strong opioids (morphine, fentanyl)

Specific pharmacologic agents are reviewed in the following section and in Table 14–2. Supplements can enhance the effects of analgesics and allow dose reduction of some agents.

Nonopioid Analgesics: Aspirin, acetaminophen, and NSAIDs are the principal nonopioid analgesics used to treat mild and moderate pain. NSAIDs are primarily cyclooxygenase inhibitors that prevent prostaglandin-mediated amplification of chemical and mechanical irritants of the sensory pathways. Short-term perioperative use of ketorolac (Toradol) can reduce pain medication requirement. **Side effects:** Possible hepatotoxicity (large doses of acetaminophen); stomach upset, nausea, dyspepsia, ulceration of gastric mucosa, dizziness, platelet dysfunction, exacerbation of bronchospasm, and acute renal insufficiency (aspirin and NSAIDs).

Opioids: These drugs attach to opioid receptors, which are responsible for the analgesia. **Side effects:** Sedation, dizziness, miosis, nausea, vomiting and constipation from smaller doses, to respiratory depression, apnea, cardiac arrest and circulatory collapse, coma, and death after high intravenous doses. Opioids can be taken orally, parenterally, or neuroaxially (intrathecal/epidural). They are available in short- (q4h) and long-duration forms (eg, q12h, q24h). Opioids can also be given as a patient-controlled analgesia (PCA) (see section with that title). Comparison of the different opioid narcotic can be found in Table 14–2.

Antidepressants: The analgesic effect produced by antidepressants is due to reuptake of serotonin and norepinephrine. **Side effects:** Antimuscarinic effects (dry mouth, impaired visual accommodation, urinary retention), antihistaminic (sedation), and alpha adrenergic blockage (orthostatic hypotension).

Neuroleptics: Useful in patients with agitation and psychologic symptoms. **Side effects:** Extrapyramidal, mask-like facies, festinating gait, cogwheel rigidity (bradykinesia).

Anticonvulsants: These medications act by suppressing the spontaneous neural discharge. **Side effects:** Bone marrow depression, hepatotoxicity, possible ataxia, dizziness, confusion, and sedation (at toxic doses).

Corticosteroids: These are antiinflammatory analgesics. **Side effects:** HTN, hyperglycemia, and increased tendency to infection, peptic ulcer, osteoporosis, myopathies, and Cushing's syndrome.

Systemic Local Anesthetics: These drugs produce sedation and central analgesia. **Side effects from excessive dosing:** Toxicity with cardiovascular collapse and CNS symptoms in the form of tonic–clonic seizures. Respiratory arrest usually follows.

Nonpharmacologic

- **Nerve blocks or neurolysis** (destruction of the nerve)
- **Radiation:** Useful for cancer pain (ie, bony metastasis)
- **Psychologic intervention:** Using cognitive therapy, behavioral therapy or biofeedback relaxation technique and hypnosis
- **Physical therapy:** Heat and cold can provide pain relief by alleviating muscle spasm. Heat decreases joint stiffness and increases blood flow; cold vasoconstricts and reduces tissue edema.

TABLE 14-2
Selected Agents Commonly Used in Pain

	Route	Onset	Duration	Initial Dose	Maximum Dose
NON-OPIOID					
Acetaminophen (Tylenol, Datril)	PO	0.5 h	4 h	500–1000 mg	1200 mg
Aspirin/sodium salicylate	PO	0.5–1 h	4 h	500–1000 mg	3600 mg
Celecoxib (Celebrex)	PO	3 h	12 h	100 mg	400 mg
Diclofenac sodium (Voltaren)	PO	1 h	4–6 h	25–75 mg	200 mg
Ibuprofen (Motrin, Rufen)	PO	0.5 h	4–6 h	400 mg	3200 mg
Indomethacin (Indocin)	PO	0.5 h	4–6 h	25–50 mg	200 mg
Piroxicam (Feldene)	PO	1 h	48–72 h	10–20 mg	20 mg
Rofecoxib (Vioxx)	PO	2–3 h	24 h	12.5 mg	50 mg
OPIOID					
Codeine	IM	0.25–0.5 h	4–6 h	15 mg	60 mg
	PO	0.25–1 h	3–4 h	15 mg	60 mg
Fentanyl	IV	1.7–2.3 h	1 h	1–1.5 µg/kg	150
	TD	1.7–2.3 h	1 h	25 mg/h	100 µg/h
Meperidine (Demorol)	PO	0.5–1 h	2–3 h	1–1.5 mg/kg	50–100 mg
	IM	0.12–0.5 h	2–4 h	1–1.5 mg/kg	50–100 mg
Methadone (Dolophine)	PO	0.5–1 h	4–8 h	2.5–10 mg	160 mg
	IM	0.25 h	4–6 h	2.5–10 mg	160 mg
Morphine (various)	IV	Rapid	1–2 h	0.1–15 mg/kg	2.5–15 mg
	IM	0.3 h	3–4 h	0.1–0.15 mg/kg	10–15 mg

(*continued*)

14

**TABLE 14–2
(Continued)**

	Route	Onset	Duration	Initial Dose	Maximum Dose
Nalbuphine (Nubain)	IV	—	—	1–5 mg	160 mg
	IM	0.25 h	3–6 h	10–20 mg	160 mg
OTHER/SUPPLEMENTS					
Amitriptyline	PO	7–21 d	—	25–150 mg	300 mg
Carbamazepine	PO	—	—	200 mg	1600 mg
Dexamethasone	PO	—	—	0.5–9 mg/kg	20–100 mg
	IV	—	—	0.5–9 mg/kg	20–100 mg
Haloperidol (Haldol)	PO	—	—	0.5–5 mg	100 mg
	IV	1 h	3 wk	0.5–5 mg	100 mg

Abbreviations: PO = by mouth; IV = intravenous; IM = intramuscular; TD = transdermal.

- **Acupuncture:** Needles inserted into discrete anatomically defined points and stimulated by mild electric current. Believed to release endogenous opioids
- **Electrical stimulation of the nervous system:** Can produce analgesia. The three methods are
1. Transcutaneous electrical stimulation (TENS) with electrodes applied to skin
2. Spinal cord stimulation by inserting electrodes epidurally connected to external generator
3. Intracerebral stimulation with electrodes implanted in the periaqueductal or periventricular area

PATIENT-CONTROLLED ANALGESIA

Most commonly used after surgery, allows the patient to self-administer the dose of narcotic via an IV pump. The patient treats the pain as soon as he or she feels necessary, thus avoiding the peak and trough of a narcotic dosing regimen that may lead to extremes of pain and potential oversedation. The pain management team can titrate the dose of the drug as required using a computerized system that controls the total dose and the interval between each dose with the use of a continuous basal infusion dosage. PCA duration varies based on procedure and patient response (eg, gyn 1–2 d, bowel 2–5 d, thoracotomy 4–6 d). Reduce dose in elderly ($\frac{1}{3}$–$\frac{2}{3}$). Consider discontinuation of PCA when patients are able to take analgesics PO.

PCA Parameters

- **Dose:** Number of mL (typically morphine concentration, page 321) given on activation of button by patient
- **Lockout:** Minimum interval of time in minutes between PCA doses
- **Hourly Max:** Maximum volume (mL) that machine administers in an hour
- **Basal Rate:** Continuous infusion rate (not required on all patients)

The following table shows examples of PCA orders:

Typical Procedure	Dose (mL)	Lockout (min)	Hourly Max (mL)	Basal
Moderately painful (lower abdominal, incisions, minor orthopedic procedures)	1	6	8	None
Fairly painful (upper abdominal incisions)	1.5	6	10	None–1 mL/h
Very painful (thoracotomy, total knee replacement)	1.5	6	10	0.5–1.5 mL

IMAGING STUDIES

X-Ray Preparations
Common X-Ray Studies: Noncontrast
Common X-Ray Studies: Contrast
Ultrasound
CT Scans

Spiral (Helical) CT Scan
Magnetic Resonance Imaging (MR or MRI)
Nuclear Scans
How to Read a Chest X-Ray

X-RAY PREPARATIONS

In general, follow this rubric: plain films before contrast, contrast before barium. Each hospital has its own guidelines for patient x-ray preps. Consult the radiology department prior to ordering. Examinations that require no specific bowel preparation include routine chest x-rays, flat and upright abdominal films, T-tube cholangiograms, cystograms, C-spines, skull series, extremity films, CT scan of the head or chest, and many others.

Studies that usually require such preps as enemas, laxatives, oral contrast agents, or those that require that the patient be NPO prior to the examination include oral cholecystogram, upper GI series, SBFT, barium enema, IVP, CT scan of the abdomen or pelvis, and many others.

COMMON X-RAY STUDIES: NONCONTRAST
Chest

Chest X-Ray (Routine):   Includes PA and lateral chest films. Used in the evaluation of pulmonary, cardiac and mediastinal diseases, and traumatic injury. See page 335 on How to Read a Chest X-Ray.

Expiratory Chest: Used to help visualize a small pneumothorax

Lateral Decubitus Chest: Allows small amounts of pleural effusion or suspected subpulmonary effusion to layer out and permits diagnosis of as little as 175 mL of pleural fluid

Lordotic Chest: Allows better visualization of apices and lesions of the right and left upper lobes. Often used in the evaluation of TB

Portable Chest and AP Films: Cannot be used to accurately evaluate heart size or widened mediastinum but can be used to detect effusions, pneumonia, edema, and to verify line or tube placement

Rib Details: Special views that more clearly delineate rib pathology; useful when plain chest radiogram or bone scan suggests fractures or other metastatic lesions.

Abdominal

Abdominal Decubitus: Used in debilitated patients instead of an upright abdominal film. The left side should be down to find free air outlining the liver and right lateral gutter.

Acute Abdominal Series ("obstruction series"):   Includes a flat and upright abdominal (KUB) and chest x-ray. Good for initial evaluation of an acute abdomen (See KUB.)

Cross-Table Lateral Abdominal: Used in debilitated patients to look for free air or to identify an aortic aneurysm.

KUB, Supine and Erect: Short for "kidneys, ureter, and bladder" and also known as **"flat and upright abdominal," "scout film,"** or **"flat plate."** Useful when the patient complains of abdominal pain or distension, and for initial evaluation of the urinary tract (80% of kidney stones and 20% of gallstones are visualized on these films). To read, look for calcifications, foreign bodies, the gas pattern, psoas shadows, renal and liver shadows, flank stripes, the vertebral bodies, and pelvic bones. On the upright, look for air–fluid levels of an adynamic ileus or mechanical obstruction and for free air under the diaphragm, which suggests a perforated viscus or recent surgery; however, the upright chest x-ray (especially the lateral view) is often best to spot a pneumoperitoneum.

Other Noncontrast X-Rays

C-Spine: Usually includes PA, lateral, and oblique films. Useful for the evaluation of trauma, neck pain, and neurologic evaluation of the upper extremities. All seven cervical vertebrae must be seen for this study to be acceptable.

DEXA: Measures bone mineral density at a variety of sites (femur/lumbar spine); used in the diagnosis and monitoring of response to treatment of osteoporosis

Mammography: Detects cancers greater than 5 mm in size. Two forms equal in diagnostic quality:

- **Screen film.** Produces standard black and white x-ray via a specially designed mammographic machine; 3–5× smaller radiation dose
- **Xeromammography.** Blue and white paper image using a general x-ray machine. Delivers a higher radiation dose. Current American Cancer Society screening guidelines for asymptomatic women: 35–39 baseline, 40–49 every 1–2 years, >50 every year.

Sinus Films (Paranasal Sinus Radiographs):   Used to evaluate sinus trauma, sinusitis, neoplasms, or congenital disorders

Skull Films: Used to detect fractures and aid in the identification of pituitary tumors or congenital anomalies

Vertebral Radiography: Used to evaluate fractures, dislocations, subluxations, disk disease, and the effects of arthritic and metabolic disorders of the spine

COMMON X-RAY STUDIES: CONTRAST

An agent, such as barium or Gastrografin, or an intravenous contrast agent is used for these studies. If a GI tract fistula or perforation is suspected, inform the radiologist because this may affect the choice of contrast agent (ie, water-soluble contrast [eg, Gastrografin] instead of barium). Standard IV contrast media are ionic and may be associated with rare contrast reaction when administered systemically (see following section). The use of nonionic contrast media may limit these side effects.

Ionic Contrast Media

- Oral cholecystographic agents: Telepaque etc
- GI contrast agents: Barium sulfate—Baro-CAT, Tomocat, etc
- Injection: Diatrizoate meglumine—Hypaque Meglumine, Urovist Meglumine, Angiovist, etc
     Diatrizoate sodium: Hypaque Sodium, Urovist Sodium, etc

     Gadopentetate dimeglumine: Magnevist, etc
     Iodamide meglumine: Renovue, etc
     Iothalamate meglumine: Conray, etc
     Iothalamate sodium: Angio Conray, etc
     Diatrizoate meglumine and diatrizoate sodium: Angiovist, Hypaque-M, etc

- Not for intravascular use, for instillation into cavities:

Diatrizoate meglumine, Cystografin, etc
Diatrizoate meglumine and diatrizoate sodium Gastrografin, etc
Diatrizoate sodium: Oral or rectal (Hypaque sodium oral)
Iothalamate meglumine: Cysto-Conray urogenital
Diatrizoate meglumine and iodipamide meglumine: Sinografin intrauterine instillation

Nonionic Contrast Media

Injectable

- Iohexol: Omnipaque
- Iopamidol: Isovue
- Ioversol: Optiray
- Metrizamide: Amipaque

Contrast reactions to IV agents may occur; severe reaction occurs 1/1000 and death due to anaphylaxis 1/40,000. Reactions include hives, bronchospasm, or pulmonary edema. (Premedication with steroids may not prevent a reaction.) Vagal reactions (hypotension and bradycardia) are another adverse effect. A history of asthma is a risk factor and a previous reaction to contrast does not necessarily preclude using IV contrast (allergy to seafood or iodine is no longer considered an important risk factor). Premedication with two doses of PO methylprednisolone, once at 12 h prior and then 2 h prior to IV contrast, is effective in reducing the incidence of reactions. Alternatively, use of new and more expensive (up to 10× the cost) nonionic contrast agents, lessens pain and cardiac dysfunction, with a possible overall decrease in adverse reactions.

Angiography: A rapid series of films obtained after a bolus contrast injection via percutaneous catheter. Used to image the aorta, major arteries and branches, tumors, and venous drainage via late "run-off" films. Helical CT scans are now capable of generating angiographic images.

- **DSA.** This is the latest enhancement of this study, allows reverse negative views and requires less contrast load

- **Cardiac angiography.** Definitive study for diagnosis and assessment of severity of CAD. Significant (>70% occlusion) stenotic lesions seen: 30% involve single vessels, 30% involve two, and 40%, three vessels. Can discriminate angina secondary to aortic valve disease and that from CAD
- **Cerebral angiography.** Evaluation of intra- and extracranial vascular disease, atherosclerosis, aneurysms, and A-V malformations. Not used for detection of cerebral structural lesions (use MRI or CT instead)
- **Pulmonary angiography.** Visualization of emboli, intrinsic or extrinsic vascular abnormalities, A-V malformations, and bleeding due to tumors. Most accurate diagnostic procedure for PE but only used if lung V/Q scan is not diagnostic

BE: Examining the colon and rectum. Indications include diarrhea, crampy abdominal pain, heme-positive stools, change in bowel habits, and unexplained weight loss

- **Air-contrast BE.** Done with the "double contrast" technique (air and barium) to better delineate the mucosa. More likely to show polyps
- **Gastrografin enema.** Similar to the barium enema, but water-soluble contrast is used (clears colon more quickly than barium). If the Gastrografin leaks from the GI tract, it is less irritating to the peritoneum (does not cause "barium peritonitis"). Therapeutic in the evaluation of severe obstipation, colonic volvulus, perforation, diverticulitis, or postop anastomotic leak

Barium Swallow (Esophagogram): Evaluating the swallowing mechanism and investigating esophageal lesions or abnormal peristalsis

Cystogram: Bladder filled and emptied and a catheter in place. Used to evaluate bladder filling defects (tumors, diverticulum) and bladder perforation. Can also be done using CT scanning (see also VCUG)

Enteroclysis: Selective intubation of the proximal jejunum and rapid infusion of contrast. Better than an SBFT in evaluating polyps or obstruction (adhesions, internal hernia, etc). May be used to evaluate small-bowel sources of chronic bleeding after negative upper and lower endoscopy

ERCP: Contrast endoscopically injected into the ampulla of Vater to visualize the common bile and pancreatic ducts in evaluating obstruction, stones, and ductal pattern

Fistulogram (Sinogram): Injection of water-soluble contrast media into any wound or body opening to determine the connection of the wound or opening with other structures

HSG: Evaluating uterine anomalies (congenital, fibroids, adhesions) or tubal abnormalities (occlusion or adhesion) often as part of infertility evaluation. Contraindicated during menses, undiagnosed vaginal bleeding, acute PID, or if pregnancy suspected. Patient in pelvic exam position, speculum placed and uterine os cannulated; then contrast injected

ExU or IVP: Contrast study of the kidneys and ureters. Limited usefulness for evaluating bladder abnormalities. Indications include flank pain, kidney stones, hematuria, UTI, trauma, and malignancy. Bowel prep helpful but not essential. Verify recent creatinine level. **Nephrotomograms** often included that include cuts of the kidney to further define the three-dimensional location or nature of renal lesions or stones

Lymphangiography. Iodinated oil injected to opacify lymphatics of the leg, inguinal, pelvic, and retroperitoneal areas. Used to test the integrity of the lymphatic system or evaluate for metastatic tumors (testicular, etc) or lymphoma

15

Myelogram: Evaluating the subarachnoid space for tumors, herniated disks, or other cause of nerve root injury. Using LP technique, contrast injected in the subarachnoid space

OCG: Visualizing gallbladder in the evaluation of cholelithiasis or cholecystitis. Patient given oral contrast pills 12–24 h before the study. Serum bilirubin should be <2 mg/100 mL. Used infrequently

PTHC: Visualizing biliary tree in a patient unable to concentrate the contrast media (bilirubin >3 mg/100 mL). Percutaneous needle inserted into a dilated biliary duct; contrast injected.

Percutaneous Nephrostogram: In the management of renal obstruction, percutaneous placement through the renal parenchyma and into the collecting system to relieve and or evaluate the level and cause of obstruction

RPG: Contrast material injected into the ureters through a cystoscope. Indications include allergy to IV contrast, a kidney or ureter that cannot be visualized on an IVP, filling defects in the collecting system, renal mass, and ureteral obstruction

RUG: Demonstrates traumatic disruption of the urethra and urethral strictures

SBFT: Usually done after a UGI series. A delayed film shows the jejunum and ileum. Used in the work-up of diarrhea, abdominal cramps, malabsorption, and UGI bleeding

T-Tube Cholangiogram: Resolution of swelling in some patients who have a T-tube placed in the common bile duct for drainage after gallbladder and common bile duct surgery. To evaluate the degree of swelling, look for residual stones, and evaluate patency of bile duct drainage

UGI Series: Includes the esophagogram plus the stomach and duodenum. Useful for visualizing ulcers, masses, hiatal hernias, and in the evaluation of heme-positive stools and upper abdominal pain

VCUG: Bladder filled with contrast through a catheter, then catheter is removed, and the patient allowed to void. Used for diagnosis of vesicoureteral reflux and urethral valves and in the evaluation of UTI

Venography, Peripheral: Contrast slowly injected into small foot or ankle vein to evaluate patency of deep veins of leg and calf. Look for a filling defect or outline of a thrombus. Noninvasive exams for DVT, such as Doppler ultrasound and impedance plethysmography, often used together before invasive venography and are highly sensitive (>90%) for proximal thrombi. A radionuclide scan with technetium-99-labeled RBCs sometimes used but is less sensitive and specific than the previously mentioned tests.

ULTRASOUND

Abdominal: Gallbladder (95% sensitivity in diagnosing stones), thickening of wall, biliary tree (obstruction), pancreas (pseudo-cyst, tumor, pancreatitis), aorta (aneurysm), kidneys (obstruction, tumor, cyst), abscesses, ascites

Endovaginal: Most useful in the diagnosis of gynecologic pathology (uterus, ovaries)

Pelvic (A full bladder is desirable)

- **Pregnancy.** Fetal dating (biparietal diameters); diagnosis of multiple gestations; determination of intrauterine growth retardation, hydrocephalus, and hydronephrosis; localization of the placenta
- **Gynecology.** Ovarian and uterine masses (tumors, cysts, fibroids, etc.), ectopic pregnancy, abscesses

Thyroid: Evaluate thyroid nodules (cyst versus solid) and to direct biopsies. Ultrasound alone cannot usually differentiate benign from malignant lesions.

Transrectal: Most useful in the diagnosis of prostate pathology and directing prostate biopsies

Echocardiograms

- **M-mode.** Valve mobility, chamber size, pericardial effusions, septal size
- **Two-dimensional.** Valvular vegetations, septal defects, wall motion, chamber size, pericardial effusion, valve motion, wall thickness
- **Doppler.** Cross-valvular pressure gradients, blood flow patterns, and valve orifice areas in the work-up of cardiac valvular disease

Other Ultrasound Uses

Testicular (identify and characterize masses, eg, hydrocele versus tumor), intraoperative, determine bladder emptying

CT SCANS

Computerized tomography (also called CAT for computerized axial tomography) can be performed with or without intravenous contrast. A dilute oral contrast agent administered prior to abdominal or pelvic scans helps delineate the bowel. IV contrast is used to provide vascular and tissue enhancement for some CT scans; a current creatinine level should be available to determine suitability of IV contrast administration. Virtually any body part can be scanned depending on the indications, but it is most helpful in evaluating the brain, lung, mediastinum, retroperitoneum (pancreas, kidney, nodes, aorta), and liver, and to a lesser extent in the pelvis, colon, or bone. CT scans allow for the use of density measurements (also known as **Hounsfield units**) to differentiate cysts, lipomas, hemochromatosis, vascular ("enhancing") and avascular ("nonenhancing") lesions. In Hounsfield units, bone is +1000, water is 0, fat is −1000, and other tissues fall within this scale, depending on the machine settings. Metal and barium can cause distortion of the image.

Head: Evaluation of tumors, subdural and epidural hematomas, atrioventricular (A-V) malformations, hydrocephalus, and sinus and temporal bone pathology. Initial test of choice for trauma; may be superior to MRI in detecting hemorrhage within first 24–48 h

Abdomen: Images virtually all intraabdominal and retroperitoneal organs or disease processes. Good accuracy with abscesses, but ultrasound may show smaller collections adjacent to the liver, spleen, or bladder. Surgical clips or barium in the gut may cause artifacts. IV contrast usually given, so check creatinine level; when using a water-soluble contrast (Tomocat, others) to visualize the gut, the patient must receive an oral contrast beforehand.

Retroperitoneum: Useful for evaluating pancreatitis and its complications; pancreatic masses; nodal metastasis from colon, prostate, renal, or testicular tumors; adrenal masses (>3 cm suggestive of carcinoma); psoas masses; aortic aneurysms

Pelvis: Staging and diagnosis of bladder, prostate, rectal, and gynecological carcinoma

Mediastinum: Masses, ectopic parathyroids

Neck: Work-up of neck masses, abscesses, and other diseases of the throat and trachea

Chest: Able to find 40% more nodules than whole lung tomograms, which demonstrate 20% more nodules than plain chest x-ray. Although calcification is suggestive of benign disease (eg, granuloma), no definite density value can reliably separate malignant from benign lesions. Useful in differentiating hilar adenopathy from vascular structures seen on plain chest x-ray

Spine: MRI generally preferred over CT. However, rare conditions, contraindication to MRI, or artifact from metal may make the CT the preferred test.

SPIRAL (HELICAL) CT SCAN

Spiral CT can be used for any type of imaging (not commonly used for brain). It relies on rapid scan acquisition (ie, >8 frames/s). This minimizes motion artifact and allows for capturing a bolus of contrast at peak levels in the region being scanned. Standard CT is too slow to capture this peak flow. These contrast-enhanced scans allow detailed 3-D reconstruction and angiographic evaluations. Bony structures can also be visualized and do not require contrast. The term *spiral/helical* is derived from the fact that the tube spins around the patient while the table moves. Spiral CT can compensate for "streak" artifact due to implanted metallic devices. Examples for uses of this technology include diagnosis of PE, pretransplant angiography, evaluation of flank pain and determination of kidney stones (largely replacing emergency IVP), and rapid evaluation of trauma.

MAGNETIC RESONANCE IMAGING (MR OR MRI)
How It Works

Although the physics of MRI is beyond the scope of this section, certain key concepts are essential to interpreting studies generated by this technology. MRI uses measurements of the magnetic movements of atomic nuclei to delineate tissues. Specifically, when nuclei, such as hydrogen, are placed in a strong magnetic field, they resonate and emit radio signals when pulsed with radio waves. A defined sequence of magnetic pulses and interval pauses produces measured changes in the tissue's magnetic vectors, which results in an MRI image. T1, or longitudinal relaxation time, is the measurement of magnetic vector changes in the z axis during the relaxation pause. T2, or transverse relaxation time, is the magnetic vector changes in the x-y plane.

Each tissue, normal or pathologic, has a unique T1 and T2 for a given MRI field strength. In general T1 > T2. T1 = 0.1–2 s and T2 = 0.03–0.6 s. The inherent tissue differences between various T1's and T2's give the visual contrast seen between tissues on the MRI image. An image is **T1-weighted** if it depends on the differences in T1 measurements for visual contrast, or **T2-weighted** if the image depends on T2 measurements.

The most common pulse sequence is called spin echo (SE). Partial saturation (PS) and inversion recovery (IR) are two newer pulse sequences. Available MRI views are transverse, sagittal, oblique, and coronal.

How to Read an MRI

SE T1-Weighted Images: Provide good anatomic planes due to the wide variances of T1 values among normal tissues.

15

- Brightest (high signal intensity): Fat
- Dark or black: Pathological tissues, tumor or inflammation, fluid collections
- Black (low signal intensity): Respiratory tract, GI tract, calcified bone and tissues, blood vessels, heart chambers, and pericardial effusions

SE T2-Weighted Images: Pathology prolongs T2 measurements, and normal tissues have a very small range of T2 values. T2-weighted images provide the best detection of pathology and a decreased visualization of normal tissue anatomy. Tumor surrounded by fat may be lost on T2 imaging.

- Brightest : Fat and fluid collections
- Bright : Pheochromocytomas

When to Use MRI

In general, MRI imaging is at least equal to CT imaging. MRI is superior to CT for imaging of brain, spinal cord, musculoskeletal soft tissues, adrenal and renal masses, and areas of high CT bony artifact. However, spiral CT may now have overcome some of these disadvantages.
   Advantages

- No ionizing radiation
- Display of vascular anatomy without contrast
- Visualization of linear structures: Spine and spinal cord, aorta, and cava
- Visualization of posterior fossa and other hard to see CT areas
- High-contrast soft tissue images

Disadvantages

- Claustrophobia due to confining magnet (Newer **open MRI** scanners may obviate this problem.)
- Longer scanning time resulting in motion artifacts
- Unable to scan critically ill patients requiring life support equipment
- Metallic foreign bodies: Pacemakers, shrapnel, CNS vascular clips, metallic eye fragments, and cochlear implants are contraindications

15

MRI Contrast: Gadolinium (gadopentetic dimeglumine) is an ionic contrast agent that acts as a paramagnetic agent and enhances vessels or lesions with abnormal vascularity.

Uses of MRI

MRI is very sensitive to motion artifact; anxious or agitated patients may require sedation. Intramuscular glucagon may be used to suppress intestinal peristalsis on abdominal studies. If metallic eye fragments are possible, a screening CT of the orbits should be obtained prior to any MRI examination. It is generally contraindicated in patients with intracranial aneurysm clips, intraocular metallic fragments, and pacemakers. Dental fillings and dental prostheses have thus far not been a problem.

Abdomen: Useful for differentiating adrenal lesions, staging tumors (renal, GI, pelvic), evaluation of abdominal masses, and virtually all intraabdominal organs and retroperitoneal structures. Useful in differentiating benign adenomas from metastasis

Chest: Mediastinal masses, differentiates nodes from vessels, cardiac diseases, tumor staging, aortic dissection or aneurysm

Head: Analysis of all intracranial pathology may identify demyelinating diseases; some conditions are better evaluated by CT (see previous section), including acute trauma. **MRS** may increase the sensitivity of diagnosis of many neurologic diseases by providing a biochemical "fingerprint" of tissues in the brain. Performed in conjunction with an MRI equipped with the MRS capability. Some uses include differentiating dementias, tumors, MS, and many others.

Musculoskeletal System: Bone tumors, bone and soft tissue infections, evaluation of joint spaces (except if a prosthesis is in place), marrow disorders, aseptic necrosis of the femoral head

Pelvis: Evaluation of all pelvic organs in males and females. Differentiates endometrium from myoma and adenomyosis. Diagnosis of congenital uterine anomalies (eg, bicornuate, septate). Endorectal surface coil allows enhanced imaging of structures such as the prostate.

Spine: Diseases of the spinal column (herniated discs, tumors, etc)

NUCLEAR SCANS

The following is a listing of some of the more commonly used nuclear scans and their purposes. Most are contraindicated in pregnancy; check with your nuclear medicine department.

Adrenal Scan: Used to accurately localize a pheochromocytoma when MRI or CT is equivocal. Uses labeled **MIBG** ; patient must return several days later for imaging after administration.

Bleeding Scan: Used to detect the source of GI tract bleeding.

- ^{99m}TC **(technetium-99m) sulfur colloid scan.** Used to detect bleeding of 0.05–0.1 mL/min.
- ^{99m}TC **(technetium-99m)-labeled red cell scan.** Same as sulfur colloid scan, but may be superior for localizing intermittent bleeding

Bone Scan: Metastatic work-ups (cancers most likely to go to bone: prostate, breast, kidney, thyroid, lung); evaluation of delayed union of fractures, osteomyelitis, avascular necrosis of the femoral head, evaluation of hip prosthesis, to distinguish pathological fractures from traumatic fractures

Brain Scan: Metastatic work-ups, determination of blood flow (in brain death or atherosclerotic disease), evaluation of space-occupying lesions (tumor, hematoma, abscess, [A-V] malformation), and encephalitis

Cardiac Scans: Diagnosis of MI, stress testing, ejection fractions, measurement of cardiac output, diagnosis of ventricular aneurysms

- **Thallium-201 (^{201}Tl).** Examines myocardial perfusion via uptake of ^{201}Tl by normal myocardium. Normal myocardium appears hot, and ischemic or infarcted areas cold. AMI (<12 h) seen as a hotspot, old MI (scar) seen as cold on both resting and exercise scans, and ischemia is cold on exercise scan and returns to normal after rest.
- **Technetium-99m pyrophosphate.** Recently damaged myocardium concentrates ^{99m}Tc pyrophosphate, producing a myocardial hotspot. Most sensitive 24–72 h after AMI
- **Technetium-99m ventriculogram.** ^{99m}Tc-labeled serum albumin or RBCs are used. Demonstrates abnormal wall motion, cardiac shunts, size and function of heart

15

chambers, cardiac output, and ejection fraction. Another form of this study is **MUGA scan,** data collection from which is synchronized to ECG, and selected aspects are used to create a "moving picture" of cardiac function. May be done at rest or during exercise stress test.

Gallium Scans: Location of abscesses (5–10 d old), chronic inflammatory lesions, original lymphoma staging or follow-up for disease detection, lung cancer, melanoma, other neoplastic tissues

Hepatobiliary Scans (HIDA-Scan, BIDA-Scan):   Differential diagnosis of biliary obstruction (when bilirubin >1.5 and <7 mg/100 mL), acute cholecystitis, diagnosis of biliary atresia; NOT good for stones unless cystic duct is completely occluded and acute cholecystitis present

Indium-111 octreotide (OctreoScan):   Imaging method for tumors with somatostatin receptors (pheochromocytoma, gastrinomas, insulinomas, small-cell lung cancer)

I^{125} (Iodine-125) Fibrinogen Scanning: Used to detect venous thrombosis in the lower extremities. After injection of the tracer, the patient is scanned several hours and for several days after. Most useful to identify clot at or below the knees. False-positives with varicosities, cellulitis, incisions, arthritis, hematomas and with recent venography. Product availability is a problem at present.

Liver–Spleen Scan: Estimation of organ size, parenchymal diseases (hepatitis, etc), abscess, cysts, primary and secondary tumors

Lung Scan (V/Q Scan):   Used along with a chest x-ray for evaluation of PE (a normal scan rules out a PE, an indeterminate scan requires further study via a pulmonary angiogram, and a clear perfusion deficit coupled with a normal ventilation scan is highly probable for a PE). V/Q scans can provide evidence of pulmonary disease, COPD, and emphysema.

Renal Scans: Agents are generally classified as functional tracers or morphologic tracers.

- ^{131}I **Hippuran.** Primarily a renal function agent; useful in renal insufficiency for evaluation of function; visualization is poor, and radiation dose can be high
- **Technetium-99m glucoheptonate.** Useful as a combination renal cortical imaging agent and renal function agent; primarily used to evaluate overall function, but can be used to determine vascular flow and to visualize the renal parenchyma and collecting system
- **Technetium-99m DMSA** (dimercaptosuccinic acid). Used only as a renal cortical imaging agent
- **Technetium-99m DTPA** (diethylenetriamine pentaacetic acid). Primarily a renal function agent; useful for renal blood flow studies, estimation of GFR, evaluation of the collecting system
- **Technetium-99m mercaptoacetyltriglycine (MAG3).** A relatively new agent, primarily a functional agent, very good imaging of the renal parenchyma can be obtained within minutes of injection and a low radiation dose. May eventually replace all other renal agents.

Strontium-89 (Metastron):   Not technically an imaging agent, but used in the palliative therapy of multiple painful bony metastasis (ie, prostate or breast cancer). Because this is a pure beta emitter, the radioactivity remains in the body so no special precautions (other than blood and urine analysis) are needed.

SPECT Scan: **S**ingle-**p**hoton **e**mission-**c**omputed **t**omography, a technique whereby multiple nuclear images are sequentially displayed similar to a CT scan; can be applied to many nuclear scans.

Thyroid Scan: Most commonly with technetium-99m pertechnetate. Useful for evaluation of nodules (solitary cold nodules require a tissue diagnosis because 25% are cancerous). Scan patterns in correlation with lab tests may help diagnose hyperfunctioning adenomas, Plummer's and Graves' diseases, and multinodular goiters; localize ectopic thyroid tissues (especially after thyroidectomy for cancer); and identify superior mediastinal thyroid masses

HOW TO READ A CHEST X-RAY
Determine the Adequacy of the Film

- Inspiration: Diaphragm below ribs 8–10 posteriorly and 5–6 anteriorly
- Rotation: Clavicles are equidistant from the spinous processes
- Penetration: Disc spaces are seen but bony details of spine cannot be seen

PA Film

Remember, the film is on the patient's chest and the x-rays are passing from back (posterior) to front (anterior). The structures described in the following material are shown in Figure 15–1.

Soft Tissues: Check for symmetry, swelling, loss of tissue planes, and subcutaneous air.

Skeletal Structures: Examine the clavicles, scapulas, vertebrae, sternum, and ribs. Look for symmetry. In a good x-ray, the clavicles are symmetrical. Check for osteolytic or osteoblastic lesions, fractures, or arthritic changes. Look for rib-notching.

Diaphragm: Sides should be equal and slightly rounded, although the left may be slightly lower. Costophrenic angles should be clear and sharp. Blunting suggests scarring or fluid. It takes about 100–200 mL of pleural fluid to cause blunting. Check below the diaphragm for the gas pattern and free air. A unilateral high diaphragm suggests paralysis (either from nerve damage, trauma, or an abscess), eventration or loss of lung volume on that side because of atelectasis or pneumothorax. A flat diaphragm suggests COPD.

Mediastinum and Heart: The aortic knob should be visible and distinct. Widening of the mediastinum is seen with traumatic disruption of the thoracic aorta. In children, do not mistake the normally prominent thymus for widening. Mediastinal masses can be associated with Hodgkin's disease and other lymphomas. The trachea should be in a straight line with a sharp carina. Tracheal deviation suggests a mass (tumor), goiter, unilateral loss of lung volume (collapse), or tension pneumothorax. The heart should be less than one-half the width of the chest wall on a PA film. If greater than one-half, think of CHF or pericardial fluid.

Hilum: The left hilum should be up to 2–3 cm higher than the right. Vessels are seen here. Look for any masses, nodes, or calcifications.

Lung Fields: Note the presence of any shadows from CVP lines, NG tubes, pulmonary artery catheters, etc. The fields should be clear with normal lung markings all the way to the periphery. The vessels should taper to become almost invisible at the periphery.

15

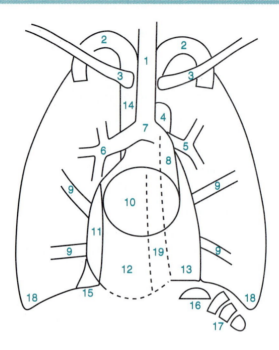

Posteroanterior Chest X-ray

1. Trachea
2. First rib
3. Clavicle
4. Aortic knob
5. Left pulmonary artery
6. Right pulmonary artery
7. Carina
8. Pulmonary trunk
9. Pulmonary veins
10. Left atrium
11. Right atrium
12. Right ventricle
13. Left ventricle
14. Superior vena cava
15. Inferior vena cava
16. Gastric air bubble
17. Splenic flexure air
18. Costophrenic angles
19. Descending aorta

FIGURE 15-1 Structures seen on a posteroanterior (PA) chest x-ray film.

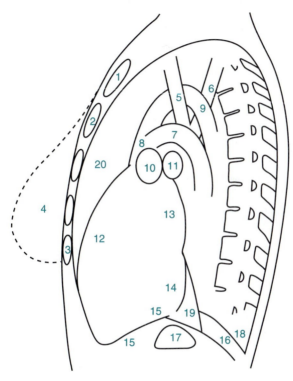

Lateral Chest X-ray

1. Manubrium
2. Body of sternum
3. Xiphoid process
4. Breast shadow
5. Trachea
6. Scapula
7. Left pulmonary artery
8. Ascending aorta
9. Aortic arch
10. Right pulmonary artery
11. Left mainstem bronchus
12. Right ventricle
13. Left atrium
14. Left ventricle
15. Right diaphragm
16. Left diaphragm
17. Gastric air bubble
18. Costophrenic angles
19. Inferior vena cava
20. Retrosternal clear space

FIGURE 15–2   Structures seen on a lateral chest x-ray film.

15

Vessels in the lower lung should be larger than those in the upper lung. A reversal of this difference (called cephalization) suggests pulmonary venous hypertension and heart failure. **Kerley's B lines,** small linear densities found usually at the lateral base of the lung, are associated with CHF. Check the margins carefully; look for pleural thickening, masses, or pneumothorax.

If the lungs appear hyperlucent with a relatively small heart and flattening of the diaphragms, COPD is likely. Thin plate-like linear densities are associated with atelectasis.

To locate a lesion, do not forget to check a lateral film and remember the "silhouette sign." Obliteration of all or part of a heart border means the lesion is anterior in the chest and lies in the right middle lobe, lingula, or anterior segment of the upper lobe. A radiopacity that overlaps the heart but does not obliterate the heart border is posterior and lies in the lower lobes.

Examine carefully for the following:

1. Coin lesions: Causes are granulomas (50% which are usually calcified), (histoplasmosis 25%, TB 20%, coccidioidomycosis 20%, varies with locale); primary carcinoma (25%), hamartoma (<10%), and metastatic disease (<5%).
2. Cavitary lesions: Causes are abscess, cancer, TB, coccidioidomycosis, Wegener's granulomatosis.
3. Infiltrates: Two major types
   a. **Interstitial pattern.** "Reticular." Causes are granulomatous infections, miliary TB, coccidioidomycosis, pneumoconiosis, sarcoidosis, CHF. "Honeycombing" represents end-stage fibrosis caused by sarcoid, RA, and pneumoconiosis.
   b. **Alveolar pattern.** Diffuse, quick progression and regression. Can see either "butterfly" pattern or air bronchograms. Causes are PE, pneumonia, hemorrhage or PE associated with CHF.

Lateral Film

Examine the structures shown in Figure 15–2. Use this study to check for the three-dimensional location of lesions. Pay close attention to the retrosternal clear space, costophrenic angles, and the path of the aorta.

16

INTRODUCTION TO THE OPERATING ROOM

Sterile Technique
Entering the OR
The Surgical Hand Scrub
Preparing the Patient
Gowning and Gloving

Draping the Patient
Finding Your Place
Universal Precautions
Latex Allergy

Working in the OR can be the best or worst experience of a clinical rotation. However, familiarity with OR procedure is crucial to the success of any such experience. Preparing yourself before you get to the OR by knowing the patient thoroughly and having a basic understanding of what is planned will greatly enhance your OR experience. Don't fall into the trap of stereotyping the nurses as cranky, the surgeons as egotistical, and the medical students as stupid. Avoid this by learning the routine of the OR. Be alert, attentive, and, above all, patient. Soon, the routine should become second nature. Most importantly, don't be afraid to admit to the scrub nurse and the circulating nurse that you're new at this. They are usually more than happy to help you follow correct procedures.

STERILE TECHNIQUE

Members of the OR team, which includes the surgeon, assistants, students, and scrub nurse (the one who is responsible for passing the instruments and gowning the OR team), maintain a sterile field. The circulating nurse acts as a go-between between the sterile and nonsterile areas.

Sterile areas include

- Front of the gown to the waist
- Gloved hands and arms to the shoulder
- Draped part of the patient down to the table level
- Covered part of the Mayo stand
- Back table where additional instruments are kept

The sides of the back table are not considered sterile, and anything that falls below the level of the patient table is considered contaminated.

ENTERING THE OR

From the moment you enter the OR, everything is geared toward maintaining a sterile field. The use of sterile technique begins in the locker room. Change into scrub clothing (remember to remove T-shirts and tuck the scrub shirt into the pants). Be sure that the ties of the scrub pants are also tucked inside the pants. Scrub clothes may occasionally be worn on the wards, provided that they are covered by a clinic coat or some other form of gown, but you

16

need to check your hospital or departmental requirements on this. If you do wear scrub clothing out of the OR, be sure that it is not bloodstained.

Pass into the anteroom to get your mask, cap, and shoe covers. The mask should cover your entire nose and mouth. Full hoods are necessary for men with a beard. The cap must cover all of your hair. Because of universal precautions, OR staff are now required to use protective eyewear while at the operative field. While wearing glasses, it is helpful to tape the mask to the bridge of your nose to prevent fogging during the surgery. Special masks are also available with self-adhesive strips to help prevent fogging of glasses. Tape the glasses to your forehead if you think they may be loose enough to fall onto the table during the operation! Do not wear nail polish, and remove any loose jewelry, watches, and rings before scrubbing. Make sure that shoelaces are tucked inside the shoe covers.

The mask does not need to be worn in the hall of the OR suite (but everything else does) at most hospitals. The mask must be worn in the OR itself, near the scrub sinks, and in the substerile room between ORs.

Find the operating room where the patient is located, and assist in transport, if necessary. Introduce yourself to the intern or resident and nurse, and try to get an idea of when to begin scrubbing (usually when the first surgeon starts to scrub). If you have a pager, follow the OR procedures and remove the pager if you are going to be scrubbed into the case.

THE SURGICAL HAND SCRUB

The purpose of a surgical hand scrub is to decrease the bacterial flora of the skin by mechanically cleansing the arms and hands before the operation. Key points to remember: (1) If contamination occurs during the scrub, it is necessary to start over, and (2) In emergency situations exceptions are made to the time allowed for scrubbing (as in obstetrics, when the baby is brought out from the delivery room and the student is still scrubbing!). Caps and masks should be properly positioned before the start of the scrub.

Povidone–Iodine (Betadine) Hand Scrub

Scrubbing technique depends somewhat on local custom. Some ORs want a timed scrub in which the duration of scrubbing is determined by watching the clock. Other ORs use an "anatomic" scrub in which the duration of scrubbing is determined by counting strokes. Either is acceptable, and you should find out what the custom is at your institution.

Timed Scrub

1. Perform a general prewash, with surgical soap and water, up to 2 in. above the elbows.
2. Use disposable brushes if available. Aseptically open one brush and place it on the ledge above the sink for the second half of the scrub. Open another brush and begin the scrub with Betadine. Use the nail cleaner to clean under all fingernails.
3. Scrub both arms during the first 5 min. Start at the fingertips and end 2 in. above the elbows; pay close attention to the fingernails and interdigital spaces. Discard the brush and rinse from fingertips to elbows.
4. Take the second brush and repeat step 3. Always start at the fingertips and work up to the elbows.
5. Always allow water to drip off the elbows by keeping the hands above the level of the elbows.
6. Move into the OR to dry your hands and arms (back into the room to push the door open).
7. Scrubbing times:
    a. Ten minutes at the start of the day or with no previous scrub within the last 12 h and on all orthopedic cases

b. Five minutes with a previous scrub or between cases if you have not been out of the OR working with other patients

Chlorhexidine (Hibiclens) 6-Min Hand Scrub (Timed)

1. Wet your hands and forearms to the elbows with water.
2. Dispense about 5 mL of Hibiclens into your cupped hands and spread it over both hands and arms to the elbows.
3. Scrub vigorously for 3 min without adding water. Use a sponge or brush for scrubbing, and pay particular attention to fingernails, cuticles, and interdigital spaces.
4. Rinse thoroughly with running water.
5. Dispense another 5 mL of Hibiclens into your cupped hands.
6. Wash for an additional 3 min. There is no need to use a brush or sponge at this point. Rinse thoroughly. Move into the OR back first to dry your hands.

Anatomic Scrub

1. Perform a general prewash, with surgical soap and water, up to 2 in. above the elbows.
2. Use disposable brushes if available. Aseptically open one brush and place it on the ledge above the sink for the second half of the scrub. Open another brush and begin the scrub with Betadine. Use the nail cleaner to clean under all fingernails.
3. Each surface is to be scrubbed vigorously 10 times. Start with each finger (each of which has four surfaces), proceeding to the hand, the forearm, and the arm above the elbow. After finishing one extremity, do the other from fingers to above the elbow. Be sure to include all parts of your hand, especially the interdigital spaces.
4. Rinse both arms thoroughly.
5. Now rescrub each extremity, this time not going above the elbow. This is done in a similar fashion, 10 times on each surface from fingers to elbow.
6. Rinse thoroughly and proceed into the OR.

PREPARING THE PATIENT

The exact technique may vary in different medical centers, but the patient prep involves mechanically cleansing the patient's skin in the region of the surgical site to reduce bacterial flora. Ask the intern or resident to guide you through the procedure the first time, and consider doing it yourself thereafter. It is always better to prep a wider area than you think necessary. For example, for a midline laparotomy, the patient is prepped from nipples to pubis, and from the flank at table level on one side to the table level on the other side.

16

Materials

Usually, a small prep table is present containing the following:

- Gloves
- Towels
- Betadine or other scrub soap (optional)
- Betadine or other paint solution
- 4 × 4 gauze squares or sponges
- Ring forceps (optional)

Technique

1. Patient prep is usually done before putting on the sterile gown. Don a pair of gloves, and scrub the area designated by the intern or resident for 4–6 min. Use the $4 \times 4s$ (or sponges) and the soap solution. This is generally done three times with a gauze or sponge in each hand for a total of 4–6 min. Note, however, many times this traditional wound scrubbing is no longer performed routinely and is used only in specific circumstances, such as, contaminated wounds.

2. Drape the area with a towel, and then gently pat the area dry if the wound was scrubbed. Taking care not to contaminate the area, gently peel off the towel from one side, being careful not to allow the towel to fall back on the prepped area. Also be careful not to contaminate your own arms, so that you do not have to rescrub before gowning.

3. Use $4 \times 4s$ or sponges to paint the exposed area with the Betadine or other provided solution, using the proposed incision site as the center. Move circumferentially away from the incision site. Never bring the $4 \times 4s$ back to the center after they have painted more peripheral areas. This is done as a series of concentric circles. Some centers will only "paint" and not "scrub" with the soap solution. Some surgeons want the paint dried with a towel at the end, and others like to leave it "wet." Check with the resident or attending physician before you start, to find out exactly what is wanted.

4. When you are finished with the prep, remove your gloves in a sterile manner and proceed to get your gown on.

GOWNING AND GLOVING

1. If you have just completed the hand scrub, back into the room to push the door open; keep your hands above your elbows.

2. Ask the scrub nurse for a towel. Do not be impatient because the scrub nurse is often very busy. Stick out one hand, palm up and well away from the body. The nurse will drape the towel over your hand.

3. Bend at the waist to maintain sterility of the towel. It should never touch your clothing.

4. With one-half of the towel, dry one arm, beginning at the fingers; change hands and dry the other arm with the remaining half of the towel. Never go back to the forearm or hands after drying your elbows.

5. Drop the towel in the hamper. Again, remember to keep your hands above your elbows.

6. Ask for a gown and hold your arms out straight. The scrub nurse will place the gown on you, and the circulator will tie the back for you.

7. The nurse will usually hold out a right glove with the palm toward you. Push your hand through the glove. Gloves come in different sizes–small (5½–6½), medium (7–7½), and large (8–8½)–and different materials: standard latex gloves, hypoallergenic (powder-free), reinforced (orthopedic), and latex-free. Ask the resident or scrub nurse for guidance on the type of glove to request. It is good form to ask the circulating nurse to open your gloves before you actually begin to scrub.

8. Repeat the procedure with the left glove. It is easier if you use two fingers of your gloved right hand to help hold the left glove open.

9. Visually inspect the gloves for any holes.

10. Give the scrub nurse the long string of your front gown-tie. Hold the other string yourself and turn around in place. Tie the strings.

11. The nurse may offer you a damp sponge to clean the powder off the gloves (the powder has been implicated in some postoperative complications, eg, adhesions). This varies by locale.

12. Now wait patiently; stay out of the way, and keep your hands above your waist. Hold them together to prevent yourself from accidentally dropping them or touching your mask. This is one of the most difficult things for the neophyte to remember. Be attentive. The only things that are sterile are your chest to your waist in the front and your hands to the shoulders. Your back is not sterile, nor is your body below the waist. Avoid crossing your arms.

DRAPING THE PATIENT

Draping the patient is usually done by the surgeon and assistants. Watch how they do it, and consider helping at a later date. It is harder to keep sterile than it looks.

FINDING YOUR PLACE

The medical student is often the "low man or woman on the totem pole" and, initially, usually stands down by the patient's feet. Ask the senior surgeon where you should stand.

The first thing to remember is that once you are scrubbed, you must not touch anything that is not sterile. Put your hands on the sterile field and do not move about unnecessarily. If you need to move around someone else, pass back to back. When passing by a sterile field, try to face it. When passing a nonsterile field, pass it with your back toward it. If you are observing a case and are not scrubbed in, do not go between two sterile fields, and stay about 1 ft away from all sterile fields to avoid contamination (and condemnation!). When not scrubbed in, it often helps to keep your hands behind your back, being careful not to back into the instrument table.

Do not drop your hands below your waist or the table level. Do not grab at anything that falls off the side of the table–it is considered contaminated. If something falls, you can quietly inform the circulating nurse. Do not reach for anything on the scrub nurse's small instrument stand (the Mayo stand). You may ask for the instrument to be given to you.

If someone says that you have contaminated a glove or anything else, do not move and do not complain or disagree. Remember that the focus of the OR is maintaining a sterile field, so if anyone says, "You're contaminated," accept the statement and change gloves, gown, or whatever is needed. If a glove alone is contaminated, hold the hand out away from the sterile field, fingers extended and palms up, and a circulating nurse will pull the glove off. The same is true if a needle sticks you or if a glove tears. Tell the surgeon and scrub nurse that you are contaminated and change gloves.

If you have to change your gown, step away from the table. The circulator will remove first the gown and then the gloves. This procedure prevents the contaminated inside of the gown from passing over the hands. Regown and reglove without scrubbing again.

Always be aware of "sharps" on the field. When passing a potentially injurious instrument, always make the other members of the team aware that you are passing a sharp (ie, "needle back," "knife back," etc). Attempt to learn the names and functions of the common instruments. A knowledgeable student may be more likely to actively participate in the case.

At the end of the case (once the dressing is on the wound), you may remove the gown and gloves but not the mask, cap, or shoe covers. To protect yourself, remove your gown first, and remove your own gloves last. This keeps your hands clean of any blood or fluids that got onto your gown during the procedure. Assist in the transfer of the patient to the postoperative recovery room. Postop orders and a brief operative note are written immediately. See Chapter 2 (page 36) on how to write postop notes and orders. It is good form to offer to write the postop note and orders if you are comfortable with the process. Due to governmental regulations that affect attending physicians at teaching hospitals, the attending must often write the note him or herself. At the very least, the attending of record will

16

annotate an "attestation" to your note saying that the surgeon was "personally present during the critical portions of the procedure."

UNIVERSAL PRECAUTIONS

All operating room personnel are at risk for infection with blood-borne agents responsible for such diseases as AIDS and hepatitis. To reduce the incidence of such transmission, a set of guidelines called Universal Precautions has been developed by the CDC. The underlying principle is that, because patients cannot be routinely tested for HIV and are rarely tested preoperatively for hepatitis, the safest policy is to treat all patients as though they are infected with these agents. This approach ensures evenhanded treatment of all patients and the safest work environment for those who are exposed to the blood of others.

Minimizing the risks to all who are in the OR requires constant vigilance. Movements must be coordinated among surgeon, assistant, and technician. Fingers are never used to pick up needles; this is done only with another instrument. Fingers and hands should not be used as retractors. Two people should never be holding the same sharp instrument. Placing a sharp instrument down or handing it to another member of the team is always preceded by a verbal warning that notifies the recipient that a sharp object is about to be passed. Protective eyewear must be worn by all members of the operating team.

The practice of "double gloving" is often reserved for cases in which the patient is known to carry a transmissible agent. This technique definitely reduces the incidence of blood–skin contact, especially in light of the extraordinarily high incidence of unrecognized glove perforations. Until puncture-resistant gloves are developed, this is the best approach we have.

LATEX ALLERGY

Individuals with certain medical conditions or occupations that are heavily exposed to products containing natural rubber latex may became sensitized to it and develop allergic reactions. Up to 7% of health care workers can have allergic reactions. Certain conditions (ie, spina bifida, cerebral palsy) predispose patients to an 18–40% incidence of allergy. Reactions can vary from mild rash and itching to anaphylaxis. Latex products are found in a wide array of products, from gloves and drapes, to IV tubing. Occasionally patients will have documented latex allergy. Hospitals have latex allergy protocols, and hospitals maintain an inventory of latex-free products.

17

SUTURING TECHNIQUES AND WOUND CARE

Wound Healing
Suture Materials
Suturing Procedure
Suturing Patterns

Surgical Knots
Suture Removal
Tissue Adhesives

WOUND HEALING

The process of wound healing is generally divided into four stages: inflammation, fibroblast proliferation, contraction, and remodeling. There are three different types of wound healing: primary intent (routine primary suturing); secondary intent (the wound is not closed with suture and closes by contraction and epithelialization, most often used for wounds that are infected and packed open); and tertiary intent (also called delayed primary closure; the wound is left open for a time and then sutured at a later date, used often with grossly contaminated wounds).

SUTURE MATERIALS

Suture materials can be broadly defined as absorbable and nonabsorbable. **Absorbable sutures** can be thought of as temporary; these include plain gut; chromic gut; and synthetic materials such as polyglactin 910 (Vicryl), polyglycolic acid (Dexon), and poliglecaprone (Monocryl). These are resorbed by the body when left internally after a variable period (Table 17–1). Polydioxanone (PDS) is a long-lasting absorbable suture. Nonabsorbable sutures can be thought of as "permanent" unless they are removed; these include silk, stainless steel wire, polypropylene (Prolene), and nylon (see Table 17–1).

The size of a suture is defined by the number of zeros. The more zeros in the number, the smaller the suture. For example, a 5-0 suture (00000) is much smaller than a 2-0 (00) suture.

Most sutures come prepackaged and mounted on needles ("swaged on"). Cutting needles are used for tough tissues such as skin, and tapered needles are used for more delicate tissues such as the intestine. The most common needle for skin closure is the ⅜ in. circle cutting needle.

SUTURING PROCEDURE

The following guidelines cover the repair of lacerations in the emergency setting. Similar principles hold true for closure of wounds in the operating room. The choice of appropriate suture material is based on many factors, including location, extent of the laceration, strength of the tissues, and preference of the physician.

TABLE 17–1
Common Suture Materials

ABSORBABLE

Suture (Brand Name)	Description	Tensile Strength*	Absorbed†	Common Uses
Fast catgut	Twisted/Fast absorption	3–5 d	30 d	Facial lacerations in children
Plain catgut	Twisted/Rapidly absorbable	7–10 d	70 d	Vessel ligation, subcutaneous tissues
Chromic catgut	Twisted/absorbable	10–14 d	90 d	Mucosa
Polyglycolic acid (Dexon)	Braided/Absorbable	14–21 d	60–90 d	GI, subcutaneous tissues
Polyglactin 910 (Vicryl Rapide)	Braided/Absorbable	5 d	42 d	Skin repair needing rapid absorption
Polyglactin 910 (Vicryl)	Braided/Absorbable	21 d	56–70 d	Bowel, deep tissue
Poliglecaprone 25 (Monocryl)	Monofilament/Absorbable	7–14 d	91–119 d	Skin, bowel
Polydioxanone (PDS)	Monofilament/Absorbable	28 d	6 mo	Fascia, vessel anastomosis
Polyglyconate (Maxon)	Braided/Absorbable	28 d	6 mo	GI, muscle, fascia
Panacryl	Braided/Absorbable	>6 mo	>24 mo	Fascia, tendons

(continued)

TABLE 17–1
(Continued)

NONABSORBABLE

Suture (Brand Name)	Description	Common Uses
Nylon (Dermalon, Ethilon)	Monofilament	Skin, drains
Nylon (Nurolon)	Braided	
Polyester (Ethibond, Tycron)	Braided	Tendon repair Cardiac, tendon
Polypropylene (Prolene)	Monofilament	Vessel, fascia, skin
Silk		GI, vessel ligation, drains
Stainless steel	Monofilament	Fascia, sternum

*When suture looses approximately 50% strength.
†Approximate.

17

347

- **Face:** 5-0 and 6-0 nylon or polypropylene where cosmetic concerns are important
- **Scalp:** 3-0 nylon or polypropylene
- **Trunk or extremities:** 4-0 or 5-0 nylon or polypropylene

Use 3-0 and 4-0 absorbable sutures such as Dexon or Vicryl to approximate deep tissues. Skin is usually best closed by using interrupted sutures placed with good approximation with a minimum amount of tension or by a running subcuticular suture. Tissue adhesives may be used selectively (see page 358). Suture patterns are discussed in the next section. Suture marks ("tracks") are the result of excessive tension on the tissue or leaving the sutures in for too long. Thus, the length of time and the technique used are probably more important in determining the final result than is the suture used in most cases.

1. Remove all foreign materials and devitalized tissues by sharp excision (debridement). Clean the wound with plain saline (antiseptic solutions used on wound cleansing should be discouraged because they can be toxic to viable cells). A useful technique involves irrigation with at least 200 mL of saline through a 35-mL syringe and a 19-gauge needle. Anesthesia may be necessary before any of this is done. If all the debris is not removed, traumatic "tattooing" of the skin may result.
2. In general, do not suture infected or contaminated wounds, lacerations more than 6–12 h old (24 h on the face), missile wounds, and human or animal bites without surgical consultation.
3. Anesthetize the wound by infiltrating it with an agent such as 0.5% or 1% lidocaine (Xylocaine). The maximum safe dosage is 4.5 mg/kg (about 28 mL of a 1% solution in an adult). Lidocaine and the other local anesthetic agents are available with epinephrine (1:100,000 or 1:200,000) added to produce local vasoconstriction that prolongs the anesthetic effect and helps decrease systemic side effects and bleeding. Epinephrine should be used with caution, particularly in patients with a history of hypertension, and should not be used on the digits, toes, or penis. 1 mL of 1:10 $NaHCO_3$ can be mixed with 9 mL of lidocaine to help minimize the discomfort of the injection. Commonly used local anesthetics are compared in Table 17–2.
4. When using local anesthetics, always aspirate before injecting to prevent intravascular injection of the drug. Anesthetize with a 26–30-gauge needle. Symptoms of toxicity from local anesthetics includes twitching, restlessness, drowsiness, light-headedness, and seizures.
5. Close the wound using one of the suturing patterns discussed in the next section. Use fine-toothed forceps (Adson or Brown-Adson) with gentle pressure to handle skin edges to decrease trauma. The toothed forceps are less traumatic to the skin than other forceps with flat surfaces that may crush the tissue.
6. Cover the wound and keep it dry for at least 24–48 h. Dry gauze or Steri-Strips are sufficient. On the face, simply covering with antibiotic ointment is often used, especially around the eyes or mouth. After that, the patient may shower and wet the wound. This will not increase the risk of infection.
7. Finally, keep tetanus and antibacterial prophylaxis in mind, particularly for contaminated wounds (Table 17–3, page 350).

SUTURING PATTERNS

Opinions vary greatly on the ideal technique for skin closure. The following are the common techniques used for approximation of skin. Critical to any suturing technique is making certain that the edges of the wound closely approximate without overlapping or inversion and that there is no tension. Remember "approximation without strangulation" or eversion

TABLE 17-2
Local Anesthetic Comparison Chart for Commonly Used Injectable Agents

Agent	Proprietary Names	Onset	Duration	Maximum Dose	
				mg/kg	Volume in 70-kg Adult*
Bupivacaine	Marcaine, Sensoricaine	7–30 min	5–7 h	3	70 mL of 0.25% solution
Lidocaine	Xylocaine, Anestacon	5–30 min	2 h	4	28 mL of 1% solution
Lidocaine with epinephrine (1:200,000)		5–30 min	2–3 h	7	50 mL of 1% solution
Mepivacaine	Carbocaine	5–30 min	2–3 h	7	50 mL of 1% solution
Procaine	Novocaine	Rapid	30 min–1 h	10–15	70–105 mL of 1% solution

*To calculate the maximum dose if the patient is not a 70-kg adult, use the fact that a 1% solution has 10 mg of drug per milliliter.

17

TABLE 17–3
Tetanus Prophylaxis

History of Absorbed Tetanus Toxoid Immunization	Clean, Minor Wounds		All Other Wounds*	
	Td[†]	TIG[‡]	Td[†]	TIG[‡]
Unknown or <3 doses	Yes	No	Yes	Yes
<3 doses[§]	No**	No	No[††]	No

*Such as, but not limited to, wounds contaminated with dirt, feces, soil, saliva, etc; puncture wounds; avulsions; and wounds resulting from missiles, crushing, burns, and frostbite.
[†]Td = tetanus-diphtheria toxoid (adult type), 0.5 mL IM.
• For children <7 y of age, DPT (DT, if pertussis vaccine is contraindicated) is preferred to tetanus toxoid alone.
• For persons >7 years of age, Td is preferred to tetanus toxoid alone.
• DT = diphtheria-tetanus toxoid (pediatric), used for those who cannot receive pertussis.
[‡]TIG = tetanus immune globulin, 250 U IM.
[§]If only three doses of fluid toxoid have been received, then a fourth dose of toxoid, preferably an absorbed toxoid, should be given.
**Yes, if >10 y since last dose.
[††]Yes, if >5 y since last dose.
Source: Based on guidelines from the Centers for Disease Control and reported in *MMWR.*

of the skin edges gives the best results (Figure 17–1). Figures 17–2 through 17–6 illustrate the commonly used suturing patterns. These include the simple interrupted suture (Fig. 17–2), running (locked or unlocked) suture (Fig. 17–3), vertical mattress suture (Fig. 17–4), horizontal mattress suture (Fig. 17–5), and subcuticular suture (Fig. 17–6).

SURGICAL KNOTS

There are two basic knot-tying techniques: the handed tie and the instrument tie. The two-handed tie is easier to learn than the one-handed tie, although one-handed ties may be more useful in certain situations (eg, with deep cavities or where speed is essential). Some programs frown on one-handed tying, especially for physicians early in their careers. Instrument ties are more useful for closing skin and for emergency room laceration repair. Figures 17–7, page 355, and 17–8, page 356, show the technique for tying a two-handed square knot. This is the standard surgical knot that should be learned first. Figure 17–9, page 357, shows the technique for an instrument tie.

SUTURE REMOVAL

The longer that suture material is left in place, the more scarring it will produce. Using a topical antibiotic (Polysporin, others) ointment on the wound is helpful in decreasing suture tract epithelialization. This epithelialization results from crusting around the suture that increases suture marks and subsequent scarring. Sutures can be safely removed when a wound has developed sufficient tensile strength. Situations vary greatly, but general guidelines for

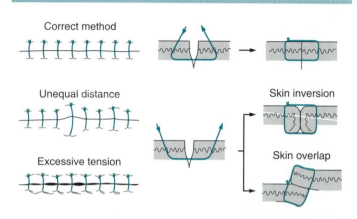

FIGURE 17-1 Proper method for simple interrupted suturing of a skin wound compared with incorrect techniques that result in poor scars from skin overlap, skin inversion, or necrosis of the skin edges because of excessive tension. (Reprinted, with permission from: Stillman RM [ed]: *Surgery: Diagnosis and Therapy*, Appleton & Lange, Stamford CT, 1989.)

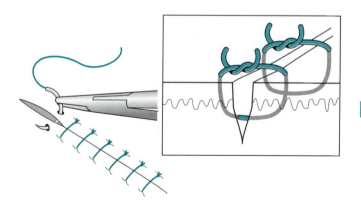

FIGURE 17-2 Simple interrupted suture. "Bites" are taken through the thickness of the skin, and the width of each stitch should equal the distance between sutures to avoid inverting the skin edges.

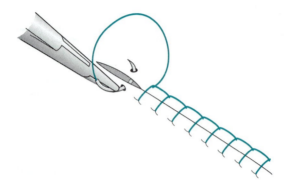

FIGURE 17-3 Continuous running suture. It allows rapid closure, but depends on only two knots for security and may not allow precise approximation of the skin edges. "Locking" each stitch, as shown, may increase scarring.

17

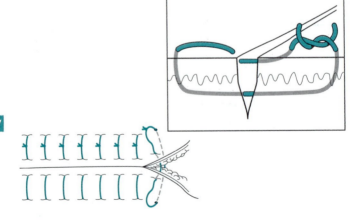

FIGURE 17-4 Vertical interrupted mattress suture. It allows precise approximation of the skin edges with little tension, but may result in more scarring than a simple stitch. The needle is placed in the skin in a "far, far, near, near" sequence.

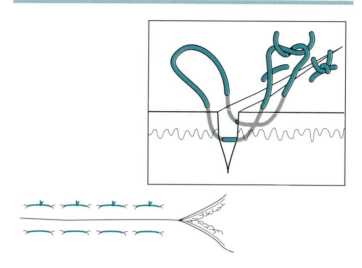

FIGURE 17–5 Horizontal interrupted mattress suture. This is an everting stitch that is more frequently used in fascia than in skin. It is often used in calloused skin such as the palms and soles.

removing sutures from different areas of the body are: face and neck, 3–5 d; scalp and body, 5–7 d; and extremities, 7–12 d. Any suture material or skin clips can be removed earlier if they have been reinforced with a deep absorbable suture or with the application of Steri-Strips after the suture is removed. Steri-Strips will stay in place more securely if tincture of benzoin (spray or solution) is applied to the skin and allowed to dry before the Steri-Strips are applied. The length of time absorbable sutures remain in tissues is shown in Table 17–1.

Suture Removal Procedure

1. Gently clear away any dried blood with saline and gauze. Verify that the wound is sufficiently healed to allow suture removal. Use a forceps to gently elevate the knot off the skin. This can be uncomfortable for the patient.
2. Cut the suture as close to the skin as possible so that a minimal amount of "dirty suture" is dragged through the wound. When removing continuous sutures, cut and pull out each section individually. Never pull a knot through the skin.
3. The use of skin staples is commonplace in the operating room because of the rapidity of closure and the nonreactive nature of the steel staples. These are typically removed 3–5 d after surgery (abdominal incisions) as shown in Figure 17–10. Because these are removed fairly quickly, reinforce the incision with Steri-Strips. When removing skin staples, make sure that the staple is completely reformed (see Figure 17–10) before removal to decrease patient discomfort.

17

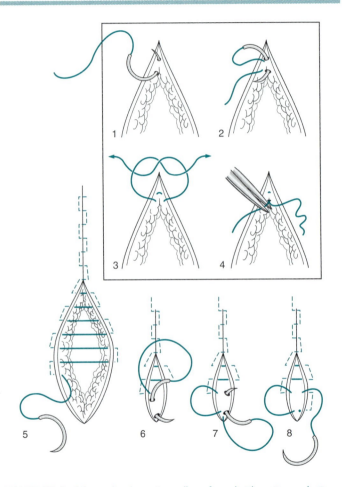

FIGURE 17–6 Subcuticular closure is usually performed with continuous, horizontally applied intradermal sutures. These are ideal for linear cosmetic closures because they eliminate possible cross-hatching deformities. If nonabsorbable suture material (eg, 5-0 or 6-0 Prolene) is used, the knot is placed on the skin and pulled taut. If absorbable (5-0 or 6-0 Dexon or Vicryl) is used, the knot is usually buried as shown. (Reprinted, with permission from: Stillman RM [ed]: *Surgery: Diagnosis and Therapy,* Appleton & Lange, Stamford CT, 1989.)

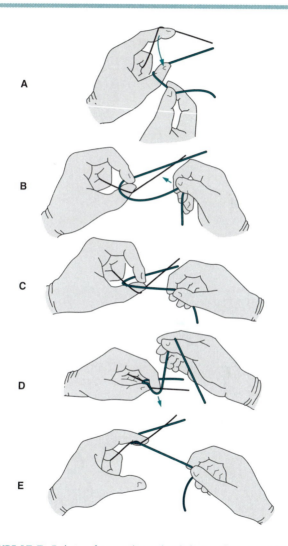

A

B

C

D

E

FIGURE 17–7 Technique for tying the two-handed square knot. Suture ends are uncrossed as step A begins (continued in Figure 17–8).

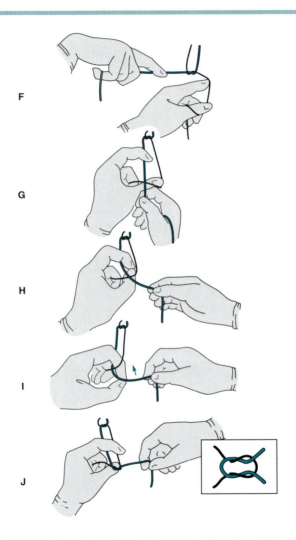

F

G

H

I

J

FIGURE 17-8 The two-handed square knot (continued from Figure 17–7). Hands must be crossed at the end of the first loop tie (step F) to give a flat knot; hands are not crossed at the end of the second loop tie (step J).

17

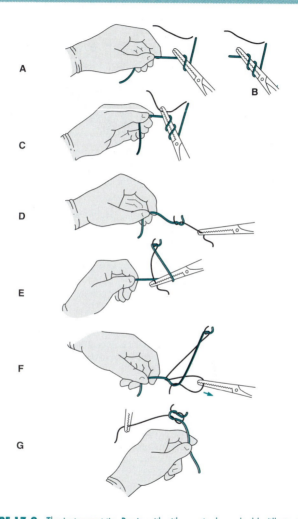

FIGURE 17-9   The instrument tie. Begin with either a single or double (illustrated) looping of the lower end of the suture around the needle holder. The first loop is laid flat without crossing the hands. Hands must be crossed after the second loop tie (step G) to produce a flat square knot.

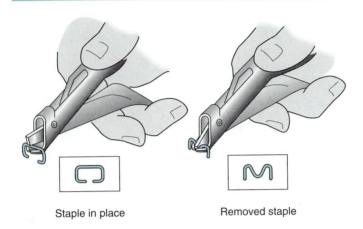

Staple in place   Removed staple

FIGURE 17–10   Removal of skin staples. The staple removal instrument is passed beneath the staple and completely closed. Be sure that the staple is completely "reformed" before removal to decrease patient discomfort. (Courtesy of Ethicon, Inc.)

TISSUE ADHESIVES

Octyl cyanoacrylate (Dermabond) is a topical skin adhesive (very similar to cyanoacrylate glue) that holds wound edges together. It is useful in wounds that are clean and easily opposed and for young children, for whom suture removal may be a problem. The wound should be nonmucosal on the face, torso, or extremity. It is recommended for wounds <8 cm with minimal tension (skin gap should be <0.5 cm). It is also useful for stabilizing wounds if the sutures were removed very early in order to minimize suture marks. It should not be used for puncture wounds, bites or wounds that need debridement, or in regions subjected to frequent movement (ie, hand or finger).

Gently approximate the wound edges with fingers or a forceps and place a small coating of the glue directly on the wound. After 2–3 min (after the glue has dried), an additional one or two coats may be applied. The glue will spontaneously separate in approximately 5–10 d. Once the glue is in place and stable, it is not necessary to use any topical medication or ointment. The patient may shower for brief periods. If the adhesive is too tacky, too much glue has been applied.

17

RESPIRATORY CARE

Respiratory Therapy
Pulmonary Function Tests
Differential Diagnosis of PFTs
Oxygen and Humidity Supplements

Bronchopulmonary Hygiene
Topical Medications
Metered-Dose Inhalers

RESPIRATORY THERAPY

Respiratory therapy is a vital component of health care. The objective is the treatment and care of all types of patients with cardiopulmonary diseases. Functions of the respiratory therapist include emergency care, ventilatory support, airway management, oxygen therapy, humidity and aerosol therapies, chest physiotherapy, physiologic monitoring, and pulmonary diagnostics.

PULMONARY FUNCTION TESTS

PFTs are useful in diagnosing a variety of pulmonary disorders. Common PFTs include spirometry, lung volume determinations, and diffusing capacity. Important measures include the FVC and the FEV_1. Spirometry may identify obstructive airway diseases such as asthma or emphysema when the ratio of FEV_1/FVC is less than 70%, or restrictive lung diseases such as sarcoidosis or ankylosing spondylitis when both the FVC and FEV_1 are reduced. Spirometry may also be an important part of a preoperative evaluation. Spirograms can be obtained before and after the administration of bronchodilators if they are not contraindicated (ie, history of intolerance). Bronchodilator responsiveness will help in predicting the response to treatment and in identifying asthma.

Lung volumes commonly determined by helium dilution must be ordered to definitively diagnose restrictive lung disease. This is usually indicated by TLC less than 80% of predicted normal. Diffusion capacity is important in the diagnosis of interstitial lung disease or pulmonary vascular disease, where it is reduced. It is also frequently followed to determine the response to therapy in interstitial diseases.

Obstructive pulmonary diseases include asthma, chronic bronchitis, emphysema, bronchiectasis, and lower airway obstruction. Restrictive pulmonary disease includes interstitial pulmonary diseases, diseases of the chest wall, and neuromuscular disorders. Interstitial disease may be due to inflammatory conditions [usual interstitial pneumonitis (UIP)], inhalation of organic dusts (hypersensitivity pneumonitis), inhalation of inorganic dusts (asbestosis), or systemic disorders with lung involvement (sarcoidosis).

Normal PFT values vary with age, sex, race, and body size. Normal values for a given patient are established from studies of normal populations and are provided along with the results. Arterial blood gases should be included in all PFTs.

Typical volumes and capacities are illustrated in Figure 18–1.

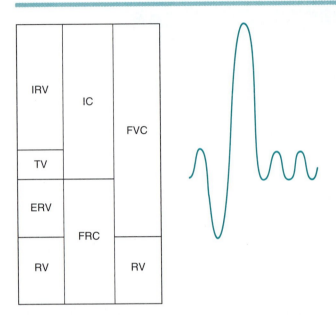

FVC = Forced vital capacity
 RV = residual volume
FRC = functional residual capacity
 TV = tidal volume

ERV = expiratory reserve volume
IRV = inspiratory reserve volume
 IC = inspiratory capacity

FIGURE 18–1   Lung volumes in the interpretation of pulmonary function tests.

Tidal Volume (TV):   Volume of air moved during a normal breath on quiet respiration

Forced Vital Capacity (FVC):   Maximum volume of air that can be forcibly expired after full inspiration

Functional Residual Capacity (FRC):   Volume of air in the lungs after a normal tidal expiration (FRC = reserve volume + expiratory reserve volume)

Total Lung Capacity (TLC):   Volume of air in the lungs after maximal inspiration

Forced Expired Volume in 1 Second (FEV$_1$):   Measured after maximum inspiration, the volume of air that can be expelled in 1 s

Vital Capacity (VC):   Maximum volume of air that can be exhaled from the lungs after a maximal inspiration

Residual Volume (RV):   The volume of air remaining in the lungs at the end of a maximal exhalation

DIFFERENTIAL DIAGNOSIS OF PFTS

Table 18–1 shows the differential diagnosis of various PFT patterns. When interpreting PFTs, remember that some patients may have combined restrictive and obstructive diseases such as emphysema and asbestosis.

OXYGEN AND HUMIDITY SUPPLEMENTS

Table 18–2 describes various methods of oxygen and humidity supplementation.

TABLE 18–1
Differential Diagnosis of Pulmonary Function Tests

Test	Restrictive Disease	Obstructive Disease
FVC	↓	N or ↓
TLC	↓	↑
FEV$_1$/FVC	N or ↑	↓
FEV$_1$	↓	↓

OBSTRUCTIVE AIRWAYS DISEASE (COPD)

Test	Normal	Mild	Moderate	Severe
FEV$_1$ (% of VC)	>75	60–75	40–60	<40
RV (% of predicted)	80–120	120–150	150–175	>200

RESTRICTIVE LUNG DISEASE

Test	Normal	Mild–Moderate	Severe	
FVC (% of predicted)	>80	60–80	50–60	<50
FEV$_1$ (% of VC)	>75	>75	>75	>75
RV (% of predicted)	80–120	80–120	70–80	70

Abbreviations: N = normal; ↑ = increased, ↓ = decreased; FVC = forced vital capacity; TLC = total lung capacity; RV/FRC = residual volume/functional residual capacity; FEV$_1$ = forced expiratory volume in 1s; VC = vital capacity.

18

TABLE 18–2
Various Methods of Oxygen and Humidity Supplementation

Device	O_2 Range	L/min	F_iO_2	Uses
Nasal cannula	Low	1–6	0.24–0.5	COPD, general oxygen needs
Simple face mask	Medium	6–8	0.5–0.6	General oxygen needs
Partial rebreathing face mask	High	8–12	0.6–0.7	High oxygen emergency needs
Nonrebreathing face mask	High	8–12	0.7–0.95	High oxygen emergency needs
Venturi mask	Low–medium	—	0.24–0.50	COPD (can specify exact F_iO_2)

Note: F_iO_2 may vary with fluctuations in the patient's minute ventilation when using a nasal cannula. This is not true when using the Venturi mask because it is a "high-flow oxygen enrichment system" that supplies three times the patient's minute ventilation, thus providing an exact F_iO_2.
Abbreviation: COPD = chronic obstructive pulmonary disease.

Humidity Therapy

Humidity generators are divided into humidifiers and nebulizers. Patients with intact upper airways do not need as high a percentage of relative humidity (% RH) as do patients with artificial airways (endotracheal tubes or tracheostomy tubes). Artificial airways require higher humidity to prevent secretions from obstructing the tubes. To bring the % RH of the inspired gas up to room humidity (30–40% RH) when using the nasal cannula, simple oxygen mask, partial rebreathing mask, or nonrebreathing mask, the bubble-diffuser humidifier is the device of choice.

To provide medium to high levels of % RH, aerosol devices such as the face tent, aerosol mask, aerosol T piece, and aerosol collar are the devices of choice. The humidity generator for these devices is the aerosol-jet nebulizer, which can provide cool or heated mist. The gas that powers the nebulizer may be blended to any desired inspired oxygen concentration (F_iO_2).

BRONCHOPULMONARY HYGIENE

The following is a listing of the modalities available through the respiratory care or nursing services of most hospitals. All are designed to help patients with their bronchopulmonary hygiene, more commonly referred to as "pulmonary toilet." Bronchopulmonary hygiene is defined as maintenance of clear airways and removal of secretions from the tracheobronchial tree. This is important for routine postoperative surgical patients, medical patients with obstructive pulmonary diseases, or any patient with excessive respiratory secretions.

Aerosol (Nebulizer) Therapy

Aerosolized medications such as bronchodilators and mucolytic agents can be delivered via nebulizer for spontaneously breathing, awake patients or intubated patients.

Indications

- Treatment of COPD, acute asthma, cystic fibrosis, and bronchiectasis
- Help in inducing sputum for diagnostic tests

Goals

- Relief of bronchospasm
- Help in decreasing the viscosity and in clearing of secretions

To Order: Specify the following:

- Frequency
- Heated or cool mist
- Medications: In sterile water or NS
- F_iO_2
- *Example.* Albuterol 2.5 mg in 3 mL of sterile saline, F_iO_2 0.28.

Chest Physiotherapy

This technique uses P&PD along with coughing and deep breathing exercises (TC&DB). P&PD is performed by positioning the patient so that the involved lobes of the lung are placed in a dependent drainage position and then using a cupped hand or vibrator to percuss the chest wall. Nasotracheal suctioning is quite uncomfortable for the patient but is still useful in the appropriate clinical setting in the absence of significant coagulopathy.

Indication

- Treatment of pneumonia, atelectasis, and diseases resulting in weak or ineffective coughing

To Order

1. **P&PD:** Specify the following:
   - Frequency
   - Segments or lobes involved (RUL, etc)
   - Duration
   - Drainage only
2. **TC&DB:** Ordered on a timed schedule or as needed
   - *Example.* P&PD qid of RUL and RML 5 min/lobe or TC&DB q4h.

Incentive Spirometry

This method encourages patients to make a maximal and sustained inspiratory effort to help reinflate the lungs or prevent atelectasis.

Indications

- Treatment of patients at risk for developing postoperative pulmonary complications
- Treatment and prevention of atelectasis, especially in postoperative setting

Goals

Set for the patient depending on the device available:

- Lighting lights
- Moving Ping-Pong balls
- Moving colored fluids in "blow bottles"

To Order

Specify the following:

- Frequency (such as 10 min q1–2h while awake)
- Device (if you have a preference)

Example. Incentive spirometry 10 min every hour with blow bottle.

TOPICAL MEDICATIONS

The following agents can be added to aerosol therapy to prevent or treat pulmonary complications caused by bronchoconstriction, mucosal congestion, or inspissated secretions. Remember, even though these are primarily topical agents, some systemic absorption can often occur.

Acetylcysteine (Mucomyst): A mucolytic agent useful for treating retained mucoid secretions; inspissated secretions; and impacted mucoid plugs seen in diseases such as COPD, cystic fibrosis, and pneumonia. A bronchodilator should be given along with Mucomyst.

Usual Adult Dosage. 1–3 mL of 20% acetylcysteine in 0.5 mL (2–10 mg) of Bronkosol

Albuterol (Ventolin, Proventil): A short-acting selective bronchodilator with principally beta-2 activity; can cause tachycardia. Onset 15 min. Peak effect at 0.5–1 h, duration 3–5 h

Usual Dosage. 2.5 mg in 3 mL NS q4h

Metaproterenol (Alupent, Metaprel): A short-acting bronchodilator with both beta-1 and beta-2 activity; can cause tachycardia. Peak effect at 0.5–1 h, duration 3–5 h.

Usual Dosage. 0.3 mL (10–15 mg) of a 5% solution in 2.5 mL NS bid–qid

Racemic Epinephrine: Contains both d and l forms of epinephrine. Useful because the alpha effects result in mucosal vasoconstriction that reduces mucosal engorgement and the bronchodilation lessens the risk of hypoxemia. Most useful for laryngotracheobronchitis and immediately after extubation in children.

Usual Dosage. 0.125–0.5 mL (3–10 mg) in 2.5 mL NS

Ipratropium Bromide (Atrovent): A parasympatholytic bronchodilating agent that causes bronchodilation and a decrease in secretions with "drying" of the respiratory mucosa. This is minimally absorbed and rarely results in tachycardia. Onset 45 min, duration 4–6 h

Usual Dosage. 0.5 mg in 3 mL NS qid

Atropine: A parasympatholytic agent that causes bronchodilation and a decrease in secretions with "drying" of the respiratory mucosa. This is readily absorbed and, therefore has cardiac effects (tachycardia).

Usual Dosage. 0.025–0.05 mg/kg of a 1% solution

18

METERED-DOSE INHALERS

All bronchodilating agents can be effectively delivered by metered-dose inhaler as long as proper technique is used. For these devices to be successful, in-patients must be well trained or have the assistance of a nurse or respiratory therapist. Albuterol and ipratropium bromide (Atrovent) can each be delivered two puffs q4h. A combination bronchodilator (Combivent) containing the equivalent of one puff of each is also available and provides synergistic bronchodilatation.

19

BASIC ECG READING

Introduction
Basic Information
Axis Deviation
Heart Rate
Rhythm

Cardiac Hypertrophy
Myocardial Infarction
Electrolyte and Drug Effects
Miscellaneous ECG Changes

INTRODUCTION

The formal procedure for obtaining a readable ECG is given in Chapter 13, page 266. Every electrocardiogram should be approached in a systematic, stepwise fashion. Many automated ECG machines can give a preliminary interpretation of a tracing; however, all automated interpretations require analysis and sign-off by a physician. Determine each of the following:

- **Standardization.** With the ECG machine set on 1 mV, a 10-mm standardization mark (0.1 mV/mm) is evident (Figure 19–1).
- **Axis.** If the QRS is upright (more positive than negative) in leads I and aVF, the axis is normal. The normal axis range is –30 degrees to +105 degrees.
- **Intervals.** Determine the PR, QRS, and QT intervals (Figure 19–2). Intervals are measured in the limb leads. The PR should be 0.12–0.20 s, and the QRS, <0.12 s. The QT interval increases with decreasing heart rate, usually <0.44 s. The QT interval usually does not exceed one half of the RR interval (the distance between two R waves).
- **Rate.** Count the number of QRS cycles in a 6-s strip and multiply it by 10 to roughly estimate the rate. If the rhythm is regular you can be more exact in determining the rate by dividing 300 by the number of 0.20-s intervals (usually depicted by darker shading) and then extrapolating for any fraction of a 0.20-s segment.
- **Rhythm.** Determine whether each QRS is preceded by a P wave, look for variation in the PR interval and RR interval (the duration between two QRS cycles), and look for ectopic beats.
- **Hypertrophy.** One way to determine LVH is to calculate the sum of the S wave in V_1 or V_2 plus the R wave in V_5 or V_6. A sum >35 indicates LVH. Some other criteria for LVH are R >11 mm in aVL or R in I + S in aVF >25 mm.
- **Infarction or Ischemia.** Check for the presence of ST-segment elevation or depression, Q waves, inverted T waves, and poor R-wave progression in the precordial leads.

A more detailed discussion of each of these categories is presented in the following sections.

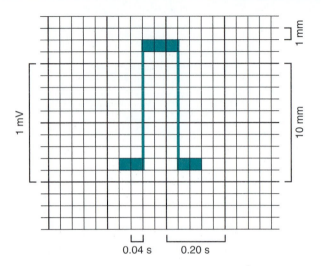

FIGURE 19–1 Examples of a 10-mm standardization mark and time marks and standard electrocardiogram paper running at 25 mm/s.

BASIC INFORMATION

Equipment

Bipolar Leads

- Lead I: Left arm to right arm
- Lead II: Left leg to right arm
- Lead III: Left leg to left arm

Precordial Leads: V_1 to V_6 across the chest, as shown in the section on electrocardiograms in Chapter 13 (see Figure 13–9, page 267).

ECG Paper: With the ECG machine set at 25 mm/s, each small box represents 0.04 s and each large box 0.2 s (see Figure 19–1, above). Most ECG machines automatically print a standardization mark.

Normal ECG Complex

Note: A small amplitude in the Q, R, or S wave is represented by a lowercase letter; a large amplitude by an uppercase letter. The pattern shown in Figure 19–2 could also be noted as qRs.

- **P Wave.** Caused by depolarization of the atria. With normal sinus rhythm, the P wave is upright in leads I, II, aVF, V_4, V_5, and V_6 and inverted in aVR.

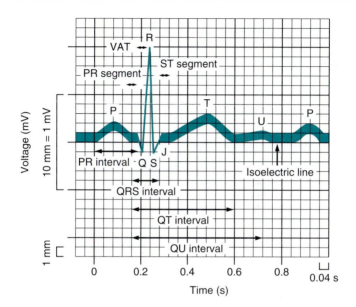

FIGURE 19–2 Diagram of the electrocardiographic complexes, intervals, and segments. The U wave is normally not well seen. (Reprinted, with permission, from: Goldman MJ [ed]: *Principles of Clinical Electrocardiography*, 12th ed. Lange Medical Publications, Los Altos CA, 1986.)

- **QRS Complex.** Represents ventricular depolarization
- **Q Wave.** The first negative deflection of the QRS complex (not always present and, if present, may be pathologic)
- **R Wave.** The first positive deflection (R) is the positive deflection that sometimes occurs after the S wave)
- **S Wave.** The negative deflection following the R wave
- **T Wave.** Caused by repolarization of the ventricles and follows the QRS complex. Normally upright in leads I, II, V_3, V_4, V_5, and V_6 and inverted in aVR

AXIS DEVIATION

The term *axis,* which represents the sum of the vectors of the electrical depolarization of the ventricles, gives some idea of the electrical orientation of the heart in the body. In a healthy person, the axis is downward and to the left, as shown in Figure 19–3.

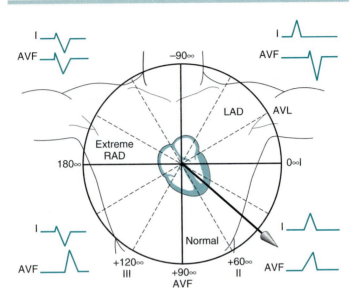

FIGURE 19–3 Graphic representation of the "axis deviation." Electrocardiographic representations of each type of axis are shown in each quadrant. The large arrow is the normal axis.

The QRS axis is midway between two leads that have QRS complexes of equal amplitude, or the axis is 90 degrees to the lead in which the QRS is isoelectric, that is, the amplitude of the R wave equals the amplitude of the S wave.

- **Normal Axis.** QRS positive in I and aVF (0–90 degrees). Normal axis is actually –30 to 105 degrees
- **LAD.** QRS positive in I and negative in aVF, –30 to –90 degrees
- **RAD.** QRS negative in I and positive in aVF, +105 to +180 degrees
- **Extreme Right Axis Deviation.** QRS negative in I and negative in aVF, +180 to +270 or –90 to –180 degrees

Clinical Correlations

- **RAD.** Seen with RVH, RBBB, COPD, and acute PE (a sudden change in axis toward the right), as well as in healthy individuals (occasionally)
- **LAD.** Seen with LVH, LAHB (–45 to –90 degrees), LBBB, and in some healthy individuals

HEART RATE

Bradycardia: Heart rate <60 bpm

Tachycardia: Heart rate >100 bpm

Rate Determination: Figure 19–4.

- **Method 1.** Note the 3-s marks along the top or bottom of the ECG paper (15 large squares). The approximate rate equals the number of cycles (ie, QRSs) in a 6-s strip × 10.
- **Method 2.** (for regular rhythms). Count the number of large squares (0.2-s boxes) between two successive cycles. The rate is equal to 300 divided by the number of squares. Extrapolate if the QRS complex does not fall exactly on the 0.2-s marks (eg, if each QRS complex is separated by 2.4 0.20-s segments, the rate is 120 bpm. The rate between two 0.20-s segments is 150 bpm, and between three 0.20-s segments is 100 bpm.

RHYTHM

Sinus Rhythms

Normal: Each QRS preceded by a P wave (which is positive in II and negative in aVR) with a regular PR and RR interval and a rate between 60 and 100 bpm (Figure 19–5)

Sinus Tachycardia: Normal sinus rhythm with a heart rate >100 bpm and <180 bpm (Figure 19–6)

Clinical Correlations. Anxiety, exertion, pain, fever, hypoxia, hypotension, increased sympathetic tone (secondary to drugs with adrenergic effects [eg, epinephrine]), anticholinergic effect (eg, atropine), PE, COPD, AMI, CHF, hyperthyroidism, and others

Sinus Bradycardia: Normal sinus rhythm with a heart rate <60 bpm (Figure 19–7)

Clinical Correlations. Well-trained athlete, normal variant, secondary to medications (eg, beta-blockers, digitalis, clonidine), hypothyroidism, hypothermia, sick sinus syndrome (tachy–brady syndrome), and others

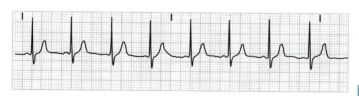

19

FIGURE 19–4   Sample strip for rapid rate determination (see text for procedure). Estimating the rate by counting the number of beats (eight) in the two 3-s intervals. The rate is 8 × 10, or 80 bpm (method 1). Using method 2, each beat is separated from another beat by four 0.20-s intervals, so you divide 300 by 4, and the rate is 75 bpm. Because the beats are separated by exactly four beats, you do not need to extrapolate.

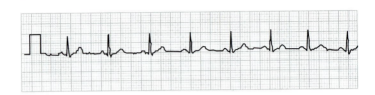

FIGURE 19–5   Normal sinus rhythm.

Treatment

- If asymptomatic (good urine output, adequate BP, and normal sensorium), no therapy needed.
- If hypotensive or disoriented: See Chapter 21, page 460

Sinus Arrhythmia: Normal sinus rhythm with a somewhat irregular heart rate. Inspiration causes a slight increase in rate; expiration decreases the rate. Normal variation between inspiration and expiration is 10% or less.

Atrial Arrhythmias

PAC: Ectopic atrial focus firing prematurely followed by a normal QRS (Figure 19–8). The compensatory pause following the PAC is partial; the RR interval between beats 4 and 6 is less than between beats 1 and 3 or 6 and 8.

    Clinical Correlations. Usually not of clinical significance; can be caused by stress, caffeine, and myocardial disease

PAT: A run of three or more consecutive PACs. The heart rate is usually between 140 and 250 bpm. The P wave may not be visible, but the RR interval is very regular (Figure 19–9).

    Clinical Correlations. Can be seen in healthy individuals but also occurs with a variety of heart diseases. Symptoms include palpitations, light-headedness, and syncope.

    Treatment

- **Increase Vagal Tone.** Valsalva maneuver or carotid massage

19

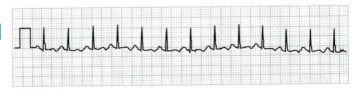

FIGURE 19–6   Sinus tachycardia. The rate is 120–130 bpm.

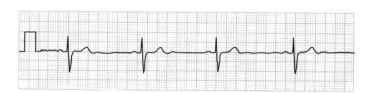

FIGURE 19–7   Sinus bradycardia. The rate is approximately 38 bpm.

- **Medical Treatment.** Can include adenosine, verapamil, digoxin, edrophonium, or beta-blockers (propranolol, metoprolol, and esmolol). Verapamil and beta-blockers should be used cautiously at the same time because asystole can occur.
- **Cardioversion with Synchronized DC Shock.** Particularly in the hemodynamically unstable patient (see Chapter 21, page 467)

MAT: An atrial arrhythmia that originates from ectopic atrial foci. It is characterized by varying P-wave morphology and PR interval and is irregular (Figure 19–10).
   Clinical Correlations. Most commonly associated with COPD, also seen in elderly patients, CHF, diabetes, or use of theophylline. Antiarrhythmics are often ineffective. Treat the underlying cause.

AFib: Irregularly irregular rhythm with no discernible P waves. The ventricular rate usually varies between 100 and 180 bpm (Figure 19–11). The ventricular response is slower with digoxin, verapamil, or beta-blocker therapy and with AV nodal disease.
   Clinical Correlations. Seen in some healthy individuals but commonly associated with organic heart disease (CAD, hypertensive heart disease, or rheumatic mitral valve disease), thyrotoxicosis, alcohol abuse, pericarditis, PE, and postoperatively.
   Treatment

- **Pharmacologic Therapy.** Intravenous adenosine, verapamil, digoxin, and beta-blockers (propranolol, metoprolol, and esmolol) can be used to slow down the ventricular response, and quinidine, procainamide, propafenone, ibutilide, and

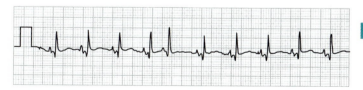

FIGURE 19–8   Premature atrial contraction (PAC). The fifth beat is a PAC.

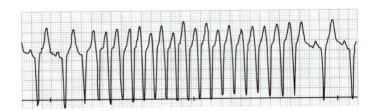

FIGURE 19–9 Paroxysmal atrial tachycardia.

amiodarone can be used to maintain or convert to sinus rhythm (see individual agents in Chapter 21)
- **DC-Synchronized Cardioversion.** Indicated if associated with increased myocardial ischemia, hypotension, or pulmonary edema (see Chapter 21, page 467)

Atrial Flutter: Characterized by sawtooth flutter waves with an atrial rate between 250 and 350 bpm; the rate may be regular or irregular depending on whether the atrial impulses are conducted through the AV node at a regular interval or at a variable interval (Figure 19–12).

Example: One ventricular contraction (QRS) for every two flutter waves = 2:1 flutter.

Clinical Correlations. Seen with valvular heart disease, pericarditis, ischemic heart disease, pulmonary disease including PE, and alcohol abuse

Treatment. Do **NOT** use quinidine or procainamide (atrial conduction may decrease to the point where 1:1 atrial:ventricular conduction can occur and the ventricular rate will increase and hemodynamic compromise can occur), otherwise, similar to treatment of atrial fibrillation. Ibutilide (a new Class III antiarrhythmic) is very effective.

Nodal Rhythm

AV Junctional or Nodal Rhythm: Rhythm originates in the AV node. Often associated with retrograde P waves that may precede or follow the QRS. If the P wave is present, it is negative in lead II and positive in aVR (just the opposite of normal sinus rhythm) (Fig-

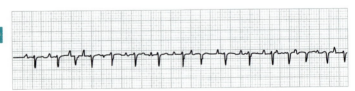

FIGURE 19–10 Multifocal atrial tachycardia.

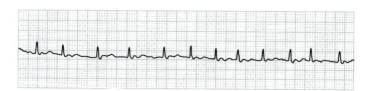

FIGURE 19–11   Atrial fibrillation.

ure 19–13). Three or more premature junctional beats in a row constitute a junctional tachy-cardia, which has the same clinical significance as PAT.

Ventricular Arrhythmias

PVC: As implied by the name, a premature beat arising in the ventricle. P waves may be present but have no relation to the QRS of the PVC. The QRS is usually >0.12 s with a left bundle branch pattern. A compensatory pause follows a PVC that is usually longer than after a PAC (Figure 19–14). The RR interval between beats 1 and 3 is equal to that between beats 3 and 5. Thus, the pause following the PVC (the fourth beat) is fully compensatory. The fol-lowing patterns are recognized:

- **Bigeminy.** One normal sinus beat followed by one PVC in an alternating fashion (Figure 19–15)
- **Trigeminy.** Sequence of two normal beats followed by one PVC
- **Unifocal PVCs.** Arise from one site in the ventricle. Each has the same configura-tion in a single lead. (See Figure 19–14.)
- **Multifocal PVCs.** Arise from different sites; therefore, have different shapes (Figure 19–16)

Clinical Correlations. PVCs occur in healthy persons and with excessive caffeine ingestion, anemia, anxiety, organic heart disease (ischemic, valvular, or hypertensive), secondary to medications (epinephrine and isoproterenol; from toxic level of digitalis and theophylline),

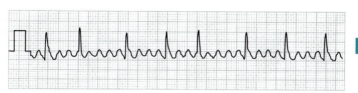

19

FIGURE 19–12   Atrial flutter with atrioventricular (AV) block (3:1 to 5:1 conduc-tion).

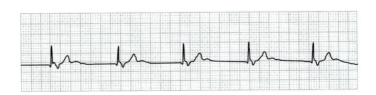

FIGURE 19–13 Junctional rhythm with retrograde P waves (inverted) following the QRS complex.

or predisposing metabolic abnormalities (hypoxia, hypokalemia, acidosis, alkalosis, or hypomagnesemia)

Criteria for Treatment. In the setting of an AMI:

- >5 PVCs in 1 min (many clinicians would treat any PVC associated with an MI or injury pattern on ECG)
- PVCs in couplets (two in a row)
- Numerous multifocal PVCs
- PVC that falls on the preceding T wave (R on T)

Treatment. See also Chapter 21, page 459.

- **Lidocaine.** Most commonly used; other antiarrhythmics include procainamide, and amiodarone.
- Treatment of aggravating cause often sufficient (eg, treat hypoxia, hypokalemia, or acidosis)

Ventricular Tachycardia: By definition, three or more PVCs in a row (Figure 19–17). Appears as a wide QRS usually with an LBBB pattern (as opposed to a narrow complex seen with supraventricular tachycardia). May occur as a short paroxysm or as a sustained run with a rate between 120 and 250 bpm. Can be life-threatening because of associated hypotension and has a tendency to degenerate into ventricular fibrillation. Treatment of nonsustained ventricular tachycardia is controversial.

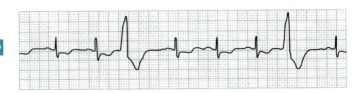

FIGURE 19–14 Premature ventricular contractions (PVCs). The fourth and eighth beats are PVCs.

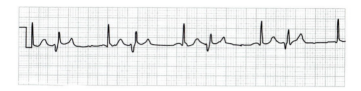

FIGURE 19–15 Ventricular bigeminy.

Clinical Correlations. See the section on PVCs. Patients with ventricular aneurysm are more susceptible to developing ventricular arrhythmias.

Treatment. See Chapter 21, page 459.

Ventricular Fibrillation: Erratic electrical activity from the ventricles, which fibrillate or twitch asynchronously. No cardiac output occurs with this rhythm (Figure 19–18).

Clinical Correlations. One of two patterns seen with cardiac arrest (the other would be asystole or flat line)

Treatment. See Chapter 21, page 252.

Heart Blocks

First-Degree Block: PR interval >0.2 s (or five small boxes). Usually not clinically significant (Figure 19–19). Drugs such as beta-blockers, digitalis, and calcium channel blockers (especially verapamil) can cause first-degree block.

Second-Degree Block

Mobitz Type I (Wenckebach). Progressive prolongation of the PR interval until the P wave is blocked and not followed by a QRS complex (Figure 19–20). May occur as a 2:1, 3:2, or 4:3 block. The ratio of the atrial:ventricular beats can vary. With a 4:3 block, every fourth P wave is not followed by a QRS.

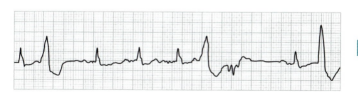

FIGURE 19–16 Multifocal PVCs. The second, sixth, seventh, and ninth beats are PVCs. Only the second and sixth PVCs have the same morphology.

19

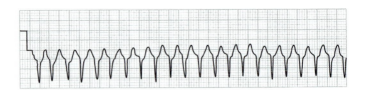

FIGURE 19–17   Ventricular tachycardia.

Clinical Correlations. Seen with acute myocardial ischemia such as inferior MI, ASDs, valvular heart disease, rheumatic fever, or digitalis or propranolol toxicity. Can be transient. May progress to bradycardia (rare)

Treatment. Usually expectant; if bradycardia occurs: atropine, isoproterenol, or a pacemaker

Mobitz Type II. A series of P waves with conducted QRS complexes followed by a nonconducted P wave. The PR interval for the conducted beats remains constant. May occur as a 2:1, 3:2, or 4:3 block. The ratio of the atrial:ventricular beats can vary. With a 4:3 block, every fourth P wave is not followed by a QRS. (*Note:* AV block that is 2:1 can be either Mobitz type I or type II and may be difficult to differentiate. In general, Mobitz I has a prolonged PR with a narrow QRS; Mobitz II has a normal PR interval with a bundle branch pattern [wide QRS]).

Clinical Correlations. Implies severe conduction system disease that can progress into complete heart block. May be seen in acute anterior MI and cardiomyopathy.

Treatment. Use of a temporary cardiac pacemaker, particularly when associated with an acute anterior MI

Third-Degree Block: Complete AV block with independent atrial and ventricular rates. The ventricular rate is usually 20–40 bpm (Figure 19–21).

Clinical Correlations. May occur as the result of degenerative changes in the conduction system in the elderly, from digitalis toxicity, transiently with an acute inferior MI (due

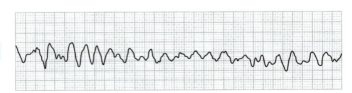

FIGURE 19–18   Ventricular fibrillation.

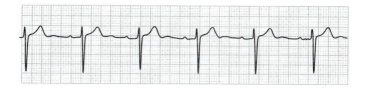

FIGURE 19–19   First-degree AV block. The PR interval is 0.26 s.

to temporary ischemia of the AV junction), and after acute anterior MI (much higher probability of mortality than after inferior MI); can result in syncope or CHF

   Treatment. Usually requires placement of a temporary or permanent pacemaker

BBB: Complete BBB is present when the QRS complex is >0.12 s (or three small boxes on the ECG strip). Look at leads I, V_1, and V_6. Degenerative changes and ischemic heart disease are the most common causes.

RBBB: The RSR′ pattern seen in V_1 and or V_2. Also a wide S in leads I and V_6 (Figure 19–22)

   Clinical Correlations. May be seen in healthy persons but usually associated with diseases affecting the right side of the heart (pulmonary hypertension, ASD, or ischemia); sudden onset is associated with pulmonary embolism or acute exacerbation of COPD.

LBBB: The RR′ in leads I and/or V_6. The QRS complex may actually be more slurred than double-peaked as in the RBBB. A wide S wave is seen in V_1 (Figure 19–23).

   Clinical Correlations. Associated with organic heart disease (hypertensive, valvular, and ischemic) as well as severe aortic stenosis. Development of a new LBBB after an AMI may be an indication for inserting a temporary cardiac pacemaker.

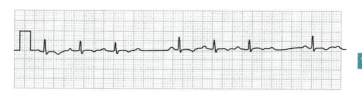

19

FIGURE 19–20   Second-degree AV block, Mobitz type I (Wenckebach), with 4:3 conduction.

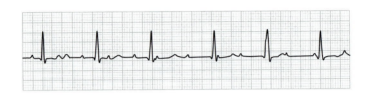

FIGURE 19–21 Third-degree AV block (complete heart block). The atrial rate is 100 bpm; the ventricular rate is 47 bpm.

CARDIAC HYPERTROPHY
Atrial Hypertrophy

Atrial Hypertrophy: P wave >2.5 mm in height and >0.12 s wide (three small boxes on the ECG paper)

RAE: Tall, slender, peaked P waves in leads II, III, aVF (may also be seen in V_1 and V_2. (Figure 19–24)
    Clinical Correlations. Seen with chronic diffuse pulmonary disease, pulmonary hypertension, and congenital heart disease (ASD)

LAE: Notched P wave ("P mitral pattern") seen in leads I and II. A wide (0.11 s or greater), slurred biphasic P in V_1 with a wider terminal than initial component (negative deflection) (Figure 19–25)
    Clinical Correlations. Seen with mitral stenosis or mitral regurgitation or secondary to LVH with hypertensive cardiovascular disease

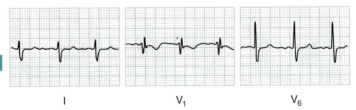

I V_1 V_6

FIGURE 19–22 Leads I, V_1, and V_6 demonstrate the right bundle branch block (RBBB) pattern.

19

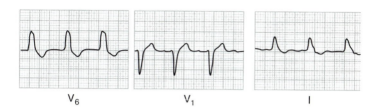

FIGURE 19–23 Leads I, V$_1$, and V$_6$ demonstrate the left bundle branch block (LBBB) pattern.

Ventricular Hypertrophy

RVH: Tall R wave in V$_1$ (R wave >S wave in V$_1$), persistent S waves in V$_5$ and V$_6$, progressively smaller R wave from V$_1$ to V$_6$, slightly widened QRS intervals (Figure 19–26), and strain pattern with ST-segment depression and T-wave inversion in V$_1$ to V$_3$. May also see a pattern of small R waves with relatively large S waves in V$_1$ to V$_6$. Invariably right axis deviation (>105 degrees) is present.

Clinical Correlations. Associated with mitral stenosis, chronic diffuse pulmonary disease, chronic recurrent PE, congenital heart disease (eg, tetralogy of Fallot), and biventricular hypertrophy (VH and RVH, with LVH findings often predominating).

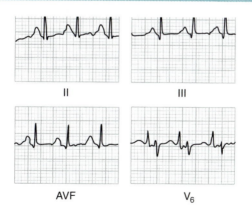

FIGURE 19–24 Right atrial enlargement, leads II, III, aVF, and V$_1$. Note the tall P waves in II, III, and aVF and the tall slender P waves in V$_1$.

19

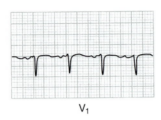

V_1

FIGURE 19–25 Left atrial enlargement.

LVH: Voltage criteria (patients >age 35): S in V_1 or V_2 plus an R in V_5 or V_6 >35 mm, or R wave in aVL >11 mm, or R wave in I plus S wave in III >25 mm, or an R in V_5 or V_6 >26 mm. The QRS complex may be >0.10 s wide in V_5 or V_6. ST-segment depression and T-wave inversion in the anterolateral leads (I, aVL, V_5, and V_6) suggest LVH with strain (Figure 19–27).

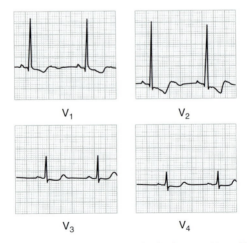

V_1 V_2

V_3 V_4

FIGURE 19–26 Right ventricular hypertrophy, leads V_1, V_2, V_3, and V_4. Note the tall R waves in V_1 and V_2, greater than the R waves in V_3 and V_4.

19

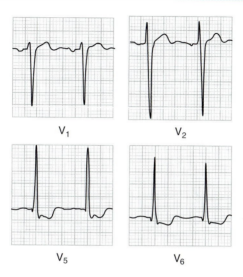

FIGURE 19–27   Left ventricular hypertrophy, leads V_1, V_2, V_5, and V_6. The S wave in the V_2 + R wave in V_5 is 55 mm. Note the ST changes and T-wave inversion in V_5 and V_6, suggesting "strain."

Clinical Correlations. Hypertension, aortic stenosis or insufficiency, long-standing CAD, and some forms of congenital heart disease

MYOCARDIAL INFARCTION

(See also Chapter 21, page 459.)

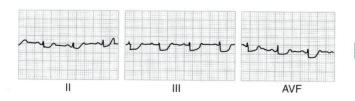

FIGURE 19–28   ST-segment depression in leads II, III, and aVF in a patient with acute inferior subendocardial ischemia/infarction.

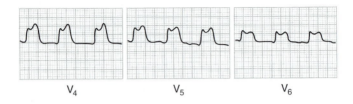

FIGURE 19–29　ST elevation in leads V_4, V_5, and V_6 in a patient with acute anterolateral transmural ischemia/infarction.

Myocardial Ischemia:　Inadequate oxygen supply to the myocardium because of blockage or spasm of the coronary arteries. The ECG can show ST-segment depression (subendocardial ischemia) (Figure 19–28), ST elevation (transmural ischemia) (Figure 19–29), or symmetrically inverted ("flipped") T waves (Figure 19–30) in the area of ischemia (eg, inferior ischemia in II, III, and F; anterior ischemia in V_1 to V_6; lateral ischemia in I, aVL; anterolateral ischemia in I, aVL, V_5, and V_6; anteroseptal ischemia in V_1, V_2, V_3, and V_4.

MI:　Refers to myocardial necrosis caused by severe ischemia. Can be transmural (ST elevation early, T-wave inversion, and Q waves late) or subendocardial (ST depression and T-wave inversion without evidence of Q waves). Table 19–1 outlines the localization of MIs.

- **Acute Injury Phase.** Hyperacute T waves, then ST-segment elevation. Hyperacute T waves return to normal in minutes to hours. ST elevation usually regresses after hours to days. Persistent ST elevation suggests a left ventricular aneurysm.
- **Evolving Phase.** Occurs hours to days after an MI. Deep T-wave inversion occurs and then replaces ST-segment elevation, and the T wave may return to normal.
- **Q Waves.** Occur hours to days after a transmural MI. A Q wave is the initial negative deflection of the QRS complex. A "significant" Q wave is 0.04 s in duration and >25% the height of the R wave (Figure 19–31). May regress to normal after years.

19

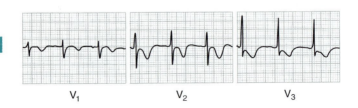

FIGURE 19–30　Inverted T waves.

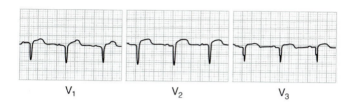

FIGURE 19-31   Q waves in leads V_1, V_2, and V_3 in a patient with an acute anteroseptal transmural myocardial infarction. Note the ST elevation in helping to determine the acute nature of the infarction.

ELECTROLYTE AND DRUG EFFECTS

Electrolytes

Hyperkalemia: Narrow, symmetrical, diffuse, peaked T waves. With severe hyperkalemia, PR prolongation occurs, the P wave flattens and is lost, and the QRS widens and can progress to ventricular fibrillation (Figure 19–32).

Hypokalemia: ST-segment depression with the appearance of U waves (a positive deflection after the T wave) (Figure 19–33)

TABLE 19–1
Localization of Transmural Myocardial Infarction on ECG

Location of MI	Presence of Q Wave or ST-Segment Elevation	Reciprocal ST Depression
Anterior	V_1 to V_6 (also poor R-wave progression in leads V_1 to V_6)*	II, III, aVF
Lateral	I, aVL, V_5, V_6	V_1, V_3
Inferior	II, III, aVF	I, aVL, possibly anterior leads
Posterior	Abnormally tall R and T waves in V_1 to V_3	V_1 to V_3
Subendocardial	No abnormal Q wave. ST-segment elevation in the anterior, lateral, or inferior leads	

*Normally in V_1 to V_6, the R-wave amplitude gradually increases and the S wave decreases with a "biphasic" QRS (R = S) in V_3 or V_4. With an anterior MI, there will be a loss of R-wave voltage and the biphasic QRS will appear more laterally in V_4 to V_6, hence the term *poor R-wave progression.*

19

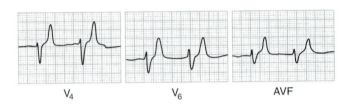

FIGURE 19–32   Diffuse tall T waves in leads V_4, V_6, and aVF with widened QRS and junctional rhythm (loss of P waves), representing hyperkalemia.

Hypercalcemia: Short QT interval

Hypocalcemia: Prolonged QT interval

Drugs

Digitalis Effect: Downsloping ST segment

Digitalis Toxicity

- **Arrhythmias.** PVCs, bigeminy, trigeminy, ventricular tachycardia, ventricular fibrillation, PAT, nodal rhythms, and sinus bradycardia.
- **Conduction Abnormalities.** First-degree, second-degree, and third-degree heart blocks

Quinidine and Procainamide: With toxic levels, prolonged QT, flattened T wave, and QRS widening

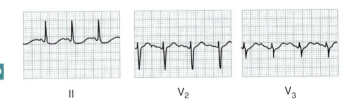

FIGURE 19–33   Leads II, V_2, and V_3 in a patient with hypokalemia. A U wave is easily seen in V_2 and V_3, but difficult to distinguish from the T wave in II.

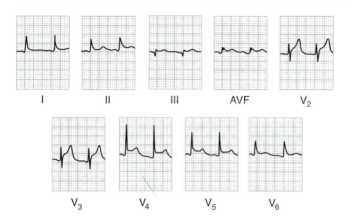

FIGURE 19–34   Acute pericarditis.

MISCELLANEOUS ECG CHANGES

Pericarditis: Diffuse ST elevation concave upward and/or diffuse PR depression and/or diffuse T-wave inversion (Figure 19–34)

   Clinical Correlations. Idiopathic, viral infections, as well as other infections, including bacterial, fungal, and TB, AMI, collagen–vascular diseases, uremia, cancer, Dressler's syndrome, and postpericardiotomy syndrome

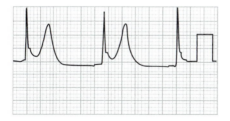

FIGURE 19–35   Sinus bradycardia, J-point elevation with ST-segment elevation and prolonged QT interval (0.56 s) in a patient with hypothermia.

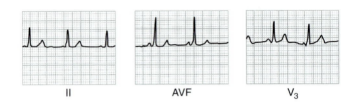

FIGURE 19–36 Short PR interval and delta waves in leads II, aVF, and V$_3$ in a patient with Wolff–Parkinson–White syndrome.

Hypothermia: Sinus bradycardia, AV junctional rhythm, or ventricular fibrillation common. Classically, J point (the end of the QRS complex and the beginning of the ST segment) elevated and an intraventricular conduction delay and a prolonged QT interval possible (Figure 19–35)

WPW Syndrome: A preexcitation syndrome caused by conduction from the SA node to the ventricle through an accessory pathway that bypasses the AV node. Classically, a short PR interval occurs along with a delta wave (a delay in the initial deflection of the QRS complex). Clinically, these patients commonly have tachyarrhythmias, such as atrial fibrillation (Figure 19–36).

CRITICAL CARE

Treatment of the Critically Ill Patient
ICU Progress Note
Cardiovascular System
Cardiovascular Physiology
Central Venous Pressure
Pulmonary Artery Catheters
Determinations of Cardiac Output
Shock States
Clinical Pulmonary Physiology

Indications for Intubation
Mechanical Ventilators
Specific Problems in Critically Ill
    Patients
Quick Reference to Critical Care
    Formulas/ICU Formulas
Guidelines for Adult Critical Care Drug
    Infusions

TREATMENT OF THE CRITICALLY ILL PATIENT

Patients in the ICU setting typically have multisystem disease or injuries. The interactions between different dysfunctional organ systems is complicated and often overwhelming for the student or junior house officer.

This chapter describes a system-by-system approach to dealing with the critically ill patient. This approach forces the clinician to focus sequentially on each major organ system and to evaluate each system's function and interaction with other organ systems. This approach also allows the physician to integrate abnormalities within each system into a strategy for treating the patient as a whole. A complete but concise daily progress note will document this critical evaluation and integration process.

ICU PROGRESS NOTE

The ICU progress note is a concise, well-organized means of documenting the events of the past 24 h. The organization of a daily progress note is outlined here. The most important parts of this note are the assessment and the plan. Although the collected data can be found elsewhere in the chart, the physician's written assessment and interpretation of these data and events communicate the medical decision-making process to all who read the chart.

A simple organizational approach to the daily ICU progress note:

A. Outline the patient's problem list and/or injury summary.
    1. Include all active problems, major inactive problems, significant past medical history.
B. Outline events and procedures of the past 24 h.
C. List current medications.
D. Flow sheet data..

    1. Include vital signs, pulmonary artery catheter data, ventilator settings, laboratory and culture data.

    2. Also include radiographic data.

E. List physical exam findings.

F. Provide impression and assessment. Each of the following systems should be addressed daily.

    1. Neurologic function

    2. Pulmonary function, including mechanical ventilator

    3. Cardiovascular function

    4. Gastrointestinal function

    5. Genitourinary function

    6. Metabolic and nutritional status

    7. Hematologic function

    8. Infectious disease status

    9. Prophylaxis (ie, DVT, ETOH, stress ulcer, etc)

       With each of the areas listed in item 9, try to anticipate and avoid complications

G. Outline therapeutic plan for the day.

The following is an example of an ICU progress note that uses this approach. It is written for a trauma patient but can easily be modified for any clinical setting.

Sample ICU Progress Note

PROBLEM LIST:

- S/P MVA
- Left pulmonary concussion
- Left hemopneumothorax S/P left chest tube
- Grade 4 splenic injury S/P splenectomy
- Acute renal failure
- ARDS
- Complex past medical history:
    - Hypertension
    - Gout
- *Allergic:* Morphine sulfate

EVENTS OF PAST 24 HOURS:

- Increasing FiO_2 and PEEP
- Renal Consult

CURRENT MEDICATIONS

- Dopamine
- Fentanyl infusion
- Ativan infusion
- Pepcid
- Vancomycin

FLOW SHEET DATA:

- P 150 (NSR), BP 110/65, I/O: 3400/2210,

(continued)

20

Sample ICU Progress Note (continued)

- PAP 45/20, PCWP 14, CO 3.78, CI 2.54, EDVI 89
- Ventilator Setting: SIMV rate 16/4, 75%, PEEP 12, PS 10
- *Lab data:* Hct 30%, WBC 17.5

PHYSICAL EXAM:

- *Neurologic:* Intubated, sedated, moves all 4 extremities to painful stimuli
- HEENT pupil equal and reactive EOM intact
- Neck immobilized
- *Cardiovascular:* RRR, no increased JVD, 2+ capillary refill, toes warm
- *Pulmonary:* Coarse BS bilat., decreased on left. Chest tube in place
- *Gastrointestinal:* Midline incision healing well, soft, nondistended, no guarding, + bowel sounds
- *Extremities:* Warm well perfused

ASSESSMENT:

- *Neurologic:* Stable, continue sedation while on ventilator.
- *Cardiovascular:* Continues to require intermittent fluid challenge to maintain BP, this may be the cause of acute renal failure. Will continue fluids and may add dopamine to improve CO.
- *Pulmonary:* Worsening FiO$_2$ and PEEP requirements overnight, likely ARDS complicated by pulmonary contusion. Will obtain CXR this AM and wean FiO$_2$ and increase PEEP as tolerated by BP and CO.
- *Gastrointestinal:* S/P splenectomy, ileus continues, will place feeding tube today.
- *Renal:* Acute renal failure continues. Will proceed with renal ultrasound to R/O postrenal cause.
- *Hematologic:* S/P splenectomy HCT stable, will give postsplenectomy vaccines.

Abbreviations: See Abbreviations list at the beginning of the book.

CARDIOVASCULAR SYSTEM

Cardiovascular instability is one of the most common problems faced in the ICU. Understanding the approach to the evaluation of the cardiovascular system is essential to treating any critically ill patient.

Inspection

Inspection of the cardiovascular system is divided into three main areas:

Jugular Venous Distention

- Daily examination of the patient in the ICU should include examination of neck veins to look for JVD. A patient sitting at a 45-degree angle who has distended neck veins has a CVP of 12–15 cm H$_2$O or higher.

20

- Distended neck veins in the face of systemic hypotension in the acutely ill or injured patient suggest:

   Tension pneumothorax
   Pericardial tamponade
   Cardiac dysfunction

Precordial Contusion
- Bruising of the anterior chest wall is commonly associated with blunt trauma from a steering wheel. Such an injury pattern should alert the physician to the possibility of a myocardial contusion. Treatment of this condition consists of continuous ECG monitoring and vigorous correction of arrhythmias.

Extremity Perfusion
- Check all four extremities for distal perfusion, including pulses, color, temperature, and capillary refill.
- Pay special attention to the following areas:

   Sites distal to long bone fractures or dislocations
   Sites distal to indwelling arterial catheters

Blood Pressure

Blood pressure over the short term is considered adequate if renal perfusion is maintained. In a young, previously healthy individual, an adequate BP usually corresponds to a MAP of greater than 70 mm Hg.
   Technical Tip: If the cuff is too small an obese arm will give a systolic BP 10–15 mm Hg higher than the actual pressure.

Systolic Hypertension: A systolic blood pressure >140 mm Hg with a normal diastolic pressure. In the acute care setting, systolic hypertension is thought to be secondary to increased cardiac output.
   Systolic hypertension is seen in the following situations:

- Generalized response to stress
- Pain
- Thyrotoxicosis
- Anemia

Diastolic Hypertension: A diastolic pressure >90 mm Hg.
   Isolated diastolic hypertension is associated with three general disease categories:

- Renal disease
- Endocrine disorders
- Neurologic disorders

Treatment of Hypertension: Hypertension is of concern in the ICU when confronting a new MI or a vascular anastomosis and especially following carotid artery surgery. Ideally, the systolic blood pressure in this instance is maintained above 130 and below 160. A systolic pressure >180 mm Hg usually requires immediate treatment. Several drugs are commonly used to treat acute hypertension in the ICU setting. These include nitroprusside (Nipride), hydralazine (Apresoline), labetalol (Normodyne), a beta-blocker, or nitroglycerin. Beta-blockade should be used with Nipride in treating hypertension associated with an

20

aortic aneurysm. The emergency management of hypertension is discussed in Chapter 21, page 470 and the specific agents are discussed on page 439 and in Chapter 22.

Pulse Pressure

Pulse pressure is the difference between systolic and diastolic blood pressures.

Wide Pulse Pressure: A pulse pressure >40 mm Hg.

A wide pulse pressure is associated with:

- Thyrotoxicosis
- Arterial venous fistula
- Aortic insufficiency

Narrow Pulse Pressure: A pulse pressure <25 mm Hg.

A narrow pulse pressure is associated with:

- Significant tachycardia
- Early hypovolemic shock
- Pericarditis
- Pericardial effusion or tamponade
- Ascites
- Aortic stenosis

Mean Arterial Blood Pressure

MAP is calculated by taking the diastolic pressure plus one third of the pulse pressure. MAP is used to calculate several other hemodynamic variables.

Paradoxical Pulse: Paradoxical pulse is a function of the change in intrathoracic pressures during inspiration and expiration. Normally, systolic blood pressure falls between 6 and 10 mm Hg with inspiration. This fall is reflected by a systolic blood pressure that varies with respiration. If this variation occurs over a range >10 mm Hg, the patient is said to have a paradoxical pulse (Figure 20–1). For the technique to measure the paradoxical pulse, see Chapter 13, page 298.

Conditions associated with a paradoxical pulse:

- Pericardial tamponade
- Asthma and COPD
- Ruptured diaphragm
- Pneumothorax

Heart Murmurs

Monitor the ICU patient for the development of a new murmur. Murmurs are classically described as systolic or diastolic. All new murmurs should be characterized by their intensity, location, and variation with position and respiration. Diastolic murmurs are practically always pathologic. Details on heart murmurs can be found in Chapter 1, page 14.

Systolic Murmurs: Abrupt onset caused by conditions that have clinical significance for the acutely ill patient:

20

1. **Papillary muscle injury.** Papillary muscle dysfunction following AMI is characterized by an apical systolic murmur. The injury to the papillary muscle may cause a murmur

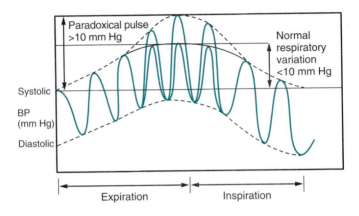

FIGURE 20–1 The paradoxical pulse.

of grade I–II/VI. After rupture of the papillary muscle, a sudden pansystolic murmur of grade II–IV/VI may appear. The diagnosis of papillary muscle rupture can be made either at cardiac catheterization or by echocardiography.

2. **Intraventricular septum rupture.** May be indicated by the appearance of a loud systolic murmur of abrupt onset. A catastrophic event that may follow MI. Usually accompanied by massive pulmonary edema. This situation is an indication for emergency cardiac catheterization.

Diastolic Murmurs: The major concern is the appearance of a diastolic murmur in the acutely injured patient is bacterial endocarditis, an entity that is becoming more common in patients who are treated in ICUs for long periods. Foreign bodies, such as central venous lines, hyperalimentation lines, and pulmonary artery catheters, all contribute to the increasing incidence of bacterial endocarditis.

1. **Gallop.** Defined as three sequential heart sounds in which the first two beats of the triplet are closer together than the third. The result is a sound that resembles the gallop of a horse.
   A newly occurring gallop may herald the onset of one or more of the following:

   - MI
   - Severe CHF
   - Mitral regurgitation secondary to injury of the papillary muscle
   - Anemia

2. **Pericardial friction rub.** Classically described as the sound of two pieces of leather rubbing together. Frequently high pitched and may be intermittent. Common following open heart surgery (in this setting, does not necessarily indicate pathologic changes).

20

Development of a pericardial friction rub should cause one to suspect one of the following:

- Pericarditis
- Pericardial effusion
- MI near the surface of the pericardium

CARDIOVASCULAR PHYSIOLOGY

Prior to a discussion of central venous pressure and pulmonary artery catheters, a brief review of cardiovascular physiology may be helpful.

Definitions

Cardiac Output: Defined as the quantity of blood pumped by the heart each minute. Normal output in an adult is 3.5–5.5 L/min.

Cardiac Index: Used to compensate for body size. Defined as the CO divided by the patient's body surface area. The normal CI is 2.8–3.2 L/min/m^2. A CI of <2.5 requires immediate assessment and treatment.

Determinants of Cardiac Output

Cardiac output is determined by heart rate and stroke volume. Stroke volume depends on the following:

- Preload
- Afterload
- Contractility

Preload: The initial length of the myocardial muscle fiber is proportional to the left ventricular end-diastolic volume. As the volume of blood remaining in the heart after each beat (end-diastolic volume) increases, the stretch on individual myocardial muscle cells increases. As the stretch increases, the energy of contraction increases proportionally until an optimal tension develops.

Starling's Law: When the myocardial muscle cell is stretched, the developed tension increases to a maximum and then declines as the stretch becomes more extreme (Figure 20–2).

Afterload: Defined as the resistance to ventricular ejection. Measured clinically by the calculation of SVR.

Contractility: The ability of the heart to alter its contractile force and velocity *independent* of fiber length. In simple terms, it represents the intrinsic strength of the individual muscle fiber cells. Contractility can be increased by stimulation of beta-receptors in the heart (see below).

Brief Review of the Adrenergic, or Sympathetic Nervous System

Cardiac output and its determinants (preload, afterload, and contractility) are all influenced by the adrenergic nervous system. The adrenergic system releases catecholamines (epinephrine and norepinephrine), which bind to end-organ receptors. These adrenergic receptors are divided into two classes, designated alpha (α) and beta (β), and their actions are summarized in Table 20–1.

20

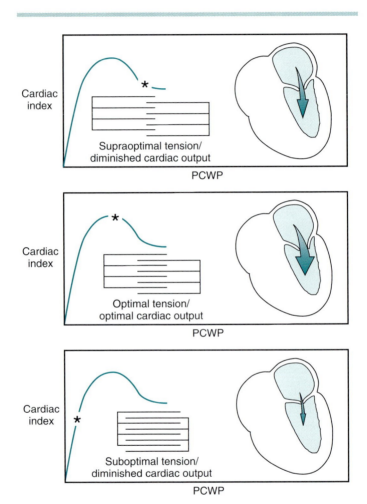

Cardiac index

Supraoptimal tension/
diminished cardiac output

PCWP

Cardiac index

Optimal tension/
optimal cardiac output

PCWP

Cardiac index

Suboptimal tension/
diminished cardiac output

PCWP

FIGURE 20–2 Representation of Starling's law. PCWP = pulmonary capillary wedge pressure.

20

TABLE 20–1
Adrenergic Receptors and Their Actions in the Cardiovascular System

Receptor	Site	Action
Beta-1	Myocardium	Increased contractility
	SA node	Increased heart rate
Beta-2	Arterioles	Vasodilation
	Lungs	Bronchodilatation
Alpha	Peripheral arterioles	Vasoconstriction

Alpha-1 Receptors: Adrenergic receptors found primarily in the peripheral arterial system. When stimulated, these receptors cause vasoconstriction and increase BP, SVR, and afterload.

Beta-1 Receptors: Found primarily on the SA node of the heart. When activated, these receptors stimulate the SA node to increase the heart rate and increase contractility. This increases CO and BP.

Beta-2 Receptors: Found in the peripheral vascular tree as well as in the bronchial wall smooth muscle. Activation causes vasodilation of the peripheral vasculature and bronchodilatation. Hemodynamically, this decreases SVR, BP, and afterload.

These adrenergic receptors are important because many of the cardiovascular drugs used in the ICU act through their sympathomimetic properties. These drugs usually have specific receptor affinity (ie, β versus α) and consequently differ in their effects. Drugs that act on alpha-1 receptors, for example, are called "vasopressors" because they cause vasoconstriction. Drugs that act on beta-1 receptors are conversely called "inotropes" because they increase contractility and heart rate. Commonly used sympathomimetics are listed in Table 20–2. A guide to administration of these agents appears in Table 20–10.

CENTRAL VENOUS PRESSURE

The CVP catheter is one of two major devices used in cardiovascular instrumentation. The other major device, the pulmonary artery catheter (often called the Swan–Ganz catheter), is considered in the next section.

The CVP reading reflects the right ventricular filling pressure. This filling pressure defines the ability of the right side of the heart to accept and pump blood.

Method

A 14-gauge intravenous catheter is inserted into the internal jugular or subclavian vein (see Chapter 13). A pressure transducer connected to the monitor provides the recordings. A chest x-ray is required to confirm the position of the catheter in the superior vena cava. The zero point for the manometer is usually 5 cm below the sternal notch, in the midaxillary line.

20

TABLE 20–2
Actions of Sympathomimetic Drugs

Drug	Effect on		
	Beta-1	Beta-2	Alpha
Dopamine	++++	++	++++
Dobutamine	++++	++	+
Isoproterenol	++++	+++	0
Norepinephrine	++	0	++++
Phenylephrine	0	0	++++
Epinephrine	++++	++	++++

Key: + = Relative effect; 0 = no clinically significant effect.

Implications

More important than the actual isolated measurements of CVP are the relative changes that take place as a patient's fluid or cardiac status changes. Therefore, serial readings are made. The implications of CVP readings are given in Table 20–3.

CVP Limitations

- CVP does not reflect total blood volume or left ventricular function.
- CVP will be altered by changes in pulmonary artery resistance and compliance of the right ventricle.
- Use may be limited by changes in intrathoracic pressure, such as those that occur during positive pressure ventilation or pneumothorax or in the presence of tumors.
- CVP may be normal in the face of sepsis or hypovolemia accompanied by compromised myocardial function.

TABLE 20–3
Interpretation of CVP Readings

Reading (cm H_2O)	Description	Implications
<4	Low	Fluids may be pushed
4–10	Midrange	Not clinically useful
>10	High	Suspect CHF, cor pulmonale, COPD, tension pneumothorax, cardiac tamponade

Abbreviations: CVP = central venous pressure; CHF = congestive heart failure; COPD = chronic obstructive pulmonary disease.

20

- Occult left ventricular failure may occur in the presence of normal CVP.
- Patients with COPD may require an elevated CVP to optimize their cardiac output.
- Pulmonary artery catheter readings are more accurate measurements of a patient's fluid and cardiac status than is the CVP.

Technical Tips

- If CVP readings do not fluctuate with respiration, the readings are inaccurate.
- If appropriate, remove the patient from the ventilator when taking a CVP reading.
- Have the head of the bed flat when taking readings, so that serial readings are comparable.
- Always use the same zero point (5 cm below the sternum in the midaxillary line) so that serial readings are comparable.

PULMONARY ARTERY CATHETERS

The pulmonary artery (PA or Swan–Ganz) catheter is a device that allows the measurement of central circulatory parameters useful in the treatment of the acutely ill patient. Volume status, vascular tone (both pulmonary and peripheral), and the heart's pumping ability are all monitored with the PA catheter. The catheter actually passes through the heart; its distal end is in the pulmonary artery (Figure 20–3). It allows the measurement of the pulmonary artery pressure (PAP), the pulmonary artery occlusion pressure (PAOP, also known as the pulmonary capillary wedge pressure, PCWP), the CO, and the CVP. Newer technology also allows for the continuous monitoring of mixed venous oxygen saturation (SvO_2), measurement of the right ventricular ejection fraction (REF), and the right ventricular end-diastolic volume index (RVEDVI).

Indications

Common clinical conditions requiring PA catheter monitoring include:

- Acute heart failure
- Complex circulatory and fluid conditions (massive resuscitation)
- Shock states
- Diagnosis of pericardial tamponade
- Intraoperative management (aneurysm repair, elderly patient undergoing major surgery)
- Complicated MI

Catheter Description

The original PA catheter, still commonly called the Swan–Ganz catheter after its inventors, consists of three lumens and a thermistor at the tip (Figure 20–4). It is typically marked in 10-cm increments and is radiopaque.

Lumens

- **Balloon port.** Usually a square white port that inflates the balloon at the tip of the catheter. Inflation of the balloon requires between 1 and 1.5 mL of air.
- **Proximal port.** Located approximately 30 cm proximal to the tip, it lies in the superior vena cava. May be used for the administration of routine IV fluids when not being used in determinations of CO.

20

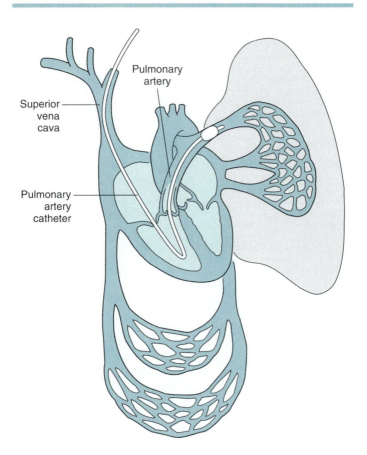

FIGURE 20–3 Relative positioning of the pulmonary artery catheter.

- **Distal port.** Lies in the pulmonary artery beyond the balloon. This port is attached to a pressure transducer that provides continuous PAP tracings and allows intermittent PAOP monitoring.

Thermistor. A temperature sensor. Provides continuous measurements of core temperature as well as measurements used in the thermal dilation method for determination of CO. (This method is described later in this chapter.)

Modifications of Pulmonary Artery Catheter: Several modifications of the original Swan–Ganz catheters allow for additional functions and measurement capabilities.
These modifications include additional ports for administration of IV medication or parenteral nutrition.

- **Pacing Swans** have extra ports (approximately 19 cm from the tip) through which
  pacing wires are passed into the right ventricle. Other models contain electrodes
  along the surface of the catheter, capable of pacing both the right atrium and ventricle.
- **Oximetric PA catheter** includes the standard ports of the Swan–Ganz type with
  fiberoptic components that emit light impulses to and from the distal end of the
  catheter. These light impulses are then reflected back by hemoglobin to monitors
  that continuously calculate O_2 saturation (See Figure 20–4).
- **Right ventricular ejection catheter** is capable of determining the right ventricular
  ejection fraction, which is then used to calculate the EDVI. The EDVI is the best indicator of preload in the shock state.

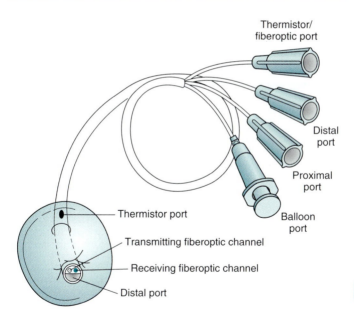

FIGURE 20–4   An example of a pulmonary artery catheter. This one features an
oximetric measuring feature (see text for a complete description).

Contraindications: If a PA catheter is needed to treat a patient in a critical care setting, there are no absolute contraindications. Patients with LBBB may experience complete heart block and may require placement of a temporary pacemaker prior to catheter placement. As with all indwelling catheters that are frequently manipulated, PA catheters increase the risk of infection.

Materials: In most institutions, a single brand of a flow-directed, balloon-tipped PA catheter is available (See Figure 20–4). An insertion kit provides the catheter as well as an introducer sheath; flexible J-tip guidewire; vessel dilator; catheter contamination shield; and the various syringes, needles, preparation material, local anesthetic, and other items needed to insert the catheter (Figure 20–5). The monitoring system (transducers, pressure tubing, stopcocks) and heparinized, pressurized flush system are usually set up by the nursing staff.

Pulmonary Artery Catheterization Procedure

1. Informed consent is usually required. The patient should be closely monitored with an ECG. Emergency resuscitation medications must be on hand in the event of an arrhythmia.
2. Choose a site and prep and drape the area. A widely draped field is needed because of the length of the tubing and guidewire. The choice of site is dictated by patient variables and operator experience. The easiest sites to place a PA catheter without fluoroscopic guidance are the right internal jugular vein and the left subclavian vein. In a patient who may receive thrombolytic therapy or who has a coagulopathy, femoral and median basilic veins are better routes.
3. Use a strict sterile approach with gown, gloves, and mask.

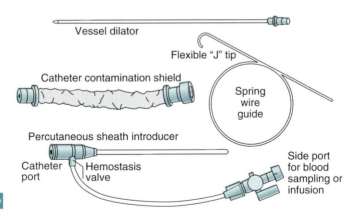

FIGURE 20–5   Additional items used for pulmonary artery catheter placement. (Reprinted, with permission, from: Chesnutt MS, et al [eds]: *Office & Bedside Procedures.* Appleton & Lange, Stamford CT, 1992.)

4. Prepare the PA catheter by attaching it to the monitor and flushing the lumens with heparinized saline solution (1 mL of 1:100 U heparin in 10 mL of NS). Check the balloon's function, and gently tap the catheter to ensure that an appropriate waveform is present on the monitor. Set the pressure transducer level to the middle of the patient's chest. This is approximately the level of the left atrium (midpoint of the chest wall at the fourth intercostal space). Some clinicians advocate checking the balloon for leaks by placing it in a container of sterile saline. *Note:* **Never fill the balloon with fluid; use air or CO_2.** The volume is typically 1–1.5 mL, depending on the catheter size. Place the catheter through the contamination shield and lay it on the sterile field.

5. The central vein is cannulated. (See Central Venous Catheterization, Chapter 13, page 253, for details.) Pass the flexible end of the J-wire (standard size is 45 cm long and 0.035 in. in diameter) into the vein through the needle. In general, **never** push a guidewire where it does not want to go and **always** keep one hand on the guidewire. Make sure the flexible tip is passed, *not* the more rigid end. The stiff end can more easily perforate a vessel.

6. Mount the introducer sheath on the vessel dilator. Pass the guidewire through the vessel dilator. If the skin site is insufficient, nick it with the No. 11 blade provided in the set.

7. Pass the vessel dilator into the vessel first. A slight twisting motion may be necessary to then advance the sheath into the vessel (Figure 20–6). Slowly remove the guidewire and the vessel dilator. Most PA catheter sheaths have a hemostatic valve mechanism that prevents air from entering the central system and blood from pouring out. If no valve mechanism is present, place a finger over the end of the sheath to prevent excessive blood loss or air embolization. It is handy to mount a syringe on the side port to aspirate blood to confirm proper intravascular positioning of the sheath. After the position is confirmed, flush with heparinized flush solution.

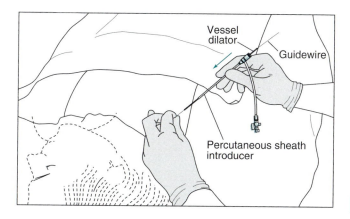

FIGURE 20–6   The introducer sheath and the vessel dilator are passed into the vessel. (Reprinted, with permission, from: Chesnutt MS, et al [eds]: *Office & Bedside Procedures.* Appleton & Lange, Stamford CT, 1992.)

20

8. Once the sheath is in place, the prepared catheter (fluid-filled, contamination sheath in place) can be advanced into the sheath (Figure 20–7). Once you have advanced it approximately 15 cm, the balloon will clear the tip of the sheath and can be gently inflated with 1.5 mL of air, using the volume-limiting syringe provided with the set (for a No. 7 or 7.5 French catheter). The maximum amount of air to be used with smaller catheters (No. 5 French) is 1.0 mL. If you encounter resistance to full inflation, consider that the balloon may not have yet cleared the sheath or that it may be in an extravascular location.

9. Once the balloon is inflated, advance the catheter to the level of the right atrium under the guidance of the pressure waveform and the ECG. Monitor the waveform and ECG at all times while advancing the balloon catheter. Figure 20–8 displays the normal pressures that can be seen as the catheter is advanced. Advance the catheter with the balloon inflated, and withdraw it with the balloon deflated. PA catheters usually come with a preformed curve on the tip. The catheter should be inserted pointing the catheter tip anteriorly and to the left. Positioning in the right atrium is probably best determined by watching for the characteristic waveform. The right atrium is generally located approximately 20 cm from the right internal jugular or subclavian vein insertion site and approximately 25–30 cm from the left subclavian vein insertion site. Advance the catheter steadily. An abrupt change in the pressure tracing occurs as the catheter enters the right ventricle. There is generally little ectopy on entry into the right ventricle; however, as the catheter advances into the right ventricular outflow tract, PVCs may occur. Keep advancing the catheter until the ectopy disappears and the pulmonary artery tracing is obtained. If this does not occur, deflate the balloon, withdraw the catheter, and

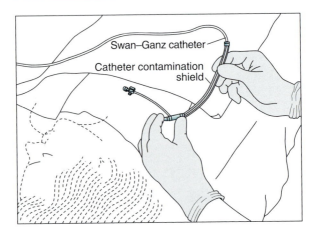

20

FIGURE 20–7 The fluid-filled pulmonary artery catheter is passed into the introducer sheath. (Reprinted, with permission, from: Chesnutt MS, et al [eds]: *Office & Bedside Procedures*. Appleton & Lange, Stamford CT, 1992.)

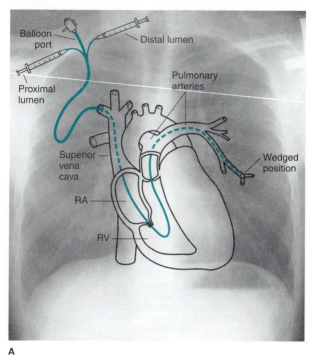

A

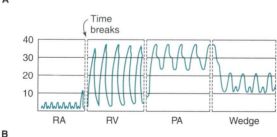

B

FIGURE 20–8 Positioning and pressure waveforms seen as the pulmonary artery catheter is advanced. (Reprinted, with permission, from: Haist SA, et al [eds]: *Internal Medicine on Call*, 2nd ed. Appleton & Lange, Stamford CT, 1996.)

20

make another attempt with the balloon inflated after slightly rotating the catheter. Obtain the PCWP after advancing the catheter another 10–15 cm. The catheter's final position should be such that the PCWP is obtained with full balloon inflation and the PAP tracing is present with the balloon deflated. In the "ideal position," transition from PAP to PCWP (and vice versa) occurs within three or fewer heart beats. In an adult, the typical length to the pulmonary artery position is 40–45 cm. **Never withdraw the catheter with the balloon inflated.** (See Figure 20–8 for normal waveforms seen as the catheter is advanced. Table 20–4 shows normal PA catheter measurements.)

10. Once the position is acceptable, lock the contamination shield onto the sheath. This allows readjustment of the catheter should this be necessary after the sterile field is taken down. Suture the sheath (using 3-0 or 4-0 nylon on a cutting needle), suture or secure the catheter in place and dress according to your institution's practice (often with a transparent dressing), and connect fluid to the inflow port on the sheath. This inflow port on the sheath can be used for IV fluid and some medication administration. Obtain a chest x-ray to document the catheter's present position as well as to rule out a pneumothorax or other complication from central venous catheterization. A properly positioned catheter should lie just beyond the vertebral bodies in the **nonwedged** position.

11. **Common problems.** Catheter placement is much more difficult if severe pulmonary artery hypertension is present. If there is significant cardiac enlargement, particularly dilation of the right heart structures, the catheter may have a propensity to coil and get lost in its path to the right ventricular outflow tract. Fluoroscopy may be required to get the catheter into the correct position and it will hold this position poorly. Placement of the catheter in the pulmonary artery may also be difficult in the setting of a low cardiac output because the balloon-tipped catheter depends on blood flow to carry it through the right heart chambers.

12. Cardiac output can be measured by thermal dilution. First, connect the thermistor to the cardiac output computer. Then rapidly inject fluid (usually 10 mL of ice-cooled NS) through the right atrial port. Have someone set the computer as you inject. The computer displays the CO. Repeat two more times. If all of these values are approximately the same, then average the readings and record. Newer continuous cardiac output monitoring PA are available in some units (see pages 401 and 412). For normal cardiac output and index, see Table 20–4.

Complications

1. Most complications that occur in the course of PA catheterization are related to central vein cannulation and include arterial puncture, placement of the wire or catheter in the extravascular space, and pneumothorax.

2. Arrhythmias are another common complication. The most common of these are transient PVCs that occur when the catheter is advanced into the right ventricular outflow tract. If a patient with a PA catheter suddenly develops frequent premature ventricular complexes, displacement of the catheter should be suspected.

3. VT and VF are rare occurrences.

4. Transient RBBB occurs occasionally as the catheter passes through the right ventricular outflow tract. In a patient with preexisting LBBB, this can result in complete heart block. In this setting, some form of backup pacing should be readily available. Complete heart block has been reported but occurs rarely.

5. Significant pulmonary infarcts and pulmonary artery rupture are serious but infrequent complications of PA catheters secondary to permanent wedge or peripheral placement of the catheter.

20

TABLE 20–4
Normal Pulmonary Artery Measurements

Parameter	Range
Right atrial pressure	1–7 mm Hg
Right ventricular pressure	
Systolic	15–25 mm Hg
Diastolic	0–8 mm Hg
PAP	
Systolic	15–25 mm Hg
Diastolic	8–15 mm Hg
Mean	10–20 mm Hg
PCWP (PAOP)	6–12 mm Hg
Cardiac output	3.5–5.5 L/min
Cardiac index	2.8–3.2 L/min/m^2
Mixed venous O_2 saturation (SvO_2)	70–80%
Right ventricular ejection fraction	80–120 mL

Abbreviations: PAP = pulmonary artery pressure; PAOP = pulmonary artery occlusion pressure; PCWP = pulmonary capillary wedge pressure.

6. Most complications and problems tend to increase with the time the catheter is in place. The risk of bacteremia and SBE is significant in severely ill patients receiving chronic instrumentation. In the setting of unexplained fever, the catheter and sheath should always be removed and cultured. The catheter and sheath should be replaced at a different site if a pulmonary catheter is still indicated.

Pulmonary Artery Catheter Measurements

Pulmonary Artery Pressure: Measured when the PA catheter is in its resting position in the pulmonary artery (balloon deflated). Measures both systolic pulmonary artery pressure and diastolic pulmonary artery pressure.

Pulmonary Artery Occlusion Pressure: (also called the "pulmonary capillary wedge pressure," or "wedge pressure"). A reflection of the left atrial pressure. Measured when the balloon at the tip of the PA catheter is slowly inflated with air (maximum 1.5 mL) and carried out, by blood flow, into one of the smaller branches of the pulmonary artery. The balloon **must** be deflated after each PAOP measurement to avoid pulmonary infarction. In the absence of mitral valvular disease, PAOP correlates closely with the LAP and with the left ventricular end-diastolic pressure. This correlation exists because of the unobstructed continuity between the pulmonary artery and the left side of the heart. As a result of this continuity, the PAOP can never be greater than the PAD. If the LVEDP increases, this should be reflected by an increase in PAOP, which, in turn, increases the PAD. Therefore, if a PA catheter monitor shows a wedge pressure higher than the PAD pressure, a technical error must exist. This is an important method to check the accuracy of the PAOP.

Left Ventricular End-Diastolic Pressure: LVEDP is a measure of preload and is used to guide fluid resuscitation and optimize cardiac output. Recall that to optimize stroke

20

volume on the Starling curve, the preload must be adequate to stretch the wall of the left ventricle. Too little volume (hypovolemia) results in too little tension and therefore a decreased CO. Conversely, too much preload volume causes overstretching beyond the point of maximum tension and causes a decrease in CO. Clinically, the PAOP is used to keep preload in an optimum range to maximize stroke volume. The normal PAOP varies between 6 and 12 mm Hg, but may be higher for different disease states.

Right Ventricular Ejection Fraction, Right Ventricular End-Diastolic Volume Index: A rapid-response thermistor and the cardiac output computer are used to calculate the REF. Once REF and CO are known, the EDVI can be calculated. The EDVI is another measure of preload, and it allows a more accurate assessment of volume status regardless of pulmonary status. For example, a patient with severe ARDS may have markedly elevated peak inspiratory pressures. Although the CVP and PAOP may be falsely elevated, the EDVI is measuring a volume, *not* a pressure, allowing a more precise determination of volume status across a wide variety of clinical situations. The normal range for EDVI is 80–120 mL.

Differential Diagnosis

Table 20–4 shows normal pulmonary artery measurements (see also Figure 20–8), and the differential diagnosis based on these and other critical care parameters is shown in Table 20–5.

Clinical Applications

The PA catheter allows the clinician to measure a patient's volume status and myocardial performance. As stated earlier, myocardial performance or CO depends on heart rate and stroke volume. Stroke volume is, in turn, dependent on preload, afterload, and contractility.

Heart Rate: Heart rate, in addition to stroke volume, determines the cardiac output. The body increases the HR to increase CO in the face of inadequate perfusion. Hence, tachycardia is an additional indicator of O_2 delivery/demand imbalance. Tachycardia >120 bpm increases myocardial O_2 demand significantly and should be promptly treated. The PA catheter allows the establishment of adequate myocardial filling pressures such that the HR may be clinically manipulated to maximize CO. In a patient with adequate filling pressures, slow HR (<80 bpm), and a low CO, drugs that speed up the heart (called "chronotropes") may be used to increase CO. Alternatively, tachycardia >120 bpm with an adequate PAOP may be pharmacologically slowed to decrease the strain on the heart.

Preload (Stroke Volume): Indicated by the PAOP or EDVI, a reflection of left ventricular end-diastolic volume. In simple terms, preload is the amount of blood in the heart prior to contraction. Consequently, preload represents the stretch placed on the individual myocardial cell. When the PAOP is optimized, myocardial performance is optimized according to the Starling curve.

1. **Clinical implications in a healthy heart.** A low PAOP or EDVI means suboptimal myocardial muscle tension and, consequently, suboptimal myocardial performance. Cardiac output may be increased by the administration of fluids. The result is an increase in left ventricular end-diastolic volume, an increase in myocardial muscle tension, and improved myocardial performance.
2. **Clinical implications in a failing heart.** Long-standing myocardial disease may shift the Starling curve to the left. Consequently, a significantly elevated PAOP may be required to optimize myocardial performance. It is common for patients who have just undergone heart valve replacement to require a PAOP of 20–25 mm Hg to optimize

TABLE 20–5
Differential Diagnosis Based on Hemodynamic Parameters*

Diagnosis	Blood Pressure	CVP	CO	PCWP/LVEDP	PAP	PVR	SVR
Cardiogenic shock	⇓	⇑	⇓	⇑	⇑	⇑	⇑
Cardiac tamponade	⇓	⇑	⇓	⇑	⇑	—	⇑
Hypovolemic shock	⇓	⇓	⇓	⇓	⇓	⇑	⇑
Septic shock	⇓	⇓	⇑	⇓	⇓	⇓	⇓
Pulmonary embolus	⇓	⇑	⇓	— or ⇓	⇑	⇑	⇑

*These trends are usually seen with the conditions noted. Clinical variables (medications, secondary conditions) can vary some of these trends.
Abbreviations: CVP = central venous pressure; CO = cardiac output; PCWP = pulmonary capillary wedge pressure; PAP = pulmonary artery pressure; PVR = peripheral vascular resistance; SVR = systemic vascular resistance; ⇑ = usually increased; ⇓ = usually decreased; LVEDP = left ventricular end-diastolic pressure; — = usually not changed.

cardiac output. Patients with a recent MI may require a PAOP of 16–18 mm Hg to optimize output.

Afterload: Defined as the resistance to ventricular ejection. Measured clinically by the calculation of systemic vascular resistance:

$$SVR = \frac{(MAP - CVP) \times 80}{Cardiac\ output\ (L\ /\ min)}$$

Normal SVR = $900 - 1200$ dynes/s/cm^3

1. **Indications for afterload reduction.**

   - Significant mitral regurgitation
   - An increased PAOP in the face of an elevated SVR and a decreased cardiac index

2. **Treatment.** Nitroprusside (Nipride) is the drug of choice.

Contractility: The ability of the heart to alter its contractile force and velocity independent of fiber length is difficult to measure clinically. Digitalis can improve contractility. Care should be maintained to ensure normal levels of serum potassium prior to the administration of digitalis.

Correctable metabolic causes for depressed contractility include:

- Hypoxia
- Acidosis (pH <7.3)
- Hypophosphatemia
- Adrenal insufficiency
- Hypothermia

The most common causes are **hypoxia and acidosis.** These must be corrected before inotropic therapy can be effective.

DETERMINATIONS OF CARDIAC OUTPUT

Several methods are currently available to determine (CO). These include:

- Thermal dilution technique
- A–Vo$_2$ difference calculation

Thermal Dilution Technique

This requires the use of a PA catheter. A measured amount of saline (usually 10 mL) at a known temperature is injected into the proximal port of the PA catheter, and a temperature-sensitive thermistor located at the distal end of the pulmonary artery senses the temperature change in the surrounding blood. The cardiac output computer then integrates the magnitude and rate of change in temperature and calculates CO.

20 Arteriovenous Oxygen (A–Vo$_2$) Difference

A reasonable estimate of cardiac output can be made on the basis of A–Vo$_2$ difference. A–Vo$_2$ difference is a measure between the oxygen content of arterial blood drawn from a peripheral artery and the oxygen content of mixed venous blood drawn from the distal lumen of a PA catheter (Table 20–6).

TABLE 20–6
Calculation of Cardiac Index Based on A–Vo$_2$ Difference

A–Vo$_2$ Difference (Vol %)	Cardiac Index* (L/min/m^2)
>6	<2
4–5	3–4
<3	>5

*Cardiac index = Cardiac output ÷ Body surface area.

A–Vo$_2$ difference = Arterial O$_2$ content − Mixed venous O$_2$ content

Concept: The A–Vo$_2$ difference measures the extraction of oxygen by the tissues during a single transit time through the circulation. Thus, the A–Vo$_2$ difference is a function of (1) Pao$_2$, (2) Hgb, (3) CO, and (4) tissue O$_2$ consumption.

- **If cardiac output is low.** Transit time is long and the tissues extract large amounts of oxygen during a single circulation time. Thus, the oxygen content of mixed venous blood is low and the A–Vo$_2$ difference is large
- **If cardiac output is high.** Circulation time is shorter and the amount of oxygen extracted is low. Consequently, the A–Vo$_2$ difference is low

Calculations: The A–Vo$_2$ difference is inversely proportional to CO. Therefore, the following approximations can be made:

1. **Determining Oxygen Content.** To calculate the A–Vo$_2$ difference, the oxygen content of both arterial and mixed venous blood must determined. *Oxygen content* describes the amount of O$_2$ the blood is able to carry. Because only a small percentage of O$_2$ is dissolved in plasma, the vast majority is carried by hemoglobin. Hence,

Oxygen content = Oxygen bound to Hgb + Oxygen dissolved in plasma

$$\text{Arterial O}_2 \text{ content (Cao}_2) = (\text{Sao}_2 \times \text{Hgb} \times 1.39) + (0.0031 \times \text{Pao}_2)$$

where Sao$_2$ is arterial O$_2$ saturation, Hgb is hemoglobin content in g/dL, and Pao$_2$ is arterial partial pressure of O$_2$. The constant 1.39 is the O$_2$-binding capacity of Hgb (mL of O$_2$/g of Hgb), and 0.0031 is mL of O$_2$ dissolved in 100 mL of plasma per mm Hg of Pao$_2$. The normal O$_2$ content of arterial blood is 16–20 mL of O$_2$/100 mL of blood.
Similarly,

$$\text{Cvo}_2 = \text{Svo}_2 \times [\text{Hgb}] \times 1.39 + (0.0031 \times \text{Pvo}_2)$$

where Cvo$_2$ is the O$_2$ content of mixed venous blood, Svo$_2$ is the mixed venous O$_2$ saturation.
Assuming that the amount of dissolved blood in plasma is small, then:

20

$$A{-}V_{O_2} = Ca_{O_2} - Cv_O = 1.39 \times Hgb \times (Sa_{O_2} - SV_{O_2})$$

2. **Calculation of A–VO_2 Difference.**

- Obtain hemoglobin concentration.
- Determine SaO_2 from heparinized peripheral arterial blood or from a pulse oximeter.
- Determine SvO_2 from a heparinized mixed venous blood sample from the distal lumen of a PA catheter or from an oximetric SvO_2 monitor (see the following discussion).
- Calculate the A–VO_2 difference according to the preceding formula, and determine the CI based on Table 20–6.

Continuous SvO_2 Monitoring

Oximetric pulmonary artery catheters house fiberoptic channels that allow direct measurement of mixed venous saturation (SvO_2). These fiberoptics carry light impulses that are reflected by hemoglobin according to its O_2 saturation. An optical microprocessor then displays a continuous graph of SvO_2 measurements. Calibration is periodically confirmed with a heparinized blood sample drawn from the oximetric catheter's distal port.

Clinical Application

- Follow trends in the O_2 supply/demand balance.
- A decrease in SvO_2 is often the first indicator of early organ dysfunction. This early warning allows correction of the problem before hemodynamic compromise.
- Treatment interventions (eg, transfusions, fluid mobilization, drugs) may be assessed by following SvO_2 changes long before other hemodynamic parameters are adversely affected.
- Clinically, SvO_2 values *between 60% and 80%* represent *adequate tissue perfusion.*
- **SvO_2 of <60%** should prompt an immediate assessment of O_2 delivery or unrecognized conditions causing increased O_2 demand. As O_2 delivery falls, SvO_2 falls because there is less O_2 for the tissues to consume. Similarly, if O_2 consumption increases, then SvO_2 also falls. A decline of SvO_2 should therefore prompt a review of the parameters describing O_2 delivery (ie, CO, Hgb, SaO_2) and consumption (SaO_2 − SvO_2). These parameters identify the causes of SvO_2 decline and their specific treatments:

  - SaO_2 <90% demands increased ventilatory support.
  - Decreased CO requires optimizing myocardial function.
  - Low Hgb requires transfusion.

- **SvO_2 of >80%** indicates increased metabolic demands, requires evaluation for conditions such as unrecognized seizures, shivering, mobilization, and large tissue defects (Figure 20–9).
- Inaccurate readings of SvO_2 may occur as a result of fibrin buildup on the tip of the catheter, fiberoptic fracture (rare), and impingement of the tip of the catheter on the vessel wall. Overall, however, these catheters are accurate and sensitive with daily calibration.

20

Continuous Cardiac Output

This technology allows measurement of the CO on a continuous basis. The specially designed PA catheter emits small pulses of energy that heat the surrounding blood. The cardiac

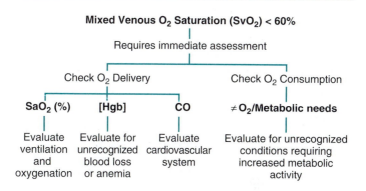

FIGURE 20–9 Algorithm for assessment of decreased SvO_2.

output computer then calculates the CO based on the magnitude and the rate of temperature change.

Continuous Sao_2 Monitoring (Pulse Oximeter)

The same fiberoptic technology used to measure mixed venous O_2 saturation is also used to measure arterial O_2 saturation (Sao_2). A light-emitting external probe is placed around a well-perfused appendage such as a digit, earlobe, lip, or bridge of the nose. The light is transmitted through the appendage to be reflected by hemoglobin according to its O_2 saturation (recall that the hemoglobin molecule absorbs different wavelengths of light at different O_2 saturations). The oximeter, in addition to calculating Hgb O_2 saturation, can also determine the pulse rate and is referred to as the "pulse oximeter." An Sao_2 of <90% implies inadequate oxygenation and requires immediate intervention. However, an Sao_2 >90% does not necessarily imply adequate O_2 delivery (see following section). **Pulse oximeter is not useful in the setting of smoke inhalation and CO poisoning.**

SHOCK STATES

Shock is defined as inadequate perfusion or oxygen delivery to meet metabolic demand.

Types of Shock

Shock can be divided into four major classes. Specific therapeutic interventions are also discussed in this chapter on page 431 and in Chapter 21 (page 460).

- Hypovolemic (low or high hematocrit)
- Cardiogenic
- Septic
- Neurogenic

20

Hypovolemic Shock: Is due to acute loss of extracellular volume. Most often due to hemorrhage in the setting of trauma but may also be due to diarrhea, vomiting, or thermal injury. Characterized by a low cardiac output, low PAOP, and elevated SVR. Svo_2 is decreased.

Therapy. Should be directed toward volume replacement and increased hemoglobin concentration to improve myocardial performance.

Cardiogenic: May be due to intrinsic pump failure, dysrhythmia, or compression (ie, tamponade). Characterized by a low cardiac output, high PAOP, and elevated SVR. The basic defect is one of myocardial performance. Svo_2 is decreased.

Therapy. Should be aimed at optimizing PAOP and increasing contractility, while decreasing SVR.

Septic (Systemic Inflammatory Response Syndrome): Sepsis implies that the shock state is due to an infectious cause. The SIRS has similar hemodynamic characteristics but is not due to an infectious agent (ie, sterile pancreatitis). Characterized by a high CO, low PAOP, and low SVR. Septic shock is characterized by prearteriolar shunting, which results in a false increase in Svo_2, despite tissue hypoxia.

Therapy. Should be aimed at increasing PAOP and increasing SVR simultaneously. In true septic shock the primary treatment is therapy directed against the infectious cause (ie, drainage of abscess).

Neurogenic: Is typically due to high cervical spine injuries or high spinal anesthetics. Characterized by a low cardiac output, low PAOP, and low SVR. Svo_2 is decreased.

Therapy. Should be aimed at increasing SVR. In the setting of acute trauma with spinal cord injury **always assume hemorrhage** is the cause of hypotension and **treat with fluid resuscitation before using vasoactive agents to raise SVR.**

Summary

Shock describes states of inadequate tissue perfusion and O_2 delivery. Svo_2 is decreased in all shock states except septic shock. The goal in all shock states is to improve myocardial performance by effecting changes in preload, afterload, contractility, and systemic vascular resistance. The PA catheter is used to guide these cardiovascular manipulations.

CLINICAL PULMONARY PHYSIOLOGY

The goal of treating any critically ill patient is to optimize both oxygenation and tissue perfusion. Pulmonary and cardiovascular physiology are intimately interwoven to achieve this goal. It does little good to optimize cardiovascular function if, because of poor pulmonary function, there is no oxygen for the hemoglobin to transport (ie, low Sao_2). *Ventilation* refers to the mechanical movement of air into and out of the respiratory system. *Oxygenation* refers to the diffusion of oxygen from the alveoli to the blood in the pulmonary capillaries and from there to the tissues. Figure 20–10 shows ventilation and oxygenation in typical alveoli.

20 Ventilation

Several parameters, such as volumes and capacities, are important in assessing the adequacy of ventilation. Spirometry provides both dynamic information (patient's ability to move air into and out of the lungs) as well as static volume measurements. The subdivisions of the lung capacities are shown on a spirometric graph in Figure 20–11.

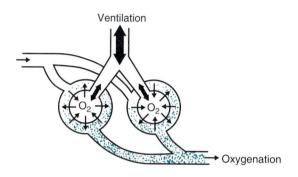

FIGURE 20–10   Ventilation and oxygenation in typical alveoli.

Basic Lung Volumes: Four basic lung volumes that together make up the total lung capacity (See Figure 20–11):

1. **Tidal volume.** The volume of inspired gas during a normal breath. In healthy individuals at rest, the tidal volume is 6–10 mL/kg.

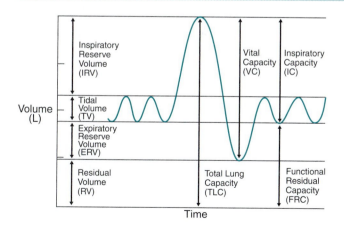

FIGURE 20–11   Spirometric graph with volumes and capacities of the lung.

2. **Inspiratory reserve volume.** The volume of gas that can be maximally inspired beyond the amount inspired during a tidal volume breath
3. **Expiratory reserve volume.** The volume of gas that can be maximally expired beyond the amount expired at the end of a tidal volume breath
4. **Residual volume.** The volume of gas that remains in the lung after a maximal expiratory effort

Lung Capacity: The sum of two or more of these lung volumes make up four divisions called lung capacities (See Figure 20–11).

1. **Total lung capacity.** The total amount of gas in the lung at the end of maximal inspiration
2. **Vital capacity.** The volume of gas expired after a maximal inspiration followed by maximal expiration. Frequently used in determining whether a patient can successfully be weaned from the ventilator. Normal vital capacity is 65–75 mL/kg. A vital capacity of <15 mL/kg is an indication for continued ventilatory support. VC = ERV + TV + IRV (Figure 20–12).
3. **Inspiratory capacity.** The volume of gas expired from maximal inspiration to end TV. IC = TV + IRV.
4. **Functional residual capacity.** The gas remaining in the lung following normal expiration (tidal volume). Acts as a buffer against extreme changes in alveolar P_{O_2} and consequent dramatic changes in arterial P_{O_2} with each breath. FRC = ERV + RV (Figure 20–13).

Clinical Implications

These volumes and capacities are important parameters for assessing ventilation because they may change under different conditions (ie, atelectasis, obstruction, consolidation, small airway collapse). For example, the ERV decreases with small airway collapse, thus decreasing FRC. These alterations in lung volumes consequently affect respiratory reserve and the

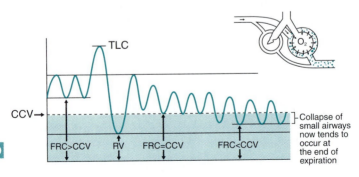

FIGURE 20–12   Functional residual capacity (FRC) and critical closing volume (CCV). TLC = total lung capacity; RV = residual volume.

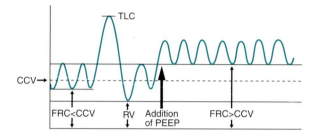

FIGURE 20–13   The effect of positive end-expiratory pressure (PEEP) is to increase the functional residual capacity (FRC); CCV = critical closing volume; TLC = total lung capacity; RV = residual volume.

patient's ability to ventilate and oxygenate. The contributing factors and the point at which they influence such volume changes must be understood to optimize support. The critical closing volume is an expression that describes the minimum volume and pressure necessary to keep small airways from collapsing during expiration.

Critical Closing Volume: The volume of gas and, consequently, pressure in the lung during expiration at which small airway collapse occurs. When collapse occurs, blood is shunted around nonventilated alveoli, thus decreasing the available surface area for gas exchange. The critical closing volume is greatly affected by compliance. Therefore, different minimum volumes and pressures may be required to prevent collapse under varying lung conditions. If the CCV is greater than the FRC (air in the lung after tidal expiration), collapse tends to occur (see Figure 20–12).

One method to overcome the CCV is to increase the amount of **positive end-expiratory pressure** in the lung (see the following discussion on PEEP). The effect of PEEP is to increase FRC by preventing small airway collapse at the end of expiration. This improves alveolar ventilation, decreases shunting and improves oxygenation (see Figure 20–13).

Lung compliance. Relates the *change* in lung volume and the *change* in pressure required to produce volume change (Figure 20–14). May be measured at the bedside and is a reflection of FRC and CCV.

$$\text{Compliance} = \frac{\Delta V}{\Delta P}$$

Dynamic compliance is determined by measuring the tidal volume and dividing it by the peak inspiratory pressure.

$$\text{Dynamic compliance} = \frac{\text{Tidal volume}}{\text{Peak inspiratory pressure} - \text{PEEP}}$$

20

Normal   **Less compliant**

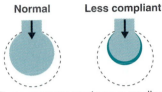

Same pressure produces a smaller
volume in the less compliant lung.

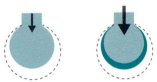

Increasing positive pressure maintains
volume in the less compliant lung.

FIGURE 20–14   Concept of pulmonary compliance.

Normal > 80–100 mL/cm H_2O

Static compliance is similarly calculated by substituting static peak pressure for peak inspiratory pressure. Static peak pressure is measured by occluding the exhalation port at the beginning of exhalation (no flow = static pressure).

Comparing dynamic with static compliance may indicate the type of processes causing changes in the elasticity of the lung. Dynamic compliance is affected by both elasticity and airway resistance. Static compliance, in contrast, is not affected by airway resistance because there is no flow. Hence, a reduction in dynamic compliance without a change in static compliance indicates an airway resistance problem such as obstruction, bronchospasm, or collapse of the small airways. A reduction in both static and dynamic compliance may indicate a decrease in lung elasticity such as pulmonary edema, atelectasis, or excessive PEEP.

Oxygenation

Oxygenation is the process of transporting oxygen from the alveolus across the capillary membrane into the pulmonary circulation and subsequently distributing that oxygen to the body's tissues.

Tests for the assessment of oxygenation include

- Measurement of arterial O_2 saturation (SaO_2) with pulse oximetry
- Calculation of oxygen delivery (or carrying capacity)
- Calculation of right-to-left shunt fraction (Qs/Qt)

Arterial Oxygen Saturation: See page 162.

Oxygen Delivery: Delivery of O_2 to the tissue, also called the O_2 carrying capacity, depends on CO in addition to the oxygen content of blood (Cao_2).

$$O_2 \text{ delivery} = CO \times Cao_2 = CO \text{ (L/min)} \times Sao_2 \times 1.39 \text{ [Hgb]} \times 10$$

Normal delivery is around 800 mL of O_2/min, with an average normal O_2 uptake of 250 mL of O_2/min.

Note that this equation simplifies O_2 delivery to three parameters: CO, Sao_2, and [Hgb]. These are measured with a PA catheter, pulse oximeter, and spun hematocrit, respectively.

Calculating the A–a Gradient: To calculate the alveolar-to-arterial gradient:

1. Place the patient on 100% oxygen (F_iO_2) for 20 min.
2. Next obtain a peripheral arterial blood gas measurement.
3. Calculate the alveolar Po_2. After breathing 100% oxygen for 20 min, the only gases other than oxygen within the alveoli are H_2O and excreted CO_2 from tissue metabolism. Thus, the partial pressure of oxygen within the alveoli is easily calculated. The alveolar Po_2 equals

    760 Barometric pressure (in torr)
    −47 Partial pressure H_2O
    −40 Pco_2 from peripheral sample
    673 Alveolar Po_2 (PAO_2)

4. Subtract the peripheral arterial oxygen content (Pao_2) from the alveolar Po_2
Example:

    673 Alveolar Po_2 (PAO_2)
    −200 Peripheral Pao_2
    473 A-a gradient

Rule: *The larger the gradient, the more serious the degree of respiratory compromise.* Any A–a gradient >400 torr indicates severe respiratory distress resulting from a process interfering with oxygen transfer (low Pao_2). (Normal A–a gradient = 20–65 torr)

Shunt Fraction: In clinical practice, the A–a gradient is calculated primarily because it may be used to calculate the shunt fraction equation. The shunt fraction (normal = <5%) reflects the ratio of ventilated alveoli to perfused capillaries. A shunt fraction of 5% (assuming normal perfusion) means that 5% of the blood leaving the pulmonary capillaries has passed without being oxygenated. In an ideal state, the volume of lung ventilation equals the volume of pulmonary capillary blood flow (Figure 20–15). Alterations in these ventilation–perfusion relationships result from two causes:

*   Relative obstruction of alveolar ventilation
*   Relative obstruction of pulmonary blood flow

1. **Perfusion greater than ventilation:** Figure 20–16 depicts the extreme situation in which alveolus A receives no ventilation, but perfusion continues. Therefore, a complete pulmonary A–V shunt exists with respect to that alveolus.
2. **Ventilation greater than perfusion:** Figure 20–17 depicts uniform ventilation to A and B, but no blood flow to the alveolus. This situation increases physiologic dead space and increases the shunt equation.
3. **Compensation mechanism:** Figure 20–18 represents the compensatory change that occurs when an alveolus is partially occluded. Blood flow is preferentially shunted to other, more efficiently ventilated alveolar units.

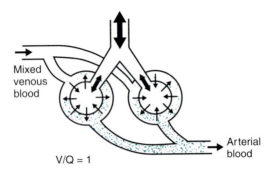

FIGURE 20–15   Ventilation–perfusion (V/Q) ratio.

Principle. It is important to recognize that at any given time, even in the normal state, gradations of all these situations exist simultaneously within the lung. The normal shunt fraction is approximately 5%. Alterations in either ventilation or perfusion can seriously affect oxygenation.

1. **Decreased lung-to-blood transfer.** Associated factors are

   - Pulmonary edema
   - ARDS
   - Atelectasis
   - Pneumonia

20

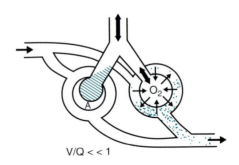

FIGURE 20–16   Perfusion greater than ventilation.

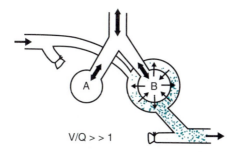

FIGURE 20–17   Ventilation greater than perfusion.

2. **Decreased perfusion.** Associated factors are

   • Massive PE
   • Continued micropulmonary embolization

Calculation of the Shunt Fraction. Q is the mathematical symbol for flow. Therefore, Qs is the symbol for the amount of flow through the pulmonary shunt. Qs is defined as that portion of the cardiac output that does not participate in gas exchange, that is, the volume of blood that is shunted past nonventilated alveoli. Qt is the symbol for total cardiac output. Therefore, the volume of blood shunted past nonventilated alveoli divided by the total cardiac output (shunted plus nonshunted blood) is Qs/Qt (Figure 20–19).

The shunt fraction is defined as

$$\frac{Qs\,(\%)}{Qt} = \frac{Cco_2 - Cao_2 \times 100}{Cco_2 - Cvo_2}$$

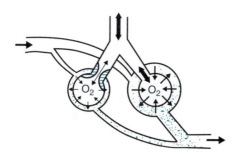

FIGURE 20–18   Compensation for ventilation–perfusion mismatching.

20

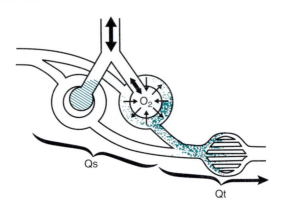

FIGURE 20–19   Representation of the shunt fraction.

where Cc_{O_2} is O_2 content (mL/100 mL) of blood leaving the alveolar capillary bed, Ca_{O_2} is arterial O_2 content (mL/100mL), and Cv_{O_2} is mixed venous O_2 content (mL/100mL) in the pulmonary artery.

The oxygen content of the capillary blood (Cc_{O_2}) is calculated using the alveolar P_{O_2} (PA_{O_2}) from the alveolar–arterial gradient calculation.

$$Cc_{O_2} = [Hgb]\,(1.39)\,(1.0) + PA_{O_2}\,(0.0031)$$

where Ca_{O_2} is measured when the patient should be on and Fi_{O_2} of 1.0 (100% O_2).

Similarly, the O_2 content of mixed venous blood found in the pulmonary artery may be calculated as follows:

$$Cv_{O_2} = [Hgb]\,(1.39)\,(Sv_{O_2}) + Pv_{O_2}\,(0.0031)$$

where Sv_{O_2} is the O_2 saturation of mixed venous blood.

Concept of the Shunt Fraction. Qs/Qt represents the amount of pulmonary flow "shunted," or not participating in gas exchange over the total cardiac output. For example, a shunt fraction of 0.25 indicates that 25% of the pulmonary blood flow is shunted. Thus, the equation serves as a useful index of ventilation–perfusion inequality. The normal value is <5%.

Breaking the equation down reveals that the numerator reflects lung-to-blood transfer (ie, A–a gradient), or "ventilation." The denominator describes O_2 consumption (ie, A–VO_2 difference), which, in turn, reflects CO, or "perfusion." Simplifying the denominator further illustrates that this equation is also a function of the four basic measured parameters describing O_2 delivery and demand: Sa_{O_2}, CO, Hgb, and Sv_{O_2}. Knowledge of these four measurements along with the alveolar–arterial gradient allows for early recognition and treatment of ventilation–perfusion mismatching.

20

Alveolar-to-Arterial Gradient [P(A–a)O₂] Provides an assessment of alveolar–capillary gas exchange

- Alveolar P_{O_2} (P_{AO_2}) minus calculated
- Arterial P_{O_2} (P_{aO_2}) minus measured

Calculating the A–a Gradient. To calculate the alveolar-to-arterial gradient:

1. Place the patient on 100% oxygen (F_{iO_2}) for 20 min.
2. Next obtain a peripheral ABG measurement.
3. Calculate the alveolar P_{O_2}. After breathing 100% oxygen for 20 min, the only gases other than oxygen within the alveoli are H_2O and excreted CO_2 from tissue metabolism.

$$[(713) \times F_{iO_2} - (P_{aCO_2})] - \frac{P_{aO_2}}{0.8}$$

INDICATIONS FOR INTUBATION

The decision to intubate a patient for prolonged ventilator support is one of the most difficult decisions for clinicians. It is easy for the physician to be lulled into a false sense of security by marginal blood gases. The following indications can be used as a basic checklist for respiratory support:

- Inability to adequately ventilate (eg, chest trauma, sedation, paralyzed or fatigued respiratory muscles)
- Inability to adequately oxygenate (eg, pulmonary edema, ARDS)
- Excessive work of breathing (eg, prophylaxis for impending collapse)
- Protection of airway (eg, unconscious, altered mental status, massive resuscitation, facial trauma)

These basic indications should be used in conjunction with **clinical judgment** in the final decision for mechanical ventilation. The decision to intubate, if made in a timely and appropriate fashion, can turn an otherwise traumatic intubation into a controlled and elective procedure. Table 20–7 lists some common parameters used to evaluate the need for respiratory support in adults.

MECHANICAL VENTILATORS

Classes of Ventilators

The two classic types of ventilator are the pressure-limited and the volume-limited ventilators. Although newer ventilators combine many of the qualities of both classes, it is conceptually advantageous to discuss the two types separately. Additionally, several other types of ventilators are occasionally used.

Pressure Limited: These ventilators deliver a volume of air until a preset pressure is reached. They are used in some neonatal units. They are not generally used to ventilate adult patients, because changes in airway pressure and in lung and chest wall compliance may result in an inadequate minute ventilation. This technique is reserved for patients who fail to respond to traditional modes of ventilation.

Volume Limited: A preset volume of air is delivered regardless of the opposing pressure. This is the most common class of ventilator used. (*Note:* A pressure limit setting usually allows the venting of excessive pressure to prevent barotrauma.)

20

TABLE 20–7
Indicators of Respiratory Failure

Condition	Normal Range (adults)
$PaCO_2$ >60 mm Hg	35–45 mm Hg
PaO_2 <70 mm Hg on 50% mask	80–100 mm Hg on room air
Tachypnea >30 breaths/min	10–20 breaths/min
Altered mental status such that the patient is unable to protect the airway against aspiration	

High-Frequency Ventilation: Rapid oscillations of breath (60–1200 cycles) used with or without the bulk delivery of gases to the lung. Several forms of this type of ventilation exist, including high-frequency jet ventilation, high-frequency positive pressure ventilation, and high-frequency oscillation.

Ventilator Modes

Ventilator modes are represented in Figure 20–20.

Controlled Ventilation: The patient gets a breath only when it is delivered by the machine. The patient cannot initiate any of his or her own breaths. Used in the past on patients who were intentionally paralyzed by drugs.

Assist Controlled: The patient gets a full mechanical tidal volume each time he or she attempts an inspiratory effort. The respiratory frequency is determined by the patient, although a backup rate is set to ensure a minimum minute ventilation.

- Advantages of AC is that patients can easily increase their minute ventilation even if they are weak and have a poor inspiratory effort.
- Disadvantage is the predisposition to hyperventilation if the patient becomes agitated or has an altered respiratory drive because of neurologic injury. Agitation may also lead to "breath stacking," in which the ventilator delivers a second tidal volume before completing the expiratory phase of the first breath. Fortunately, this is rarely a clinical problem because the patient often feels more comfortable and consequently less agitated because of the decreased work of breathing on AC.

Synchronous IMV: The respirator delivers a set number of breaths each minute and allows the patient to supplement ventilation with his or her own inspiratory efforts between machine breaths. This allows the patient to use the respiratory muscles. As the ventilator rate decreases progressively, the patient assumes more of the work of breathing. The ventilator also senses when the patient is taking a breath and will not deliver the mandatory breath until after the patient's own breath is completed. This was developed to prevent the patient's working against the ventilator or receiving a double tidal volume (ie, a mechanical tidal volume on top of a spontaneous breath). This is the most commonly used type of ventilatory mode in conjunction with pressure support and PEEP.

20

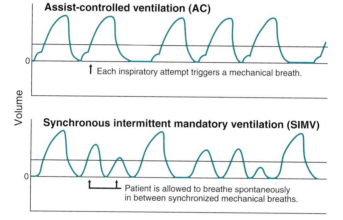

Controlled ventilation (CV)

← Mechanical ventilation

Rate is fixed by ventilator.   ↑ Patient is not allowed to
                                       breathe spontaneously
                                       in between mechanical breaths.

Assist-controlled ventilation (AC)

↑ Each inspiratory attempt triggers a mechanical breath.

Volume

Synchronous intermittent mandatory ventilation (SIMV)

↑___↑ Patient is allowed to breathe spontaneously
      in between synchronized mechanical breaths.

Pressure support ventilation (PSV) + SIMV

↑___↑ Patient triggers positive pressure support
      during inspiration of spontaneous breath - -
      in between SIMV mechanical breaths.

Time

FIGURE 20–20   Representation of different ventilator modes.

20

Pressure Support Ventilation: A preset level of positive pressure is turned on only during the inspiratory phase and is turned off during expiration. The patient controls the rate and inspiratory time while augmenting tidal volume and inspiratory flow. The higher the pressure support, the less work the patient expends to take a breath. Thus, PSV is comfortable because the patient has more control of his or her ventilation. PSV serves as an ideal weaning mode because the pressure can be turned down slowly, with changes as small as 1 cm H_2O. This allows the patient to assume the workload of breathing in small increments. PSV is often integrated with SIMV as a backup to ensure a minimum minute ventilation.

Positive End-Expiratory Pressure: Positive pressure applied during expiration. It represents the supraatmospheric pressure remaining in the airways at the end of expiration. PEEP increases alveolar ventilation by preventing small airway collapse, thereby increasing FRC. PEEP also is often used prophylactically against atelectasis, particularly in the postoperative period. It has become a standard modality to treat pulmonary edema. Increasing levels of PEEP is typically used to decrease the Fio_2, in an attempt to limit oxygen toxicity. One disadvantage of PEEP, however, is that it may decrease the cardiac index by decreasing left ventricular end-diastolic volume and should be used cautiously in patients at risk for myocardial ischemia.

Pressure Regulated Volume Control: This mode of ventilation is used in the setting of increased airway pressure. A microprocessor in the ventilator adjusts the pressure needed to achieve the proper tidal volume.

Continuous Positive Airway Pressure: Positive pressure throughout inspiration and expiration without mechanical assistance during ventilation. This is equivalent to PS plus PEEP at a constant pressure level. The patient does all the breathing on his or her own. Often used as a last step before extubation. A CPAP trial may be performed at room air or an Fio_2 of 40%. (See the discussion on extubation-weaning trials page 427.)

High-Frequency Ventilation: The physiologic explanation of HFV defies conventional teaching and is under current study. Despite the marked reduction in flow rates, oxygenation and CO_2 exchange are still achieved. HFV may be ideally suited to treat such conditions as bronchopleural fistulas or may serve as a more desirable form of ventilation during surgeries requiring a minimum of lung movement.

Ventilator Management

Ventilator Orders

Once the decision has been made to place a patient on a ventilator, the patient must be intubated with an appropriate endotracheal tube (see Chapter 13, page 268). The following is a sample of typical initial ventilator orders for an adult:

- Mode (ie, AC, SIMV)
- Fio_2 30–100%
- Rate 8–12/min
- Tidal volume 5–7 mL/kg
- Pressure support (level depends on the clinical situation)
- PEEP (5 cm H_2O or higher, if needed)

Ventilator Setting Changes

The following four **basic** respiratory parameters can be changed to improve ventilation, oxygenation, and compliance, and to prevent ventilator induced lung injury:

20

- Fio_2
- Minute volume (tidal volume X rate)
- Pressure support
- PEEP

1. **Fio_2.** Initially, an Fio_2 that ensures a saturation (Sao_2) >90% is set on the ventilator. Once adequate oxygenation is established, the Fio_2 is decreased to avoid oxygen toxicity. Because of the danger of oxygen toxicity, an Fio_2 >50% is to be avoided. Increasing the level of PEEP is often a helpful means of decreasing the Fio_2 requirement while maintaining adequate oxygenation.

2. **Minute volume.** Adjust to maintain Pco_2 within a normal range (35–45 mm Hg). Usually done by increasing tidal volume. Changes in rate are usually limited by a decrease in Pco_2, with a resultant respiratory alkalosis.

3. **Pressure support.** After the patient's respiratory pattern is established on SIMV, pressure support may be added initially at a level of 5–8 cm H_2O. Pressure support may then be turned up to a level that allows the patient to breathe at a comfortable rate (eg, <30 bpm). Depending on the stability and mental status of the patient, the number of SIMV backup breaths may be turned down to allow the patient more control of his or her ventilation. PS rarely needs to be turned up beyond 35 cm H_2O.

4. **PEEP.** Added to decrease Fio_2 while maintaining Pao_2. Five centimeters of PEEP is considered physiologic and is often enough to stabilize the Po_2. If the patient continues to deteriorate, PEEP is added in 2- to 3-cm increments until oxygenation is improved. This usually is at a level of 10–12 cm. Serial measurements of compliance are made to confirm improvement in pulmonary mechanics.

High-Dose PEEP. If additional PEEP is required, a pulmonary artery catheter is essential to monitor cardiac output, mixed venous saturation, pulmonary artery pressures, and the shunt fraction. Static pulmonary compliance and oxygen saturation are also followed. At high levels of PEEP, intrathoracic pressure increases to a point that **venous return is impaired.** Thus, left ventricular end-diastolic volume decreases along with cardiac output. This point defines the maximum level of PEEP and may vary considerably from patient to patient or for the same patient over time.

PEEP Side Effects

- Falsely elevated PAOP (PCWP)
- Decreased cardiac output
- Barotrauma (pneumothorax, alveolar rupture, pneumomediastinum)

Ventilator Weaning: Prior to the successful weaning of a patient from the ventilator, assess the patient's pulmonary mechanics and oxygenation. Additionally, the major problem that required the patient be placed on mechanical ventilation must have been corrected.

Pulmonary Mechanics. These provide useful information regarding a patient's ability to perform the work of respiration. Routine pulmonary mechanics consist of:

- Vital capacity
- Tidal volume
- Spontaneous respiratory rate
- Lung compliance
- Inspiratory force

Inspiratory Force. The maximum negative pressure that can be exerted against a completely closed airway. A function of respiratory muscle strength. An inspiratory force between 0 and –25 would indicate that the patient is incapable of generating adequate inspiratory effort to allow extubation.

Criteria for Weaning. These are based on the assessment of pulmonary mechanics and of oxygenation (Table 20–8).

Checklist for Weaning

- Correction of primary problem (eg, pneumonia has been treated, hemodynamic stability)
- Level of consciousness stable or improving
- Stable vital signs
- Respiratory rate <30
- Blood gases in the vicinity of:

$$Sao_2 > 90\%$$
$$Pao_2 > 70 \text{ mm Hg}$$
$$Pco_2 < 55 \text{ mm Hg}$$
$$pH > 7.35$$

- Vital capacity >15 mL/kg
- Tidal volume in adults (50–70 kg) >400 mL
- Inspiratory force > –30 cm H_2O

Weaning Modes. Modern respirators are designed to facilitate weaning. Once the preceding criteria have been met, a ventilator mode appropriate to the clinical situation, such as SIMV or PSV, is usually selected. SIMV and PSV are considered weaning modes because the patient is allowed to assume more of the workload of breathing as mechanical support is withdrawn.

Extubation Trials. Once weaning has achieved minimal ventilatory settings, various trials off mechanical support (while still intubated) may be attempted. **CPAP trials** with 5 cm of positive pressure is the most commonly used. For example, a 5-cm CPAP trial with

TABLE 20–8
Criteria for Weaning from Mechanical Ventilation

Parameter	Value
Pulmonary mechanics	
Vital capacity	>10–15 mL/kg
Resting minute ventilation	<10 L/min
(tidal volume × rate)	
Spontaneous respiratory rate	<30 breaths/min
Lung compliance	>100 mL/cm H20
Negative inspiratory forces (NIF)	> –25 cm H_2O
Oxygenation	
A-a gradient	<300–500 mm Hg
Shunt fraction	<15%
PO_2 (on 40% FiO_2)	>70 mm Hg
P_{CO_2}	<45 mm Hg

an Fio_2 at 21% (room air) or 40% should result in a Pao_2 of >50 mm Hg or 70 mm Hg, respectively. **T-piece trials,** which provide only humidified air with no pressure, are also occasionally used, but may be unnecessarily stressful to the patient. CPAP is thought to be more physiologic because positive pressure partially counterbalances the added resistance encountered by breathing through a long, narrow ET tube. These trials may vary in duration from 30 min to several hours and are used primarily as the last test prior to extubation. Patients without COPD are usually capable of going from IMV-4, Fio_2 30%, and PEEP of 5 cm H_2O to an extubation trial. The ventilator remains at the bedside in case respiratory support needs to be restarted.

Order of Weaning. The following steps are taken routinely:

1. Sequentially reduce Fio_2 by 10% until an Fio_2 of 50% is tolerated. Use pulse oximetry (Sao_2) to assist in weaning because it reduces the number of ABGs needed. Fio_2 can be decreased as long as Sao_2 >90–92% or Pao_2 >70 mm Hg.
2. Sequentially reduce the IMV rate to a level of 4 breaths per minute. Add pressure support to maintain adequate minute volume. ABGs as well as capnography are used to monitor for hypercarbia.
3. Sequentially reduce PEEP in 2- to 3-cm H_2O increments while maintaining Sao_2 >90%, until a level of 5 cm H_2O is achieved. Follow Fio_2. If a PA catheter is present, mixed venous saturation information will allow for calculation of the shunt equation. Qs/Qt should be kept below 0.25.
4. Sequentially reduce pressure support by 2- to 3-cm H_2O increments, maintaining minute volume until a pressure support of 5 cm H_2O is met. Monitor respiratory rate, work of breathing, and Pco_2.

Essential Tips in Ventilator Management

- Avoid changing more than one ventilator parameter at a time.
- A Po_2 <60 or an Sao_2 <90% requires a return to previous levels of respiratory support.
- A Po_2 of 60–70 or an Sao_2 of 90% requires a hold at the current level of respiratory support.
- A Po_2 >70 or an Sao_2 ≥92% allows for progression of weaning.

Extubation: A patient who is able to maintain a Po_2 >70, a Pco_2 <45, and a respiratory rate <25 for 1–2 h on a T piece or CPAP trial is ready for extubation.

1. Disconnect the ET tube from the ventilator or T piece.
2. Suction the patient's endotracheal tube and oral pharynx.
3. Deflate the endotracheal balloon.
4. Have the patient take a deep breath.
5. As the patient expires forcefully, remove the tube and clean any secretions.
6. Apply nasal cannula at 2–4 L/min.
7. Check postextubation blood gases.

SPECIFIC PROBLEMS IN CRITICALLY ILL PATIENTS

Adult Respiratory Distress Syndrome

ARDS, also called "wet lung" or "shock lung," is respiratory failure associated with acute pulmonary injury manifested by marked respiratory distress and hypoxia. Pulmonary capillary membranes become more permeable, resulting in pulmonary edema in the setting of low to normal pulmonary artery pressures.

Clinical Criteria for the Diagnosis of ARDS

- PaO_2: FiO_2 ratio of < 200
- Recent diffuse bilateral panlobar infiltrates on chest x-ray
- Pulmonary wedge pressure (PAOP) <18
- Lack of an alternative clinical explanation for pulmonary findings

Etiology

The cause of ARDS is multifactorial. There are three primary mechanisms of injury:

1. **Increased pulmonary vascular resistance.** Neurogenic pulmonary edema is caused by a dramatic increase in pulmonary capillary hydrostatic pressure. This increase forces fluid across the capillary membrane and results in interstitial and then alveolar edema.

2. **Permeability edema.** Circulating toxic substances within the bloodstream can cause the pulmonary capillary membrane to become leaky and allow extravasation of protein into the interstitial space. This extravasation increases the interstitial hydrostatic pressure and eventually results in injury to the alveolar membrane. At this point, fluid and protein migrate into the alveolar space and directly impede oxygen exchange. Several factors have been implicated as mediators to this increased capillary–alveolar permeability, including prostaglandins and oxygen radicals. Sepsis is often the primary cause.

3. **Injury to the alveolar membrane.** Conditions directly toxic to the alveolar membrane include

   - Smoke inhalation
   - High doses of oxygen (>60% FiO_2)
   - Aspiration

Treatment

Primary efforts are directed at treating the underlying condition while providing sufficient pulmonary support. Currently, no specific therapy is available for ARDS.

1. **Aggressive ventilatory support.** Use PEEP to maintain the FiO_2 <0.6 while maintaining a PO_2 >70 mm Hg. Use the PaO_2, volume status, and level of PEEP to guide ventilatory management. Although some may advocate increased levels of PEEP to minimize intrapulmonary shunting (Qs/Qt) without regard to PaO_2, doing so may necessitate increased intravascular volume and inotropic support of the heart. Many clinicians recommend using PaO_2 as a guide to increasing PEEP, rather than following the shunt fraction specifically.

2. **Aggressive fluid administration.** Maintain cardiac output and peripheral perfusion. The use of colloid versus crystalloid remains controversial. Many clinicians recommend the use of crystalloid (NS, lactated Ringer's) and blood to maintain the hematocrit above 30–35%.

3. **Aggressive monitoring.** Use a PA catheter to guide fluid administration (by following filling pressures), and observe the effect of added PEEP on cardiac output. Inotropic agents may be indicated if cardiac output remains low despite adequate filling pressures. Use an arterial line to obtain arterial blood for frequent ABG determinations.

4. **Pulmonary toilet.** To manage secretions

5. **Chest x-rays.** To monitor lung status

6. Watch for associated DIC (see page 434).

7. Steroids are not indicated in the treatment of ARDS.

20

Clinical Correlations

ARDS should be anticipated in the following clinical situations:

- Severe head injury
- Severe trauma with prolonged hypotension
- Massive fluid resuscitation
- Sepsis
- Necrotizing pancreatitis
- Burn of the respiratory tract or aspiration
- Severe chest contusion

Shock

(See also Algorithm, Chapter 21, page 460.)

Shock is inadequate tissue perfusion, and is a syndrome with several possible causes. All four of these have in common a resultant poor perfusion of tissues that leads to tissue injury and death if untreated. The most common classification is based on etiology and includes hypovolemic, cardiogenic, septic, and neurogenic types. Treatment of shock is *always* directed at treatment of the underlying problem, maximizing cardiac performance to restore tissue perfusion, and maintaining essential physiologic support to keep oxygenation and renal function as normal as possible.

Hypovolemic Shock: Caused by inadequate circulating blood volume

Physiology. Low cardiac output, low wedge pressure, elevated peripheral vascular resistance as a result of reflex vasoconstriction

Therapy

1. Correct source of blood loss (hemorrhage).
2. Replete intravascular volume with packed cells, isotonic crystalloid fluids (normal saline, lactated Ringer's), or colloid.

Cardiogenic Shock: Caused by primary "pump" failure

Physiology. Low cardiac output, high wedge pressure resulting from fluid accumulation in the pulmonary capillary bed, elevated peripheral vascular resistance

Therapy. Directed at improving cardiac performance

1. Optimize filling pressures (preload).
2. Decrease afterload (vasodilation with nitroglycerin, nitroprusside, etc).
3. Improve contractility (dobutamine).

Septic Shock: Decreased peripheral (systemic) resistance as a result of massive infection

Physiology. High cardiac output (until late stages), low wedge pressure, low peripheral vascular resistance

Therapy

1. Treat the cause of sepsis (parenteral antibiotics, drainage of abscess).
2. Administer fluids to increase filling pressures.
3. Increase vascular resistance (pressors such as dopamine).
4. Provide inotropic support of the heart as needed.

Neurogenic Shock: Caused by loss of sympathetic vascular tone (eg, cord injury)

Physiology. Low cardiac output, low wedge pressure, low peripheral vascular resistance

Therapy. Optimize filling pressures, increase peripheral vascular resistance (norepinephrine, phenylephrine).

20

Acute Renal Failure

Many patients in the ICU are unable to receive oral nutrition or fluid. Therefore, particular attention must be paid to fluid and electrolyte requirements in the critically ill patient. The following data provide useful information:

- **Urine output.** One of the best and simplest parameters for following fluid balance.
- **Daily weight.** Because daily changes in weight are mostly the result of loss or gain of fluid.
- **Pulmonary artery catheter data.** In a critically ill patient in whom the fluid status is not discernible, a PA catheter can be placed to determine intravascular fluid status.

Oliguria and Progressive Azotemia: These conditions are the final result of a number of pathologic processes that constitute **acute renal failure.** Once recognized, the primary goal of the clinician is to identify the cause and treat the underlying condition. To simplify the multitude of causes, renal failure is usually divided into **prerenal, renal,** and **postrenal** causes. These are outlined in Chapter 6.

Acute tubular necrosis. (eg. Nephrotoxic medications, ischemia), intravascular volume depletion, and congestive heart failure are the most common causes of renal failure in the ICU patient.

The following outline describes the general approach to the problem of oliguria or anuria in an ICU patient.

Physical Examination

1. **Vital signs.** Hypotension with or without associated tachycardia can be a sign of hypovolemia, indicating prerenal causes of oliguria. Orthostatic blood changes also point to hypovolemia.
2. **Mucous membranes.** Dry mucous membranes indicate overall fluid depletion.
3. **Lungs.** Fluid overload often manifests itself as pulmonary edema, often heard when auscultating the chest.
4. **Abdomen.** Low urine output may result from postrenal obstruction, which may be manifest as bladder distention, palpable on examination. Bladder palpation may cause pain, also indicating distention. A distended abdomen may indicate ileus with associated fluid sequestration in the bowel.
5. **Extremities.** Fluid overload may be evident as peripheral edema.

Diagnostic Studies

1. **Laboratory results**
2. **Bladder catheterization.** If a catheter is in place, irrigate it gently to confirm proper drainage.
3. **Radiographic.** Renal ultrasonography helps evaluate for possible postrenal obstruction. Avoid intravenous contrast studies if possible.

Therapeutic trials. These can be used as an adjunct to differentiate prerenal from renal azotemia. After obstruction has been ruled out, failure to respond to these measures with increased urine flow most likely indicates an intrinsic renal cause of azotemia. Furosemide has little effect in ATN.

20

- Fluid challenge (1000 mL of NS infusion, rapid)
- Furosemide 80 mg IV push
- Mannitol 25 g IV
- Dopamine infusion

Management. As a general approach, daily intake and output should be closely reviewed, and daily weights are very useful. Follow electrolytes, particularly potassium, closely. Many clinicians remove potassium from the IV fluids immediately in cases of renal failure to prevent accumulation of deadly potassium levels.

Prerenal

1. Optimize hemodynamic status to maximize cardiac output and, hence, renal perfusion.
2. Replete fluids. Use blood in anemic patients; otherwise, use isotonic fluid or albumin.
3. Once you are sure that fluid status is optimal and urine output is still suboptimal, use low-dose dopamine (2–5 mg/kg/min) to dilate the renal vessels. A PA catheter is usually needed to monitor the patient at this point.

Renal

1. Optimize fluid status, keeping cardiac filling pressures in the normal range.
2. Try furosemide (20–40 µg) once fluid status is optimal.
3. If there is no response to furosemide, try mannitol 12.5–25 g IV.
4. Metolazone can be given if there is still no response (5–10 mg PO).
5. If the patient is fluid-overloaded, use furosemide in increasing doses to diurese fluid.
6. Restrict fluids, salt, and particularly potassium.
7. Treat the usual metabolic acidosis with sodium bicarbonate.
8. Dialysis may be necessary.

Postrenal

1. Check the Foley catheter for patency, replacing it immediately if there is any question.
2. Obtain a urologic consultation. Prostatic obstruction in men can be easily corrected with a Foley catheter. Decompression of the upper urinary tracts may require stents or percutaneous drainage.

Stress Ulceration

The development of stress ulceration in the ICU patient is a serious complication. Most importantly, it is a largely preventable problem. It is common in neurosurgical (**Cushing's ulcers**) and burn (**Curling's ulcers**) patients. The pathophysiology is related to diminished blood flow to the viscera in stress situations, leading to alterations in the mucosal barrier to the effects of gastric acid.

Prophylaxis

- Routine cardiovascular support of perfusion
- Routine use of H_2 blockers (Pepcid, etc)
- Antacid administration (eg, Maalox 30 mL per NG tube q2h). In patients with renal failure, use aluminum hydroxide, avoid magnesium-containing antacids
- Enteral feedings, when tolerated, remain a good method to neutralize gastric acid.

Treatment of Ulceration

1. Early endoscopy is indicated in upper GI bleeding.
2. A clearly visible lesion (bleeding vessel) warrants operative intervention, but diffuse gastritis is best treated initially with aggressive antacid and H_2 blocker therapy. Persistent bleeding from gastritis may warrant total gastrectomy.

20

Acalculous Cholecystitis

Cholecystitis in the absence of stones is not uncommon in the ICU patient, and is probably related to diminished blood flow in the critically ill patient, although the exact pathophysiology remains unclear. First and foremost in the treatment of this potentially fatal condition is to remain vigilant for its development in the critically ill patient. Presenting signs are similar to those in healthy patients with cholecystitis and include right upper quadrant pain, fever, leukocytosis, and elevated liver chemistries (especially bilirubin or alkaline phosphatase). The most valuable test is an HIDA scan. Nonvisualization of the gallbladder is clear evidence of cholecystitis. Treatment is surgical (cholecystectomy), and should be done as early as possible to avoid perforation.

Nutrition

The nutritional needs of the critically ill patient are of major significance in overall patient care. Restoring the patient to an anabolic state will hasten recovery. The details of TPN, or hyperalimentation, as well as enteral feedings are covered in Chapters 11 and 12. Remember the following two rules:

1. The "5-day" rule applies to most patients. If you do not think the critically ill patient can take nutrition for 5 days because of postoperative ileus, intubation, etc, be sure to start nutritional support by the fifth day.
2. "If the gut works, use it." That is, do not use parenteral nutrition if the GI tract is functioning. Enteral nutrition (eg, oral, NG tube, jejunostomy tube) should be used in all patients with a functioning intestinal tract. The enteral feeding is reviewed in Chapter 11.

Disseminated Intravascular Coagulation

DIC is a complex management problem that often presents in the critically ill patient. This clinical syndrome may accompany a number of disease states, including shock syndromes, sepsis, malignancy, and some obstetric conditions. As with many of the pathologic conditions that accompany major illness (eg, ARDS), the successful treatment of DIC depends on treating the **underlying condition.**

Diagnosis: The diagnosis of DIC is usually contemplated in the critically ill patient who develops thrombocytopenia, and occasionally an elevated PT. The following list details other laboratory findings that are caused by the effect of plasmin on fibrinogen. They result in increased levels of fibrin monomers and feedback stimulation of the fibrinolytic system, yielding fibrin degradation products *and* increased plasmin formation.

- Low fibrinogen level
- Elevated FSP level
- Elevated PTT
- Microangiopathic RBC morphology

Treatment: The treatment of this disease is controversial.

1. The most important element of therapy is to identify and treat the underlying cause.
2. Treat associated shock appropriately to maintain cardiovascular stability.
3. If there is evidence of thrombosis (eg, PE), begin heparin therapy with a loading dose of 100 U/kg followed by a drip at 10–15 U/kg/h (see Chapter 22).
4. Administer FFP to replenish fibrinogen.

5. If the patient is bleeding severely, despite replacement therapy with FFP and platelets, begin antifibrinolytic therapy with epsilon–aminocaproic acid (Amicar). Use a loading dose of 4 g, followed by 1 g/h, for a total of 12 g. In general, if there is no improvement after 12 h, therapy should be stopped.

Line Sepsis

Indwelling catheters not only provide a convenient means of infusing fluids and medications, but also act as a portal of entry for bacteria. With the widespread use of indwelling intravenous catheters (eg, central venous lines), the diagnosis of infection from the catheter itself must be considered when evaluating a febrile patient in the ICU. As a general rule, fever in a person with a central line should be attributed to the line until proven otherwise.

The most common mechanism of line sepsis is entry of skin flora along the catheter tract. The use of clear polyurethane dressings left in place for prolonged periods has been associated with increased risk of infection and should be avoided. Some institutions have a policy of routine line changes, over a guidewire, every 3–4 d. Little objective data support this practice; in fact, some evidence suggests that this practice is associated with an increased rate of complications. Prevention of line sepsis is best accomplished by meticulous aseptic technique during placement and meticulous care of the line once in place.

Treatment: A presumed episode of line sepsis is treated by determining whether the line is actually responsible. Erythema at the entry site may suggest the cause. Short-term central venous catheters that may be infected are best treated by removing the line. The catheter may be changed over a guidewire, but some centers do not advocate this practice. Cultures of the intracutaneous segment are essential.

In the absence of florid sepsis, or if placement of a new line would jeopardize the ability to obtain vascular access, then quantitative cultures of blood from a peripheral site and the line may be obtained and treatment may be based on the results of these cultures, once available. Empiric antimicrobial therapy may be started in the interim. Using isolator tubes (Dupont), colony counts are performed 16–18 h after obtaining the culture. If the colony count from the catheter is equal to or greater than five times the count from the peripheral culture, the result is interpreted as probable catheter infection.

Pulmonary Embolism

PE is a major cause of death in the United States (approximately 150,000 deaths annually) and the world. Deep venous thrombosis is known to be responsible for a majority of PE in hospitalized patients. It is estimated that about 90% of all PE originate in the femoral–iliac–pelvic veins. DVT is caused by the classical causes of thromboses: vessel injury, hypercoagulability, or stasis.

Prevention of DVT: Prevention is especially important in "high-risk" patients (those with malignancy, obesity, previous history, age >40 years, extensive abdominal/pelvic surgery, immobilization). For patients undergoing surgery, prevention should be initiated in the operating room. Intermittent compression stockings and the selected use of heparin have greatly reduced the incidence of DVT in the postoperative patient. Remember that prophylaxis against DVT is effective **only when started preoperatively** for those patients undergoing surgery.

Physical Methods. These include leg elevation, intermittent compression devices, early postoperative ambulation.

Pharmacologic Methods

- Heparin 5000 U SQ q12h. Check the platelet count (eg, every 3 days) because of risk of thrombocytopenia.
- Coumadin for chronic therapy
- Enoxaparin is now the drug of choice in many institutions for high-risk patients, despite the high cost of therapy.

Diagnosis of Pulmonary Embolus

- Maintain a high index of suspicion.
- **Signs and symptoms.** *None* is diagnostic, but may include dyspnea, tachypnea, tachycardia, chest pain (usually pleuritic), Po_2 <80 (compare with baseline).
- Routine chest x-ray may show localized volume loss or **Hampton's hump** due to pulmonary infarction.
- **Nuclear V/Q scan.** A normal scan effectively rules out PE, and a positive scan is sufficient evidence to treat the patient. An indeterminate scan in a symptomatic patient with a high index of suspicion necessitates angiography.
- **Spiral CT scan.** This scan is helpful in identifying proximal pulmonary emboli.
- **Pulmonary angiogram.** The "gold standard."

Treatment

1. **Support oxygenation.** Monitor ABGs, and support as indicated. Intubation may be necessary.
2. **Use intravenous heparin.** Prevents clot propagation, decreases inflammation, and allows intrinsic fibrinolysis to lyse the clot.
   a. Bolus with 80–100 U/kg and start an intravenous drip at 10–15 U/kg/h. Adjust the drip to keep the PTT at 2–2.5 × control values. The half-life of heparin is 1.5 h, so check the PTT at 3–6 h after adjusting the rate of heparin administration.
   b. Monitor the platelet count because some patients can manifest "heparin-induced thrombocytopenia."
   c. Start oral warfarin (Coumadin) by day 7 of heparin therapy, to maintain a therapeutic ratio. (See Chapter 22, page 637.)
   d. In cases of massive embolus, thrombolytic therapy (streptokinase) can be used in the absence of contraindications.
   e. Open embolectomy, using cardiopulmonary bypass, has been effective in some cases of massive PE.
3. In patients who cannot undergo systemic anticoagulation (those with recent surgery, stroke, GI bleeding, etc) or patients with recurrent emboli despite adequate therapy, vena caval interruption may be indicated using an intracaval filter or a caval clip (placed transabdominally).

QUICK REFERENCE TO CRITICAL CARE/ICU FORMULAS

See Table 20–9

GUIDELINES FOR ADULT CRITICAL CARE DRUG INFUSIONS

See Table 20–10

TABLE 20-9
Quick Reference to Common ICU Equations

Determination	Derivation	Normal
RAP, CVP	Measured	2–10 mm Hg
RVP	Measured	15–30/0–5 mm Hg
PAS/PAD	Measured	15–30/8–15 mm Hg
PCWP	Measured	5–11 mm Hg
CO	Measured (CO = SV × HR)	3.5–5.5 L/min
CI	CO × BSA	2.8–4.2 L/min/m²
MAP	$DBP \times \dfrac{(SBP - DBP)}{3}$	85–90 mm Hg
MPAP	$PAD \times \dfrac{(PAS - PAD)}{3}$	11–18 mm Hg
SVR	$\dfrac{(MAP - CVP)}{CO} \times 80$	770–1500 dynes/s/cm⁵
PVR	$\dfrac{(MPAP - PCWP)}{CO} \times 80$	20–120 dynes/s/cm⁵
A–a gradient	$\left[(713 \times FiO_2 - \dfrac{(PaCO_2)}{0.8}) \right] - PaO_2$	Room air 2–22 mmHg 100% FiO_2 10–60 mmHg
CaO_2 (arterial O_2 content)	$(Hgb \times 1.39)\, SaO_2 + (PaO_2 \times 0.0031)$	16–22 mL O_2/dL blood
CvO_2 (mixed venous O_2 content)	$(Hgb \times 1.39)\, SvO_2 + (PvO_2 \times 0.0031)$	12–17 mL O_2/dL blood
$C(a\text{-}v)O_2$ (A–VO_2 difference)	$CaO_2 - CvO_2 = (Hgb \times 1.39)\,(SaO_2 - SvO_2)$	3.5–5.5 mL O_2/dL blood
O_2 carrying capacity	$Hgb \times SaO_2 \times CO \times 10$	700–1400 mL/min delivery

(continued)

20

437

TABLE 20-9
(Continued)

Determination	Derivation	Normal
O_2 consumption	$(CaO_2 - CvO_2) \times CO \times 10$	180–280 mL/min
Qs/Qt (shunt fraction)	$\dfrac{(CcO_2 - CvO_2) \times CO \times 10}{(CcO_2 - CvO_2)}$	0.05
ICP	Measured	0–20 mmHg
CPP	MAP – ICP	keep >70 mmHg

Abbreviations: RAP = right atrial pressures; CVP = central venous pressure; RVP = right ventricular pressure; PAS = pulmonary artery systolic; PAD = pulmonary artery diastolic; PCWP = pulmonary capillary wedge pressure; CO = cardiac output; CI = cardiac input; MAP = mean arterial pressure; MPAP = mean pulmonary artery pressure; SVR = systemic vascular resistance; PVR = pulmonary vascular resistance; ICP = intracranial pressure; CPP = cerebral perfusion pressure; FiO$_2$ = inhaled O$_2$; Hgb = hemoglobin; SaO$_2$ = arterial oxygen; BSA = body surface area; DBP = diastolic blood pressure; SBP = systolic blood pressure; FiO$_2$ = inhaled O$_2$; Hgb = hemoglobin; SaO$_2$ = arterial oxygen, SvO$_2$ = mixed venous oxygen saturation; Qs = volume of shunted blood (ie, blood shunted past nonventilated alveoli, not participating in gas exchange); Qt = total cardiac output; CcO$_2$ = O$_2$ content of alveolar-capillary blood; CvO$_2$ = mixed venous O$_2$ content of pulmonary artery blood.

TABLE 20-10
Guidelines for Adult Critical Care Drug Infusions*

Drug	Dilution	(Final Concentration) Flow Rate = mL/h	Usual Dose Range
Amrinone (Inocor)	$\dfrac{500 \text{ mg}}{250 \text{ mL}}$ (150 mL PSS+ 100 mL drug) PSS only	(2 mg/ml) 1500 µg/min = 45 1000 µg/min = 30 750 µg/min = 22.5 500 µg/min = 15 350 µg/min = 10.5	LD = 0.75 µg/kg MD = 5–20 µg/kg/min
Diliazem (Cardizem)	$\dfrac{125 \text{ mg}}{125 \text{ mL}}$ (100 mL diluent +25 mL drug) D_5W or PSS	(1 mg/ml) 5 mg/h = 5 10 mg/h = 10 15 mg/h = 15	Bolus = 0.25 mg/kg over 2 min; may give second bolus 0.35 mg/kg 15 min after initial bolus MD = 5–15 mg/h
Dobutamine (Dobutrex)	$\dfrac{500 \text{ mg}}{250 \text{ mL}}$	(2000 µg/ml) 1500 µg/min = 45	2.5–20 µg/kg/min

(continued)

20

TABLE 20–10
Continued

Drug	Dilution	(Final Concentration) Flow Rate = mL/h	Usual Dose Range
Dobutamine (continued)	D_5W or PSS	1250 µg/min = 37.5 1000 µg/min = 30 750 µg/min = 22.5 500 µg/min = 15 250 µg/min = 7.5	
Dopamine	$\frac{400 \text{ mg}}{250 \text{ mL}}$ D_5W or PSS	(1600 µg/ml) 1400 µg/min = 52.5 1200 µg/min = 45 1000 µg/min = 37.5 800 µg/min = 30 600 µg/min = 22.5 400 µg/min = 15 200 µg/min = 7.5	0.5–2.0 µg/kg/min (renal) 2.0–10 µg/kg/min (inotropic) 10–20 µg/kg/min (vasopressor)
Epinephrine	$\frac{3 \text{ mg}}{250 \text{ mL}}$ D_5W or PSS	(12 µg/ml) 4 µg/min = 20 3 µg/min = 15 2 µg/min = 10 1 µg/min = 5	Initially 1 µg/min Titrate to response
Esmolol (Brevibloc)	$\frac{5000 \text{ mg}}{500 \text{ mL}}$ D_5W or PSS	(10 mg/ml) 5000 µg/min = 30 4000 µg/min = 24 3000 µg/min = 18	LD = 500 µ/kg/min over 1 minute MD = 50 µ/kg/min, titrate to response. Increase by 50 µ/kg/min increments every 5 minutes

(continued)

TABLE 20-10
(Continued)

Drug	Dilution	(Final Concentration) Flow Rate = mL/h	Usual Dose Range
Isoproterenol (Isuprel)	2 mg 500 mL D$_5$W or PSS	(8 µg/mL) 10 µg/min = 75 6 µg/min = 45 4 µg/min = 30 2 µg/min = 15 1 µg/min = 7.5	Initially: 1–4 µg/min Titrate up to 20 µg/min
Labetalol (Trandate)	200 mg 200 mL (160 mL diluent +40 mL drug) D$_5$W or PSS	(1 mg/mL) 2 mg/min = 120	Bolus = 20 mg over 2 min Additional 20–80 mg may be given every 10 min until response or maximum of 300 mg **or** Initially 2 mg/min Titrate to response
Lidocaine (Xylocaine)	2 g 250 mL D$_5$W or PSS	(8 mg/mL) 4 mg/min = 30 3 mg/min = 22.5 2 mg/min = 15 1 mg/min = 7.5	LD = 1–1.5 mg/kg over 2 min MD = 1–4 mg/min Maximum 4 mg/min
Nicardipine (Cardene)	25 mg 250 mL	(0.1 mg/mL) 5 mg/h = 50 7.5 mg/h = 75	Initially: 5 mg/h Titrate to BP: increase rate by 2.5 mg/h every 5–15 min

(continued)

TABLE 20–10
(Continued)

Drug	Dilution	(Final Concentration) Flow Rate = mL/h	Usual Dose Range
Nicardipine (continued)	D_5W or PSS	10 mg/h = 100 12.5 mg/h = 125 15 mg/h = 150	Maximum: 15 mg/h MD 3 mg/h
Nitroglycerin (Tridil)	$\dfrac{100\ mg}{250\ mL}$ D_5W or PSS (glass bottle)	(400 µg/mL) 80 µg/min = 12 60 µg/min = 9 40 µg/min = 6 20 µg/min = 3 10 µg/min = 1.5	Initially 5–10 µg/min Titrate up by 10–20 µg/min every 5 min based on current dose and patient condition
Nitroprusside (Nipride)	$\dfrac{100\ mg}{250\ mL}$ D_5W	(400 µg/mL) 300 µg/min = 45 200 µg/min = 30 150 µg/min = 22.5 100 µg/min = 15 70 µg/min = 10.5 50 µg/min = 7.5	Initially: 0.3–0.5 µg/kg/min Titrate to response every few minutes Maximum: 10 µg/kg/min
Norepinephrine (Levophed)	$\dfrac{4\ mg}{250\ mL}$ D_5W or PSS	(16 µg/mL) 12 µg/min = 45 8 µg/min = 30 6 µg/min = 22.5 4 µg/min = 15 2 µg/min = 7.5	Initially: 8–12 µg/min Titrate to response

(continued)

TABLE 20-10 (Continued)

Drug	Dilution	(Final Concentration) Flow Rate = mL/h	Usual Dose Range
Phenylephrine (Neo-Synephrine)	$\dfrac{50\ mg}{250\ mL}$ D₅W or PSS	(200 μg/mL) 100 μg/min = 30 80 μg/min = 24 60 μg/min = 18 50 μg/min = 15	Initially: 10–50 μg/min Titrate to response
Procainamide (Procan)	$\dfrac{2\ g}{250\ mL}$ D₅W or PSS	(8 mg/mL) 4 mg/min = 30 3 mg/min = 22.5 2 mg/min = 15 1 mg/min = 7.5	LD = 17 mg/kg over 1 h, or 100 mg every 5 min up to 1 g MD = 1–4 mg/min
Vasopressin (Pitressin)	$\dfrac{100\ units}{250\ mL}$ D₅W or PSS	(0.4 units/mL) 0.4 units/min = 60 0.3 units/min = 45 0.2 units/min = 30 0.1 units/min = 15	0.1–0.4 units/min Maximum 0.9 units/min

Abbreviation: LD = loading dose; MD = maintenance dose; BP = blood pressure; PSS = physiologic saline solution; D₅W = dextrose 5% in water

*These agents must be administered in the appropriately monitored clinical setting.

Source: Reprinted, with permission, from Thomas Jefferson University Pharmacy and Therapeutic Committee, Philadelphia, PA.

20

21

EMERGENCIES

Cardiopulmonary Resuscitation
Advanced Cardiac Life Support
and Emergency Cardiac Care*
Advanced Cardiac Life Support
Drugs

Electrical Defibrillation
and Cardioversion
Other Common Emergencies

CARDIOPULMONARY RESUSCITATION

Emergency cardiac care guidelines from the American Heart Association now recommend that health care providers have the following items readily available: gloves, a barrier device or bag mask, and an automated defibrillator to handle cardiac emergencies. In cardiopulmonary resuscitation, remember there are now **two** sets of **ABCDs:**

Primary Survey

- **A**irway: Assess and manage noninvasively.
- **B**reathing: Use positive pressure ventilations.
- **C**irculation: Perform chest compressions as needed.
- **D**efibrillation: Assess for VT/VF and defibrillate using an AED. These are also called PADs and are becoming widely available in public areas such as airports, stadiums, health clubs, and shopping malls.

Secondary Survey: Uses advanced medical techniques

- **A**irway: Assess and manage with airway device (eg, endotracheal intubation, etc).
- **B**reathing: Verify tube function and placement, use positive pressure ventilation system through tube.
- **C**irculation: Start IV, attach ECG, use rhythm-based ACLS medications.
- **D**ifferential Diagnosis: Search for, find, and treat problems according to AHA algorithms presented in this chapter.

Adult CPR

(Victim's age ≥8 y)

One Rescuer

1. Determine unresponsiveness (shake and shout). If the patient is unresponsive, call for help (activate EMS system, eg, call "code," dial 911). In trauma situation do not move

---

* The section on basis CPR and ACLS are based on guidelines from the American Heart Association and the International Liaison Committee on Resuscitation [*Circulation* 2000;**102** (Sup 1)] and the Guidelines 2000 for Cardiopulmonary Resuscitation and Emergency Cardiovascular Care by the American Heart Association in Collaboration with the International Liaison Committee on Resuscitation (ILCOR).

the victim unless in immediate danger. Roll victim on to back as a unit if lying face down. Protect the neck.

2. Kneel at the level of the victim's shoulder. Open the airway (head-tilt, chin-lift,), determine breathlessness ("**look** [chest movement], **listen** [for air escaping], **feel** [for air movement]") for no more than 10 s. In the unresponsive victim with spontaneous respiration, place the victim in the recovery position. Jaw thrust maneuver recommended as alternative for health care providers especially if neck injury is suspected. If the victim is breathing, place in the **RECOVERY POSITION** (see page 449).

3. If not breathing, give patient two slow ventilations (2 s/inspiration) while maintaining airway. Use pocket mask or bag mask. Volume should be between 0.8–1.2 L. A barrier device (face shield or mask with one-way valve) is recommended if mouth-to-mouth or mouth-to-nose contact is necessary. Ventilate 10–12 breaths/min. If unable to ventilate, reposition head and try again. If unsuccessful, perform the **FOREIGN BODY OB-STRUCTION AIRWAY SEQUENCE** (see page 448).

4. Check for circulation (breathing, coughing, movement). Palpate the carotid artery no more than 10 s to determine lack of a pulse. If pulse is present, perform rescue breathing: 1 ventilation every 5 s (10–12 ventilation/min).

5. If no pulse, use four cycles of 15 compressions and two ventilations (compression rate 100/min, two ventilations 1.5–2 s each). Depth of compression 1.5–2 in. or slightly greater to generate carotid pulse. Apply compressions to lower half of sternum using the heels of both hands placed on top of each other.

6. After the four cycles (approximately 1 min of CPR), pause and check for return pulse and spontaneous respirations.

7. If no pulse or respiration, resume cycles with two ventilations, then compressions, as noted earlier.

8. Incorporate appropriate ACLS management guidelines.

Two-Rescuer Adult CPR
For laypersons

1. Second rescuer identifies him or herself. Verify that EMS has been notified. If so, second rescuer gets into position opposite first rescuer. If EMS not notified, the second rescuer does so before assisting first rescuer.

2. First rescuer continues CPR.

3. If and when first rescuer tires, second rescuer takes over one-person CPR as described in the preceding section.

For health care professionals

1. Sequence to continue from one-rescuer CPR as mentioned in previous section. Second rescuer identifies him or herself and gets into position for compressions.

2. First rescuer completes compression and ventilation cycle (15 compression and two ventilations).

3. First rescuer then checks for spontaneous pulse and breathing, states: "No pulse...continue CPR," then ventilate once (1.5–2 s).

4. Second rescuer resumes compressions at same rate of 80–100/min.("1 & 2 & 3 & 4 & 5 & pause," ventilate) Ratio of five compressions to one breath. If airway is protected, do not pause for ventilations.

5. When ready to switch, rescuer doing compressions says "switch & 2 & 3 & 4 & 5 &."

6. Both rescuers change position simultaneously immediately after ventilation.

7. Rescuer who will perform ventilations opens airway and performs a 5-s pulse check.

8. If no pulse, give ventilation. Rescuer states "No pulse...continue CPR."

9. In patient with unprotected airway, cricoid pressure may be applied (Sellick's maneuver) by a third rescuer (if health care professional) to help limit gastric distention.

Child CPR
(Victim's age 1–8 y)

1. Determine unresponsiveness, and shout for help. Activate EMS system (call code or 911).
2. Open airway (head-tilt, chin-lift; jaw thrust if neck trauma is suspected), determine breathlessness (follow "look, listen, feel" rubric as for adult). If victim is breathing, place in **RECOVERY POSITION** (see page 449).
3. If victim not breathing, give two ventilations (1–1.5 s). If unable to ventilate, perform the **FOREIGN BODY OBSTRUCTED AIRWAY SEQUENCE** (see page 448).
4. Check for circulation (breathing, coughing, movement). Palpate the carotid artery for no more than 10 s to determine presence of a pulse. If pulse is present, perform rescue breathing using pocket mask or bag-mask device (20 breaths/min).
5. If no pulse, or if pulse is <60 bpm and perfusion is poor, begin cardiac compressions at five compressions to one ventilation at rate of 100/min. Depth of compressions less than for an adult (1–1.5 in. or one third to one half the depth of chest).Use the heel of one hand at the lower half of the sternum. Pause compressions for ventilations until patient is intubated.
6. Check for return of pulse and spontaneous breathing after 20 cycles (approximately 1 min).
7. Resume cycles with one ventilation (1–1.5 s each), then resume compressions.

Infant CPR
(Victim's age, ≤1 y)

1. Determine unresponsiveness, and shout for help. Activate EMS system (call code or 911).
2. Open airway (head-tilt, chin-lift). Do not hyperextend head; however, create adequate head-tilt to accomplish chest rise with breath. If neck trauma suspected, use jaw thrust. If victim is breathing, place in **RECOVERY POSITION** (see page 449).
3. If patient is not breathing, give two ventilations (1–1.5 s) using pocket mask or bag-mask device. If unable to ventilate, perform the **FOREIGN BODY OBSTRUCTED AIRWAY SEQUENCE** using back blows and chest thrusts as noted on page 448.
4. Check for circulation (breathing, coughing, movement). Palpate the femoral or brachial artery for no more than 10 s to determine presence of a pulse. If pulse is present, continue rescue breathing (20 breaths/min).
5. If no pulse or if pulse is <60 bpm and perfusion is poor, begin cardiac compressions. Draw an imaginary line between the nipples and identify where this line crosses the sternum (intermammary line). The site of compression is one finger breadth below this intersection. Use a compression depth of ½–1 in., using the middle and ring fingers. Use five compressions to one ventilation (rate of compression is 100/min or 120 min for newborns).
6. Use the mnemonic: ("1 & 2 & 3 & 4 & 5 & pause, head-tilt, chin-lift, ventilate–continue compressions"). When patient is intubated, no need to pause.
7. Check for return of pulse and spontaneous breathing after 20 cycles (1 min).

Neonatal CPR

1. The newborn should be dried, placed head down, gently suctioned and stimulated.
2. Supplemental oxygen is useful. If baby is not breathing, ventilate 40–60 breaths/min with gentle puff of air or with bag mask.

21

3. Check apical pulse. If absent or if <60 bpm and perfusion is poor, compress at a rate of 120/min. Wrap your hands around infant's chest and compress ½–¾ in. with thumbs side by side at the midsternum.
4. The compression/ventilation ratio is 3:1 for intubated newborn with two rescuers. Discontinue compressions when rate reaches 80 bpm or greater.

Foreign Body Obstructed Airway Sequence

Adult (≥8) and Child (1–8 y)

A. **Conscious victim *can* cough, speak, breath.** Do not interfere and reassure patient. Stand by and allow patient to clear partial obstruction.
B. **Conscious victim *cannot* cough, speak, breath.**
   1. Ask "Are you choking" or "Can you speak?" Observe for "universal distress signal" for choking (hands clutched at neck).
   2. Give abdominal thrusts/Heimlich maneuver. Stand behind victim. Using arms wrapped around victim, place thumb side of fist above umbilicus but below xiphoid. Give up to five subdiaphragmatic thrusts (Heimlich maneuver).
   3. Reassess victim's status, repeat Heimlich maneuvers as needed. If not improved by 1 min, activate EMS.
C. **Victim becomes unconscious.**
   1. Place in supine (face up) position. Activate EMS or if second rescuer becomes available have that person activate EMS.
   2. Open airway with tongue-jaw lift; finger sweep to clear airway, open airway (head-tilt, chin-lift).
   3. Give five abdominal thrusts/Heimlich maneuver astride victim.
D. **Victim found unconscious: Cause unknown**
   1. Determine unresponsiveness, call for help (activate EMS).
   2. Open airway (head-tilt, chin-lift), determine breathlessness (look, listen, feel).
   3. Attempt to ventilate. If unsuccessful, reposition head and reattempt.
   4. If unsuccessful:
      a. Perform up to five Heimlich maneuvers astride victim.
      b. Open mouth (tongue-jaw lift); finger sweep; open airway (head-tilt, chin-lift)
   5. Attempt to ventilate, if unsuccessful, repeat sequence until ventilations are effective.

Infant
(Victim's age, <1 y)

Victim conscious

1. Verify airway obstruction (ineffective cough, no strong cry).
2. Hold child with head lower than body, give five back blows or five gentle abdominal thrusts. Repeat until victim becomes responsive.

Victim becomes unconscious

1. If second rescuer is available, have that person activate EMS.
2. Open airway with tongue-jaw lift, remove foreign body if visualized. Attempt to ventilate.
3. If still obstructed, reposition head and attempt to ventilate. Give five back blows and five abdominal thrusts. Repeat step 2 until ventilation is effective.
4. If obstruction still not relieved after 1 min, activate EMS system.

21

Recovery Position

Place an unconscious person who is still breathing and who has not suffered a traumatic neck injury in this position.

1. Kneel alongside the victim and straighten the legs.
2. Place victim's arm that is closest to you in the "waving goodbye" position and place the other arm across the victim's chest.
3. Grasp the far side leg above the knee and pull the thigh up toward the body. With the other hand, grasp the shoulder on the same side as the thigh.
4. Gently roll the patient toward you. Adjust the leg you are holding until both the thigh and knee are at right angles to the body. Tilt the patient's head back and use the patient's uppermost hand to support the head and maintain a head-tilt position.
5. Continue to monitor for breathing, and call for EMS.
6. If patient stops breathing, roll on back and follow basic CPR guidelines.

ADVANCED CARDIAC LIFE SUPPORT AND EMERGENCY CARDIAC CARE

ACLS includes the use of advanced airway management (See Endotracheal Intubation, Chapter 13, page 268), defibrillation, and drugs along with basic CPR. Most cardiac arrests are due to VF and are unwitnessed outside the hospital setting. ACLS protocols incorporating all these emergency cardiac care techniques are reviewed in the following algorithms for adults:

- Universal/International ACLS algorithm (Figure 21–1)
- Comprehensive emergency cardiac care algorithm (Figure 21–2)
- Ventricular fibrillation and pulseless VT algorithm (Figure 21–3)
- Pulseless electrical activity algorithm (Figure 21–4)
- Asystole: The silent heart algorithm (Figure 21–5)
- Bradycardia algorithm (Figure 21–6)
- Tachycardia overview algorithm (Figure 21–7)
- Narrow complex SVT algorithm (Figure 21–8)
- Stable VT algorithm (Figure 21–9)
- Acute coronary syndromes algorithm (Figure 21–10)
- Acute pulmonary edema, hypotension, and shock (Figure 21–11)

Advanced Cardiac Life Support Drugs

The most commonly used agents are listed on the inside covers for quick reference.

ACE Inhibitors
INDICATIONS: These agents improve the outcome in post-MI patients.

- Enalapril (Enalaprilat IV)
   SUPPLIED: Tabs 2.5, 5, 10, 20 mg; IV 1.25 mg/mL (1- and 2-mL vial)
   DOSAGE: .2.5 mg PO single dose, increase to 20 mg PO bid; 1.25 mg IV over 5 min, then 1.25–5.0 mg IV q6h

- Captopril
   SUPPLIED: Caps 12.5, 25, 50, 100 mg
   DOSAGE: 6.25 mg PO, increase to 25 mg tid and the 50 mg PO tid as tolerated

21

(continued on page 461)

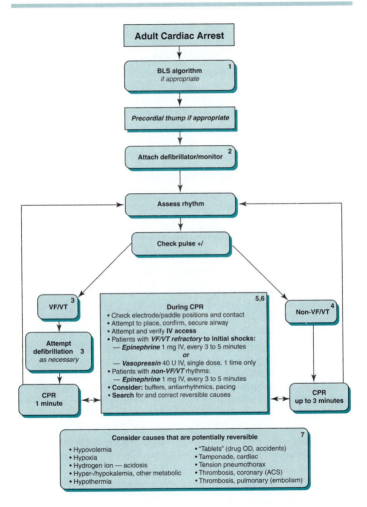

FIGURE 21–1 Universal/international advanced cardiac life support algorithm. *Abbreviations:* VF = ventricular fibrillation; VT = ventricular tachycardia; BLS = basic life support. (Reproduced, with permission, from: *Circulation* 2000;**102** supplement 1, part 6.)

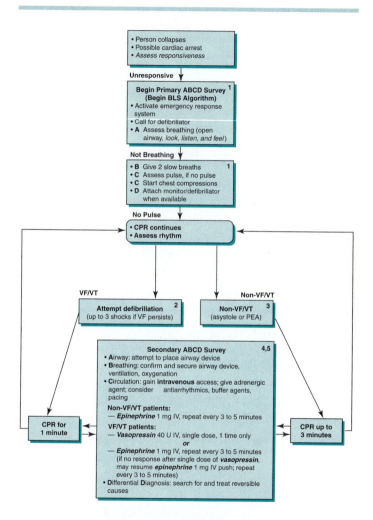

FIGURE 21–2 Comprehensive emergency cardiac care (ECC) algorithm. *Abbreviations:* VF = ventricular fibrillation; VT = ventricular tachycardia; BLS = basic life support; PEA = pulseless electrical activity. (Reproduced, with permission, from: *Circulation* 2000;**102** supplement 1, part 6.)

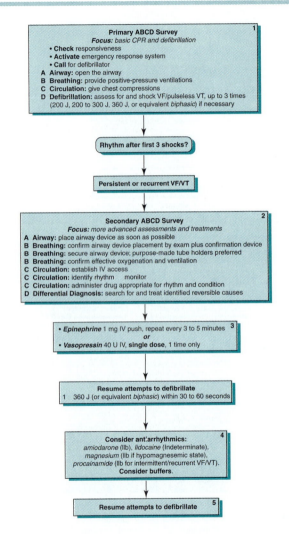

FIGURE 21–3 Ventricular fibrillation and pulseless ventricular tachycardia algorithm. *Abbreviations:* VF = ventricular fibrillation; VT = ventricular tachycardia. (Reproduced, with permission, from: *Circulation* 2000;**102** supplement 1, part 6.)

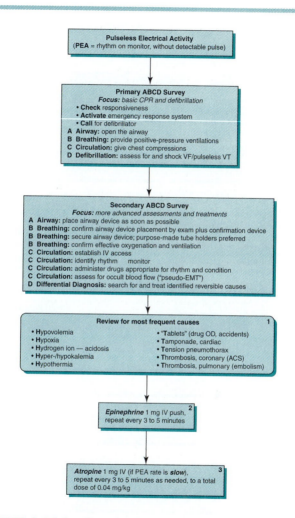

Pulseless Electrical Activity
(**PEA** = rhythm on monitor, without detectable pulse)

Primary ABCD Survey
Focus: basic CPR and defibrillation
- **Check** responsiveness
- **Activate** emergency response system
- **Call** for defibrillator
- **A Airway:** open the airway
- **B Breathing:** provide positive-pressure ventilations
- **C Circulation:** give chest compressions
- **D Defibrillation:** assess for and shock VF/pulseless VT

Secondary ABCD Survey
Focus: more advanced assessments and treatments
- **A Airway:** place airway device as soon as possible
- **B Breathing:** confirm airway device placement by exam plus confirmation device
- **B Breathing:** secure airway device; purpose-made tube holders preferred
- **B Breathing:** confirm effective oxygenation and ventilation
- **C Circulation:** establish IV access
- **C Circulation:** identify rhythm   monitor
- **C Circulation:** administer drugs appropriate for rhythm and condition
- **C Circulation:** assess for occult blood flow ("pseudo-EMT")
- **D Differential Diagnosis:** search for and treat identified reversible causes

Review for most frequent causes 1
- Hypovolemia
- Hypoxia
- Hydrogen ion — acidosis
- Hyper-/hypokalemia
- Hypothermia
- "Tablets" (drug OD, accidents)
- Tamponade, cardiac
- Tension pneumothorax
- Thrombosis, coronary (ACS)
- Thrombosis, pulmonary (embolism)

Epinephrine 1 mg IV push, 2
repeat every 3 to 5 minutes

Atropine 1 mg IV (if PEA rate is *slow*), 3
repeat every 3 to 5 minutes as needed, to a total
dose of 0.04 mg/kg

FIGURE 21–4 Pulseless electrical activity algorithm. *Abbreviations:* VF = ventricular fibrillation; VT = ventricular tachycardia; EMT = emergency medical treatment; ACS = acute coronary syndrome; PEA = pulseless electrical activity. (Reproduced, with permission, from: *Circulation* 2000;**102** supplement 1, part 6.)

21

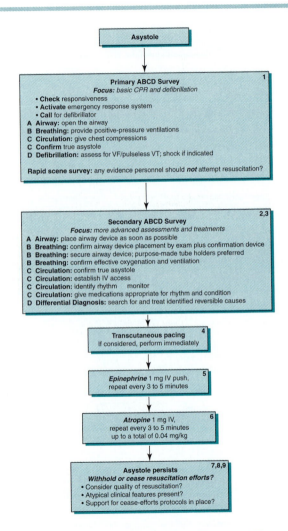

FIGURE 21-5 Asystole: the silent heart algorithm. *Abbreviations:* VF = ventricular fibrillation; VT = ventricular tachycardia. (Reproduced with permission from Circulation 2000;**102** supplement 1, part 6)

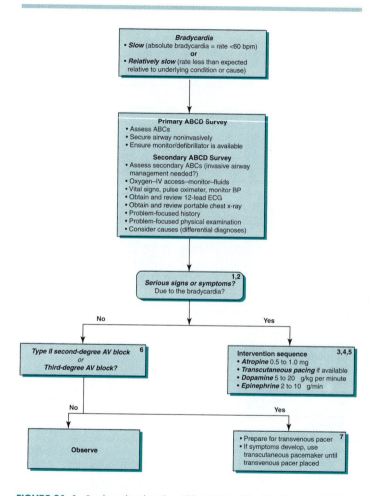

Bradycardia
- *Slow* (absolute bradycardia = rate <60 bpm)
  or
- *Relatively slow* (rate less than expected relative to underlying condition or cause)

↓

Primary ABCD Survey
- Assess ABCs
- Secure airway noninvasively
- Ensure monitor/defibrillator is available

Secondary ABCD Survey
- Assess secondary ABCs (invasive airway management needed?)
- Oxygen–IV access–monitor–fluids
- Vital signs, pulse oximeter, monitor BP
- Obtain and review 12-lead ECG
- Obtain and review portable chest x-ray
- Problem-focused history
- Problem-focused physical examination
- Consider causes (differential diagnoses)

↓

Serious signs or symptoms?[1,2]
Due to the bradycardia?

No → | Yes →

No

Type II second-degree AV block[6]
or
Third-degree AV block?

Yes

Intervention sequence[3,4,5]
- *Atropine* 0.5 to 1.0 mg
- *Transcutaneous pacing* if available
- *Dopamine* 5 to 20 g/kg per minute
- *Epinephrine* 2 to 10 g/min

No

Observe

Yes

- Prepare for transvenous pacer[7]
- If symptoms develop, use transcutaneous pacemaker until transvenous pacer placed

FIGURE 21–6 Bradycardia algorithm. Abbreviations: BP = blood pressure; ECG = electrocardiogram; AV = atrioventricular. (Reproduced, with permission, from: *Circulation* 2000;**102** supplement 1, part 6.)

21

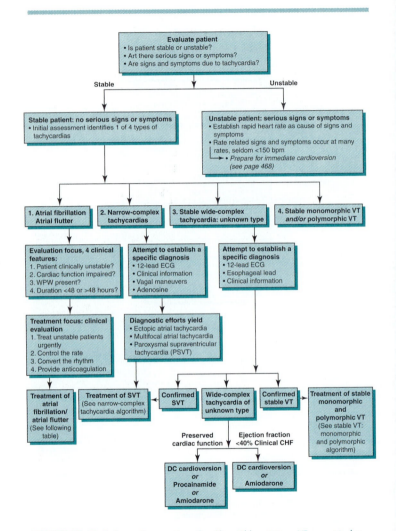

FIGURE 21–7 Tachycardia overview algorithm. *Abbreviations:* VF = ventricular fibrillation; ECG = electrocardiogram; PSVT = paroxysmal supraventricular tachycardia; SVT = supraventricular tachycardia. (Reproduced, with permission, from: *Circulation* 2000;**102** supplement 1, part 6.)

21

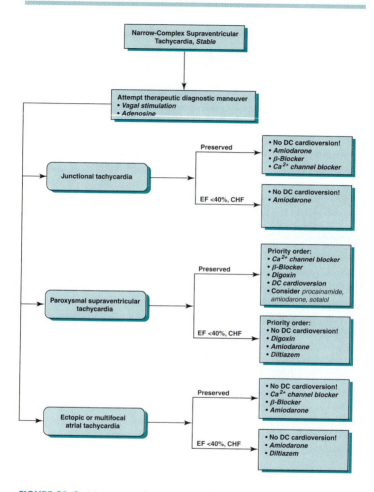

FIGURE 21–8 Narrow complex SVT algorithm. *Abbreviations:* EF = ejection fraction; CHF = congestive heart failure. (Reproduced, with permission, from: *Circulation* 2000;**102** supplement 1, part 6.)

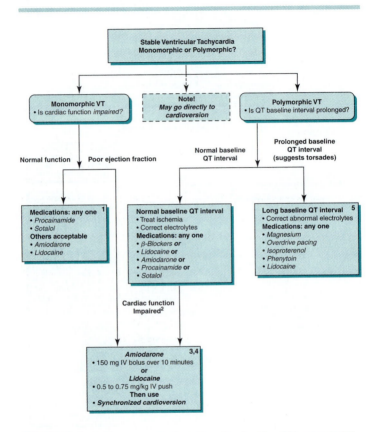

FIGURE 21–9   Stable supraventricular tachycardia algorithm. *Abbreviations:* VT =
ventricular tachycardia. (Reproduced, with permission, from: *Circulation* 2000;**102**
supplement 1, part 6.)

21

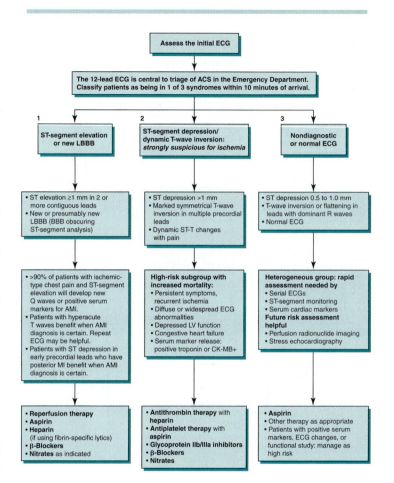

FIGURE 21–10 Acute coronary syndromes algorithm. *Abbreviations:* ECG = electrocardiogram; LBBB = left bundle branch block; BBB = bundle branch block; AMI = acute myocardial infarction; MI = myocardial infarction; LV = left ventricle; CK-MB+ = positive for myocardial muscle creatine kinase isoenzyme. (Reproduced, with permission, from: *Circulation* 2000;**102** supplement 1, part 6.)

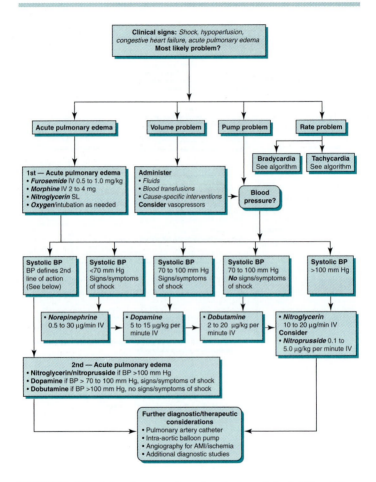

FIGURE 21–11 Acute pulmonary edema, hypotension and shock. *Abbreviations:* BP = blood pressure; AMI = acute myocardial infarction. (Reproduced, with permission, from: *Circulation* 2000;**102** supplement 1, part 7)

- Lisinopril

  SUPPLIED: Caps 2.5, 5, 10, 20, 30, 40 mg
  DOSAGE: 5 mg PO within 24 h of symptoms, 5 mg after 24 h, then 10 mg over 48 h, then 10 mg PO daily for 6 wk

- Ramipril

  SUPPLIED: Caps 1.25, 2.5, 5, 10 mg
  DOSAGE: 2.5 mg PO single dose, increase to 5 mg PO bid

Adenosine (Adenocard)

INDICATIONS: First drug for narrow-complex PSVT (not for AF or VT)
SUPPLIED: 2 mg/mL in 2-mL vial
DOSAGE: *Adults.* Put patient in reverse Trendelenburg position before administering dose; initial 6 mg over 1–3 s followed by NS bolus of 20 mL, then elevate extremity. Repeat 12 mg in 1–2 min PRN. A third dose of 12 mg in 1–2 min PRN. *Peds.* 0.1 mg/kg rapid IV push with continuous ECG monitoring. Follow with >5 mL NS flush. May double (0.2 mg/kg for second dose). Max: first dose: 6 mg; second dose:12 mg; single dose:12 mg

Amiodarone

INDICATIONS: Atrial and ventricular tachyarrhythmias and for rate control of rapid atrial arrhythmias in patients with impaired LV function when digoxin is ineffective
SUPPLIED: 50 mg/mL in 3-mL vial
DOSAGE: *Adults.* Max cumulative dose: 2.2 g IV/24 h. *Cardiac arrest.* 300 mg IV push. Consider repeating 150 mg IV push in 3–5 min. *Wide-complex tachycardia (stable)*: Rapid inf: 150 mg IV over 10 min (15 mg/min), every 15 min PRN. Slow inf: 360 mg IV over 6 h (1 mg/min). Maintenance inf: 540 mg IV over 18 h (0.5 mg/min). *Peds. Refractory pulseless VT, VF:* 5 mg/kg rapid IV bolus. *Perfusing supraventricular and ventricular arrhythmias:* Loading dose: 5 mg/kg IV/IO over 20–60 min (repeat, max 15 mg/kg/day).

Amrinone

INDICATIONS: CHF refractory to conventional agents
SUPPLIED: 0.5 mg/mL in 20-mL vial
DOSAGE: *Adults.* 0.75 mg/kg, over 10–15 min (Do NOT mix with dextrose.). Then 5–15 µg/kg/min titrated to effect. Hemodynamic monitoring preferred. *Peds.* Loading dose: 0.75–1.0 mg/kg IV over 5 min; may repeat twice (Max: 3 mg/kg). Cont inf: 5–10 µg/kg/min IV

Aspirin

INDICATIONS: In the acute setting, administer to all patients with acute coronary syndrome (ACS)
SUPPLIED: Tabs 160, 325 mg
DOSAGE: 160–325 mg PO (chewing preferred ASAP onset of ACS)

Atropine Sulfate

INDICATIONS: First drug for symptomatic bradycardia (but not Mobitz II). Second drug (after epinephrine or vasopressin) for asystole or bradycardic PEA
SUPPLIED: 0.1 mg/mL in 10-mL syringe (total = 1 mg).
DOSAGE: *Adults. Asystole or PEA:* 1 mg IV push. Repeat every 3–5 min (if asystole persists) to 0.03–0.04 mg/kg max. *Bradycardia:* 0.5–1.0 mg IV every 3–5 min as needed; max 0.03–0.04 mg/kg. *Endotracheal administration:* 2–3 mg in 10 mL NS. *Peds.* IV administration: 0.02 mg/kg. Min single dose: 0.1 mg, max: 0.5 mg. Max adolescent single dose: 1.0 mg. May double for second IV dose. Max child total dose: 1.0 mg. Max adolescent total dose: 2.0 mg. Endotracheal administration: 0.02 mg/kg (larger doses than IV may be required)

Beta Blockers

INDICATIONS: All patients with suspected MI; may reduce chance of VF and reduce damage. Second line agents after adenosine, diltiazem, or digoxin to slow ventricular response in supraventricular tachyarrhythmias. Antihypertensive for hemorrhagic and ischemic stroke. Do NOT administer along with calcium channel blockers due to risk of hypotension.

- Metoprolol (Lopressor)

  SUPPLIED: 1 mg/mL in 5-mL vial
  DOSAGE: *Adults.* 5 mg slow IV q 5 min, total 15 mg

- Atenolol (Tenormin)

  SUPPLIED: 0.5 mg/mL in 10-mL amp
  DOSAGE: *Adults.* 5 mg slow IV (over 5 min). In 10 min, second dose 5 mg slow IV. In 10 min, if tolerated, start 50 mg PO, then 50 mg PO bid

- Propanolol (Inderal)

  SUPPLIED: 1.0 mg/mL in 1 amp, 4 mg/mL in 5-mL
  DOSAGE: *Adults.* 0.1 mg/kg slow IV push, divided 3 equal doses 2–3 min intervals, max 1 mg/min. Repeat after 2 min, PRN

- Esmolol (Brevibloc)

  SUPPLIED: 10 mg/mL in 10-mL amp
  DOSAGE: *Adults.* 0.5 mg/kg over 1 min, then 0.05 mg/kg/min

- Labetalol

  SUPPLIED: 5 mg/mL (Amps 20, 40, 60 mL)
  DOSAGE: 10 mg IV push over 1–2 min. Repeat or double dose every 10 min (max: 150 mg); or initial bolus, then 2–8 µg/min

Calcium Chloride

INDICATIONS: Known/suspected hyperkalemia, hypocalcemia (eg, multiple transfusions), antidote for calcium channel blocker overdose, prophylactically before IV calcium channel blockers (prevent hypotension)
SUPPLIED: 100 mg/mL in 10-mL vial (total = 1 g; 10% solution)
DOSAGE: *Adults.* 8–16 mg/kg (usually 5–10 mL) IV slow push for hyperkalemia and calcium channel blocker overdose. 2–4 mg/kg (usually 2 mL) IV before IV calcium blockers. *Peds.* 20 mg/kg (0.2–0.25 mL/kg) slow push. Repeat PRN

Calcium Gluconate

SUPPLIED: 10% = 100 mg/10 mL = 9 mg/mL Ca
DOSAGE: *Peds.* 60–100 mg/kg (0.6–1.0 mL/kg) IV slow push. Repeat for documented conditions

Digibind

Digoxin-specific antibody therapy
INDICATIONS: Digoxin toxicity with uncontrolled life-threatening arrhythmias, shock, CHF; hyperkalemia >5 mEq/L with serum dig levels above 10–15 ng/mL
SUPPLIED: 40-mg vial (each vial binds about 0.6 mg digoxin)
DOSAGE: *Adults. Chronic intoxication:* 3–5 vials may be effective. *Acute overdose:* See Chapter 22; based on dose ingested (average dose is 10 vials (400 mg), but may require up to 20 vials (800 mg).

Digoxin

21

SUPPLIED: 0.15 mg/mL or 0.1 mg/mL in 1- or 2-mL amp
INDICATIONS: Slow ventricular response in AF or atrial flutter. Second-line for PSVT
DOSAGE: *Adults.* Loading 10–15 µg/kg. Maintenance dose see Chapter 22.

Diltiazem (Cardizem)

INDICATIONS: Control ventricular rate in AF and atrial flutter. Use after adenosine to treat refractory PSVT in patients with narrow QRS complex and adequate BP.
SUPPLIED: 5 mg/mL in 5- or 10-mL vial (total = 25 or 50 mg)
DOSAGE: *Adults. Acute rate control:* 15–20 mg (0.25 mg/kg) IV over 2 min. Repeat in 15 min at 20–25 mg (0.35 mg/kg) over 2 min. *Maintenance:* 5–15 mg/h, titrated to heart rate

Dobutamine (Dobutrex)

INDICATIONS: Pump problems with BP 70–100 mm Hg and no signs of shock
SUPPLIED: 12.5 mg/mL in 20-mL vial (total = 250 mg). IV inf: Dilute 250 mg (20 mL) in 250 mL NS or D_5W
DOSAGE: *Adults.* 2–20 µg/kg/min; titrate heart rate not >10% of baseline. Hemodynamic monitoring recommended. *Peds.* Cont IV inf: Titrate to effect (initial dose 5–10 µg/kg/min). Typical inf dose: 2–20 µg/kg/min

Dopamine (Intropin)

INDICATIONS: Second line for symptomatic bradycardia. Hypotension (BP <70–100 mm Hg) with signs of symptoms of shock
SUPPLIED: 40 mg/mL or 160 mg/mL. *IV inf:* Mix 400–800 mg in 250 mL NS or D_5W.
DOSAGE: *Adults.* Titrate to response. *Low:* 1–5 µg/kg/min ("renal doses"). *Moderate:* 5–10 µg/kg/min ("cardiac doses"). *High:* 10–20 µg/kg/min ("vasopressor doses"). *Peds.* Titrate to effect. Initial, 5–10 µg/kg/min; typical: 2–20 µg/kg/min
Note: If >20 µg/kg/min is required, consider use of alternative adrenergic agent (eg, epinephrine)

Epinephrine

INDICATIONS: *Cardiac arrest:* VF, pulseless VT, asystole, PEA. *Symptomatic bradycardia:* After atropine and transcutaneous pacing. *Anaphylaxis, severe allergic reactions:* Combine with large fluid volumes, corticosteroids, antihistamines.
SUPPLIED: 1.0 mg/10 mL in preloaded 10-mL syringe (total = 1 mg), 1 mg/mL in glass 1-mL amp (total = 1 mg)
DOSAGE: *Adults. Cardiac arrest:* IV dose: 1.0 mg IV push, repeat every 3–5 min; doses up to (0.2 mg/kg) if 1 mg dose fails. Inf: 30 mg epinephrine (30 mL of 1:1000 solution) to 250 mL NS or D_5W, run at 100 mL/h, titrate. Endotracheal: 2.0–2.5 mg in 20 mL NS. *Profound bradycardia/hypotension:* 2–10 µg/min (1 mg of 1:1000 in 500 mL NS, infuse 1–5 mL/min). *Peds. Asystole, pulseless arrest:* First dose: 0.1 mg/kg IV (0.1 mL/kg of 1:10,000 "standard concentration"). Second and subsequent doses: 0.1 mg/kg IV (0.1 mL/kg of 1:1000 "High" concentration. Administer every 3–5 min during arrest; up to 0.2 mg/kg may be effective. Endotracheal: 0.1 mg/kg (0.1 mL/kg of 1:1000 ["high"] concentration) continue q3–5 min of arrest until IV access is achieved; then begin with first IV dose. *Symptomatic bradycardia:* 0.01 mg/kg IV (0.1 mL/kg of 1:10,000 ["standard"] concentration). Endotracheal doses: 0.1 mg/kg (0.1 mL/kg of 1:1000 ["high"] concentration). Cont IV inf: Begin with rapid infusion; then titrate to response. Typical inf: 0.1–1.0 µg/kg/min (Higher doses may be effective)

Flumazenil (Romazicon)

INDICATIONS: Reverse benzodiazepine toxicity (do NOT use in tricyclic overdose or in unknown poisoning)
SUPPLIED: 0.1 mg/mL in 5- and 10-mL vials
DOSAGE: *Adults.* 0.2 mg IV over 15 s then 0.3 mg IV over 30 s, if no response, give third dose. Third dose: 0.5 mg IV given over 30 s, repeat once per min until response, or total of 3 mg.

Furosemide (Lasix)

INDICATIONS: Acute pulmonary edema in BP >90–100. Hypertensive emergencies or increased intracranial pressure
SUPPLIED: 10 mg/mL in 2-, 4-, and 10-mL amp or vials

21

DOSAGE: *Adults.* 0.5–1.0 mg/kg over 1–2 min. If no response, double the dose to 2.0 mg/kg over 1–2 min

Glucagon

INDICATIONS: Reverse effects of calcium channel blocker or beta-blocker
SUPPLIED: 1- and 10-mg vials
DOSAGE: *Adults.* 1–5 mg over 2–5 min

Glucoprotein IIb/IIIa inhibitors

INDICATIONS: Acute coronary syndromes without ST elevation. Do NOT use with history of active bleeding or surgery within 30 d or if platelets <150,000/mm^3. Note that optimum dosing and duration not established; check package insert.

- Abciximab (ReoPro)

  SUPPLIED: 2 mg/mL in 5-mL vial
  DOSAGE: ACS with planned PCI within 24 h: 0.25 mg/kg IV bolus up to 1 h before procedure, then 0.125 μg/kg/IV; must use with heparin. Platelet recovery within 48 h; redosing may cause hypersensitivity reaction.

- Eptifibatide (Integrilin)

  SUPPLIED: 0.75 and 2 mg/mL in 10-mL vial
  DOSAGE: *ACS:* 180 μg/kg IV bolus then 2 μg/kg/min infusion
  PCI: 135 μg/kg IV bolus then 0.5 μg/kg/min infusion; repeat bolus in 10 min.

- Tirofiban (Aggrastat)

  SUPPLIED: 250 μg/mL in 50 mL or premixed 50 μg/mL
  DOSAGE: *ACS or PCI:* 0.4 μg/kg/min IV for 30 min, then 0.1 μg/kg/min inf

Heparin (Unfractionated)

INDICATIONS: Adjuvant therapy in AMI. Begin heparin with fibrinolytics.
SUPPLIED: 0.5–1.0 mL amp, vials, and prefilled syringes. Multidose vials 1, 2, 5 and 30 mL. Concentrations range from 1000 to 40,000 IU/mL.
DOSAGE: *Adults.* Bolus 60 IU/kg (max bolus: 4000 IU). Continue 12 IU/kg/h (max 1000 IU/h for patients >70 kg) round to the nearest 50 IU. Adjust to maintain PTT 1.5–2.0 × control values for 48 h or until angiography.

Heparin (Low Molecular Weight) (Fragmin, Lovenox)

INDICATIONS: ACS with non-Q wave or unstable angina
SUPPLIED: Dalteparin (Fragmin), Enoxaparin (Lovenox)
DOSAGE: 1 mg/kg bid SQ for 2–8 d with aspirin

Ibutilide

INDICATIONS: Supraventricular arrhythmias (AFiB, A flutter); short-acting
SUPPLIED: 1 mg/10 mL
DOSAGE: 1 mg IV over 10 min (if <60 kg 0.01 mg/kg)

Isoproterenol (Isuprel)

INDICATIONS: Torsades de pointes unresponsive to magnesium sulfate. Temporary control of bradycardia in heart transplant patients. Class IIb at low doses for symptomatic bradycardias
SUPPLIED: 0.1 mg/mL in 1-mL vial. IV inf: Mix 1 mg in 250 mL NS or D$_5$W.
DOSAGE: *Adults.* 2–10 μg/min. Titrate to effect.

21

Lidocaine

INDICATIONS: Cardiac arrest from VF/VT. Stable VT, wide-complex tachycardias of uncertain type, wide-complex PSVT
SUPPLIED: 20 mg/mL in preloaded 5-mL syringe, 10 mg/mL in 5-mL vial. Can be given via endotracheal tube.
DOSAGE: *Adults. Cardiac arrest from VF/VT:* Initial dose: 1.0–1.5 mg/kg IV. For refractory VF may give additional 0.5–0.75 mg/kg IV push, repeat in 5–10 min, max total dose is 3 mg/kg. A single dose of 1.5 mg/kg IV in cardiac arrest is acceptable. Endotracheal administration: 2–4 mg/kg. *Perfusing arrhythmia:* For stable VT, wide-complex tachycardia or uncertain type, significant ectopy, use as follows: 1.0–1.5 mg/kg IV push. Repeat 0.5–0.75 mg/kg every 5–10 min; max total dose, 3 mg/kg. Maintenance inf: 1–4 mg/min (30–50 µg/min)

Magnesium Sulfate

INDICATIONS: Cardiac arrest associated with torsades de pointes or suspected hypomagnesemic state, refractory VF, life-threatening ventricular arrhythmias due to digitalis toxicity, tricyclic overdose. Consider prophylactic administration in hospitalized patients with AMI.
SUPPLIED: Amps 2 and 10 mL of 50% MgSO$_4$ (total = 1 g and 5 g). 10 mL in preloaded syringe (total = 5 g/10 mL)
DOSAGE: *Adults. Cardiac arrest:* 1–2 g IV push (2–4 mL of a 50% solution) diluted in 10 mL of D$_5$W. *AMI:* Loading dose of 1–2 g, mixed in 50–100 mL of D$_5$W, over 5–60 min IV. Follow with 0.5–1.0 g/h IV for up to 24 h. *Torsades de pointes:* Loading dose of 1–2 g mixed in 50–100 mL of D$_5$W, over 5–60 min IV. Follow with 1–4 g/h IV (titrate dose to control the torsades).

Mannitol

INDICATIONS: Increased intracranial pressure in management of neurologic emergencies
SUPPLIED: 150-, 250-, and 1000-mL IV containers (strengths: 5%, 10%, 15%, 20%, and 25%).
DOSAGE: *Adults.* Administer 0.5–1.0 g/kg over 5–10 min. Additional doses of 0.25–2g/kg can be given every 4–6 h as needed. Use in conjugation with oxygenation and ventilation.

Morphine Sulfate

INDICATIONS: Chest pain and anxiety associated with AMI or cardiac ischemia, acute cardiogenic pulmonary edema (if blood pressure is adequate)
SUPPLIED: 2–10 mg/mL in a 1-mL syringe
DOSAGE: *Adults.* 2–4 mg IV (over 1–5 min) every 5–30 min

Naloxone (Narcan)

INDICATIONS: To reverse effects of narcotic toxicity, including respiratory depression, hypotension, and hypoperfusion
DOSAGE: *Adults.* 0.4–2.0 mg IV every 2 min; up to 10 mg over <30 min. *Peds.* Bolus IV dose: For total reversal of narcotic effects (smaller doses may be used if total reversal not required), as follows: *Birth–5 y* (≤ 10 kg): 0.1 mg/kg. *≥5 y* (>20 kg): 2.0 mg. May be necessary to repeat doses frequently. Cont inf: 0.04–0.16 mg/kg/h

Nitroglycerin

INDICATIONS: Chest pain of suspected cardiac origin; unstable angina; complications of AMI, including CHF, left ventricular failure; HTN crisis or urgency with chest pain
SUPPLIED: *Parenteral:* Amps: 5 mg in 10 mL, 8 mg in 10 mL, 10 mg in 10 mL, vials: 25 mg in 5 mL, 50 mg in 10 mL, 100 mg in 10 mL. *SL tabs:* 0.3 and 0.4 mg. *Aerosol spray:* 0.4 mg/dose
DOSAGE: *Adults.* IV bolus: 12.5–25 µg. Infuse at 10–20 µg/min. Route of choice for emergencies. Use IV sets provided by manufacturer. *SL route:* 0.3–0.4 mg, repeat every 5 min. *Aerosol spray:* Spray for 0.5–1.0 s at 5-min intervals.

Nitroprusside (Sodium Nitroprusside, Nipride)

INDICATIONS: HTN crisis, reduce afterload in CHF and acute PE

21

SUPPLIED: 50-mg amp, mix in 250 mL D_5W only (keep covered with opaque material)
DOSAGE: 0.10 μg/kg/min, titrate up to 5.0 μg/kg/min. Use infusion pump; hemodynamic monitoring for optimal safety

Norepinephrine

INDICATIONS: Severe cardiogenic shock and significant hypotension. Last resort for ischemic heart disease and shock
SUPPLIED: 1 mg/mL in 4-mL amp. Mix 4 mg in 250 mL of D_5W or D_5NS
DOSAGE: *Adults.* 0.5–1.0 μg/min titrated to 30 μg/min. *Peds.* IV inf: Initial 0.1–2 μg/kg/min to effect. Do NOT administer with alkaline solutions.

Procainamide (Pronestyl)

INDICATIONS: Recurrent VT not controlled by lidocaine, refractory PSVT, refractory VF/pulseless VT, stable wide-complex tachycardia of unknown origin, AF with rapid rate in WPW
SUPPLIED: 100 mg/mL in 10-mL vial, 500 mg/mL in 2-mL vial
DOSAGE: *Adults. Recurrent VF/VT:* 20 mg/min IV (max total 17 mg/kg). In urgent situations up to 50 mg/min to a total dose of 17 mg/kg. *Other indications:* 20 mg/min IV until one of the following occurs: arrhythmia suppression, hypotension, QRS widens by more than 50%, total dose of 17 mg/kg is given. *Maintenance:* 1–4 mg/min

Sodium Bicarbonate

INDICATIONS: Specific indications for bicarbonate use are as follows: Class I (usually indicated) if known preexisting hyperkalemia. Class IIa (accepted, possibly controversial) if known preexisting bicarbonate-responsive acidosis (eg, DKA); tricyclic antidepressant overdose; alkalinize urine in aspirin overdose. Class IIb (accepted, but may not help, probably not harmful) if prolonged resuscitation with effective ventilation; on return of spontaneous circulation after long arrest interval. Class III (harmful) in hypoxic lactic acidosis (eg, cardiac arrest and CPR without intubation)
SUPPLIED: 50-mL syringe (8.4% sodium bicarbonate provides 50 mEq/50 mL)
DOSAGE: *Adults.* IV inf: 1 mEq/kg IV bolus. Repeat half this dose every 10 min thereafter. If rapidly available, use ABG analysis to guide therapy.

Sodium Bicarbonate (Pediatric)

INDICATIONS: Severe metabolic acidosis (documented or following prolonged arrest) unresponsive to oxygenation and hyperventilation, hyperkalemia, tricyclic antidepressant toxicity
DOSAGE: *Adults.* 8.4% 1 mEq/mL in 10- or 50-mL syringe, 4.2% 0.5 mEq/mL in 10-mL syringe. *Peds.* 1 mEq/kg. Dose may be calculated to correct ¼–½ of base deficit.

Thrombolytic Agents (Fibrinolytic Agents)

INDICATIONS: *AMI in adults:* ST-segment elevation of 1 mm or more in at least two contiguous leads in the setting of AMI. *Adjuvant therapy:* 60–325 mg aspirin chewed as soon as possible. Begin heparin immediately and continue for 48 h if alteplase is used.

- Alteplase, Recombinant

   SUPPLIED: Vials 20, 50, and 100 mg, reconstituted with sterile water to 1 mg/mL
   DOSAGE: *Adults.* Recommended dose based on patient's weight, not to exceed 100 mg. *AMI:* Accelerated inf: Give 15 mg bolus. Then 0.75 mg/kg over next 30 min (not to exceed 50 mg). Then 0.50 mg/kg over next 60 min (not to exceed 35 mg). 3-h inf: 60 mg in first hour (initial 6–10 mg as a bolus). Then 20 mg/h for 2 additional hours. *Acute ischemic stroke:* 0.9 mg/kg (max 90 mg) infused over 60 min. 10% of total dose as initial IV bolus over 1 min. Give the remaining 90% over the next 60 min.

- Streptokinase

   SUPPLIED: Reconstitute to 1 mg/mL
   DOSAGE: *Adults.* 1.5 million IU in a 1-h infusion

21

- Anistreplase APSAC

    SUPPLIED: Reconstitute 30 U in 50 mL water or D_5W. Use two peripheral IV lines, one exclusively for thrombolytic administration.
    DOSAGE: *Adults.* 30 IU IV over 2–5 min

- Reteplase, recombinant (Retavase)

    SUPPLIED: 10-U vials reconstituted with sterile water to 1 U/mL
    DOSAGE: *Adults.* 10 U IV bolus over 2 min. 30 min later, give second 10 U IV bolus over 2 min. NS flush before and after each bolus

Verapamil (Colan, Isoptin)

INDICATIONS: Second line for PSVT with narrow QRS complex and adequate BP
SUPPLIED: 2.5 mg/mL in 2-, 4-, and 5-mL vials (totals = 5, 10, and 12.5 mg)
DOSAGE: *Adults.* 2.5–5.0 mg IV over 1–2 min. Repeat 5–10 mg, if needed, in 15–30 min (30 mg max). Alternative: 5 mg bolus every 15 min to total dose of 30 mg

Electrical Defibrillation and Cardioversion

Although the defibrillator is the basic piece of equipment for both defibrillation and cardioversion, they are two distinctly different procedures. New devices include shock advisory defibrillators (automated external defibrillators). The energy level is the watt-second or joule.

Standard Defibrillation Procedure (conventional device)

1. This is the primary therapy for VF or pulseless VT. Asystole is not now routinely defibrillated.
2. Use paste or pads on skin (see step 3 for location).
3. **Shout "Charging defibrillator-stand clear," synchronization switch off** (if **on,** the defibrillator may not fire). In *adults,* energy levels begin at 200 J. In *children,* use 2 J/kg advance to 6 J/kg max.
4. Place paddles as directed on the handles: one at the right upper sternum and one at the left anterior axillary line (apex).
5. Apply paddles with firm pressure (approximately 25 lb).
6. Shout "I am going to shock on three. Stand clear!" and make sure no one is touching the patient or bed *including yourself.*
7. Shout "Clear," and visually check for other team members.
8. Shout three times "Everybody clear," and press both paddle buttons simultaneously to fire the unit, and observe for any change in the dysrhythmia.
9. Defibrillate up to three times with increasing joules (200, >200–300, >360). If these fail to convert, continue full output (360 J) for all future shocks. If VT recurs, shock again at last energy level.
10. If a patient is **HYPOTHERMIC** (Core temperature < 30 °C) shock only three times as in step 8. Resume shocks only after temperature rises above 30 °C.
11. If patient has automated implantable defibrillator and device is delivering shocks, wait 60 s for cycle to complete. If defibrillation attempted, place paddles several inches from the implanted pacer unit.

Automated External Defibrillator (AED)

1. Familiarize yourself with the features of the unit well in advance of using it. These computerized devices "analyze" the rhythm and indicate if a shock is appropriate.

21

2. Place the pads on the patient (upper right sternum and cardiac apex). Press the "analyze" button.
3. If appropriate (VT or VF), the unit charges and the "shock" sign is given.
4. Announce "Shock is indicated . . . Stand clear," and verify that no one is touching patient. Depress "shock" button to administer shock.
5. Repeat until arrhythmia is cleared ("no shock indicated" signal will flash). In general, shock in sets of three without interposing CPR. After three shocks, do 1 min of CPR.

Cardioversion

Used for VT with a pulse, atrial arrhythmias with rapid ventricular response (PAT, AF, or atrial flutter); an attempt to slow the heart or convert rhythm. Procedure is like that for defibrillation, **except:**

1. **Consider sedation because most of these patients are conscious.** Agents can include diazepam, midazolam with or without a narcotic such as morphine, or fentanyl. Anesthesia support is helpful if readily available.
2. **Start with lower energy levels than for defibrillation. Start at 100 J and increase to 200, 300, and finally 360.**
3. **Keep the synchronizer switch on** (prevents shocking during vulnerable part of QRS complex when shock may cause VF, so-called R-on-T phenomenon). Observe for the markers on the R waves indicating that the synch mode is engaged.
4. Place paddles, apply pressure, and verify area is cleared as for the defibrillation steps.
5. Most defibrillators default back to the unsynchronized mode to allow rapid shock in case of VF. Reset synch mode if multiple cardioversions needed.

Transcutaneous Pacing

Primarily used for hemodynamically unstable bradycardia. External pacemakers can be set in the asynchronous (nondemand or fixed mode) or demand mode in the range of 30–180 bpm with current outputs from 0–200 mA.

1. Place electrode pads on chest as per unit's instructions.
2. Turn unit on and set pacer to 80 bpm initially.
3. Adjust current upward until capture is achieved (ie, wide QRS after each pacer spike on ECG for bradycardia.
4. For asystole (not routinely used) begin at full output. If capture occurs, decrease to threshold and increase by 2 mA.

OTHER COMMON EMERGENCIES

The following material gives the treatment for other common emergencies. Dosages are for *adult*s unless stated otherwise.

Anaphylaxis

Systolic BP <90 mm Hg

Epinephrine

DOSAGE: *Adults.* IV bolus: 100 μg of 1:10,000 over 5–10 min. IV inf: 1–4 μg/min. *Peds.* IV inf: 0.1–0.3 μg/kg/min, max 1.5 μg/kg/min

Systolic BP >90 mm Hg

- Epinephrine
  DOSAGE: 1:1000 soln SQ. *Adults.* 0.3–0.5 mL. *Peds.* 0.01 mL/kg, max 0.5 mL

Supplemental drugs for anaphylaxis include:

- Diphenhydramine
  DOSAGE: *Adults.* IV/IM/PO 50 mg. *Peds.* IV/IM/PO 1 mg/kg
- Methylprednisolone
  DOSAGE: 1–2 mg/kg IV
- Ranitidine (Zantac)
  DOSAGE: *Adults.* IV 50 mg over 5 min. *Peds.* IV 0.5mg/kg over 5 min
- Albuterol
  DOSAGE: *Adults.* 2.5 mg nebulized. *Peds.* 1.25 mg nebulized

Asthmatic Attack

Mild

Albuterol (Nebulized)
DOSAGE: *Adults.* 2.5–5.0 mg at 20 min for 3 doses. *Peds.* 1.25–2.5 mg at 20 min for 3 doses

Moderate to Severe

Ipratropium Bromide (nebulized)
DOSAGE: *Adults.* 0.5 mg with first albuterol treatment. *Peds.* 250 µg with first albuterol treatment.

Methylprednisolone
DOSAGE: *Adults.* 1 mg/kg IV. *Peds.* 2 mg/kg IV

Severe

Epinephrine
NOTE: Administer SQ or aerosolized beta agonists as for mild to moderate cases

Aminophylline
NOTE: Administer as for mild to moderate cases.
Give early consideration to

Hydrocortisone sodium
DOSAGE: 4 mg/kg IV q2–4h
or

Methylprednisolone
DOSAGE: 2–4 mg/kg IV q4h

Anticholinergic Crisis

Usually related to drug overdose. Patients present "red as a beet, mad as a hatter, hot as a furnace, dry as a bone, blind as a bat."

21

Physostigmine

DOSAGE: 0.5–2.0 mg IV
NOTE: Administer S-L-O-W-L-Y (may cause seizures if given rapidly). Have cardiac monitor attached and resuscitation equipment at the bedside.

Coma

1. Establish/secure airway.
2. Protect cervical spine.
3. Assess for respiratory failure and shock (ACLS).
4. Supply oxygen, IV access, cardiac monitor, and pulse oximetry.
5. Administer 1 amp (50 mL) of D_{50} IV manually; some recommend checking a stat glucose first
6. Administer 100 mg thiamine IV.
7. Give naloxone (Narcan) (see following section on Narcotics Overdose).
8. Obtain fingerstick glucose, SMA, CBC, urinalysis, and ABG.

Dental Emergencies

Not including facial fractures, there are generally two major categories of dental emergencies: toothaches with associated abscesses and avulsed (knocked-out) teeth. Most toothaches may be managed with antibiotics (usually penicillin-V 500 mg, q6h) and analgesics until proper dental attention can be obtained. Fluctuant abscesses may be drained if convenient. The exception to this rule is submandibular or infraorbital swelling. With submandibular infections, Ludwig's angina may develop, a life-threatening occurrence. These patients should be held for observation with special attention to maintaining the airway until a dental consult can be obtained. Infraorbital infections can lead to a cavernous sinus thrombosis if allowed to progress.

Avulsed teeth may or may not have an associated dentoalveolar fracture. The best treatment is to reposition the displaced tooth back in the socket within 30 min or as soon as possible. If the tooth root is dirty, wash it gently with sterile saline. Do not scrub or scrape the root. Get a dental consult to arrange to have the tooth splinted back in the socket.

Hypercalcemia

See Chapter 9, page 188

Hyperkalemia

See Chapter 9, page 186

Hypertensive Crisis

1. Treat only if signs of end organ damage.
2. MAP should not be reduced more than 20–25% over 30–60 min.

$$MAP = [\frac{1}{3} (SBP - DBP) + DBP]$$

- Labetalol
  DOSAGE: 20 mg IV bolus then 2 mg/min IV to target BP or

- Sodium Nitroprusside
  DOSAGE: 0.5 μg /kg/min $\uparrow$ to max (10 μg/kg) min

Hypoglycemia

1. Draw a STAT serum glucose. **Do not wait for result before treating if hypoglycemia is strongly suspected. A finger Dextro stick can usually be quickly checked.**
2. Give orange juice with sugar if the patient is awake and alert; if not, give 1 amp of D_{50} IV (*Peds.* 1 mL/kg).
3. If IV access is not possible, give glucagon 1 mg IM or SC.

Narcotics Overdose

Naloxone (Narcan)

DOSAGE: *Adults.* 0.4–0.8 mg IV or IM, repeat as needed. (*Note:* if you suspect the patient is a narcotic addict give 0.4 mg instead and repeat as needed to avoid precipitating severe withdrawal. *Peds.* 0.01–0.02 mg/kg IV or IM, repeat as needed. Observe patient for at least 6 h after treatment.

Poisoning

1. Support airway, respiration, and circulation, as needed.
2. Determine ingested substance; give specific antidote, if available. The following is a list of some common poisons with their antidotes (Dosages for *adults,* unless otherwise specified):

Acetaminophen	*N*-acetylcysteine, 140 mg/kg
Anticholinesterases	Atropine 0.5–2 mg IV; may need up to
(organophosphates, physostigmine)	5 mg IV q 15 min if severe, then 70 mg/kg
	× 17 more doses; 0.05 mg/kg IV
	in children
Benzodiazepines	Flumazenil (see page 463)
Beta-blockers	Glucagon 0.05 mg/kg IV bolus for BP
	<90, then infusion of 75–150 mg/kg/h
Carbon monoxide	High-flow oxygen
Calcium channel blockers	Calcium chloride 10–20 mL/kg of
	1% solution then 20 mg/kg/h
Cyanide	Amyl nitrate pearls inhale every 2 min then
	sodium nitrite 10 mL 3% IV over 3 min
	(0.33 mL/kg of 3% solution in children) or
	sodium thiosulfate 50 mL of 25% solution
	over 10 min or 1.65 mL/kg in children
Cyclic antidepressants	$NaHCO_3$ 3 amps (50 mg/50 mL) in
	1 L D_5W @ 2–3 mL/kg/h
Digoxin	Digoxin-specific Fab

$$\text{Number of vials} =$$
$$\text{Serum digoxin level} \times \frac{\text{Patient's weight (kg)}}{100}$$

Methanol, ethylene glycol	Loading dose 1 g/kg of a 10% solution slowly
	IV, followed by an infusion of 130 mg/kg/h.
	If patient is on dialysis give 250–300 mg/kg/h
	to maintain levels.
Opiates, narcotics	Naloxone see page 465.

3. Prevent further absorption as described if conscious/unconscious

21

Unconscious Patient

- Protect airway with an endotracheal tube.
- Lavage with an Ewald tube or 28 French or larger NG tube, if ingestion occurred, 1 h.
- Use 300 mL NS boluses at a time through the NG or Ewald tube for adults and 20 mL/kg in children.
- Activated charcoal can be added, unless an oral antidote is to be given.
- Cathartics (sorbitol or magnesium citrate) promote GI elimination.

Conscious Patient

- Activated charcoal 1 g/kg, Contraindicated for iron, lithium, lead, alkali, acid. Also give 70% sorbitol solution (2 mL/kg body weight). Anyone given sorbitol should be monitored for hypokalemia and hypomagnesemia.
- Attempt to promote excretion through IV hydration.
- Alkalinization (0.5–1 mEq/kg/L in IV fluids) for salicylates, barbiturates, tricyclics

Shock

See also Chapter 20, page 431, and this chapter, page 460.

Hypovolemic: Initially, use isotonic fluids such as NS or lactated Ringer's, blood, albumin, Plasmanate, or hetastarch.

Seizures/Status Epilepticus

Status epilepticus refers to >1 min of continuous seizure activity or back-to-back seizures without recovery in between.

Initial Supportive Care

- Maintain airway with C-spine precautions.
- Deliver oxygen by nasal cannula.
- Monitor ECG and blood pressure.
- Maintain normal temperature.

Pharmacologic Therapy
See Table 21–1.

- Establish IV.
- Administer thiamine 100 mg IV.
- Administer 1 amp of D_{50} IV in an adult (2 mL/kg D_{25} in children) unless obviously hyperglycemic.
- Administer lorazepam or diazepam initially (see Table 21–1) (midazolam 0.2 mg/kg) can be given IM in children if no IV.
- If seizures persist, give fosphenytoin or phenytoin (see Table 21–1).
- If seizures persist, administer phenobarbital, paraldehyde.
- If still no response, obtain emergency neurosurgical and anesthesiology consultation.

TABLE 21–1
Drugs for the Emergency Treatment of Seizures

Drug	Pediatric Dose (mg/kg)	Adult Dose	Maximum Rate (mg/min)
Diazepam (Valium)	0.10–0.20 IV	5–10 mg IV (up to 30 mg)	3–5
Fosphenytoin	N/A	20 mg/kg IV	150
Paraldehyde	0.15–0.3 mL/kg PR*	30 mL PR*	NA
Phenytoin (Dilantin)[†]	15 IV	Same as for child	50
Phenobarbital[‡]	10 IV or IM	120–140 mg IV	100

*When given rectally, mix 2:1 with cottonseed or olive oil.
[†]When given IV, use a maximum dose of 50 mg/min and monitor ECG and vital signs closely. Can cause severe hypotension and bradycardia. Mix with NS to prevent precipitation.
[‡]Indicated when the patient is allergic to phenytoin. Patients may require intubation.

22

COMMONLY USED MEDICATIONS

Introduction
Classification
    Allergy Treatments
    Antidotes
    Antimicrobial Agents
    Antineoplastic Agents
    Cardiovascular Agents
    Central Nervous System Agents
    Dermatologic Agents
    Dietary Supplements
    Ear (Otic) Agents
    Endocrine System
    Eye (Ophthalmic) Agents
    Gastrointestinal Agents

Hematologic Agents
Immune System Agents
Musculoskeletal Agents
OB/GYN Agents
Pain Relievers
Respiratory Agents
Urinary/Genitourinary Agents
Wound Care
Miscellaneous Agents
Generic Drug Listing and Data
Aminoglycoside Dosing
Immunization Schedule

INTRODUCTION

This section is a quick reference of commonly used medications with selected key data listed for each drug. Be familiar with all the indications, contraindications, adverse effects, and drug interactions of any medication you prescribe. Such detailed information is beyond the scope of this manual but can be found in the package insert, the *Physicians' Desk Reference* (*PDR*), or from the American Hospital Formulary Service.

Medications are listed by class, and then the individual medications are listed in alphabetical order by generic name. Some of the more common trade names are listed (in parentheses after the generic name) for each medication. Because many medications are used to treat various conditions based on the medical literature and not listed in their package insert, we list common uses of the medication rather than the official "labeled indications" (FDA approved). If no pediatric dosage is provided, we assume the agent is not well established for this age group.

Medications under the control of the U.S. Drug Enforcement Agency (Schedule I–V controlled substances) are indicated by the symbol [C]. The following is a general description for the schedules of controlled substances:

- **Schedule I:** All nonresearch use forbidden (eg, heroin, LSD, mescaline, etc)
- **Schedule II:** High addictive potential; medical use accepted. No telephone call-in prescriptions; no refills. Some states require special prescription form (eg, cocaine, morphine, methadone)
- **Schedule III:** Low to moderate risk of physical dependence, high risk of psychological dependence; prescription must be rewritten after 6 months or five refills (eg, acetaminophen plus codeine)

- **Schedule IV:** Limited potential for dependence; prescription rules same as for Schedule III (eg, benzodiazepines)
- **Schedule V:** Very limited abuse potential; prescribing regulations often same as for uncontrolled medications, some states have additional restrictions

CLASSIFICATION

Allergy Treatments

Antihistamines

Cetirizine
Chlorpheniramine
Clemastine fumarate

Cyproheptadine
Diphenhydramine
Fexofenadine

Hydroxyzine
Loratadine

Miscellanous Agents

Budesonide
Cromolyn

Antidotes

Acetylcysteine
Amifostine
Charcoal
Dexrazoxane

Digoxin immune FAB
Flumazenil
Ipecac syrup
Mesna

Naloxone
Physostigmine
Succimer

Antimicrobial Agents

Antibiotics

Aminoglycosides

Amikacin
Gentamicin

Neomycin
Streptomycin

Tobramycin

Cephalosporins, First-Generation

Cefadroxil
Cefazolin

Cephalexin
Cephalothin

Cephapirin
Cephradine

Cephalosporins, Second-Generation

Cefaclor
Cefmetazole
Cefonicid

Cefotetan
Cefoxitin
Cefprozil

Cefuroxime
Loracarbef

Cephalosporins, Third-Generation

Cefdinir
Cefixime
Cefoperazone

Cefotaxime
Cefpodoxime
Ceftazidime

Ceftizoxime
Ceftriaxone

Cephalosporins, Fourth-Generation

Cefepime

Fluoroquinolones

Ciprofloxacin
Gatifloxacin
Levofloxacin

Lomefloxacin
Moxifloxacin
Norfloxacin

Ofloxacin

Macrolides

Azithromycin
Clarithromycin

Dirithromycin
Erythromycin

Erythromycin and sulfi-
soxazole

Penicillins

Amoxicillin
Amoxicillin-clavulanate
Ampicillin
Ampicillin-sulbactam
Cloxacillin
Dicloxacillin

Mezlocillin
Nafcillin
Oxacillin
Penicillin G aqueous
Penicillin G benzathine
Penicillin G procaine

Penicillin V
Piperacillin
Piperacillin-tazobactam
Ticarcillin
Ticarcillin-clavulanate

Tetracyclines

Doxycycline
Tetracycline

Miscellaneous agents

Aztreonam
Clindamycin
Fosfomycin
Imipenem-cilastatin

Linezolid
Meropenem
Metronidazole
Quinupristin/dalfopristin

Trimethoprim-sulfamethoxazole (co-trimoxazole)
Vancomycin

Antifungals

Amphotericin B
Amphotericin B cholesteryl
Amphotericin B lipid com-
plex
Amphotericin B liposomal
Clotrimazole

Clotrimazole and betametha-
sone
Econazole
Fluconazole
Itraconazole
Ketoconazole

Miconazole
Nystatin
Terbinafine
Triamcinolone and nystatin

Antimycobacterials

Clofazimine
Dapsone
Ethambutol

Isoniazid
Pyrazinamide
Rifabutin

Rifampin
Rifapentine

Antiretrovirals

Abacavir
Amprenavir
Delavirdine
Didanosine
Efavirenz

Indinavir
Lamivudine
Nelfinavir
Nevirapine
Ritonavir

Saquinavir
Stavudine
Zalcitabine
Zidovudine
Zidovudine and lamivudine

Antivirals

Acyclovir
Amantadine
Cidofovir
Famciclovir
Foscarnet

Ganciclovir
Interferon Alfa-2b and rib-
avirin combination
Oseltamivir
Penciclovir

Ribavirin
Rimantadine
Valacyclovir
Zanamivir

Miscellaneous Agents

Atovaquone

Pentamidine
Permethrin

Trimetrexate

Antineoplastic Agents

Alkylating Agents

Altretamine
Busulfan

Carboplatin
Cisplatin

Procarbazine
Triethylene-triphosphoramide

Nitrogen Mustards

Chlorambucil
Cyclophosphamide

Ifosfamide
Mechlorethamine

Melphalan

Nitrosoureas

Carmustine

Lomustine

Streptozocin

Antibiotics

Bleomycin sulfate
Dactinomycin
Daunorubicin

Doxorubicin
Idarubicin
Mitomycin

Pentostatin
Plicamycin
Valrubicin

Antimetabolites

Cytarabine
Cytarabine liposomal
Floxuridine

Fludarabine
Fluorouracil (5-FU)
Gemcitabine

Mercaptopurine
Methotrexate
6-Thioguanine

Hormones

Anastrozole
Bicalutamide
Estramustine phosphate
Fluoxymesterone

Flutamide
Goserelin
Leuprolide acetate
Megestrol acetate

Nilutamide
Tamoxifen acetate

Mitotic Inhibitors

Etoposide
Teniposide

Vinblastine
Vincristine

Vinorelbine

Miscellaneous Agents

Aldesleukin
Altretamine
Aminoglutethimide
L-Asparaginase

BCG (bacillus Calmette-
Guérin)
Cladribine
Dacarbazine

Docetaxel
Hydroxyurea
Interferon Alfa
Irinotecan

Letrozole
Levcovorin
Levamisole
Mitotane

Mitoxantrone
Paclitaxel
Pentostatin

Procarbazine
Topotecan
Tretinoin (retinoic acid)

Cardiovascular Agents

α_1-(Alpha) Blockers

Doxazosin

Prazosin

Terazosin

Angiotensin-converting Enzyme Inhibitors

Benazepril
Captopril
Enalapril and enalaprilat
Fosinopril

Lisinopril
Moexipril
Perindopril
Quinapril

Ramipril
Trandolapril

Angiotensin II Receptor Antagonist

Candesartan
Eprosartan

Irbesartan
Losartan

Telmisartan
Valsartan

Antiarrhythmic Agents

Adenosine
Amiodarone
Atropine
Bretylium
Digoxin
Disopyramide

Esmolol
Flecainide
Ibutilide
Lidocaine
Methoxamine
Mexiletine

Moricizine
Procainamide
Propafenone
Quinidine
Sotalol
Tocainide

β-(Beta) Blockers

Acebutolol
Atenolol
Atenolol and chlorthalidone
Betaxolol
Bisoprolol

Carteolol
Carvedilol
Labetalol
Metoprolol
Nadolol

Penbutolol
Pindolol
Propranolol
Timolol

Calcium Channel Antagonists

Amlodipine
Bepridil
Diltiazem
Felodipine

Isradipine
Nicardipine
Nifedipine
Nimodipine

Nisoldipine
Verapamil

Centrally Acting Antihypertensive Agents

Clonidine
Guanabenz

Guanadrel
Guanethidine

Guanfacine
Methyldopa

Diuretics

Acetazolamide
Amiloride
Bumetanide
Chlorothiazide
Chlorthalidone

Ethacrynic acid
Furosemide
Hydrochlorothiazide
Hydrochlorothiazide and
    amiloride

Hydrochlorothiazide and
    spironolactone
Hydrochlorothiazide and tri-
    amterene
Indapamide

Mannitol
Metolazone
Spironolactone
Torsemide
Triamterene

Inotropic/Pressor Agents

Amrinone
Digoxin
Dobutamine
Dopamine
Epinephrine
Isoproterenol
Methoxamine
Milrinone
Norepinephrine
Phenylephrine

Lipid-Lowering Agents

Atorvastatin
Cerivastatin
Cholestyramine
Colesevelam
Colestipol
Fenofibrate
Fluvastatin
Gemfibrozil
Lovastatin
Niacin
Pravastatin
Simvastatin

Vasodilators

Alprostadil
Epoprostenol
Fenoldopam
Hydralazine
Isosorbide dinitrate
Isosorbide mononitrate
Minoxidil
Nitroglycerin
Nitroprusside
Tolazoline

Central Nervous System Agents

Antianxiety

Alprazolam
Buspirone
Chlordiazepoxide
Clorazepate
Diazepam
Doxepin
Hydroxyzine
Lorazepam
Meprobamate
Oxazepam
Prazepam

Anticonvulsants

Carbamazepine
Clonazepam
Diazepam
Ethosuximide
Fosphenytoin
Gabapentin
Lamotrigine
Levetiracetam
Lorazepam
Oxcarbazepine
Pentobarbital
Phenobarbital
Phenytoin
Tiagabine
Topiramate
Valproic acid
Zonisamide

Antidepressants

Amitriptyline
Amoxapine
Bupropion
Citalopram
Desipramine
Doxepin
Fluoxetine
Fluvoxamine
Imipramine
Maprotiline
Mirtazapine
Nefazodone
Nortriptyline
Paroxetine
Phenelzine
Sertraline
Trazodone
Trimipramine
Venlafaxine

Antiparkinson Agents

Amantadine
Benztropine
Bromocriptine
Carbidopa/levodopa
Entacapone
Pergolide
Pramipexole
Procyclidine
Selegiline
Trihexyphenidyl

22

Antipsychotics

Chlorpromazine
Clozapine
Fluphenazine
Haloperidol
Lithium carbonate

Mesoridazine
Molindone
Olanzapine
Perphenazine
Prochlorperazine

Quetiapine
Risperidone
Thioridazine
Thiothixene
Trifluoperazine

Sedative Hypnotics

Chloral hydrate
Diphenhydramine
Estazolam
Flurazepam
Hydroxyzine

Midazolam
Pentobarbital
Phenobarbital
Propofol
Quazepam

Secobarbital
Temazepam
Triazolam
Zaleplon
Zolpidem

Miscellaneous Agents

Nimodipine

Rivastigmine

Tacrine

Dermatologic Agents

Acitretin
Acyclovir
Amphotericin B
Anthralin
Bacitracin
Bacitracin, topical
Bacitracin, neomycin and
    polymyxin B, topical
Bacitracin, neomycin,
    polymyxin B and hydro-
    cortisone, topical
Bacitracin, neomycin,
    polymyxin B and lido-
    caine, topical
Bacitracin and polymyxin B,
    topical
Calcipotriene
Capsaicin
Ciclopirox
Ciprofloxacin
Clindamycin, topical

Clotrimazole and betametha-
    sone
Dibucaine
Doxepin
Econazole
Erythromycin, topical
Finasteride
Gentamicin, topical
Haloprogin
Imiquimod
Isotretinoin (13-*cis* retinoic
    acid)
Ketoconazole
Lactic acid and ammonium
    hydroxide
Lindane
Metronidazole
Miconazole
Minoxidil
Mupirocin
Naftifine

Nystatin
Nystatin and triamcinolone
Oxiconazole
Penciclovir
Permethrin
Pramoxine
Pramoxine and hydrocorti-
    sone
Podophyllin
Selenium sulfide
Silver sulfadiazine
Steroids, topical (Table 22–6,
    pages 628–630)
Tazarotene
Terbinafine
Tolnaftate
Tretinoin, topical (retinoic
    acid)
Witch hazel

Dietary Supplements

Calcium acetate
Calcium glubionate
Calcium gluceptate
Calcium salts (chloride and
    gluconate)
Cholecalciferol
Cyanocobalamin (vitamin B_{12})

Ferric gluconate complex
Ferrous gluconate
Ferrous sulfate
Folic acid
Iron dextran
Magnesium oxide
Magnesium sulfate

Phytonadione (vitamin K)
Potassium supplements
    (Table 22–4, page 626)
Pyridoxine (vitamin B_6)
Sodium bicarbonate (bicar-
    bonate)
Thiamine (vitamin B_1)

Ear (Otic) Agents

Acetic acid and aluminum acetate
Benzocaine and antipyrine
Ciprofloxacin and hydrocortisone
Neomycin, colistin, and hydrocortisone
Neomycin, colistin, hydrocortisone, and thonzonium
Neomycin, polymyxin, and hydrocortisone
Polymyxin B and hydrocortisone
Sulfacetamide and prednisolone
Triethanolamine

Endocrine System

Antidiabetic Agents

Acarbose
Acetohexamide
Chlorpropamide
Glimepiride
Glipizide
Glyburide
Insulins (Table 22–2, page 622)
Metformin
Miglitol
Pioglitazone
Repaglinide
Rosiglitazone
Tolazamide
Tolbutamide

Hormone and Synthetic Substitutes

Calcitonin
Calcitriol
Cortisone
Desmopressin
Dexamethasone
Fludrocortisone acetate
Glucagon
Hydrocortisone
Methylprednisolone
Metyrapone
Prednisolone
Prednisone
Vasopressin

Hypercalcemia Agents

Etidronate
Gallium nitrate
Pamidronate
Plicamycin

Obesity

Sibutramine

Osteoporosis Agents

Alendronate
Raloxifene
Risedronate

Thyroid/Antithyroid

Levothyroxine
Liothyronine
Methimazole
Propylthiouracil

Miscellanous Agents

Demeclocycline
Diazoxide
Metyrosine

Eye (Ophthalmic) Agents

Glaucoma Agents

Acetazolamide
Apraclonidine
Betaxolol
Brimonidine
Brinzolamide
Carteolol
Dipivefrin
Dorzolamide
Dorzolamide and timolol
Echothiophate iodine
Latanoprost
Levobunolol

22

Levocabastine
Lodoxamide

Metipranolol
Timolol

Ophthalmic Antibiotics

Bacitracin
Bacitracin, neomycin and
   polymyxin B
Bacitracin, neomycin,
   polymyxin B and hydro-
   cortisone
Bacitracin and polymyxin B
Ciprofloxacin
Erythromycin

Gentamicin
Neomycin and dexametha-
   sone
Neomycin, polymyxin B and
   dexamethasone
Neomycin, polymyxin B and
   prednisolone
Ofloxacin
Silver nitrate

Sulfacetamide
Sulfacetamide and pred-
   nisolone
Tobramycin
Tobramycin and dexametha-
   sone
Trifluridine

Other Agents

Artificial tears
Cromolyn
Cyclopentolate

Dexamethasone (ophthalmic)
Ketorolac
Naphazoline and antazoline

Naphazoline and pheniramine

Gastrointestinal Agents

Antacids

Alginic acid
Aluminum carbonate
Aluminum hydroxide
Aluminum hydroxide with
   magnesium carbonate

Aluminum hydroxide with
   magnesium hydroxide
Aluminum hydroxide with
   magnesium hydroxide and
   simethicone

Aluminum hydroxide with
   magnesium trisilicate
Calcium carbonate
Magaldrate
Simethicone

Antidiarrheal

Bismuth subsalicylate
Diphenoxylate with atropine
Kaolin/pectin

Lactobacillus
Loperamide
Octreotide

Paregoric

Antiemetic

Buclizine
Chlorpromazine
Dimenhydrinate
Dolasetron
Dronabinol

Droperidol
Granisetron
Meclizine
Metoclopramide
Ondansetron

Prochlorperazine
Promethazine
Scopolamine
Thiethylperazine
Trimethobenzamide

Antiulcer

Cimetidine
Famotidine
Lansoprazole

Nizatidine
Omeprazole
Pantoprazole

Rabeprazole
Ranitidine
Sucralfate

Cathartics/Laxatives

Bisacodyl
Docusate calcium
Docusate potassium
Docusate sodium
Glycerin suppositories

Lactulose
Magnesium citrate
Magnesium hydroxide
Mineral oil

Polyethylene glycol-elec-
   trolyte (PEG) solution
Psyllium
Sorbitol

Enzymes

Pancreatin
Pancrelipase

Miscellaneous Agents

Alosetron
Dexpanthenol
Dibucaine
Dicyclomine
Hydrocortisone, rectal
Hyoscyamine
Hyoscyamine, atropine,
  scopolamine, and pheno-
  barbital

Infliximab
Mesalamine
Metoclopramide
Misoprostol
Olsalazine
Pramoxine
Pramoxine with hydrocorti-
  sone

Propantheline
Sulfasalazine
Vasopressin

Hematologic Agents

Anticoagulants

Ardeparin
Dalteparin

Enoxaparin
Heparin

Protamine
Warfarin

Antiplatelet Agents

Abciximab
Aspirin
Clopidogrel

Eptifibatide
Dipyridamole
Reteplase

Ticlopidine
Tirofiban

Antithrombic Agents

Alteplase, recombinant (TPA)
Aminocaproic acid
Anistreplase

Aprotinin
Dextran 40
Reteplase

Streptokinase
Tenecteplase
Urokinase

Hemopoietic Stimulants

Epoetin alfa (erythropoietin)
Filgrastim (G-CSF)

Oprelvekin
Sargramostim (GM-CSF)

Volume Expanders

Albumin
Dextran 40

Hetastarch
Plasma protein fraction

Miscellaneous Agents

Antihemophilic factor VIII
Desmopressin

Lepirudin
Pentoxifylline

Immune System Agents

Immunomodulators

Interferon alfa
Interferon alfacon-1

Interferon beta-1b
Interferon gamma-1b

Immunosuppressive Agents

Antithymocyte globulin (ATG)
Azathioprine
Basiliximab

Cyclosporine
Dacliximab
Muromonab-CD3
Mycophenolate mofetil

Sirolimus
Steroids, systemic (See Table 22–5, page 627
Tacrolimus

Vaccine/Serums/Toxoids

CMV Immune globulin
Haemophilus B conjugate
Hepatitis A vaccine
Hepatitis B immune globulin
Hepatitis B vaccine

Immune globulin
Influenza vaccine
Lyme disease vaccine
Pneumococcal vaccine, polyvalent

Pneumococcal 7-valent conjugate
Tetanus immune globulin
Tetanus toxoid
Varicella virus vaccine

Musculoskeletal Agents

Antigout Agents

Allopurinol
Colchicine

Probenecid
Sulfinpyrazone

Muscle Relaxants

Baclofen
Carisoprodol
Chlorzoxazone

Cyclobenzaprine
Dantrolene
Diazepam

Metaxalone
Methocarbamol
Orphenadrine

Neuromuscular Blockers

Atracurium
Mivacurium

Pancuronium
Pipecuronium

Succinylcholine
Vecuronium

Miscellaneous Agents

Edrophonium

Leflunomide

Methotrexate

OB/GYN Agents

Contraceptives

Levonorgestrel implants
Oral contraceptives monophasic (Table 22–3, pages 623–625)

Oral contraceptives biphasic (Table 22–3, pages 623–625)
Oral contraceptives triphasic (Table 22–3, pages 623–625)

Oral contraceptives progestin only (Table 22–3, pages 623–625)
Norgestrel

Estrogen Supplementation

Esterified estrogens
Esterified estrogens with methyltestosterone
Estradiol

Estradiol transdermal
Estrogen, conjugated
Estrogen, conjugated with methylprogesterone

Estrogen, conjugated with methyltestosterone
Ethinyl estradiol

Vaginal Preparations

Amino-Cerv pH 5.5 cream
Miconazole

Nystatin
Terconazole

Tioconazole

22

Miscellaneous Agents

Gonadorelin
Leuprolide
Magnesium sulfate

Medroxyprogesterone
Methylergonovine
Mifepristone (RU486)

Oxytocin
Terbutaline

Pain Relievers

Local Anesthetics

Benzocaine and antipyrine
Bupivacaine
Capsaicin

Cocaine
Dibucaine
Lidocaine

Lidocaine and prilocaine
Pramoxine

Migraine Headache Agents

Acetaminophen with butal-
   bital ±/– caffeine
Aspirin with butalbital and
   caffeine

Naratriptan
Rizatriptan
Sumatriptan
Zolmitriptan

Narcotics

Acetaminophen with codeine
Alfentanil
Aspirin with codeine
Buprenorphine
Butorphanol
Codeine
Dezocine
Fentanyl
Fentanyl transdermal
Fentanyl transmucosal
Hydrocodone and aceta-
   minophen

Hydrocodone and aspirin
Hydrocodone and ibuprofen
Hydromorphone
Levorphanol
Meperidine
Methadone
Morphine
Nalbuphine
Oxycodone
Oxycodone and aceta-
   minophen

Oxycodone and aspirin
Oxymorphone
Pentazocine
Propoxyphene
Propoxyphene and aceta-
   minophen
Propoxyphene and aspirin
Sufentanil

Nonnarcotic Agents

Acetaminophen

Tramadol

Nonsteroidal Antiinflammatory Agents

Aspirin
Celecoxib
Diclofenac
Diflunisal
Etodolac
Fenoprofen
Flurbiprofen

Ibuprofen
Indomethacin
Ketoprofen
Ketorolac
Meloxicam
Nabumetone
Naproxen

Naproxen sodium
Oxaprozin
Piroxicam
Rofecoxib
Sulindac
Tolmetin

Miscellanous Agents

Amitriptyline

Imipramine

Tramadol

Respiratory Agents

Antitussives and Decongestants

Acetylcysteine
Benzonatate
Codeine
Dextromethorphan
Guaifenesin
Guaifenesin and codeine

Guaifenesin and dextromethorphan
Hydrocodone and guaifenesin
Hydrocodone and homatropine
Hydrocodone and pseudoephedrine
Hydrocodone, chlorpheniramine, phenylephrine, acetaminophen, and caffeine
Pseudoephedrine

Bronchodilators

Albuterol
Albuterol and ipratropium
Aminophylline
Bitolterol
Ephedrine

Epinephrine
Isoetharine
Isoproterenol
Levalbuterol
Metaproterenol

Pirbuterol
Salmeterol
Terbutaline
Theophylline

Respiratory Inhalants

Acetylcysteine
Beclomethasone
Beractant
Calfactant

Colfosceril palmitate
Cromolyn sodium
Dexamethasone, nasal
Flunisolide

Fluticasone, oral, nasal
Ipratropium
Nedocromil
Triamcinolone

Miscellanous Agents

Alpha$_1$ protease inhibitor
Dornase alfa

Montelukast
Zafirlukast

Zileuton

Urinary/Genitourinary Agents

Alprostadil intracavernosal
Alprostadil urethral suppository
Ammonium aluminum sulfate (alum)
Belladonna and opium supp
Bethanechol
Dimethyl sulfoxide (DMSO)
Flavoxate

Hyoscyamine
Methenamine
Nalidixic acid
Neomycin–polymyxin bladder irrigant
Nitrofurantoin
Oxybutynin
Pentosan polysulfate

Phenazopyridine
Potassium citrate
Potassium citrate and citric acid
Sildenafil
Sodium citrate
Trimethoprim
Tolterodine

Benign Prostatic Hyperplasia

Doxazosin
Finasteride

Tamsulosin
Terazosin

Wound Care

Silver nitrate
Becaplermin

Miscellaneous Agents

Megestrol acetate
Metaraminol
Naltrexone

Nicotine gum
Nicotine nasal spray
Nicotine transdermal

Potassium iodide
Sodium polystyrene sulfonate
Triethanolamine

GENERIC DRUG LISTING AND DATA

Abacavir (Ziagen)

COMMON USES: HIV infection
ACTIONS: Nucleoside reverse transcriptase inhibitor
DOSAGE: *Adults.* 300 mg bid. *Peds.* 8 mg/kg bid
SUPPLIED: Tabs 300 mg; soln 20 mg/mL
NOTES: Fatal hypersensitivity reactions possibly manifested as respiratory symptoms. Discontinue immediately if hypersensitivity symptoms arise (fever, skin rash, fatigue, nausea, vomiting, diarrhea or abdominal pain). Lactic acidosis and hepatomegaly with steatosis also possible

Abciximab (ReoPro)

COMMON USES: Prevent acute ischemic complications in PTCA
ACTIONS: Inhibits platelet aggregation (GPII b/IIIa inhibitor)
DOSAGE: 0.25 mg/kg bolus 10–60 min prior to PTCA, then 0.125 µg/kg/min (max = 10 µg/min) cont inf for 12 h
SUPPLIED: Inj 2 mg/mL
NOTES: Used with heparin; allergic reactions possible

Acarbose (Precose)

COMMON USES: Type 2 DM
ACTIONS: α-Glucosidase inhibitor; delays digestion of carbohydrates, resulting in lower plasma glucose levels
DOSAGE: 25–100 mg PO tid at the start of each main meal
SUPPLIED: Tabs 25, 50, 100 mg
NOTES: May be taken with sulfonylureas

Acebutolol (Sectral)

COMMON USES: HTN
ACTIONS: Competitively blocks β-adrenergic receptors, β_1 and ISA
DOSAGE: 200–800 mg/d
SUPPLIED: Caps 200, 400 mg

Acetaminophen (Tylenol, others)

COMMON USES: Mild pain, headache, and fever
ACTIONS: Nonnarcotic analgesic; inhibits synthesis of prostaglandins in the CNS and inhibits hypothalamic heat-regulating center
DOSAGE: *Adults.* 650 mg PO or PR q4–6h or 1000 mg PO q6h; do not exceed 4 g/24h. *Peds <12 y.* 10–15 mg/kg/dose PO or PR q4–6h; do not exceed 2.6 g/24h. See quick dosing information in Table 22–1 (page 621).
SUPPLIED: Tabs 160, 325, 500, 650 mg; chewable tabs 80, 160 mg; liq 100 mg/mL, 120 mg/2.5 mL, 120 mg/5 mL, 160 mg/5 mL, 167 mg/5 mL, 325 mg/5 mL, 500 mg/5 mL; gtt 48 mg/mL, 60 mg/0.6 mL; supp 80, 120, 125, 300, 325, 650 mg
NOTES: No antiinflammatory or platelet-inhibiting action; ↓ dose with alcohol use; overdose causes hepatotoxicity, which is treated with *N*-acetylcysteine; charcoal not usually recommended

Acetaminophen + Butalbital +/– Caffeine (Fioricet, Medigesic, Repan, Sedapap-10, Two-Dyne, Triapin, Axocet, Phrenilin Forte, others) [C-III]

COMMON USES: Mild pain; headache, especially associated with stress
ACTIONS: Nonnarcotic analgesic with barbiturate
DOSAGE: 1–2 tabs or caps PO q4–6h PRN
SUPPLIED: Caps *Medigesic, Repan, Two-Dyne:* Butalbital 50 mg, caffeine 40 mg, + acetaminophen 325 mg. Caps *Axocet, Phrenilin Forte:* Butalbital 50 mg and acetaminophen 650 mg; *Triaprin:* Butalbital 50 mg + acetaminophen 325 mg. Tabs *Esgic, Fioricet, Repan:* Butalbital 50 mg, caffeine

22

40 mg, + acetaminophen 325 mg; *Phrenilin:* Butalbital 50 mg and acetaminophen 325 mg; *Seda-pap-10:* Butalbital 50 mg + acetaminophen 650 mg
NOTES: Butalbital habit-forming

Acetaminophen + Codeine (Tylenol No. 1, No. 2, No. 3, No. 4) [C-II]

COMMON USES: No. 1, No. 2, and No. 3 for mild to moderate pain; No. 4 for moderate to severe pain
ACTIONS: Combined effects of acetaminophen and a narcotic analgesic
DOSAGE: *Adults.* 1–2 tabs q3–4h PRN. (Max dose acetaminophen = 4 g/d). *Peds.* Acetaminophen 10–15 mg/kg/dose; codeine 0.5–1.0 mg/kg dose q4–6h (useful dosing guide: 3–6 y, 5 mL/dose; 7–12 y, 10 mL/dose)
SUPPLIED: Tabs 300 mg of APAP + codeine; caps 325 mg of APAP + codeine; liq acetaminophen 120 mg + codeine 12 mg/5 mL
NOTES: Codeine in No. 1 = 7.5 mg, No. 2 = 15 mg, No. 3 = 30 mg, No.4 = 60 mg

Acetazolamide (Diamox)

COMMON USES: Diuresis, glaucoma, acute mountain sickness, and refractory epilepsy
ACTIONS: Carbonic anhydrase inhibitor; $\downarrow$ renal excretion of hydrogen ions, and $\uparrow$ renal excretion of sodium, potassium, bicarbonate, and water
DOSAGE: *Adults.* Diuretic: 250–375 mg IV or PO q24h. *Glaucoma:* 250–1000 mg PO q24h in ÷ doses. *Epilepsy:* 8–30 mg/kg/d PO in ÷ doses. *Altitude sickness:* 250 mg PO q8–12h or SR 500 mg PO q12–24h. *Peds.* Epilepsy: 8–30 mg/kg/24h PO in ÷ doses; max 1 g/d. *Diuretic:* 5 mg/kg/24h PO or IV. *Alkalinization of urine:* 5 mg/kg/dose PO bid–tid. *Glaucoma:* 5–15 mg/kg/24h PO in ÷ doses; max 1 g/d
SUPPLIED: Tabs 125, 250 mg; SR caps 500 mg; inj 500 mg/vial
NOTES: Contra in renal and hepatic failure, sulfa hypersensitivity; follow Na^+ and K^+; watch for metabolic acidosis; SR dosage forms not recommended for use in epilepsy

Acetic Acid And Aluminum Acetate (Otic Domeboro)

COMMON USES: Otitis externa
ACTIONS: Antiinfective
DOSAGE: 4–6 gtt in ear(s) q2–3h
SUPPLIED: Otic soln

Acetohexamide (Dymelor)

COMMON USES: Type 2 DM
ACTION: Sulfonylurea. Stimulates release of insulin from pancreas; increases insulin sensitivity at peripheral sites; reduces glucose output from liver
DOSAGE: 250–1500 mg/d
SUPPLIED: Tabs 250, 500 mg

Acetylcysteine (Mucomyst, Mucosil)

COMMON USES: Mucolytic agent as adjuvant Rx for chronic bronchopulmonary diseases and CF; antidote to acetaminophen hepatotoxicity within 24 h of ingestion
ACTIONS: Splits disulfide linkages between mucoprotein molecular complexes; protects the liver by restoring glutathione levels in acetaminophen overdose
DOSAGE: *Adults & Peds.* Nebulizer: 3–5 mL of 20% soln diluted with an equal vol of water or NS tid–qid. *Antidote:* PO or NG: 140 mg/kg loading dose, then 70 mg/kg q4h for 17 doses. Dilute 1:3 in carbonated beverage or orange juice
SUPPLIED: Soln 10%, 20%
NOTES: Watch for bronchospasm when used by inhalation in asthmatics; activated charcoal adsorbs acetylcysteine when given PO for acute APAP ingestion

Acitretin (Soriatane)

COMMON USES: Severe psoriasis and other keratinization disorders (lichen planus, etc)

ACTIONS: Retinoid-like activity
DOSAGE: 25–50 mg/d PO, with main meal; can ↑ if no response by 4 wk to 75 mg/d
SUPPLIED: Caps 10, 25 mg
NOTES: Teratogenic, contra in PRG; Use with caution in women of reproductive potential; check LFTs, can be hepatotoxic; response often takes 2–3 mo

Acyclovir (Zovirax)

COMMON USES: Herpes simplex and herpes zoster viral infections
ACTIONS: Interferes with viral DNA synthesis
DOSAGE: *Adults.* Oral: Initial genital herpes: 200 mg PO q4h while awake, total of 5 caps/d for 10 d or 400 mg PO tid for 7–10 d. *Chronic suppression:* 400 mg PO bid. *Intermittent Rx:* As for initial treatment, except treat for 5 d, or 800 mg PO bid, initiated at the earliest prodrome. *Herpes zoster:* 800 mg PO 5×/d for 7–10 d. *IV.* 5–10 mg/kg/dose IV q8h. *Topical initial herpes genitalis:* Apply q3h (6×/d) for 7 d. *Peds.* 5–10 mg/kg/dose IV or PO q8h or 750 mg/m^2/24h ÷ q8h. *Chickenpox:* 20 mg/kg/dose PO qid
SUPPLIED: Caps 200 mg; tabs 400, 800 mg; susp 200 mg/5 mL; inj 500 mg/vial; oint 5%
NOTES: Adjust dose in renal insufficiency; oral better than topical for herpes genitalis

Adenosine (Adenocard)

Used for emergency cardiac care (see Chapter 21).
COMMON USES: PSVT, including that associated with Wolff-Parkinson-White syndrome
ACTIONS: Class IV antiarrhythmic; slows conduction time through the AV node
DOSAGE: *Adults.* 6 mg rapid IV bolus; may be repeated in 1–2 min; max 12 mg IV. *Peds.* 0.05 mg/kg IV bolus; may repeat q 1–2 min to a max of 0.25 mg/kg
SUPPLIED: Inj 6 mg/2 mL
NOTES: Doses >12 mg not recommended; caffeine and theophylline antagonize effects of adenosine

Albumin (Albuminar, Buminate, Albutein, others)

COMMON USES: Plasma volume expansion for shock resulting from burns, surgery, hemorrhage, or other trauma
ACTIONS: Maintenance of plasma colloid oncotic pressure
DOSAGE: *Adults.* Initially, 25 g IV; subsequent infusions depend on clinical situation and response. No more than 250 g/48h. *Peds.* 0.5–1.0 g/kg/dose; infuse at 0.05–0.1 g/min
SUPPLIED: Soln 5%, 25%
NOTES: Contains 130–160 meq Na$^+$/L.

Albuterol (Proventil, Ventolin)

COMMON USES: Bronchospasm in reversible obstructive airway disease; prevention of exercise-induced bronchospasm
ACTIONS: β-Adrenergic sympathomimetic bronchodilator; relaxes bronchial smooth muscle
DOSAGE: *Adults.* 2 inhal q4–6h PRN; 1 Rotacaps inhaled q4–6h; 2–4 mg PO tid–qid; *Neb:* 1.25–5 mg (0.25–1 mL of 0.5% soln) in 2–3 mL of NS tid–qid. *Peds.* 2 inhal q4–6h; 0.1–0.2 mg/kg/dose PO; max 2–4 mg PO tid; *Neb:* 0.05 mg/kg (max 2.5 mg) in a 2–3 mL of NS tid–qid
SUPPLIED: Tabs 2, 4 mg; ER tabs 4, 8 mg; syrup 2 mg/5 mL; 90 μg/dose met-dose inhaler; Rotacaps 200 μg; soln for neb 0.083, 0.5%

Albuterol and Ipratropium (Combivent)

COMMON USES: COPD
ACTIONS: Combination of β-adrenergic bronchodilator and quaternary anticholinergic compound
DOSAGE: 2 inhal qid
SUPPLIED: Met-dose inhaler, 18 μg ipratropium/103 μg Albuterol/puff

Aldesleukin [IL-2] (Proleukin)

COMMON USES: RCC, melanoma
ACTIONS: Acts via IL-2 receptor; numerous immunomodulatory effects
DOSAGE: 600,000 IU/kg q8h for 14 doses (FDA-approved dose/schedule for RCC). Multiple cont inf and SCSC dosing schedules (including "high-dose" therapy with 24×10^6 IU/m^2 IV q8h on d 1–5 and 12–16)
SUPPLIED: Inj 1.1 mg/mL (22×10^6 IU)
NOTES: *Toxicity symptoms:* flu-like syndrome (malaise, fever, chills), nausea and vomiting, diarrhea, and increased serum bilirubin. Capillary leak syndrome with hypotension, pulmonary edema, fluid retention, and weight gain. Renal toxicity and mild hematologic toxicity (anemia, thrombocytopenia, leukopenia) and secondary eosinophilia. Cardiac toxicity (myocardial ischemia, atrial arrhythmias). Neurologic toxicity (CNS depression, somnolence, rarely coma, delirium). Pruritic skin rashes, urticaria, and erythroderma common. Cont inf schedules less likely in severe hypotension and fluid retention

Alendronate (Fosamax)

COMMON USES: Rx and prevention of osteoporosis, Rx of glucocorticoid-induced osteoporosis and Paget's disease
ACTIONS: Inhibits normal and abnormal bone resorption
DOSAGE: *Osteoporosis: Rx:* 10 mg/d PO. *Glucocorticoid-induced osteoporosis: Rx:* 5 mg/d PO. *Prevention:* 5 mg/d PO. *Paget's disease:* 40 mg/d PO
SUPPLIED: Tabs 5, 10, 40 mg
NOTES: Take first thing in AM with plain water (8 oz) at least 30 min prior to the first food or beverage of the day. Do not lie down for 30 min after taking. Adequate calcium and vitamin D supplement necessary

Alfentanil (Alfenta) [C]

COMMON USES: Adjunct in the maintenance of anesthesia; analgesia
ACTIONS: Short-acting narcotic analgesic
DOSAGE: *Adults & Peds >12 y.* 3–75 µg/kg IV inf; total dose depends on duration of procedure
SUPPLIED: Inj 500 µg/mL

Alginic Acid + Aluminum Hydroxide and Magnesium Trisilicate (Gaviscon)

COMMON USES: Heartburn; pain from hiatal hernia
ACTIONS: Forms protective layer preventing reflux of gastric acid
DOSAGE: 2–4 tabs or 15–30 mL PO qid followed by water
SUPPLIED: Tabs, susp

Allopurinol (Zyloprim, Lopurin, Aloprim, others)

COMMON USES: Gout, hyperuricemia of malignancy, and uric acid urolithiasis
ACTIONS: Xanthine oxidase inhibitor, which decreases the production of uric acid
DOSAGE: *Adults.* PO: Initially, 100 mg/d; usual 300 mg/d; max 800 mg/d. *IV:* 200–400 mg/m^2/d (max 600 mg/24h). *Peds.* Use only for treating hyperuricemia of malignancy in children (*<10 y*): 10 mg/kg/24h PO or 200 mg/m^2/d IV ÷ q6–8h (max 600 mg/24h)
SUPPLIED: Tabs 100, 300 mg; inj 500 mg/30 mL
NOTES: Aggravates acute gouty attack; do not begin until acute attack resolves; administer pc. IV administration of 6 mg/mL final conc as single daily infusion or ÷ 6-, 8-, or 12-h intervals. Dosage adjustment necessary in renal impairment

Alosetron (lotronex)

COMMON USES: Irritable bowel syndrome in women, diarrhea as main symptom
ACTIONS: 5-HT$_3$ receptor antagonist
NOTES: Removed from the market

α_1-Protease Inhibitor (Prolastin)

COMMON USES: Panacinar emphysema
ACTIONS: Replacement of human α_1-protease inhibitor
DOSAGE: 60 mg/kg IV once/wk
SUPPLIED: Inj 500 mg/20 mL; 1000 mg/40 mL

Alprazolam (Xanax) [C]

COMMON USES: Anxiety and panic disorders + anxiety associated with depression
ACTIONS: Benzodiazepine; antianxiety agent
DOSAGE: *Anxiety:* Initially, 0.25–0.5 mg tid; $\uparrow$ to a max of 4 mg/d in ÷ doses. *Panic:* Initially, 0.5 mg tid; may gradually $\uparrow$ to desired response
SUPPLIED: Tabs 0.25, 0.5, 1.0, 2.0 mg
NOTES: $\downarrow$ Dose in elderly and debilitated patients; avoid abrupt discontinuation after prolonged use

Alprostadil, Intracavernosal (Caverject, Edex)

COMMON USES: Erectile dysfunction due to neurogenic, vasculogenic, or mixed cause
ACTIONS: Relaxes smooth muscles, dilates cavernosal arteries, increases lacunar spaces and entrapment of blood by compressing venules against tunica albuginea
DOSAGE: 2.5–60 µg intracavernosal; adjusted to individual needs
SUPPLIED: *Caverject:* 6–10 or 6–20 µg vials +/– diluent syringes. *Edex:* 5, 10, 20, 40 µg vials + syringes
NOTES: Penile pain common side effect; dosage must be titrated at physician's office. Patients should be informed of other side effects, including priapism, penile fibrosis, and hematoma

Alprostadil [Prostaglandin E_1] (Prostin VR)

COMMON USES: Any state in which blood flow must be maintained through the ductus arteriosus to sustain either pulmonary or systemic circulation until corrective or palliative surgery can be performed (eg, pulmonary atresia, pulmonary stenosis, tricuspid atresia, transposition, severe tetralogy of Fallot)
ACTIONS: Vasodilator, platelet aggregation inhibitor. Smooth muscle of the ductus arteriosus is especially sensitive
DOSAGE: 0.05 µg/kg/min IV. $\downarrow$ Dosage to lowest rate that maintains response
SUPPLIED: Injectable forms
NOTES: Cutaneous vasodilation, seizure-like activity, jitteriness, temperature elevation, hypocalcemia, apnea, thrombocytopenia, hypotension. May cause apnea. Have an intubation kit at bedside if patient is not intubated

Alprostadil, Urethral Suppository (Muse)

COMMON USES: Erectile dysfunction
ACTIONS: Alprostadil (PGE_1) absorbed through urethral mucosa. Portion of administered dose transported to the corpus cavernosa where it acts as vasodilator and smooth muscle relaxant
DOSAGE: 125–1000 µg system 5–10 min prior to sexual activity
SUPPLIED: 125, 250, 500, 1000 µg with a transurethral delivery system
NOTES: Hypotension, dizziness, syncope, penile pain, and priapism. Dose titration administered under physician's supervision

Alteplase, Recombinant [TPA] (Activase)

Used for emergency cardiac care (see Chapter 21)
COMMON USES: AMI, PE, and acute ischemic stroke
ACTIONS: Results in thrombolysis; inhibits local fibrinolysis by binding to fibrin in the thrombus
DOSAGE: *AMI and PE:* 100 mg IV over 3 h (10 mg over 2 min, then 50 mg over 1 h, then 40 mg over 2 h). *Stroke:* 0.9 mg/kg (max 90 mg) infused over 60 min
SUPPLIED: Powder for inj 50, 100 mg

NOTES: May cause bleeding; give heparin to prevent reocclusion. In AMI doses of >150 mg associated with intracranial bleeding

Altretamine (Hexalen)

COMMON USES: Epithelial ovarian cancer
ACTIONS: Unknown; cytotoxic agent, possibly alkylating agent; inhibits nucleotide incorporation into DNA and RNA
DOSAGE: 260 mg/m²/d in 4 ÷ doses for 14–21 d of a 28-d treatment cycle; dose ↓ to 150 mg/m²/d for 14 d in multiagent regimens. (Refer to specific protocols)
SUPPLIED: Caps 50, 100 mg
NOTES: *Toxicity symptoms:* Vomiting, diarrhea, and cramps; neurologic toxicity (peripheral neuropathy, CNS depression); minimally myelosuppressive

Aluminum Carbonate (Basaljel)

COMMON USES: Hyperacidity (peptic ulcer, GERD, etc); supplement to the Rx of hyperphosphatemia
ACTIONS: Neutralizes gastric acid; binds phosphate
DOSAGE: *Adults.* 2 caps or tabs or 10 mL (in water) q2h PRN. *Peds.* 50–150 mg/kg/24h PO ÷ q4–6h
SUPPLIED: Tabs, caps, susp

Aluminum Hydroxide (Amphojel, Alternagel)

COMMON USES: Hyperacidity (peptic ulcer, hiatal hernia, etc); supplement to Rx of hyperphosphatemia
ACTIONS: Neutralizes gastric acid; binds phosphate
DOSAGE: *Adults.* 10–30 mL or 2 tabs PO q4–6h. *Peds.* 5–15 mL PO q4–6h or 50–150 mg/kg/24h PO ÷ q4–6h (hyperphosphatemia)
SUPPLIED: Tabs 300, 600 mg; chewable tabs 500 mg; susp 320, 600 mg/5 mL
NOTES: Can be used in renal failure; may cause constipation

Aluminum Hydroxide + Magnesium Carbonate (Gaviscon)

COMMON USES: Hyperacidity (peptic ulcer, hiatal hernia, etc)
ACTIONS: Neutralizes gastric acid
DOSAGE: *Adults.* 15–30 PO pc and hs. *Peds.* 5–15 mL PO qid or PRN
SUPPLIED: Liq containing aluminum hydroxide 95 mg + magnesium carbonate 358 mg/15 mL
NOTES: Doses qid are best given pc and hs; may cause hypermagnesemia

Aluminum Hydroxide + Magnesium Trisilicate (Gaviscon, Gaviscon-2)

COMMON USES: Hyperacidity
ACTIONS: Neutralizes gastric acid
DOSAGE: Chew 2–4 tabs qid
SUPPLIED: *Gaviscon:* Aluminum hydroxide 80 mg and magnesium trisilicate 20 mg; *Gaviscon 2:* Aluminum hydroxide 160 mg and magnesium trisilicate 40 mg

Aluminum Hydroxide + Magnesium Hydroxide (Maalox)

COMMON USES: Hyperacidity (peptic ulcer, hiatal hernia, etc)
ACTIONS: Neutralizes gastric acid
DOSAGE: *Adults.* 10–60 mL or 2–4 tabs PO qid or PRN. *Peds.* 5–15 mL PO qid or PRN
SUPPLIED: Tabs, susp
NOTES: Doses qid best given pc and hs; may cause hypermagnesemia in renal insufficiency

Aluminum Hydroxide + Magnesium Hydroxide and Simethicone (Mylanta, Mylanta II, Maalox Plus)

COMMON USES: Hyperacidity with bloating

ACTIONS: Neutralizes gastric acid
DOSAGE: *Adults.* 10–60 mL or 2–4 tabs PO qid or PRN. *Peds.* 5–15 mL PO qid or PRN
SUPPLIED: Tabs, susp
NOTES: May cause hypermagnesemia in renal insufficiency; Mylanta II contains twice the aluminum and magnesium hydroxide of Mylanta

Amantadine (Symmetrel)

COMMON USES: Rx or prophylaxis for influenza A viral infections and Parkinsonism
ACTIONS: Prevents release of infectious viral nucleic acid into the host cell; releases dopamine from intact dopaminergic terminals
DOSAGE: *Adults.* Influenza A: 200 mg/d PO or 100 mg PO bid. *Parkinsonism:* 100 mg PO qd–bid. *Peds.* 1–9 y: 4.4–8.8 mg/kg/24h to a max of 150 mg/24h ÷ doses qd–bid. *10–12 y:* 100–200 mg/d in 1–2 ÷ doses
SUPPLIED: Caps 100 mg; tabs 100 mg, soln 50 mg/5 mL
NOTES: ↓ in renal insufficiency

Amifostine (Ethyol)

COMMON USES: Xerostomia prophylaxis during radiation therapy for head and neck, ovarian, or non-small-cell lung cancer. Reduction of cumulative renal toxicity associated with repeated administration of cisplatin
ACTIONS: Prodrug, dephosphorylated by alkaline phosphatase to the pharmacologically active thiol metabolite
DOSAGE: 910 mg/m^2/d as a 15-min IV inf 30 min prior to chemotherapy
SUPPLIED: Vials containing 500 mg of lyophilized drug with 500 mg of mannitol, reconstituted in sterile NS
NOTES: *Toxicity symptoms:* Transient hypotension in >60%, nausea and vomiting, flushing with hot or cold chills, dizziness, hypocalcemia, somnolence, and sneezing. Does not reduce the effectiveness of cyclophosphamide plus cisplatin chemotherapy

Amikacin (Amikin)

COMMON USES: Serious infections caused by gram (−) bacteria and mycobacterial infections
ACTIONS: Aminoglycoside antibiotic; inhibits protein synthesis
DOSAGE: See also page 620. *Adults & Peds.* 5–7.5 mg/kg/dose ÷ q8–24h based on renal function. *Neonates.* <1200 g, 0–4 wk: 7.5 mg/kg/dose q12h-18h. *Postnatal age <7 d.* 1200–2000 g: 7.5 mg/kg/dose q12h. *>2000 g:* 10 mg/kg/dose q12h. *Postnatal age >7 d.* 1200–2000 g: 7 mg/kg/dose q8h. *>2000 g:* 7.5–10 mg/kg/dose q8h
SUPPLIED: Inj 100, 500 mg/2 mL
NOTES: May be effective against gram (−) bacteria resistant to gentamicin and tobramycin; monitor renal function carefully for dosage adjustments; monitor serum levels (see Table 22–7, pages 631–634)

Amiloride (Midamor)

COMMON USES: HTN and CHF
ACTIONS: K$^+$-sparing diuretic; interferes with K$^+$/Na$^+$ exchange in the distal tubules
DOSAGE: *Adults.* 5–10 mg PO qd. *Peds.* 0.625 mg/kg/d
SUPPLIED: Tabs 5 mg
NOTES: Hyperkalemia possible; monitor serum K$^+$ levels

Aminocaproic Acid (Amicar)

COMMON USES: Excessive bleeding resulting from systemic hyperfibrinolysis and urinary fibrinolysis
ACTIONS: Inhibits fibrinolysis via inhibition of TPA substances
DOSAGE: *Adults.* 5 g IV or PO (1st h) followed by 1–1.25 g/h IV or PO. *Peds.* 100 mg/kg IV (1st h), (Max dose/d: 30 g), then 1 g/m^2/h; max 18 g/m^2/d
SUPPLIED: Tabs 500 mg; syrup 250 mg/mL; inj 250 mg/mL

NOTES: Administer for 8 h or until bleeding is controlled; contra in DIC; not for upper urinary tract bleeding

Amino-Cerv pH 5.5 Cream

COMMON USES: Mild cervicitis, postpartum cervicitis/cervical tears, postcauterization, post-cryosurgery, and postconization
DOSAGE: 1 applicator full intravaginally hs for 2–4 wk
SUPPLIED: Vaginal cream
NOTES: Contains 8.34% urea, 0.5% sodium propionate, 0.83% methionine, 0.35% cystine, 0.83% inositol, and benzalkonium chloride

Aminoglutethimide (Cytadren)

COMMON USES: Adrenal cortex carcinoma, Cushing's syndrome, breast cancer, and prostate cancer
ACTIONS: Inhibits adrenal steroidogenesis and adrenal conversion of androgens to estrogens
DOSAGE: 750–1500 mg/d in ÷ doses plus hydrocortisone 20–40 mg/d
SUPPLIED: Tabs 250 mg
NOTES: *Toxicity symptoms:* Adrenal insufficiency ("medical adrenalectomy"), hypothyroidism, masculinization, hypotension, vomiting, rare hepatotoxicity, rash, myalgia, and fever

Aminophylline

Used for emergency care (see Chapter 21)
COMMON USES: Asthma and bronchospasm
ACTIONS: Relaxes the smooth muscle of the bronchi and pulmonary blood vessels
DOSAGE: *Adults.* Acute asthma: Load 6 mg/kg IV, then 0.4–0.9 mg/kg/h IV cont inf. *Chronic asthma:* 24 mg/kg/24h PO or PR ÷ q6h. *Peds.* Load 6 mg/kg IV, then 1.0 mg/kg/h IV cont inf
SUPPLIED: Tabs 100, 200 mg; soln 105 mg/5 mL; supp 250, 500 mg; inj 25 mg/mL
NOTES: Individualize dosage. *Toxicity symptoms:* Nausea and vomiting, irritability, tachycardia, ventricular arrhythmias, and seizures; follow serum levels carefully (as theophylline, see Table 22–7, pages 631–634); aminophylline is about 85% theophylline; erratic absorption with rectal doses

Amiodarone (Cordarone) (Pacerone)

COMMON USES: Recurrent VF or hemodynamically unstable VT
ACTIONS: Class III antiarrhythmic
DOSAGE: *Adults.* Loading dose: 800–1600 mg/d PO for 1–3 wk. *Maintenance:* 600–800 mg/d PO for 1 mo, then 200–400 mg/d *IV:* 15 mg/min for 10 min, followed by 1 mg/min for 6 h, then a maintenance dose of 0.5 mg/min cont inf. *Peds.* 10–15 mg/kg/24h ÷ q12h PO for 7–10 d, then 5 mg/kg/24h ÷ q12h or qd (infants and neonates may require a higher loading dose)
SUPPLIED: Tabs 200 mg; inj 50 mg/mL
NOTES: Average half-life is 53 d; potentially toxic effects leading to pulmonary fibrosis, liver failure, and ocular opacities, as well as exacerbation of arrhythmias; IV concentrations of 0.2 mg/mL administered via a central catheter

Amitriptyline (Elavil, others)

COMMON USES: Depression, peripheral neuropathy, chronic pain, and cluster and migraine headaches
ACTIONS: Tricyclic antidepressant; inhibits reuptake of serotonin and norepinephrine by the pre-synaptic neuronal membrane
DOSAGE: *Adults.* Initially, 30–50 mg PO hs; may ↑ to 300 mg hs. *Peds.* Not recommended for children <12 y unless for chronic pain; initially, 0.1 mg/kg PO hs, then advance over 2–3 wk to 0.5–2 mg/kg PO hs
SUPPLIED: Tabs 10, 25, 50, 75, 100, 150 mg; inj 10 mg/mL
NOTES: Strong anticholinergic side effects; may cause urine retention and sedation; overdose may be fatal

22

Amlodipine (Norvasc)

COMMON USES: HTN, chronic stable angina, and vasospastic angina
ACTIONS: Calcium channel-blocking agent; produces relaxation of coronary vascular smooth muscle
DOSAGE: 2.5–10 mg/d PO
SUPPLIED: Tabs 2.5, 5, 10 mg
NOTES: May be taken without regard to meals

Ammonium Aluminum Sulfate (Alum)

COMMON USES: Hemorrhagic cystitis when bladder irrigation fails
ACTIONS: Astringent
DOSAGE: 1–2% soln used with constant bladder irrigation with NS
SUPPLIED: Powder for reconstitution
NOTES: Can be used safely without anesthesia and in the presence of vesicoureteral reflux. Encephalopathy possible; obtain aluminum levels, especially in renal insufficiency. Alum soln often precipitates and occludes catheters

Amoxapine (Asendin)

COMMON USES: Depression and anxiety
ACTIONS: Tricyclic antidepressant; reduces reuptake of serotonin and norepinephrine
DOSAGE: Initially, 150 mg PO hs or 50 mg PO tid; ↑ to 300 mg/d
SUPPLIED: Tabs 25, 50, 100, 150 mg
NOTES: ↓ in elderly; taper slowly when discontinuing therapy

Amoxicillin (Amoxil, Polymox, others)

COMMON USES: Infections resulting from susceptible gram (+) bacteria (streptococci) and gram (−) bacteria (*H. influenzae, E. coli, P. mirabilis*)
ACTIONS: β-Lactam antibiotic; inhibits cell wall synthesis
DOSAGE: *Adults.* 250–500 mg PO tid or 500–875 mg bid. *Peds.* 25–100 mg/kg/24h PO ÷ q8h. 200–400 mg PO bid (equivalent to 125–250 mg tid)
SUPPLIED: Caps 250, 500 mg; chewable tabs 125, 200, 250, 400 mg; susp 50 mg/mL, 125, 250 mg/5mL; tabs 500, 875 mg
NOTES: Cross-hypersensitivity with penicillin; may cause diarrhea; skin rash common; many hospital strains of *E. coli* resistant

Amoxicillin and Clavulanic Acid (Augmentin)

COMMON USES: Infections caused by β-lactamase-producing strains of *H. influenzae, S. aureus, and E. coli*
ACTIONS: Combination of a β-lactam antibiotic and a β-lactamase inhibitor
DOSAGE: *Adults.* 250–500 mg PO q8h or 875 mg q12h. *Peds.* 20–40 mg/kg/d as amoxicillin PO ÷ q8h or 45 mg/kg/d ÷ q12h
SUPPLIED: (Expressed as amoxicillin/clavulanic acid) Tabs 250/125, 500/125, 875/125 mg; chewable tabs 125/31.25, 200/28.5, 250/62.5, 400/57 mg; susp 125/31.25, 250/62.5, 200/28.5, 400/57 mg/5 mL
NOTES: Do not substitute two 250-mg tabs for one 500-mg tab or an overdose of clavulanic acid will occur; may cause diarrhea and GI intolerance

Amphotericin B (Fungizone)

COMMON USES: Severe, systemic fungal infections; oral and cutaneous candidiasis
ACTIONS: Binds to ergosterol in the fungal membrane, altering membrane permeability
DOSAGE: *Adults & Peds.* Test dose of 1 mg in adults or 0.1 mg/kg to 1 mg in children, then 0.25–1.5 mg/kg/24h IV over 2–6 h. Doses often range from 25 to 50 mg/d or every other day. Total dose varies with indication. *Oral:* 1 mL qid. *Topical:* Apply bid–qid for 1–4 wk depending on infection

22

SUPPLIED: Powder for inj 50 mg/vial, oral susp 100 mg/mL, cream, lotion, oint 3%
NOTES: Monitor renal function; hypokalemia and hypomagnesemia possible from renal wasting; pretreatment with acetaminophen and antihistamines (Benadryl) help minimize adverse effects associated with IV infusion

Amphotericin B Cholesteryl (Amphotec)

COMMON USES: Refractory invasive fungal infection in persons intolerant to conventional amphotericin B
ACTIONS: Binds to sterols in the cell membrane, resulting in changes in membrane permeability
DOSAGE: *Adults & Peds.* Test dose of 1.6–8.3 mg, over 15–20 min, followed by a dose of 3–4 mg/kg/d. Infuse at a rate of 1 mg/kg/h
SUPPLIED: Powder for inj 50 mg, 100 mg/vial
NOTES: Do NOT use in-line filter, final concentration 0.6 mg/mL

Amphotericin B Lipid Complex (Abelcet)

COMMON USES: Refractory invasive fungal infection in persons intolerant to conventional amphotericin B
ACTIONS: Binds to sterols in the cell membrane, resulting in changes in membrane permeability
DOSAGE: 5 mg/kg/d IV administered as a single daily dose; infuse at a rate of 2.5 mg/kg/h
SUPPLIED: Inj 5 mg/mL
NOTES: Filter soln with a 5-mm filter needle; do not mix in electrolyte-containing solns. If inf >2 h, manually mix contents of the bag

Amphotericin B Liposomal (Ambisome)

COMMON USES: Refractory invasive fungal infection in persons intolerant to conventional amphotericin B
ACTIONS: Binds to sterols in the cell membrane, resulting in changes in membrane permeability
DOSAGE: *Adults & Peds.* 3–5 mg/kg/d, infused over 60–120 min
SUPPLIED: Powder for inj 50 mg

Ampicillin (Amcil, Omnipen, others)

COMMON USES: Susceptible gram (−) (*Shigella, Salmonella, E. coli, H. influenzae,* and *P. mirabilis*) and gram (+) (streptococci) bacteria
ACTIONS: β-Lactam antibiotic; inhibits cell wall synthesis
DOSAGE: *Adults.* 500 mg to 2 g IM or IV q6h or 250–500 mg PO q6h. *Peds. Neonates <7 d:* 50–100 mg/kg/24h IV ÷ q8h. *Term infants:* 75–150 mg/kg/24h ÷ q6–8h IV or PO. *Children >1 mo:* 100–200 mg/kg/24h IM or IV; 50–100 mg/kg/24h ÷ q6h PO up to 250 mg/dose. *Meningitis:* 200–400 mg/kg/24h ÷ q4–6h IV
SUPPLIED: Caps 250, 500 mg; susp 100 mg/mL (reconstituted as drops), 125 mg/5 mL, 250 mg/5 mL, 500 mg/5 mL; powder for inj 125 mg, 250 mg, 500 mg, 1 g, 2 g, 10 g/vial
NOTES: Cross-hypersensitivity with penicillin; can cause diarrhea and skin rash; many hospital strains of *E. coli* now resistant

Ampicillin-Sulbactam (Unasyn)

COMMON USES: Infections caused by β-lactamase-producing strains of *S. aureus, Enterococcus, H. influenzae, P. mirabilis,* and *Bacteroides* spp
ACTIONS: Combination of a β-lactam antibiotic and a β-lactamase inhibitor
DOSAGE: *Adults.* 1.5–3.0 g IM or IV q6h. *Peds.* 100–200 mg ampicillin/kg/d (150–300 mg Unasyn) q6h
SUPPLIED: Powder for inj 1.5, 3.0 g/vial
NOTES: *2:1 ratio of ampicillin:* Sulbactam; adjust dose in renal failure; observe for hypersensitivity reactions

22

Amprenavir (Agenerase)

COMMON USES: HIV infection
ACTIONS: Protease inhibitor, prevents the maturation of the virion to a mature viral particle
DOSAGE: *Adults.* 1200 mg bid. *Peds.* 20 mg/kg bid or 15 mg/kg tid up to 2400 mg/d
SUPPLIED: Caps 50, 150 mg; soln 15 mg/mL
NOTES: Caps and soln contain vitamin E exceeding the reference daily intake amounts; avoid high-fat meals with administration; many drug interactions; life-threatening rash, hyperglycemia, and fat redistribution possible; use with caution in persons with known sulfa allergy

Amrinone (Inocor)

Used for emergency cardiac care (see Chapter 21)
COMMON USES: Short-term Rx low cardiac output states and pulmonary HTN
ACTIONS: Positive inotrope with vasodilator activity
DOSAGE: *Adults & Peds.* Initially, give IV bolus of 0.75 mg/kg over 2–3 min followed by a mainte-nance dose of 5–10 µg/kg/min
SUPPLIED: Inj 5 mg/mL
NOTES: Not to exceed 10 mg/kg/d; incompatible with dextrose-containing solns; monitor for fluid and electrolyte changes and renal function during therapy

Anastrozole (Arimidex)

COMMON USES: Breast cancer following tamoxifen
ACTIONS: Selective nonsteroidal aromatase inhibitor, ↓ circulating estradiol
DOSAGE: 1 mg/d
SUPPLIED: Tabs 1 mg
NOTES: No detectable effect on adrenal corticosteroids or aldosterone; may ↑ cholesterol levels

Anistreplase (Eminase)

Used for emergency cardiac care (see Chapter 21)
COMMON USES: AMI
ACTIONS: Thrombolytic agent; activates the conversion of plasminogen to plasmin, promoting thrombolysis
DOSAGE: 30 U IV over 2–5 min
SUPPLIED: Vials containing 30 U
NOTES: May not be effective if readministered >5 d after the previous dose of anistreplase, strep-tokinase, or streptococcal infection because of the production of antistreptokinase antibody

Anthralin (Anthraderm, others)

COMMON USES: Psoriasis
ACTIONS: Keratolytic
DOSAGE: Apply qd
SUPPLIED: Cream, oint 0.1; 0.2 ; 0.25; 0.4; 0.5; 1%

Antihemophilic Factor [Factor VIII] [AHF] (Monoclate)

COMMON USES: Classic hemophilia A
ACTIONS: Provides factor VIII needed to convert prothrombin to thrombin
DOSAGE: *Adults & Peds.* 1 AHF unit/kg increases factor VIII conc in the body by approximately 2%. Units required = (kg) (desired factor VIII ↑ as % normal) × (0.5). *Prophylaxis of spontaneous hemorrhage* = 5% normal. *Hemostasis following trauma or surgery* = 30% normal. *Head injuries, major surgery, or bleeding* = 80–100% normal. Patient's % of normal level of factor VIII concen-tration must be ascertained prior to dosing for these calculations
SUPPLIED: Check each vial for number of units contained
NOTES: Not effective in controlling bleeding in von Willebrand's disease

Antithymocyte Globulin [ATG] (Atgam)

COMMON USES: Allograft rejection in transplant patients
ACTIONS: Reduces the number of circulating, thymus-dependent lymphocytes
DOSAGE: *Adults & Peds.* 10–15 mg/kg/d
SUPPLIED: Inj 50 mg/mL
NOTES: Do not administer in cases of prior history of severe systemic reaction to any other equine γ-globulin preparation; discontinue treatment with severe thrombocytopenia or leukopenia

Apraclonidine (Iodipine)

COMMON USES: Glaucoma
ACTIONS: α_2-Adrenergic agonist
DOSAGE: 1–2 gtt of 0.5% tid
SUPPLIED: 0.5, 1.0% soln

Aprotinin (Trasylol)

COMMON USES: Reduction or prevention of blood loss in patients undergoing a CABG
ACTIONS: Protease inhibitor; antifibrinolytic
DOSAGE: *High-dose:* 2 million KIU load, 2 million KIU for the pump prime dose, followed by 500,000 KIU/h until surgery ends. *Low-dose:* 1 million KIU load, 1 million KIU for the pump prime dose, followed by 250,000 KIU/h until surgery ends. Max total dose of 7 million KIU
SUPPLIED: Inj 1.4 mg/mL (10,000 KIU/mL)
NOTES: 1000/KIU = 0.14 mg of aprotinin. Give all patients 1-mL IV test dose to assess for allergic reaction

Ardeparin (Normiflo)

COMMON USES: Prevention of DVT and PE following knee replacement
ACTIONS: Low-molecular-weight heparin
DOSAGE: 35–50 U/kg SC q12h. Begin the day of surgery and continue up to 14 d
SUPPLIED: Inj 5000, 10,000 IU/0.5 mL
NOTES: Laboratory monitoring not necessary

Artificial Tears (Tears Naturale, others)

COMMON USES: Dry eyes
ACTIONS: Ocular lubricant
DOSAGE: 1–2 gtt tid–qid
SUPPLIED: OTC soln

L-Asparaginase (Elspar)

COMMON USES: ALL (in combination with other agents)
ACTIONS: Protein synthesis inhibitor
DOSAGE: 500–20,000 IU/m^2/d for 1–14 d. (Refer to specific protocols)
SUPPLIED: Inj 10,000 IU
NOTES: *Toxicity symptoms:* Hypersensitivity reactions in 20–35% (spectrum of urticaria to anaphylaxis), test dose recommended; rare GI toxicity (mild nausea/anorexia, pancreatitis)

Aspirin (Bayer, St. Joseph, others)

COMMON USES: Mild pain, headache, fever, inflammation, prevention of emboli, and prevention of MI
ACTIONS: Prostaglandin inhibitor
DOSAGE: *Adults.* Pain, fever: 325–650 mg q4–6h PO or PR. *RA:* 3–6 g/d PO in ÷ doses. *Platelet inhibitory action:* 325 mg PO qd. *Prevention of MI:* 160–325 mg PO qd. *Peds.* Caution: Use linked to Reye's syndrome; avoid use with viral illness in children. *Antipyretic:* 10–15 mg/kg/dose PO or PR q4h up to 80 mg/kg/24h. *RA:* 60–100 mg/kg/24h PO ÷ q4–6h (monitor serum levels to maintain between 15 and 30 mg/dL)

SUPPLIED: Tabs 325, 500 mg; chewable tabs 81 mg; EC tabs 165, 325, 500, 650, 975 mg; SR tabs 650, 800 mg; effervescent tabs 325, 500 mg; supp 120, 200, 300, 600 mg
NOTES: GI upset and erosion common adverse reactions; discontinue use 1 wk prior to surgery to avoid postoperative bleeding complications

Aspirin and Butalbital Compound (Fiorinal, Lanorinal, others) [C]

COMMON USES: Tension headache, pain
ACTIONS: Combination barbiturate and analgesic
DOSAGE: 1–2 PO q4h PRN, max 6 tabs/d
SUPPLIED: Caps *Fiorgen PF, Fiorinal, Lanorinal, Marnal:* Aspirin 325 mg/butalbital 50 mg/ caffeine 40 mg. Tabs *Fiorinal, Lanorinal, Marnal:* Aspirin 325 mg/butalbital 50 mg/ caffeine 40 mg
NOTES: Butalbital habit-forming

Aspirin + Butalbital, Caffeine and Codeine (Fiorinal + Codeine) [C]

COMMON USES: Mild pain; headache, especially when associated with stress
ACTIONS: Sedative analgesic, narcotic analgesic
DOSAGE: 1–2 tabs (caps) PO q4–6h PRN
SUPPLIED: Each cap or tab contains 325 mg aspirin, 40 mg caffeine, 50 mg of butalbital, codeine: No. 3 = 30 mg
NOTES: Significant drowsiness associated with use

Aspirin + Codeine (Empirin No. 2, No. 3, No. 4) [C]

COMMON USES: Mild to moderate pain
ACTIONS: Combined effects of aspirin and codeine
DOSAGE: *Adults.* 1–2 tabs PO q4–6h PRN. *Peds.* Aspirin 10 mg/kg/dose; codeine 0.5–1.0 mg/kg/dose q4h
SUPPLIED: Tabs 325 mg of aspirin and codeine as in Notes
NOTES: Codeine in No. 2 = 15 mg, No. 3 = 30 mg, No. 4 = 60 mg

Atenolol (Tenormin)

Used for emergency cardiac care (see Chapter 21)
COMMON USES: HTN, angina, MI
ACTIONS: Competitively blocks β-adrenergic receptors, β_1
DOSAGE: *HTN and angina:* 50–100 mg/d PO. *AMI:* 5 mg IV ×2 over 10 min, then 50 mg PO bid if tolerated
SUPPLIED: Tabs 25, 50, 100 mg; inj 5 mg/10 mL

Atenolol and Chlorthalidone (Tenoretic)

COMMON USES: HTN
ACTION: β-Adrenergic blockade with diuretic
DOSAGE: 50–100 mg/d PO
SUPPLIED: *Tenoretic 50:* Atenolol 50 mg/chlorthalidone 25 mg; *Tenoretic 100:* Atenolol 100 mg/chlorthalidone 25 mg

Atorvastatin (Lipitor)

COMMON USES: Elevated cholesterol and triglycerides
ACTIONS: HMG-CoA reductase inhibitor
DOSAGE: Initial dose 10 mg/d, may be ↑ to 80 mg/d
SUPPLIED: Tabs 10, 20, 40, 80 mg
NOTES: May cause myopathy, monitor LFT regularly

Atovaquone (Mepron)

22

COMMON USES: Rx and prevention mild to moderate PCP

ACTIONS: Inhibits nucleic acid and ATP synthesis
DOSAGE: *Rx:* 750 mg PO bid for 21 d. *Prevention:* 1500 mg PO once/d
SUPPLIED: Suspension 750 mg/5 mL
NOTES: Take with meals

Atracurium (Tracrium)

COMMON USES: Adjunct to anesthesia to facilitate endotracheal intubation
ACTIONS: Nondepolarizing neuromuscular blocker
DOSAGE: *Adults & Peds.* 0.4–0.5 mg/kg IV bolus, then 0.08–0.1 mg/kg q 20–45 min PRN
SUPPLIED: Inj 10 mg/mL
NOTES: Patient must be intubated and on controlled ventilation. Use adequate amounts of sedation and analgesia

Atropine

Used for emergency care (see Chapter 21)
COMMON USES: Preanesthetic; symptomatic bradycardia and asystole
ACTIONS: Antimuscarinic agent; blocks acetylcholine at parasympathetic sites
DOSAGE: *Adults.* Emergency cardiac care, bradycardia (see Chapter 21). *Preanesthetic:* 0.3–0.6 mg IM. *Peds.* Emergency cardiac care: 0.01–0.03 mg/kg IV q 2–5 min max 1.0 mg; min dose 0.1 mg. *Preanesthetic:* 0.01 mg/kg/dose SC/IV (max 0.4 mg)
SUPPLIED: Tabs 0.3, 0.4, 0.6; inj 0.05, 0.1, 0.3, 0.4, 0.5, 0.8, 1.0 mg/mL
NOTES: Blurred vision, urinary retention, and dried mucous membranes

Azathioprine (Imuran)

COMMON USES: Adjunct for the prevention of rejection following organ transplantation; RA; SLE
ACTIONS: Immunosuppressive agent; antagonizes purine metabolism
DOSAGE: *Adults & Peds.* 1–3 mg/kg/d IV or PO
SUPPLIED: Tabs 50 mg; inj 100 mg/20 mL
NOTES: GI intolerance; inj should be handled with cytotoxic precautions. Interaction with allopurinol

Azithromycin (Zithromax)

COMMON USES: Acute bacterial exacerbations of COPD, mild community-acquired pneumonia, pharyngitis, otitis media, skin and skin structure infections, nongonococcal urethritis, and PID. Rx and prevention of MAC infections in HIV-infected persons
ACTIONS: Macrolide antibiotic; inhibits protein synthesis
DOSAGE: *Adults.* Oral: Respiratory tract infections: 500 mg on the first day, followed by 250 mg/d PO for 4 more d. *Nongonococcal urethritis:* 1 g as a single dose. *Prevention of MAC:* 1200 mg PO once/wk. *IV:* 500 mg for at least 2 d, followed by 500 mg PO for total of 7–10 d. *Peds.* Otitis media: 10 mg/kg PO on day 1, then 5 mg/kg/d on days 2–5. *Pharyngitis:* 12 mg/kg/d PO for 5 d
SUPPLIED: Tabs 250, 600 mg; susp 1-g single-dose packet; susp 100, 200 mg/5 mL; inj 500 mg
NOTES: Take susp on an empty stomach; tabs may be taken with or without food

Aztreonam (Azactam)

COMMON USES: Infections caused by aerobic gram (−) bacteria, including *Pseudomonas aeruginosa*
ACTIONS: Monobactam antibiotic; inhibits cell wall synthesis
DOSAGE: *Adults.* 1–2 g IV/IM q6–12h. *Peds.* Premature infants: 30 mg/kg/dose IV q12h. *Term infants, children:* 30 mg/kg/dose q6–8h
SUPPLIED: Inj 500 mg, 1 g, 2 g
NOTES: Not effective against gram (+) or anaerobic bacteria; may be given to penicillin-allergic patients; adjust dose in renal impairment

22

Bacitracin, Topical (Baciguent)

Bacitracin and Polymyxin B, Topical (Polysporin)

Bacitracin, Neomycin and Polymyxin B, Topical (Neosporin Ointment)

Bacitracin, Neomycin, Polymyxin B and Hydrocortisone, Topical (Cortisporin)

Bacitracin, Neomycin, Polymyxin B and Lidocaine, Topical (Clomycin)

COMMON USES: Prevention and Rx of minor cuts, scrapes and burns
ACTIONS: Topical antibiotic with added effects based on components (antiinflammatory and analgesic)
DOSAGE: Apply sparingly bid–qid
SUPPLIED: Bacitracin 500 U/g oint. Bacitracin 500 U/polymyxin B sulfate 10,000 U/g oint and powder. Bacitracin 400 U/neomycin/ 3.5 mg/polymyxin B 5000 U/g oint (for Neosporin Cream, see page 576). Bacitracin 400 U/neomycin 3.5 mg/polymyxin B/10,000 U/hydrocortisone 10 mg/g oint. Bacitracin 500 U/neomycin 3.5 g/polymyxin B 5000 U/lidocaine 40 mg/g oint
NOTES: Systemic and irrigation forms of bacitracin available but not generally used due to potential toxicity. *Note:* Neosporin ointment different from cream (page 576)

Bacitracin, Ophthalmic (AK-Tracin Ophthalmic)

Bacitracin and Polymyxin B, Ophthalmic (AK Poly Bac Ophthalmic, Polysporin Ophthalmic)

Bacitracin, Neomycin and Polymyxin B, Ophthalmic (AK Spore Ophthalmic, Neosporin Ophthalmic)

Bacitracin, Neomycin, Polymyxin B and Hydrocortisone, Ophthalmic (AK Spore HC Ophthalmic, Cortisporin Ophthalmic)

COMMON USES: Blepharitis, conjunctivitis, and prophylactic treatment of corneal abrasions
ACTIONS: Topical antibiotic with added effects based on components (antiinflammatory)
DOSAGE: Apply q3–4h into conjunctival sac
SUPPLIED: See Topical equivalents, above

Baclofen (Lioresal, others)

COMMON USES: Spasticity secondary to severe chronic disorders, eg, MS or spinal cord lesions, trigeminal neuralgia
ACTIONS: Centrally acting skeletal muscle relaxant; inhibits transmission of both monosynaptic and polysynaptic reflexes at the spinal cord
DOSAGE: *Adults.* Initially, 5 mg PO tid; ↑ q 3 d to max effect; max 80 mg/d. *Peds.* 2–7 y: 10–15 mg/d ÷ q8h; titrate to effect or max of 40 mg/d. >8 y: Max of 60 mg/d. *IT:* Through implantable pump
SUPPLIED: Tabs 10, 20 mg; IT inj 10 mg/20 mL, 10 mg/5 mL
NOTES: Use caution in epilepsy and neuropsychiatric disturbances, withdrawal may occur with abrupt discontinuation

Basiliximab (Simulect)

COMMON USES: Prevention of acute organ transplant rejections
ACTIONS: IL-2 receptor antagonists
DOSAGE: *Adults.* 20 mg IV 2 h prior to transplant, then 20 mg IV 4 d posttransplant. *Peds.* 12 mg/m² up to a max of 20 mg 2 h prior to transplant, then the same dose IV 4 d posttransplant
SUPPLIED: Inj 20 mg
NOTES: Murine/human monoclonal antibody

BCG [Bacillus Calmette-Guerin] (Theracys, TICE BCG)

COMMON USES: Bladder carcinoma, TB prophylaxis
ACTIONS: Immunomodulator
DOSAGE: Bladder cancer, contents of 1 vial prepared and instilled in bladder for 2 h. Repeat once weekly for 6 wk; repeat 3 weekly doses 3, 6, 12, 18, and 24 mo after the initial therapy
SUPPLIED: Inj 27 mg ($3.4 + 3 \times 10^8$ CFU)/vial (TheraCys), $1-8 \times 10^8$ CFU/vial (TICE BCG)
NOTES: *Intravesical toxicity symptoms:* Hematuria, urinary frequency, dysuria, and bacterial urinary tract infection. Routine adult BCG immunization in the U.S. no longer recommended. BCG vaccine occasionally used in high risk-children who are negative on the PPD skin test and cannot be given isoniazid prophylaxis.

Becaplermin (Regranex Gel)

COMMON USES: Adjunct to local wound care in diabetic foot ulcers
ACTIONS: Recombinant human PDGF, enhanced formation of granulation tissue
DOSAGE: Based on size of lesion; 1⅓-in. ribbon from 2-g tube, ⅔-in. ribbon from 7.5- or 15-g tube/in.^{2} of ulcer; apply and cover with moist gauze; rinse after 12 h; do not reapply; repeat process 12 h later
SUPPLIED: 0.01% gel in 2-, 7.5-, 15-g tubes
NOTES: Use along with good wound care; wound must be vascularized

Beclomethasone (Beclovent Inhaler, Vanceril Inhaler Quar)

COMMON USES: Chronic asthma
ACTIONS: Inhaled corticosteroid
DOSAGE: *Adults.* 2–4 inhal tid–qid (max 20/d); Vanceril double strength: 2 inhal bid (max 10/d); quar 1–4 inhal bid. *Peds.* 1–2 inhal tid–qid (max 10/d); Vanceril double strength: 2 inhal bid (max 5/d)
SUPPLIED: Oral met-dose inhaler; 42, 84 μg/inhal; quar HFA formulation 40, 80 μg/inhal
NOTES: Not effective for acute asthmatic attacks; may cause oral candidiasis

Beclomethasone (Beconase, Vancenase Nasal Inhaler)

COMMON USES: Allergic rhinitis refractory to conventional therapy with antihistamines and decongestants
ACTIONS: Inhaled corticosteroid
DOSAGE: *Adults.* 1 spray intranasally bid–qid; *Aqueous inhal:* 1–2 spays/nostril qd–bid. *Peds.* 6–12 y: 1 spray intranasally tid
SUPPLIED: Nasal met-dose inhaler
NOTES: Nasal spray delivers 42 μg/dose and 84 μg/dose

Belladonna and Opium Supp (B & O Supprettes) [CII]

COMMON USES: Bladder spasms; moderate to severe pain
ACTIONS: Antispasmodic
DOSAGE: Insert 1 supp PR q6h PRN. 15A = 30 mg powdered opium; 16.2 mg belladonna extract. 16A = 60 mg powdered opium; 16.2 mg belladonna extract
SUPPLIED: Supp 15A, 16A
NOTES: Anticholinergic side effects; caution patients about sedation, urinary retention, and constipation

Benazepril (Lotensin)

COMMON USES: HTN
ACTIONS: ACE inhibitor
DOSAGE: 10–40 mg/d PO
SUPPLIED: Tabs 5, 10, 20, 40 mg
NOTES: Symptomatic hypotension in patients taking diuretics; nonproductive cough

Benzocaine and Antipyrine (Auralgan)

COMMON USES: Analgesia in severe otitis media
ACTIONS: Anesthetic and local decongestant
DOSAGE: Fill the ear and insert a moist cotton plug; repeat 1–2 h PRN
SUPPLIED: Soln
NOTES: Do not use with perforated eardrum

Benzonatate (Tessalon Perles)

COMMON USES: Symptomatic relief of cough
ACTIONS: Anesthetizes the stretch receptors in the respiratory passages
DOSAGE: *Adults & Peds >10 y.* 100 mg PO tid
SUPPLIED: Caps 100 mg
NOTES: May cause sedation; do not chew or puncture the caps

Benztropine (Cogentin)

COMMON USES: Parkinsonism and drug-induced extrapyramidal disorders
ACTIONS: Partially blocks striatal cholinergic receptors
DOSAGE: *Adults.* 0.5–6 mg PO, IM, or IV in ÷ doses/d. *Peds >3 y.* 0.02–0.05 mg/kg/dose 1–2/d
SUPPLIED: Tabs 0.5, 1.0, 2.0; inj 1 mg/mL
NOTES: Anticholinergic side effects

Bepridil (Vascor)

COMMON USES: Chronic stable angina
ACTIONS: Calcium channel-blocking agent
DOSAGE: 200–400 mg/d PO
SUPPLIED: Tabs 200, 300, 400 mg
NOTES: Agranulocytosis and serious ventricular arrhythmias, including Torsades de Pointes

Beractant (Survanta)

COMMON USES: Prevention and Rx of RDS in premature infants
ACTIONS: Replacement of pulmonary surfactant
DOSAGE: 100 mg/kg administered via endotracheal tube. May be repeated 3 more × q6h for a max of 4 doses/48h
SUPPLIED: Suspension 25 mg of phospholipid/mL
NOTES: Administer via 4-quadrant method

Betaxolol (Kerlone)

COMMON USES: HTN
ACTIONS: Competitively blocks β-adrenergic receptors (β_1)
DOSAGE: 10–20 mg/d
SUPPLIED: Tabs 10, 20 mg

Betaxolol, Ophthalmic (Betoptic)

COMMON USES: Glaucoma
ACTIONS: Competitively blocks β-adrenergic receptors (β_1)
DOSAGE: 1 gtt bid
SUPPLIED: Soln 0.5%; susp 0.25%

Bethanechol (Urecholine, Duvoid, Various)

COMMON USES: Neurogenic atony of the bladder with urinary retention, acute postoperative and postpartum functional (nonobstructive) urinary retention
ACTIONS: Stimulates cholinergic receptors in the smooth muscle of the bladder and GI tract
DOSAGE: *Adults.* 10–50 mg PO tid–qid or 2.5–5 mg SC tid–qid and PRN. *Peds.* 0.6 mg/kg/24h PO ÷ tid–qid or 0.15–2 mg/kg/d SC ÷ 3–4×/d

SUPPLIED: Tabs 5, 10, 25, 50 mg; inj 5 mg/mL
NOTES: Contra in bladder outlet obstruction, asthma, and CAD; do NOT administer IM or IV

Bicalutamide (Casodex)

COMMON USES: Advanced prostate cancer (in combination with GnRH agonists such as leuprolide or goserelin)
ACTIONS: Nonsteroidal antiandrogen
DOSAGE: 50 mg/d
SUPPLIED: Caps 50 mg
NOTES: *Toxicity symptoms:* Hot flashes, loss of libido, impotence, diarrhea, nausea and vomiting, gynecomastia, and LFT elevation

Bicarbonate (see Sodium Bicarbonate page 602)

Bisacodyl (Dulcolax)

COMMON USES: Constipation; preoperative bowel preparation
ACTIONS: Stimulates peristalsis
DOSAGE: *Adults.* 5–15 mg PO or 10 mg PR PRN. *Peds.* <2 y: 5 mg PR PRN. *>2 y:* 5 mg PO or 10 mg PR PRN
SUPPLIED: EC tabs 5 mg; supp 10 mg
NOTES: Contra in acute abdomen or bowel obstruction; do NOT chew tabs; do NOT give within 1 h of antacids or milk

Bismuth Subsalicylate (Pepto-Bismol)

COMMON USES: Indigestion, nausea, and diarrhea. In combination for treatment of *H. pylori* infection
ACTIONS: Antisecretory and antiinflammatory effects
DOSAGE: *Adults.* 2 tabs or 30 mL PO PRN (max 8 doses/24h). *Peds.* 3–6 y: ⅓ tab or 5 mL PO PRN (max 8 doses/24h). *6–9 y:* ⅔ tab or 10 mL PO PRN (max 8 doses/24h). *9–12 y:* 1 tab or 15 mL PO PRN (max 8 doses/24h)
SUPPLIED: Chewable tabs 262 mg; liq 262, 524 mg/15 mL
NOTES: May turn tongue and stools black

Bisoprolol (Zebeta)

COMMON USES: HTN
ACTIONS: Competitively blocks β-adrenergic receptors (β_1)
DOSAGE: 5–10 mg/d (max dose 20 mg/d)
SUPPLIED: Tabs 5, 10 mg

Bitolterol (Tornalate)

COMMON USES: Prophylaxis and Rx of asthma and reversible bronchospasm
ACTIONS: Sympathomimetic bronchodilator; stimulates β_2-adrenergic receptors in the lungs
DOSAGE: *Adults & Children.* >12 y: 2 inhal q8h; acute 2 inhal 1–3 min apart, repeat × 1
SUPPLIED: Aerosol 0.8%

Bleomycin Sulfate (Blenoxane)

COMMON USES: Testicular carcinomas; Hodgkin's and non-Hodgkin's lymphomas; cutaneous lymphomas; and squamous cell carcinomas of the head and neck, larynx, cervix, skin, and penis
ACTIONS: Induces breakage (scission) of single- and double-stranded DNA
DOSAGE: 10–20 mg (U)/m^2 1–2/wk (Refer to specific protocols)
SUPPLIED: Inj 15 mg (15 U)
NOTES: *Toxicity symptoms:* Hyperpigmentation (skin staining) and hypersensitivity (rash to anaphylaxis); test dose of 1 mg (U) recommended, especially in lymphoma patients; fever in 50%;

lung toxicity (idiosyncratic and dose-related); pneumonitis may progress to fibrosis. Lung toxicity likely when the total dose >400 mg (U)

Bretylium

COMMON USES: Acute Rx of VF or tachycardia unresponsive to conventional therapy
ACTIONS: Class III antiarrhythmic
DOSAGE: *Adults.* 5 mg/kg IV rapid inj (1 min); may repeat q 15–30 min with 10 mg/kg (max 30 mg/kg); maintenance 1–2 mg/min IV infusion. *Peds.* Same as adults, except the maintenance dose is 5 mg/kg/dose q6–8h
SUPPLIED: Inj 50 mg/mL; premixed inf 1, 2, 4 mg/mL (limited availability)
NOTES: Nausea and vomiting associated with rapid IV bolus; gradually ↓ dose and discontinue in 3–5 d; effects seen within the first 10–15 min; transient rise in BP seen initially; hypotension most frequent adverse effect and occurs within the first hours of treatment

Brimonidine (Alphagan)

COMMON USES: Open-angle glaucoma
ACTIONS: α_2-Adrenergic agonist
DOSAGE: 1 gtt in eye(s) tid
SUPPLIED: 0.2% soln

Brinzolamide (Azopt)

COMMON USES: Open-angle glaucoma
ACTIONS: Carbonic anhydrase inhibitor
DOSAGE: 1 gtt in eye(s) tid
SUPPLIED: 1.0% susp

Bromocriptine (Parlodel)

COMMON USES: Parkinson's syndrome, hyperprolactinemia
ACTIONS: Direct-acting on the striatal dopamine receptors; inhibits prolactin secretion
DOSAGE: Initially, 1.25 mg PO bid; titrate to effect
SUPPLIED: Tabs 2.5 mg; caps 5 mg
NOTES: Nausea and vertigo common

Buclizine (Bucladin-S Softabs)

COMMON USES: Control of nausea, vomiting, and dizziness of motion sickness
ACTIONS: Centrally acting antiemetic
DOSAGE: 50 mg dissolved in the mouth bid; 50 mg PO prophylactically 30 min prior to travel
SUPPLIED: Tabs 50 mg
NOTES: NOT safe in PRG; contains tartrazine; observe the patient for allergic reactions

Budesonide (Rhinocort, Pulmicort, Pulmicort Respules)

COMMON USES: Allergic and nonallergic rhinitis, asthma
ACTIONS: Steroid
DOSAGE: *Intranasal:* 2 sprays/nostril bid or 4 sprays/nostril/d; *Aqueous:* 1 spray/nostril/d. *Oral inhaled:* 1–4 inhal bid. *Peds.* 1–2 inhal bid; *Nebulization:* 0.25–1 mg given qd or bid
SUPPLIED: Met-dose Turbuhaler, nasal inhaler and aqueous spray; respules 0.25 mg/2 mL, 0.5 mg/2 mL

Bumetanide (Bumex)

COMMON USES: Edema from CHF, hepatic cirrhosis, and renal disease
ACTIONS: Loop diuretic; inhibits reabsorption of sodium and chloride in the ascending loop of Henle and the distal renal tubule
DOSAGE: *Adults.* 0.5–2.0 mg/d PO; 0.5–1.0 mg IV q8–24h (max 10 mg/d). *Peds.* 0.015–0.1 mg/kg/d PO, IV, or IM ÷ q6–24h

SUPPLIED: Tabs 0.5, 1, 2 mg; inj 0.25 mg/mL
NOTES: Monitor fluid and electrolyte status during treatment

Bupivacaine (Marcaine)

COMMON USES: Peripheral nerve block
ACTIONS: Local anesthetic
DOSAGE: *Adults & Peds.* Dose dependent on procedure, vascularity of tissues, depth of anesthesia, and degree of muscle relaxation required (see Chapter 17)
SUPPLIED: Inj 0.25, 0.5, 0.75%

Buprenorphine (Buprenex) [C]

COMMON USES: Moderate to severe pain
ACTIONS: Opiate agonist–antagonist
DOSAGE: 0.3–0.6 mg IM or slow IV push q6h PRN
SUPPLIED: Inj 0.324 mg/mL (= 0.3 mg of buprenorphine)
NOTES: May induce withdrawal syndrome in opioid-dependent patients

Bupropion (Wellbutrin, Zyban)

COMMON USES: Depression, adjunct to smoking cessation
ACTIONS: Weak inhibitor of neuronal uptake of serotonin and norepinephrine; inhibits the neuronal reuptake of dopamine
DOSAGE: *Depression:* 100–450 mg/d ÷ bid–tid. *Smoking cessation:* 150 mg/d for 3 d, then 150 mg bid for 8–12 wk
SUPPLIED: Tabs 75, 100 mg; SR tabs 100, 150 mg
NOTES: Associated with seizures; avoid use of alcohol and other CNS depressants

Buspirone (Buspar)

COMMON USES: Short-term relief of anxiety
ACTIONS: Antianxiety agent; selectively antagonizes CNS serotonin receptors
DOSAGE: 5–10 mg PO tid. ↑ dose to desired response; usual dose 20–30 mg/d; max 60 mg/d
SUPPLIED: Tabs 5, 10, 15 mg
NOTES: No abuse potential. No physical or psychological dependence

Busulfan (Myleran)

COMMON USES: CML, preparative regimens for allogeneic and ABMT in high doses
ACTIONS: Alkylating agent
DOSAGE: 4–12 mg/d for several weeks; 16 mg/kg once or 4 mg/kg/d for 4 d in conjunction with another agent in transplant regimens. Refer to specific protocol
SUPPLIED: Tabs 2 mg
NOTES: *Toxicity symptoms:* Myelosuppression, pulmonary fibrosis, nausea (high-dose therapy), gynecomastia, adrenal insufficiency, and hyperpigmentation of the skin

Butorphanol (Stadol) [C]

COMMON USES: Moderate to severe pain and headaches
ACTIONS: Opiate agonist–antagonist with central analgesic actions
DOSAGE: 1–4 mg IM or IV q 3–4 h PRN. *Headaches:* 1 spray in 1 nostril, may be repeated once if pain not relieved in 60–90 min
SUPPLIED: Inj 1, 2 mg/mL; nasal spray 10 mg/mL
NOTES: May induce withdrawal syndrome in opioid-dependent patients

Calcipotriene (Dovonex)

COMMON USES: Plaque psoriasis
ACTIONS: Keratolytic

DOSAGE: Apply bid
SUPPLIED: Cream; oint; soln 0.005%

Calcitonin (Cibacalcin, Miacalcin)

COMMON USES: Paget's disease of bone; hypercalcemia; osteogenesis imperfecta, postmenopausal osteoporosis
ACTIONS: Polypeptide hormone
DOSAGE: *Paget's salmon form:* 100 U/d IM/SC initially, 50 U/d or 50–100 U q1–3d maintenance. *Paget's human form:* 0.5 mg/d initially; maintenance 0.5 mg 2–3×/wk or 0.25 mg/d, max 0.5 mg bid. *Hypercalcemia salmon calcitonin:* 4 U/kg IM/SC q12h; ↑ to 8 U/kg q12h, max q6h. *Osteoporosis salmon calcitonin:* 100 U/d IM/SC; Intranasal 200 U = 1 nasal spray/d
SUPPLIED: Spray, nasal 200 U/activation; inj, human (Cibacalcin) 0.5 mg/vial, salmon 200 U/mL (2 mL)
NOTES: Human (Cibacalcin) and salmon forms; human only approved for Paget's bone disease

Calcitriol (Rocaltrol)

COMMON USES: Reduction of elevated parathyroid hormone levels, hypocalcemia associated with dialysis
ACTIONS: 1,25-Dihydroxycholecalciferol, a vitamin D analogue
DOSAGE: *Adults.* Renal failure: 0.25 µg/d PO, ↑ 0.25 µg/d q 4–6 wk PRN; 0.5 µg 3×/wk IV, ↑ PRN. *Hyperparathyroidism:* 0.5–2.0 µg/d. *Peds.* Renal failure: 15 ng/kg/d, ↑ PRN; typical maintenance 30–60 ng/kg/d. *Hyperparathyroidism:* <5 y, 0.25–0.75 µg/d; >6 y, 0.5–2.0 µg/d
SUPPLIED: Inj 1, 2 µg/mL (in 1 mL volume); caps 0.25, 0.5 µg
NOTES: Monitor dosing to keep calcium levels within normal range

Calcium Acetate (Calphron, Phos-Ex, PhosLo)

COMMON USES: ESRD-associated hyperphosphatemia
ACTIONS: Ca supplement to treat ESRD hypophosphatemia without aluminum
DOSAGE: 2–4 tabs PO with meals
SUPPLIED: Caps Phos-Ex 500 mg (125 mg Ca); Tabs Calphron and Phos-Lo 667 mg (169 mg Ca)
NOTES: Can cause hypercalcemia, monitor Ca levels

Calcium Carbonate (Tums, Alka-Mints)

COMMON USES: Hyperacidity associated with peptic ulcer disease, hiatal hernia, etc
ACTIONS: Neutralizes gastric acid
DOSAGE: 500 mg–2 g PO PRN
SUPPLIED: Chewable tabs 350, 420, 500, 550, 750, 850 mg; susp

Calcium Glubionate (Neo-Calglucon) [OTC]

COMMON USES: Rx and prevention of Ca deficiency
ACTIONS: Oral Ca supplementation
DOSAGE: *Adults.* 6–18 g/d ÷ doses. *Peds.* 600–2000 mg/kg/d ÷ qid (9 g/d max)
SUPPLIED: OTC syrup 1.8 g/5 mL = Ca 115 mg/5 mL

Calcium Salts (Chloride, Gluconate, Gluceptate)

Used for emergency cardiac care (see Chapter 21)
COMMON USES: Ca replacement, VF, electromechanical dissociation, Ca blocker toxicity, Mg intoxication, tetany, hyperphosphatemia in ESRD
DOSAGE: *Adults.* Replacement: 1–2 g/d PO. *Cardiac emergencies:* CaCl 0.5–1.0 g IV q 10 min or Ca gluconate 1–2 g IV q 10 min. *Tetany:* 1 g CaCl over 10–30 min; repeat in 6 h PRN. *Peds.* Replacement: 200–500 mg/kg/24h PO or IV ÷ qid. *Cardiac emergency:* 100 mg/kg/dose IV of gluconate salt q 10 min. *Tetany:* 10 mg/kg CaCl over 5–10 min; repeat in 6 h or use inf (200 mg/kg/d max). *Adult and Peds.* Hypocalcemia due to citrated blood infusion: 0.45 meq Ca/100 mL citrated blood infused

22

SUPPLIED: CaCl inj 10% = 100 mg/mL = Ca 27.2 mg/mL = 10 mL ampule. Ca gluconate inj 10% = 100 mg/mL = Ca 9 mg/mL; tabs 500 mg = 45 mg Ca, 650 mg = 58.5 mg , 975 mg = 87.75 mg Ca, 1 g = 90 mg Ca. Ca gluceptate inj 220 mg/mL = 18 mg/mL Ca

NOTES: CaCl contains 270 mg (13.6 meq) elemental Ca/g, and calcium gluconate contains 90 mg (4.5 meq) Ca/g. RDA for Ca: Adults = 800 mg/d, Peds = <6 mo 360 mg/d, 6 mo–1 y 540 mg/d, 1–10 y 800 mg/d; 10–18 y 1200 mg/d

Calfactant (Infasurf)

COMMON USES: Prevention and Rx of RSD in infants
ACTIONS: Exogenous pulmonary surfactant
DOSAGE: 3 mL/kg instilled into lungs. May be retreated for a total of 3 doses administered 12 h apart
SUPPLIED: Intratracheal susp 35 mg/mL
NOTES: Monitor for cyanosis and airway obstruction during administration

Candesartan (Atacand)

COMMON USES: HTN
ACTIONS: Angiotensin II receptor antagonists
DOSAGE: 2–32 mg/d, usual dose is 16 mg/d
SUPPLIED: Tabs 4, 8, 16, 32 mg

Capsaicin (Capsin, Zostrix, etc) [OTC]

COMMON USES: Pain due to postherpetic neuralgia, chronic neuralgia, arthritis, diabetic neuropathy, postoperative pain psoriasis, intractable pruritus
ACTIONS: Topical analgesic
DOSAGE: Apply tid–qid
SUPPLIED: OTC creams; gel; lotions; roll-ons

Captopril (Capoten, Various)

COMMON USES: HTN, CHF, LVD, and diabetic nephropathy
ACTIONS: ACE inhibitor
DOSAGE: *Adults.* HTN: Initially, 25 mg PO bid–tid; ↑ to a maintenance dose q 1–2 wk by 25-mg increments/dose (max 450 mg/d) to desired effect. *CHF:* Initially, 6.25–12.5 mg PO tid; titrate to desired effect. *LVD:* 50 mg PO tid. *Diabetic nephropathy:* 25 mg PO tid. *Peds.* Infants <2 mo: 0.05–0.5 mg/kg/dose PO q8–24h. *Children:* Initially, 0.3–0.5 mg/kg/dose PO; ↑ to a max of 6 mg/kg/d
SUPPLIED: Tabs 12.5, 25, 50, 100 mg
NOTES: Use with caution in renal failure. Give 1 h ac; can cause rash, proteinuria, and cough; contra in 2nd or 3rd trimester of PRG.

Carbamazepine (Tegretol)

COMMON USES: Epilepsy and trigeminal neuralgia
ACTIONS: Anticonvulsant
DOSAGE: *Adults.* Initially, 200 mg PO bid; ↑ by 200 mg/d; usual 800–1200 mg/d in ÷ doses. *Peds.* <6 y: 5 mg/kg/d, ↑ to 10–20 mg/kg/d ÷ in 2–4 doses. *6–12 y:* Initially, 100 mg PO bid or 10 mg/kg/24h PO ÷ qd–bid; ↑ to a maintenance dose of 20–30 mg/kg/24h ÷ tid–qid
SUPPLIED: Tabs 200 mg; chewable tabs 100 mg; XR tabs 100, 200, 400 mg; susp 100 mg/5 mL
NOTES: Severe hematologic side effects possible; monitor CBC; monitor serum levels (see Table 22–7, pages 631–634); generic products not interchangeable

Carbidopa/Levodopa (Sinemet)

COMMON USES: Parkinson's disease
ACTIONS: Increases CNS levels of dopamine
DOSAGE: 25/100 bid–qid; ↑ as needed (max 200/2000 mg/d)

SUPPLIED: Tabs (mg of carbidopa/mg of levodopa) 10/100, 25/100, 25/250; Tabs SR (mg of carbidopa/mg of levodopa) 25/100, 50/200
NOTES: Psychiatric disturbances, orthostatic hypotension, dyskinesias, and cardiac arrhythmias

Carboplatin (Paraplatin)

COMMON USES: Ovarian, lung (small-cell and non-small-cell), head and neck, testicular, and brain cancers, and allogeneic and ABMT in high doses
ACTIONS: DNA cross-linker; forms DNA–platinum adducts
DOSAGE: 360 mg/m^2 (ovarian carcinoma); AUC dosing 4–7 mg/mL (using Calvert's formula: mg = AUC × [25 + calculated GFR]); also may be adjusted based on pretreatment platelet count, CrCl, and BSA (Egorin's formula); up to 1500 mg/m^2 used in ABMT setting (refer to specific protocols)
SUPPLIED: Inj 50, 150, 450 mg
NOTES: *Toxicity symptoms:* Myelosuppression, nausea and vomiting, diarrhea, nephrotoxicity, hematuria, neurotoxicity, and hepatic enzyme elevations; physiologic dosing based on either Calvert's or Egorin's formula allows larger doses to be given with reduced toxicity

Carisoprodol (Soma)

COMMON USES: Adjunct to sleep and physical therapy for the relief of painful musculoskeletal conditions
ACTIONS: Centrally acting muscle relaxant
DOSAGE: 350 mg PO tid–qid
SUPPLIED: Tabs 350 mg
NOTES: Avoid alcohol and other CNS depressants; available in combination with aspirin or codeine

Carmustine (BCNU, BiCNU)

COMMON USES: Primary brain tumors, melanoma, Hodgkin's and non-Hodgkin's lymphomas, multiple myeloma, and preparative regimens for allogeneic and ABMT in high doses
ACTIONS: Alkylating agent; forms DNA cross-links; inhibitor of DNA synthesis
DOSAGE: 75–100 mg/m^2/d for 2 d; 200 mg/m^2 in a single dose; 450–900 mg/m^2 in BMT regimens (refer to specific protocols)
SUPPLIED: Inj 100 mg; wafer: 7.7 mg
NOTES: *Toxicity symptoms:* Myelosuppression (especially leukocytes and platelets), phlebitis, facial flushing, hepatic and renal dysfunction, pulmonary fibrosis, and optic neuroretinitis. Hematologic toxicity may persist up to 4–6 wk after administration

Carteolol (Cartrol, Occupress Ophthalmic)

COMMON USES: HTN, increased intraocular pressure
ACTIONS: Competitively blocks β-adrenergic receptors, β$_1$, β$_2$, ISA
DOSAGE: PO 2.5–5 mg/; ophth 1 gtt in eye(s) bid
SUPPLIED: Tabs 2.5, 5 mg; ophth soln 1%

Carvedilol (Coreg)

COMMON USES: HTN and CHF
ACTIONS: Competitively blocks β-adrenergic receptors, β$_1$, β$_2$, α
DOSAGE: *HTN:* 6.25–12.5 mg bid. *CHF:* 3.125–25 mg bid
SUPPLIED: Tabs 3.125, 6.25, 12.5, 25 mg
NOTES: Take with food to slow absorption and reduce incidence of orthostatic hypotension

Cefaclor (Ceclor)

COMMON USES: Infections caused by susceptible bacteria involving the upper and lower respiratory tract, skin, bone, urinary tract, abdomen and gynecologic system
ACTIONS: 2nd-Generation cephalosporin; inhibits cell wall synthesis
DOSAGE: *Adults.* 250–500 mg PO tid. *Peds.* 20–40 mg/kg/d PO ÷ tid

SUPPLIED: Caps 250, 500 mg; ER tabs 375, 500 mg; susp 125, 187, 250, 375 mg/5 mL
NOTES: Has more gram (–) activity then 1st-generation cephalosporins

Cefadroxil (Duricef, Ultracef)

COMMON USES: Infections caused by susceptible strains of *Streptococcus, Staphylococcus, E. coli, Proteus* and *Klebsiella* involving the skin, bone, upper and lower respiratory tract, and urinary tract
ACTIONS: 1st-generation cephalosporin; inhibits cell wall synthesis
DOSAGE: *Adults.* 500–1000 mg PO bid–qd. *Peds.* 30 mg/kg/d ÷ bid
SUPPLIED: Caps 500 mg; tabs 1 g; susp 125; 250, 500 mg/5 mL

Cefazolin (Ancef, Kefzol)

COMMON USES: Infections caused by susceptible strains of *Streptococcus, Staphylococcus, E. coli, Proteus,* and *Klebsiella* involving the skin, bone, upper and lower respiratory tract, and urinary tract
ACTIONS: 1st-generation cephalosporin; inhibits cell wall synthesis
DOSAGE: *Adults.* 1–2 g IV q8h. *Peds.* 50–100 mg/kg/d IV ÷ q8h
SUPPLIED: Inj
NOTES: Widely used for surgical prophylaxis

Cefdinir (Omnicef)

COMMON USES: Infections caused by susceptible bacteria involving the respiratory tract, skin, bone, and urinary tract
ACTIONS: 3rd-Generation cephalosporin; inhibits cell wall synthesis
DOSAGE: *Adults.* 300 mg PO bid or 600 mg/d PO. *Peds.* 7 mg/kg PO bid or 14 mg/kg/d PO
SUPPLIED: Caps 300 mg; susp 125 mg/5 mL

Cefepime (Maxipime)

COMMON USES: UTI and pneumonia caused by susceptible *S. pneumoniae, S. aureus, K. pneumoniae, E. coli, P. aeruginosa,* and *Enterobacter* spp
ACTIONS: 4th-generation cephalosporin; inhibits cell wall synthesis
DOSAGE: 1–2 g IV q12h
SUPPLIED: Inj 500 mg, 1 g, 2 g

Cefixime (Suprax)

COMMON USES: Infections caused by susceptible bacteria involving the respiratory tract, skin, bone, and urinary tract
ACTIONS: 3rd-generation cephalosporin; inhibits cell wall synthesis
DOSAGE: *Adults.* 200–400 mg PO qd–bid. *Peds.* 8 mg/kg/d PO ÷ qd–bid
SUPPLIED: Tabs 200, 400 mg; susp 100 mg/5 mL
NOTES: Use susp to treat otitis media

Cefmetazole (Zefazone)

COMMON USES: Infections caused by susceptible bacteria involving the upper and lower respiratory tract, skin, bone, urinary tract, abdomen and gynecologic system
ACTIONS: 2nd-generation cephalosporin; inhibits cell wall synthesis
DOSAGE: *Adults.* 1–2 mg IV q8h
SUPPLIED: Inj
NOTES: Has more gram (–) activity than 1st-generation cephalosporins; has anaerobic activity; ↑ risk of bleeding

Cefonicid (Monocid)

COMMON USES: Susceptible bacterial infections (respiratory tract, skin, bone and joint, urinary tract, gynecologic system, sepsis)
ACTIONS: 2nd-generation cephalosporin

DOSAGE: 1 g/24h IM/IV
SUPPLIED: Injectable forms

Cefoperazone (Cefobid)

COMMON USES: Susceptible bacterial infections (respiratory, skin, urinary tract, sepsis; as a 3rd-generation cephalosporin, cefoperazone has activity against gram (–) organisms (eg, *E. coli, Klebsiella*); variable activity against *Streptococcus* and *Staphylococcus* spp.; active against *P. aeruginosa*, but less than ceftazidime
ACTIONS: 3rd-generation cephalosporin
DOSAGE: *Adults.* 2–4 g/d IM/IV ÷ q12h (12 g/d max). *Peds.* 100–150 mg/kg/d IM/IV ÷ bid–tid
SUPPLIED: Injectable forms

Cefotaxime (Claforan)

COMMON USES: Infections caused by susceptible bacteria involving the respiratory tract, skin, bone, urinary tract, meningitis, sepsis
ACTIONS: 3rd-generation cephalosporin; inhibits cell wall synthesis
DOSAGE: *Adults.* 1–2 g IV q4–12h. *Peds.* 100–200 mg/kg/d IV ÷ q6–8h
SUPPLIED: Inj

Cefotetan (Cefotan)

COMMON USES: Infections caused by susceptible bacteria involving the upper and lower respiratory tract, skin, bone, urinary tract, abdomen and gynecologic system
ACTIONS: 2nd-generation cephalosporin; inhibits cell wall synthesis
DOSAGE: *Adults.* 1–2 g IV q12h. *Peds.* 40–80 mg/kg/d IV ÷ q12h
SUPPLIED: Inj
NOTES: Has more gram (–) activity than 1st-generation cephalosporins; has anaerobic activity; contains MTT side chain, which may increase risk of bleeding

Cefoxitin (Mefoxin)

COMMON USES: Infections caused by susceptible bacteria involving the upper and lower respiratory tract, skin, bone, urinary tract, abdomen and gynecologic system
ACTIONS: 2nd-generation cephalosporin; inhibits cell wall synthesis
DOSAGE: *Adults.* 1–2 mg IV q6h. *Peds.* 80–160 mg/kg/d ÷ q4–6h
SUPPLIED: Inj
NOTES: Has more gram (–) activity than 1st-generation cephalosporins; has anaerobic activity

Cefpodoxime (Vantin)

COMMON USES: Infections caused by susceptible bacteria involving the respiratory tract, skin, and urinary tract
ACTIONS: 3rd-generation cephalosporin; inhibits cell wall synthesis
DOSAGE: *Adults.* 200–400 mg PO q12h. *Peds.* 10 mg/kg/d PO ÷ bid
SUPPLIED: Tabs 100, 200 mg; susp 50, 100 mg/5 mL
NOTES: Drug interactions with agents increasing gastric pH

Cefprozil (Cefzil)

COMMON USES: Infections caused by susceptible bacteria involving the upper and lower respiratory tract, skin, and urinary tract
ACTIONS: 2nd-generation cephalosporin; inhibits cell wall synthesis
DOSAGE: *Adults.* 250–500 mg PO qd–bid. *Peds.* 7.5–15 mg/kg/d PO ÷ bid
SUPPLIED: Tabs 250, 500 mg; susp 125, 250 mg/5 mL
NOTES: Has more gram (–) activity then 1st-generation cephalosporins; use higher doses for otitis and pneumonia

22

Ceftazidime (Fortaz, Ceptaz, Tazidime, Tazicef)

COMMON USES: Infections caused by susceptible bacteria involving the respiratory tract, skin, bone, urinary tract, meningitis, and septicemia
ACTIONS: 3rd-generation cephalosporin; inhibits cell wall synthesis
DOSAGE: *Adults.* 1–2 g IV q8h. *Peds.* 30–50 mg/kg/d IV ÷ q8h
SUPPLIED: Inj

Ceftibutin (Cedax)

COMMON USES: Infections caused by susceptible bacteria involving the respiratory tract, skin, and urinary tract
ACTIONS: 3rd-generation cephalosporin; inhibits cell wall synthesis
DOSAGE: *Adults.* 400 mg/d PO. *Peds.* 9 mg/kg/d PO
SUPPLIED: Caps 400 mg; susp 90, 180 mg/5 mL
NOTES: Take on an empty stomach; little activity against *Streptococcus*

Ceftizoxime (Cefizox)

COMMON USES: Infections caused by susceptible bacteria involving the respiratory tract, skin, bone, urinary tract, meningitis, and septicemia
ACTIONS: 3rd-generation cephalosporin; inhibits cell wall synthesis
DOSAGE: *Adults.* 1–2 g IV q 8–12h. *Peds.* 150–200 mg/kg/d IV ÷ q6–8h
SUPPLIED: Inj

Ceftriaxone (Rocephin)

COMMON USES: Infections caused by susceptible bacteria involving the respiratory tract, skin, bone, urinary tract, meningitis, and septicemia
ACTIONS: 3rd-generation cephalosporin; inhibits cell wall synthesis
DOSAGE: *Adults.* 1–2 g IV q12–24h. *Peds.* 50–100 mg/kg/d IV ÷ q12–24h
SUPPLIED: Inj

Cefuroxime (Ceftin [oral], Zinacef [parenteral])

COMMON USES: Infections caused by susceptible bacteria involving the upper and lower respiratory tract, skin, bone, urinary tract, abdomen and gynecologic system
ACTIONS: 2nd-generation cephalosporin; inhibits cell wall synthesis
DOSAGE: *Adults.* 750 mg–1.5 g IV q8h or 250–500 mg PO bid. *Peds.* 100–150 mg/kg/d IV ÷ q8h or 20–30 mg/kg/d PO ÷ bid
SUPPLIED: Tabs 125, 250, 500 mg; susp 125, 250 mg/5 mL; inj forms
NOTES: Has more gram (−) activity then 1st-generation cephalosporin; IV crosses the blood–brain barrier

Celecoxib (Celebrex)

COMMON USES: Osteoarthritis and RA
ACTIONS: NSAID, inhibits the COX-2 pathway
DOSAGE: 100–200 mg/d or bid
SUPPLIED: Caps 100, 200 mg

Cephalexin (Keflex, Keftab)

COMMON USES: Infections caused by susceptible strains of *Streptococcus, Staphylococcus, E. coli, Proteus,* and *Klebsiella* involving the skin, bone, upper and lower respiratory tract, and urinary tract
ACTIONS: 1st-generation cephalosporin; inhibits cell wall synthesis
DOSAGE: *Adults.* 250–500 mg PO qid. *Peds.* 25–100 mg/kg/d PO ÷ qid
SUPPLIED: Caps 250, 500 mg; tabs 250, 500, 1000 mg; susp 125; 250 mg/5 mL

Cephapirin (Cefadyl)

COMMON USES: Respiratory, skin, urinary tract, bone and joint infections, endocarditis, sepsis due to susceptible gram (+) cocci (not enterococcus); some gram (−) coverage (*E. coli, Proteus, Klebsiella*)
ACTIONS: 1st-generation cephalosporin; inhibits cell wall synthesis
DOSAGE: *Adults.* 1 g IM/IV q6h (12 g/d max). *Peds.* 10–20 mg/kg q6h (4 g/d max)
SUPPLIED: Powder for inj

Cephradine (Velosef)

COMMON USES: Various bacterial infections (includes group A β-hemolytic strep)
ACTIONS: 1st-generation cephalosporin; inhibits cell wall synthesis
DOSAGE: *Adults.* 2–4 g/d PO/IV ÷ qid (8 gm/d max). *Peds.* >9 mo: 25–100 mg/kg/d ÷ bid–qid (4 gm/d max)
SUPPLIED: Caps: 250, 500 mg; powder for susp 125 ,250 mg/5 mL, injectable

Cerivastatin (Baycol)

COMMON USES: Reduction of cholesterol, triglycerides and apolipoprotein B
ACTIONS: HMG-CoA reductase inhibitor
DOSAGE: 0.4 mg/d in the evening
SUPPLIED: Withdrawn by manufacturer
NOTES: May cause myopathy, monitor LFT regularly

Cetirizine (Zyrtec)

COMMON USES: Allergic rhinitis and chronic urticaria
ACTIONS: Nonsedating antihistamine
DOSAGE: *Adults & Children.* >6 y: 5–10 mg/d
SUPPLIED: Tabs 5, 10 mg; syrup 5 mg/5 mL

Charcoal, Activated (Superchar, Actidose, Liqui-Char)

COMMON USES: Emergency treatment in poisoning by most drugs and chemicals
ACTIONS: Adsorbent detoxicant
DOSAGE: See also Chapter 21. *Adults.* Acute intoxication: 30–100 g/dose. *GI dialysis:* 25–50 g q4–6h. *Peds.* Acute intoxication: 1–2 g/kg/dose. *GI dialysis:* 5–10 g/dose q4–8h
SUPPLIED: Powder, liq
NOTES: Administer with a cathartic; some liq dosage forms in sorbitol base; protect the airway in lethargic or comatose patients

Chloral Hydrate (Noctec, etc) [C]

COMMON USES: Nocturnal and preoperative sedation
ACTIONS: Sedative hypnotic
DOSAGE: *Adults.* Hypnotic: 500 mg–1 g PO or PR 30 min prior to hs or procedure. *Sedative:* 250 mg PO or PR tid. *Peds.* Hypnotic: 20–40 mg/kg/24h PO or PR 30 min prior to hs or procedure. *Sedative:* 25–50 mg/kg/d ÷ q6–8h
SUPPLIED: Caps 500 mg; syrup 250, 500 mg/5 mL; supp 324, 500, 648 mg
NOTES: Mix syrup in a glass of water or fruit juice

Chlorambucil (Leukeran)

COMMON USES: CLL, Hodgkin's disease, Waldenström's macroglobulinemia
ACTIONS: Alkylating agent
DOSAGE: 0.1–0.2 mg/kg/d for 3–6 wk or 0.4 mg/kg q 2 wk (Refer to specific protocol)
SUPPLIED: Tabs 2 mg
NOTES: *Toxicity symptoms:* Myelosuppression, CNS stimulation, nausea and vomiting, drug fever, skin rash, chromosomal damage that can result in secondary leukemias, alveolar dysplasia, and pulmonary fibrosis

Chlordiazepoxide (Librium) [C]

COMMON USES: Anxiety, tension, alcohol withdrawal, and preoperative apprehension
ACTIONS: Benzodiazepine; antianxiety agent
DOSAGE: *Adults.* Mild anxiety: 5–10 mg PO tid–qid or PRN. *Severe anxiety:* 25–50 mg IM, IV, or PO 3–4×/d or PRN. *Alcohol withdrawal:* 50–100 mg IM or IV; repeat in 2–4 h if needed, up to 300 mg in 24 h; gradually taper the daily dosage. *Peds.* >6 y: 0.5 mg/kg/24h PO or IM ÷ q6–8h
SUPPLIED: Caps 5, 10, 25 mg; tabs 10, 25 mg; inj 100 mg
NOTES: ↓ Dose in the elderly; absorption of IM doses can be erratic

Chlorothiazide (Diuril)

COMMON USES: HTN, edema, and CHF
ACTIONS: Thiazide diuretic
DOSAGE: *Adults.* 500 mg–1.0 g PO or IV qd–bid. *Peds.* 20–30 mg/kg/24h PO ÷ bid
SUPPLIED: Tabs 250, 500 mg; susp 250 mg/5 mL; inj 500 mg/vial
NOTES: Contra in anuria

Chlorpheniramine (Chlor-Trimeton, etc)

COMMON USES: Allergic reactions
ACTIONS: Antihistamine
DOSAGE: *Adults.* 4 mg PO q4–6h or 8–12 mg PO bid of SR. *Peds.* 0.35 mg/kg/24h PO ÷ q4–6h or 0.2 mg/kg/24h SR
SUPPLIED: Tabs 4 mg; chewable tabs 2 mg; SR tabs 8, 12 mg; syrup 2 mg/5 mL; inj 10, 100 mg/mL
NOTES: Anticholinergic side effects and sedation common

Chlorpromazine (Thorazine)

COMMON USES: Psychotic disorders, apprehension, intractable hiccups, and control of nausea and vomiting
ACTIONS: Phenothiazine antipsychotic; antiemetic
DOSAGE: *Adults.* Psychosis: 10–25 mg PO or PR bid–tid. (Usual dose 30–800 mg/d in ÷ doses). *Children.* Psychosis & N+V: 0.5–1 mg/kg/dose PO q or IM/IV q6–8h. *Severe symptoms:* 25 mg IM; can repeat in 1 h; then 25–50 mg PO or PR tid. *Hiccups:* 25–50 mg PO bid–tid
SUPPLIED: Tabs 10, 25, 50, 100, 200 mg; SR caps 30, 75, 150 mg; syrup 10 mg/5 mL; conc 30, 100 mg/mL; supp 25, 100 mg; inj 25 mg/mL
NOTES: Beware of extrapyramidal side effects and sedation; has α-adrenergic-blocking properties

Chlorpropamide (Diabinese)

COMMON USES: Type 2 DM
ACTION: Sulfonylurea. Stimulates the release of insulin from the pancreas; increases insulin sensitivity at peripheral sites; reduces glucose output from the liver
DOSAGE: 100–500 mg/d
SUPPLIED: Tabs 100, 250 mg
NOTES: Use with caution in renal insufficiency

Chlorthalidone (Hygroton, others)

COMMON USES: HTN, edema associated with CHF
ACTIONS: Thiazide diuretic
DOSAGE: *Adults.* 50–100 mg/d PO qd. *Peds.* 2 mg/kg/dose PO 3×/wk or 1–2 mg/kg/d PO
SUPPLIED: Tabs 15, 25, 50, 100 mg
NOTES: Contra in anuric patients

Chlorzoxazone (Paraflex, Parafon Forte DSC, others)

COMMON USES: Adjunct to rest and physical therapy for the relief of discomfort associated with acute, painful musculoskeletal conditions
ACTIONS: Centrally acting skeletal muscle relaxant

DOSAGE: *Adults.* 250–500 mg PO tid–qid. *Peds.* 20 mg/kg/d in 3–4 ÷ doses
SUPPLIED: Tabs 250, 500 mg; caps 250, 500 mg

Cholecalciferol [Vitamin D₃] (Delta-D)

COMMON USES: Dietary supplement for treatment of vitamin D deficiency
ACTIONS: Enhances intestinal calcium absorption
DOSAGE: 400–1000 IU/d PO
SUPPLIED: Tabs 400, 1000 IU
NOTES: 1 mg of cholecalciferol = 40,000 IU of vitamin D activity

Cholestyramine (Questran)

COMMON USES: Adjunctive therapy for the reduction of serum cholesterol in patients with primary hypercholesterolemia; Rx pruritus associated with partial biliary obstruction
ACTIONS: Binds bile acids in the intestine to form insoluble complexes
DOSAGE: *Adults.* Individualize the dose:4 g/d–bid (↑ to max 24 g/d and 6 doses/d). *Peds.* 240 mg/kg/d in 3 ÷ doses
SUPPLIED: 4 g of cholestyramine resin/9 g of powder; with aspartame: 4 g resin/5 g of powder
NOTES: Mix 4 g of cholestyramine in 2–6 oz of noncarbonated beverage; take other medications 1–2 h before or 6 h after cholestyramine

Ciclopirox (Loprox)

COMMON USES: Tinea pedis, tinea cruris, tinea corporis, cutaneous candidiasis, tinea versicolor
ACTIONS: Antifungal antibiotic
DOSAGE: *Adults & Peds.* >10: Massage into affected area bid
SUPPLIED: Cream; gel; lotion 1%

Cidofovir (Vistide)

COMMON USES: CMV retinitis
ACTIONS: Selective inhibition of viral DNA synthesis
DOSAGE: *Rx:* 5 mg/kg IV once/wk for 2 wk; administered with probenecid. *Maintenance:* 5 mg/kg IV once/2 wk; administered with probenecid. *Probenecid:* 2 g PO 3 h prior to Cidofovir, and then 1 g PO at 2 h and 8 h after Cidofovir
SUPPLIED: Inj 75 mg/mL
NOTES: Dose adjust in renal impairment, hydrate patient with NS prior to each infusion; causes renal toxicity

Cimetidine (Tagamet, others)

COMMON USES: Duodenal ulcer; ulcer prophylaxis in hypersecretory states, eg, trauma, burns, surgery, ZE; and GERD
ACTIONS: Histamine-2 receptor antagonist
DOSAGE: *Adults.* Active ulcer: 2400 mg/d IV cont inf or 300 mg IV q6; 400 mg PO bid or 800 mg hs. *Maintenance therapy:* 400 mg PO hs. *GERD:* 800 mg PO bid; maintenance 800 mg PO hs. *Peds.* Infants: 10–20 mg/kg/24h PO or IV ÷ q6–12h. *Children:* 20–40 mg/kg/24h PO or IV ÷ q6h
SUPPLIED: Tabs 200, 300, 400, 800 mg; liq 300 mg/5 mL; inj 300 mg/2 mL
NOTES: Extend dosing interval with renal insufficiency; ↓ dose in the elderly

Ciprofloxacin (Cipro)

COMMON USES: Broad-spectrum activity against a variety of gram (+) and gram (−) aerobic bacteria
ACTIONS: Quinolone antibiotic; inhibits DNA gyrase
DOSAGE: *Adults.* 250–750 mg PO q12h or 200–400 mg IV q12h. *Peds.* NOT recommended for children <18 y old
SUPPLIED: Tabs 100, 250, 500, 750 mg; susp 5 g/100 mL, 10 g/100 mL; inj 200, 400 mg
NOTES: Little activity against streptococci; drug interactions with theophylline, caffeine, sucralfate, and antacids; nausea, vomiting, and abdominal discomfort common side effects; contra in PRG

Ciprofloxacin, Ophthalmic (Ciloxan)

COMMON USES: Rx and prevention of ocular infections eg, conjunctivitis, blepharitis, corneal abrasions
ACTIONS: Quinolone antibiotic; inhibits DNA gyrase, antiinflammatory
DOSAGE: Instill 1–2 gtt in eye(s) q2h while awake for 2 d, then 1–2 gtt q4h while awake for 5 more d
SUPPLIED: Soln 3.5 mg/mL

Ciprofloxacin, Otic (Cipro HC Otic)

COMMON USES: Otitis externa
ACTIONS: Quinolone antibiotic; inhibits DNA gyrase
DOSAGE: *Adult and Peds >1 mo.* 1–2 gtt in ear(s) bid for 7 d
SUPPLIED: Susp ciprofloxacin 0.2% and hydrocortisone 1%

Cisplatin (Platinol)

COMMON USES: Testicular, small-cell and non-small-cell lung, bladder, ovarian, breast, head and neck, and penile cancers; osteosarcoma; and pediatric brain tumors
ACTIONS: DNA-binding; intrastrand cross-linking; formation of DNA adducts
DOSAGE: 20 mg/m^2/d for 5 d q 3 wk; 120 mg/m^2 q 3–4 wk; 100 mg/m^2 on days 1 and 8 q 20 d. (Refer to specific protocols)
SUPPLIED: Inj 1 mg/mL
NOTES: *Toxicity symptoms:* Allergic reactions, nausea and vomiting, nephrotoxicity (exacerbated by concurrent administration of other nephrotoxic drugs and minimized by saline infusion and mannitol diuresis), high-frequency hearing loss in approximately 30%, peripheral "stocking glove"-type neuropathy, cardiotoxicity (ST-T-wave changes), hypomagnesemia, mild myelosuppression, and hepatotoxicity. Renal impairment is dose-related and cumulative

Citalopram (Celexa)

COMMON USES: Depression
ACTIONS: SSRI
DOSAGE: Initial 20 mg/d, may be ↑ to 40 mg/d
SUPPLIED: Tabs 20, 40 mg

Cladribine (Leustatin)

COMMON USES: HCL
ACTIONS: Induces DNA strand breakage and interference with DNA repair enzymes and DNA synthesis
DOSAGE: 0.09 mg/kg/d cont IV inf for 7 d. (Refer to specific protocols)
SUPPLIED: Inj 1 mg/mL
NOTES: *Toxicity symptoms:* Myelosuppression; T-lymphocyte suppression may be prolonged (26–34 wk). Fever occur in 46% (probably related to tumor lysis); infections common (especially at lung and IV catheter sites); rash common (50%) in patients treated for HCL

Clarithromycin (Biaxin)

COMMON USES: Upper and lower respiratory tract infections, skin and skin structure infections, *H. pylori* infections, and infections caused by nontuberculosis (atypical) *Mycobacterium.* Prevention of MAC infections in HIV-infected individuals.
ACTIONS: Macrolide antibiotic; inhibits protein synthesis
DOSAGE: *Adults.* 250–500 mg PO bid or 1000 mg (2 × 500 mg ER tab)/d. *Mycobacterium:* 500–1000 mg PO bid. *Peds.* 7.5 mg/kg/dose PO bid
SUPPLIED: Tabs 250, 500 mg; susp 125, 250 mg/5 mL; 500 mg ER tab
NOTES: Increases theophylline and carbamazepine levels; avoid concurrent use with cisapride; causes metallic taste

Clemastine Fumarate (Tavist)

COMMON USES: Allergic rhinitis
ACTIONS: Antihistamine
DOSAGE: *Adults & Peds.* >12 y: 1.34 mg bid to 2.68 mg tid; max 8.04 mg/d. *<12 y:* 0.4 mg PO bid
SUPPLIED: Tabs 1.34, 2.68 mg; syrup 0.67 mg/5 mL

Clindamycin (Cleocin, Cleocin-T)

COMMON USES: Susceptible strains of streptococci, pneumococci, staphylococci, and gram (+) and gram (−) anaerobes; no activity against gram (−) aerobes and bacterial vaginosis; topical for severe acne and vaginal infections
ACTIONS: Bacteriostatic; interferes with protein synthesis
DOSAGE: *Adults.* 150–450 mg PO qid; 300–600 mg IV q6h or 900 mg IV q8h. *Vaginal:* 1 applicatorful hs for 7 d. *Topical:* Apply 1% gel, lotion, or soln bid. *Peds.* Neonates: 10–15 mg/kg/24h ÷ q8–12h. *Children >1 mo:* 10–30 mg/kg/24h ÷ q6–8h, to a max of 1.8 g/d oral or 4.8 g/d IV. *Topical:* Apply 1%, gel, lotion, or soln bid
SUPPLIED: Caps 75, 150, 300 mg; susp 75 mg/5 mL; inj 300 mg/2 mL; vaginal cream 2%
NOTES: Beware of diarrhea that may represent pseudomembranous colitis caused by *Clostridium difficile*

Clofazimine (Lamprene)

COMMON USES: Leprosy and as part of combination therapy for MAC in AIDS patients
ACTIONS: Bactericidal; inhibits DNA synthesis
DOSAGE: *Adults.* 100–300 mg PO qd. *Peds.* 1 mg/kg/d
SUPPLIED: Caps 50 mg
NOTES: Take with meals; may change skin pigmentation pink to brownish black; may cause skin dryness and GI intolerance

Clonazepam (Klonopin) [C]

COMMON USES: Lennox–Gastaut syndrome, akinetic and myoclonic seizures, and absence seizures
ACTIONS: Benzodiazepine; anticonvulsant
DOSAGE: *Adults.* 1.5 mg/d PO in 3 ÷ doses; ↑ by 0.5–1.0 mg/d q 3 d PRN up to 20 mg/d. *Peds.* 0.01–0.03 mg/kg/24h PO ÷ tid; ↑ to 0.1–0.2 mg/kg/24h ÷ tid
SUPPLIED: Tabs 0.5, 1.0, 2.0 mg
NOTES: CNS side effects, including sedation

Clonidine, Oral (Catapres)

COMMON USES: HTN; opioid and tobacco withdrawal
ACTIONS: Centrally acting α-adrenergic stimulant
DOSAGE: *Adults.* 0.10 mg PO bid adjusted daily by 0.1- to 0.2-mg increments (max 2.4 mg/d). *Peds.* 5–10 μg/kg/d ÷d q8–12h (max 0.9 mg/d)
SUPPLIED: Tabs 0.1, 0.2, 0.3 mg
NOTES: Dry mouth, drowsiness, and sedation frequent; more effective for HTN when combined with diuretics; rebound HTN can occur with abrupt cessation of doses >0.2 mg bid. (See TD dose.)

Clonidine, Transdermal (Catapres TTS)

COMMON USES: HTN
ACTIONS: Centrally acting α-adrenergic stimulant
DOSAGE: Apply 1 patch q 7 d to a hairless area on the upper arm or torso; titrate according to individual therapeutic requirements
SUPPLIED: TTS-1, TTS-2, TTS-3 (programmed to deliver 0.1, 0.2, 0.3 mg, respectively, of clonidine/d for 1 wk)
NOTES: Doses >2 TTS-3 usually not associated with increased efficacy

Clopidogrel (Plavix)

COMMON USES: Reduction of atherosclerotic events
ACTIONS: Inhibits platelet aggregation
DOSAGE: 75 mg/d
SUPPLIED: Tabs 75 mg
NOTES: Prolongs bleeding time, use with caution in persons at risk of bleeding from trauma, etc

Clorazepate (Tranxene) [C]

COMMON USES: Acute anxiety disorders, acute alcohol withdrawal symptoms, and adjunctive therapy in partial seizures
ACTIONS: Benzodiazepine; antianxiety agent
DOSAGE: *Adults.* 15–60 mg/d PO in single or ÷ doses. *Elderly and debilitated patients:* Initiate therapy at 7.5–15 mg/d in ÷ doses. *Alcohol withdrawal:* Day 1: Initially, 30 mg; followed by 30–60 mg in ÷ doses. Day 2: 45–90 mg in ÷ doses. Day 3: 22.5–45 mg in ÷ doses. Day 4: 15–30 mg in ÷ doses. *Peds.* 3.75–7.5 mg/dose bid, to a max of 60 mg/d ÷ bid–tid
SUPPLIED: Tabs 3.75, 7.5, 11.25, 15, 22.5 mg
NOTES: Monitor patients with renal and hepatic impairment because drug may accumulate; CNS depressant effects

Clotrimazole (Lotrimin, Mycelex)

COMMON USES: Candidiasis and tinea infections
ACTIONS: Antifungal agent; alters cell wall permeability
DOSAGE: *Oral:* One troche dissolved slowly in the mouth 5 (times)/d for 14 d. *Vaginal:* Cream 1 applicatorful hs for 7–14 d. Tabs 100 mg vaginally hs for 7 d or 200 mg (2 tabs) vaginally hs for 3 d or 500-mg tabs vaginally hs once. *Topical:* Apply bid for 10–14 d
SUPPLIED: 1% cream; soln; lotion; troche 10 mg; vaginal tabs 100, 500 mg; vaginal cream 1%
NOTES: Oral prophylaxis commonly used in immunosuppressed patients

Clotrimazole and Betamethasone (Lotrisone)

COMMON USES: Fungal skin infections
ACTIONS: Imidazole antifungal and antiinflammatory
DOSAGE: Apply and gently massage into the area bid from 2–4 wk
SUPPLIED: Cream 15, 45 g
NOTES: Contra in children and varicella

Cloxacillin (Cloxapen, Tegopen)

COMMON USES: Infections caused by susceptible strains of *S. aureus* and *Streptococcus*
ACTIONS: Bactericidal; inhibits cell wall synthesis
DOSAGE: *Adults.* 250–500 mg PO qid. *Peds.* 50–100 mg/kg/d ÷ qid
SUPPLIED: Caps 250, 500 mg; soln 125 mg/5 mL
NOTES: Take on an empty stomach

Clozapine (Clozaril)

COMMON USES: Refractory severe schizophrenia
ACTIONS: Tricyclic "atypical" antipsychotic agent
DOSAGE: Initially, 25 mg qd–bid; ↑ dose to 300–450 mg/d over 2 wk. Maintain the patient at the lowest dose possible
SUPPLIED: Tabs 25, 100 mg
NOTES: Monitor blood counts frequently (weekly for the first 6 mo; then every other week) because of the risk of agranulocytosis. Drowsiness and seizures possible

Cocaine [C]

COMMON USES: Topical anesthetic for mucous membranes
ACTIONS: Narcotic analgesic, local vasoconstrictor

22

DOSAGE: Apply topically lowest amount of topical soln that provides relief; 1 mg/kg max
SUPPLIED: Topical soln and viscous preparations 4, 10% powder, soluble tabs (135 mg) for soln

Codeine [C-II]

COMMON USES: Mild to moderate pain; symptomatic relief of cough
ACTIONS: Narcotic analgesic; depresses cough reflex
DOSAGE: *Adults.* Analgesic: 15–60 mg PO or IM qid PRN. *Antitussive:* 10–20 mg PO q4h PRN; max 12 mg/d. *Peds.* Analgesic: 0.5–1.0 mg/kg/dose PO or IM q4–6h PRN. *Antitussive:* 1.0–1.5 mg/kg/24h PO ÷ q4h; max 30 mg/24h
SUPPLIED: Tabs 15, 30, 60 mg; soln 15 mg/5 mL; inj 30, 60 mg/mL
NOTES: Most often combined with acetaminophen for pain or with agents, eg, terpin hydrate as an antitussive; 120 mg IM = to 10 mg of morphine IM

Colchicine

COMMON USES: Acute gout
ACTIONS: Inhibits migration of leukocytes; reduces production of lactic acid by leukocytes
DOSAGE: *Initially:* 0.5–1.2 mg PO, then 0.5–0.6 mg q 1–2 h until relief or GI side effects develop (max 8 mg/d). Do not repeat for 3 d. IV: 1–3 mg, then 0.5 mg q6h until relief (max 4 mg/d) do not repeat for 7 d. *Prophylaxis:* PO: 0.5–0.6 mg/d or 3–4 d/wk
SUPPLIED: Tabs 0.5, 0.6 mg; inj 1 mg/2 mL
NOTES: Use caution in elderly and in renal impairment. Colchicine 1–2 mg IV within 24–48 h of an acute attack can be diagnostic and therapeutic in monoarticular arthritis

Colesevelam (Welchol)

COMMON USES: Reduction of LDL and total cholesterol
ACTIONS: Bile acid sequestrant
DOSAGE: 3 tabs PO bid with meals
SUPPLIED: Tabs 625 mg

Colestipol (Colestid)

COMMON USES: Adjunctive for ↓ serum cholesterol in primary hypercholesterolemia
ACTIONS: Binds bile acids in the intestine to form an insoluble complex
DOSAGE: Granules: 5–30 g/d ÷ into 2–4 doses; tabs: 2–16 g/d qd–bid
SUPPLIED: Tabs 1 g; granules
NOTES: Do not use dry powder; mix with beverages, soups, cereals, etc

Colfosceril Palmitate (Exosurf Neonatal)

COMMON USES: Prophylaxis and Rx for RSD in infants
ACTIONS: Synthetic lung surfactant
DOSAGE: 5 mL/kg/dose administered through the endotracheal tube as soon after birth as possible and again at 12 and 24 h
SUPPLIED: Suspension 108 mg
NOTES: Monitor pulmonary compliance and oxygenation carefully. Pulmonary hemorrhage possible in infants weighing <700 g at birth. Mucous plugging of endotracheal tube possible

Cortisone

See Steroids pages 628–630. (See Table 22–5, page 627 and Table 22–6, page 627.)

Cromolyn Sodium (Intal, Nasalcrom, Opticrom)

COMMON USES: Adjunct to the Rx of asthma; prevention of exercise-induced asthma; allergic rhinitis; ophth allergic manifestations
ACTIONS: Antiasthmatic; mast cell stabilizer
DOSAGE: *Adults & Children >12 y.* Inhal: 20 mg (as powder in caps) inhaled qid or met-dose inhaler 2 puffs qid. *Oral:* 200 mg qid 15–20 min ac, up to 400 mg qid. *Nasal instillation:* Spray once

in each nostril 2–6 ×/d. *Ophth:* 1–2 gtt in each eye 4–6×/d. **Peds.** Inhal: 2 puffs qid of met-dose inhaler. *Oral: Infants <2 y:* 20 mg/kg/d in 4 ÷ doses. *2–12 y:* 100 mg qid ac
SUPPLIED: Oral conc 100 mg/5 mL; soln for neb 20 mg/2 mL; met-dose inhaler; nasal soln 40 mg/mL; ophth soln 4%
NOTES: No benefit in acute situations; may require 2–4 wk for maximal effect in perennial allergic disorders

Cyanocobalamin [Vitamin B$_{12}$]

COMMON USES: Pernicious anemia and other vitamin B$_{12}$ deficiency states
ACTIONS: Dietary supplement of vitamin B$_{12}$
DOSAGE: *Adults.* 100 µg IM or SC qd for 5–10 d, then 100 µg IM 2×/wk for 1 mo, then 100 µg IM monthly. **Peds.** 100 µg IM or SC for 5–10 d, then 30–50 µg IM q 4 wk
SUPPLIED: Tabs 25, 50, 100, 250, 500, 1000 µg; inj 30, 100, 1000 µg/mL
NOTES: Oral absorption highly erratic, altered by many drugs and not recommended; for use with hyperalimentation (see Chapter 12)

Cyclobenzaprine (Flexeril)

COMMON USES: Adjunct to rest and physical therapy for the relief of muscle spasm associated with acute painful musculoskeletal conditions
ACTIONS: Centrally acting skeletal muscle relaxant; reduces tonic somatic motor activity
DOSAGE: 10 mg PO 2–4×/d
SUPPLIED: Tabs 10 mg
NOTES: Do not use for longer than 2–3 wk; has sedative and anticholinergic properties

Cyclopentolate (Cyclogyl)

COMMON USES: Diagnostic procedures requiring cycloplegia and mydriasis
ACTIONS: Cycloplegia and mydriatic agent (can last up to 24 h)
DOSAGE: 1 gtt followed by another in 5 min
SUPPLIED: Soln, 0.5, 1, 2%

Cyclophosphamide (Cytoxan, Neosar)

COMMON USES: Hodgkin's and non-Hodgkin's lymphomas, multiple myeloma, breast and ovarian cancers, mycosis fungoides, neuroblastoma, retinoblastoma, acute leukemias, small-cell lung cancer, and allogeneic and ABMT in high doses; severe rheumatologic disorders
ACTIONS: Converted to acrolein and phosphoramide mustard, the active alkylating moieties
DOSAGE: 500–1500 mg/m^2 as a single dose at 2–4-wk intervals; 1.8 g/m^2 to 160 mg/kg (or ≈12 g/m^2 in a 75-kg individual) in the BMT setting. (Refer to specific protocols)
SUPPLIED: Tabs 25, 50 mg; inj 100 mg
NOTES: *Toxicity symptoms:* Myelosuppression (leukopenia and thrombocytopenia); sterile hemorrhagic cystitis, SIADH, alopecia, and anorexia; nausea and vomiting common. Hepatotoxicity and rarely interstitial pneumonitis possible. Irreversible testicular atrophy possible. Cardiotoxicity rare. Second malignancies (bladder cancer and acute leukemias); cumulative risk of 3.5% at 8 y, 10.7% at 12 y. Preventive measures to avoid hemorrhagic cystitis often applied in high-dose regimens and may include continuous bladder irrigation and MESNA uroprotection (see page 567)

Cyclosporine (Sandimmune, Neoral)

COMMON USES: Organ rejection in kidney, liver, heart, and BMT in conjunction with adrenal corticosteroids
ACTIONS: Immunosuppressant; reversible inhibition of immunocompetent lymphocytes
DOSAGE: *Adults & Peds.* Oral: 15 mg/kg/d beginning 12 h prior to transplant; after 2 wk, taper the dose by 5 mg/wk to 5–10 mg/kg/d. *IV:* If the patient is unable to take the drug orally, give ½ the oral dose IV
SUPPLIED: Caps 25, 50 mg, 100 mg; oral soln 100 mg/mL; inj 50 mg/mL

NOTES: May elevate BUN and creatinine, which may be confused with renal transplant rejection; should be administered in glass containers; many drug interactions; Neoral and Sandimmune not interchangeable. (See Table 22–7 pages 631–634.)

Cyproheptadine (Periactin)

COMMON USES: Allergic reactions; especially good for itching
ACTIONS: Phenothiazine antihistamine
DOSAGE: *Adults.* 4–20 mg PO ÷ q8h; max 0.5 mg/kg/d. *Peds.* 2–6 y: 2 mg bid–tid (max 12 mg/24h). *7–14 y:* 4 mg bid–tid
SUPPLIED: Tabs 4 mg; syrup 2 mg/5 mL
NOTES: Anticholinergic side effects and drowsiness common; may stimulate appetite in some patients

Cytarabine [Ara-C] (Cytosar-U)

COMMON USES: Acute leukemias, CML, non-Hodgkin's lymphoma; IT administration for leukemic meningitis or prophylaxis
ACTIONS: Antimetabolite; interferes with DNA synthesis
DOSAGE: 100–150 mg/m^2/d for 5–10 d (low-dose); 3 g/m^2 q12h for 8–12 doses (high-dose); 1 mg/kg 1–2×/wk (SC maintenance regimens); 5–70 mg/m^2 up to 3×/wk IT. (Refer to specific protocols)
SUPPLIED: Inj 100 mg, 500 mg, 1 g, 2 g
NOTES: *Toxicity symptoms:* Myelosuppression, nausea and vomiting, diarrhea, stomatitis, flu-like syndrome, rash of the palms and soles of the feet, and hepatic dysfunction. Toxicity of high-dose regimens (conjunctivitis) ameliorated by corticosteroid ophth soln, cerebellar dysfunction, and noncardiogenic pulmonary edema

Cytarabine Liposomal (Depocyt)

COMMON USES: Lymphomatous meningitis
ACTIONS: Antimetabolite; interferes with DNA synthesis
DOSAGE: 50 mg IT q 14 d for 5 doses; followed by 50 mg IT q 28 d for 4 doses
SUPPLIED: IT inj 50 mg/5 mL

Cytomegalovirus Immune Globulin [CMV-GIV] (Cytogam)

COMMON USES: Attenuation of primary CMV disease associated with transplantation
ACTIONS: Provides exogenous IgG antibodies to CMV
DOSAGE: Administered for 16 wk posttransplant, 15 mg/kg/hr, ↑Q30 min to 60 mg/kg/hr, max 75 mL/hr IV
SUPPLIED: Inj 50±10 mg/mL

Dacarbazine (DTIC-Dome)

COMMON USES: Melanoma, Hodgkin's disease, sarcoma
ACTIONS: Alkylating agent; antimetabolite activity as a purine precursor; inhibits synthesis of protein, RNA, and especially DNA
DOSAGE: 2–4.5 mg/kg/d for 10 consecutive d or 250 mg/m^2/d for 5 d. (Refer to specific protocols)
SUPPLIED: Inj 100, 200, 500 mg
NOTES: *Toxicity symptoms:* Moderate myelosuppression, severe nausea and vomiting, hepatotoxicity, flu-like syndrome, hypotension with high-dose therapy, photosensitivity, alopecia, facial flushing, facial paresthesias, urticaria, and phlebitis at the inj site

Daclizumab (Zenapax)

COMMON USES: Prevention of acute organ rejection
ACTIONS: IL-2 receptor antagonists
DOSAGE: 1 mg/kg IV/dose; first dose before transplant then 4 doses 14 d apart posttransplant
SUPPLIED: Inj 5 mg/mL

Dactinomycin (Cosmegen)

COMMON USES: Choriocarcinoma, Wilms' tumor, Kaposi's sarcoma, Ewing's sarcoma, rhabdomyosarcoma, testicular cancer
ACTIONS: DNA intercalating agent
DOSAGE: 0.5 mg/d for 5 d; 2 mg/wk for 3 consecutive wk; 15 µg/kg or 0.45 mg/m^2/d (max 0.5 mg) for 5 d q 3–8 wk in pediatric sarcoma. (Refer to specific protocols)
SUPPLIED: Inj 0.5 mg
NOTES: *Toxicity symptoms:* Myelosuppression, immunosuppression, nausea and vomiting, alopecia, acne-form skin changes and hyperpigmentation, radiation recall phenomenon, phlebitis and tissue damage with extravascular extravasation, and hepatotoxicity

Dalteparin (Fragmin)

COMMON USES: Unstable angina, non-Q-wave MI, prevention of ischemic complications due to clot formation in patients on concurrent aspirin, prevention of DVT following surgery
ACTIONS: Low-molecular-weight heparin
DOSAGE: *Angina/MI:* 120 IU/kg (max 10,000 IU) SC q12h with aspirin. *DVT prophylaxis:* 2500–5000 IU SC 1–2 h prior to surgery, then qd for 5–10 d. *Systemic anticoagulation:* 200 IU/kg/d SC or 100 IU/kg bid SC
SUPPLIED: Inj 2500 IU (16 mg/0.2 mL), 5000 IU (32 mg/0.2 mL), 10,000 IU (64 mg/mL)
NOTES: Predictable antithrombotic effects eliminates need for laboratory monitoring

Dantrolene (Dantrium)

COMMON USES: Clinical spasticity resulting from upper motor neuron disorders, eg, spinal cord injuries, strokes, CP, or MS; Rx of malignant hyperthermic crisis
ACTIONS: Skeletal muscle relaxant
DOSAGE: *Adults.* Spasticity: Initially, 25 mg PO qd; ↑ to effect by 25 mg to a max dose of 100 mg PO qid PRN. *Peds.* Initially, 0.5 mg/kg/dose bid; ↑ by 0.5 mg/kg to effectiveness to a max dose of 3 mg/kg/dose qid PRN. *Adults & Peds. Malignant hyperthermia: Treatment:* Continuous rapid IV push beginning at 1 mg/kg until symptoms subside or 10 mg/kg is reached. *Postcrisis follow-up:* 4–8 mg/kg/d in 3–4 ÷ doses for 1–3 d to prevent recurrence
SUPPLIED: Caps 25, 50, 100 mg; powder for inj 20 mg/vial
NOTES: Monitor ALT and AST closely

Dapsone [DDS] (Avlosulfon)

COMMON USES: Rx and prevention of PCP; toxoplasmosis prophylaxis; leprosy
ACTIONS: Unknown; bactericidal
DOSAGE: *Adults.* Prophylaxis of PCP 50–100 mg/d PO. Rx of PCP 100 mg/d PO with TMP 5 mg/kg for 21 d. *Peds.* Prophylaxis of PCP 1–2 mg/kg/24h PO qd; max 100 mg/d
SUPPLIED: Tabs 25 mg, 100 mg
NOTES: Absorption enhanced by an acidic environment; leprosy therapy in combination with rifampin and other agents

Daunorubicin (Daunomycin, Cerubidine)

COMMON USES: Acute leukemias
ACTIONS: DNA intercalating agent; inhibits topoisomerase II; generates oxygen free radicals
DOSAGE: 45–60 mg/m^2/d for 3 consecutive d; 25 mg/m^2/wk. (Refer to specific protocols)
SUPPLIED: Inj 20 mg
NOTES: *Toxicity symptoms:* Myelosuppression, mucositis, nausea and vomiting, alopecia, radiation recall phenomenon, hepatotoxicity (hyperbilirubinemia), tissue necrosis on extravascular extravasation, and cardiotoxicity (1–2% risk of CHF with a cumulative dose of 550 mg/m^2)

Delavirdine (Rescriptor)

COMMON USES: HIV infection
ACTION: Nonnucleoside reverse transcriptase inhibitor

DOSAGE: 400 mg PO tid
SUPPLIED: Tabs 100 mg
NOTES: Inhibits cytochrome P-450 enzymes. Numerous drug interactions

Demeclocycline (Declomycin)

COMMON USES: SIADH
ACTIONS: Antagonizes the action of ADH on renal tubules
DOSAGE: 300–600 mg PO q12h
SUPPLIED: Caps 150 mg; tabs 150, 300 mg
NOTES: ↓ Dose in renal failure. DI possible

Desipramine (Norpramin)

COMMON USES: Endogenous depression, chronic pain, and peripheral neuropathy
ACTIONS: Tricyclic antidepressant; increases synaptic concentration of serotonin or norepinephrine in CNS
DOSAGE: 25–200 mg/d in single or ÷ doses; usually as a single hs dose. (Max 300 mg/d)
SUPPLIED: Tabs 10, 25, 50, 75, 100, 150 mg; caps 25, 50 mg
NOTES: Many anticholinergic side effects, including blurred vision, urinary retention, and dry mouth

Desmopressin (DDAVP, Stimate)

COMMON USES: DI (intranasal and parenteral); bleeding caused by hemophilia A and type I von Willebrand's disease (parenteral), nocturnal enuresis
ACTIONS: Synthetic analogue of vasopressin, a naturally occurring human ADH; increases factor VIII
DOSAGE: *DI:* Intranasal: *Adults.* 0.1–0.4 mL (10–40 μg)/d in 1–4 ÷ doses. *Peds 3 mo–12 y.* 0.05–0.3 mL/d in 1 or 2 doses. *Parenteral: Adults.* 0.5–1 mL (2–4 μg)/d in 2 ÷ doses. If converting from intranasal to parenteral dosing, use ¹⁄₁₀ of the intranasal dose. *Oral: Adults.* 0.05 mg bid; may be ↑ to max of 1.2 mg. *Hemophilia A and von Willebrand's disease (type I): Adults & Peds >10 kg.* 0.3 μg/kg diluted to 50 mL with NS infused slowly over 15–30 min. *Peds <10 kg.* Same as above with dilution to 10 mL with NS. *Nocturnal enuresis: Peds >6 y.* 20 μg intranasally hs.
SUPPLIED: Tabs 0.1, 0.2 mg; inj 4 μg/mL; nasal soln 0.1, 1.5 mg/mL
NOTES: In very young and old patients adjust fluid intake to avoid water intoxication and hyponatremia
NOTES: Must be used in conjunction with a glucocorticoid

Dexamethasone, Nasal (Dexacort Phosphate Turbinaire)

COMMON USES: Chronic nasal inflammation or allergic rhinitis
ACTIONS: Antiinflammatory corticosteroid
DOSAGE: *Adult and Peds > 12 y.* 2 sprays/nostril bid–tid, max 12 sprays/d. *Peds 6–12 y.* 1–2 sprays/nostril, bid, max 8 sprays/d
SUPPLIED: Aerosol, 84 μg/activation

Dexamethasone, Ophthalmic (AK-Dex Ophthalmic, Decadron Ophthalmic, others)

COMMON USES: Inflammatory or allergic conjunctivitis
ACTIONS: Antiinflammatory corticosteroid
DOSAGE: Instill 1–2 gtt tid–qid
SUPPLIED: Susp and soln 0.1%; oint 0.05%

Dexamethasone, Systemic, Topical (Decadron)

See Steroids (Table 22–5, page 627 and Table 22–6, pages 628–630)

Dexpanthenol (Ilopan-Choline Oral, Ilopan)

COMMON USES: Minimize paralytic ileus, Rx postop distention
ACTIONS: Cholinergic agent
DOSAGE: *Adults.* Relief of gas: 2–3 tabs PO tid. *Prevention of postop ileus:* 250–500 mg IM stat, repeat in 2 h, then q6h PRN. *Ileus:* IM: 500 mg stat, repeat in 2 h, followed by doses q6h, if needed
SUPPLIED: Inj; tabs 50 mg; cream
NOTES: Do NOT use if obstruction is suspected

Dexrazoxane (Zinecard)

COMMON USES: Prevention of anthracycline-induced (doxorubicin) cardiomyopathy in metastatic breast cancer and other therapies
ACTIONS: Chelates heavy metals; binds intracellular iron and prevents anthracycline-induced free-radical generation
DOSAGE: 10:1 ratio of dexrazoxane to doxorubicin, 30 min prior to each dose of anthracycline
SUPPLIED: Inj 10 mg/mL
NOTES: *Toxicity symptoms:* Myelosuppression (especially leukopenia), fever, infection, stomatitis, alopecia, diarrhea, and nausea and vomiting. Mild elevations of hepatic transaminases and local pain at injection site less frequent

Dextran 40 [Low Molecular Weight Dextran] (Rheomacrodex)

COMMON USES: Plasma expander for adjunctive therapy in shock, prophylaxis of DVT and thromboembolism, adjunct in peripheral vascular surgery
ACTIONS: Expands plasma volume; ↓ blood viscosity
DOSAGE: *Shock:* 10 mL/kg infused rapidly with a max dose of 20 mL/kg in the first 24 h; max dosage beyond 24 h not to exceed 10 mL/kg; discontinue after 5 d. *Prophylaxis of DVT and thromboembolism:* 10 mL/kg IV on day of surgery followed by 500 mL/d IV for 2–3 d, then 500 mL IV q 2–3 d based on the patient's risk factors for up to 2 wk
SUPPLIED: 10% dextran 40 in 0.9% NaCl or 5% dextrose
NOTES: Observe for hypersensitivity reactions; monitor renal function and electrolytes

Dextromethorphan (Mediquell, Benylin DM, Pediacare 1)

COMMON USES: Controlling nonproductive cough
ACTIONS: Depresses the cough center in the medulla
DOSAGE: *Adults.* 10–30 mg PO q4h PRN. *Peds.* 7 mo–1 y: 2–4 mg q6–8h; *2–6 y:* 2.5–7.5 mg q4–8h (max 30 mg/24h). *7–12 y:* 5–10 mg q4–8h (max 60 mg/24/h)
SUPPLIED: Caps 30 mg; lozenges 2.5, 5, 7.5, 15 mg; syrup 15 mg/15 mL, 10 mg/5 mL; liq 10 mg/15 mL, 3.5, 7.5, 15 mg/5 mL; sustained-action liq 30 mg/5 mL
NOTES: May be found in combination products with guaifenesin

Dezocine (Dalgan)

COMMON USES: Moderate to severe pain
ACTIONS: Narcotic agonist–antagonist
DOSAGE: 5–20 mg IM or 2.5–10 mg IV q2–4h PRN
SUPPLIED: Inj 5, 10, 15 mg/mL
NOTES: Withdrawal symptoms possible in patients dependent on narcotics. NOT recommended for patients <18 y

Diazepam (Valium, others) [C$_{IV}$]

COMMON USES: Anxiety, alcohol withdrawal, muscle spasm, status epilepticus, panic disorders, amnesia, and preoperative sedation
ACTIONS: Benzodiazepine
DOSAGE: *Adults.* Status epilepticus: 5–10 mg q 10–20 min to max dose of 30 mg in 8-h period. *Anxiety, muscle spasm:* 2–10 mg PO bid–qid or IM/IV q3–4h PRN. *Preop:* 5–10 mg PO or IM 20–30 min before procedure; can be given IV just prior to procedure. *Alcohol withdrawal:* Initially,

2–5 mg IV, then 5–10 mg q 5–10 min, not to exceed 100 mg in 1 h. May require up to 1000 mg in 24-h period for severe withdrawal symptoms. Titrate to agitation; avoid excessive sedation; may lead to aspiration or respiratory arrest. **Peds.** Status epilepticus: <5 y: 0.05–0.3 mg/kg/dose IV q 15–30 min up to a max of 5 mg. >5 y: May administer up to a max of 10 mg. *Sedation, muscle relaxation:* 0.04–0.3 mg/kg/dose q2–4h IM or IV up to a max of 0.6 mg/kg in 8 h, or 0.12–0.8 mg/kg/24h PO ÷ tid–qid

SUPPLIED: Tabs 2, 5, 10 mg; soln 1, 5 mg/mL; inj 5 mg/mL; gel for rectal delivery 5 mg/mL

NOTES: Do NOT exceed 5 mg/min IV in adults or 1–2 mg/min in peds, as respiratory arrest possible; absorption of IM dose may be erratic

Diazoxide (Hyperstat, Proglycem)

COMMON USES: Hypoglycemia caused by hyperinsulinism

ACTIONS: Inhibits pancreatic insulin release

DOSAGE: *Adults & Peds.* 3–8 mg/kg/24h PO ÷ q8–12h. *Neonates.* 8–15 mg/kg/24h ÷ in 3 equal doses; maintenance 8–10 mg/kg/24h PO in 2–3 equal doses

SUPPLIED: Inj 15 mg/mL; caps 50 mg; oral susp 50 mg/mL

NOTES: Sodium retention and hyperglycemia frequent; possible thiazide diuretic cross-hypersensitivity; cannot be titrated

Dibucaine (Nupercainal)

COMMON USES: Hemorrhoids and minor skin conditions

ACTIONS: Topical anesthetic

DOSAGE: Insert PR with applicator bid and after each bowel movement; apply sparingly to skin

SUPPLIED: 1% Oint with rectal applicator; 0.5% cream

Diclofenac (Cataflam, Voltaren)

COMMON USES: Arthritis and pain

ACTIONS: NSAID

DOSAGE: 50–75 mg PO bid

SUPPLIED: Tabs 50 mg; tabs DR 25, 50, 75, 100 mg

Dicloxacillin (Dynapen, Dycill)

COMMON USES: Infections caused by susceptible strains of *S. aureus* and *Streptococcus*

ACTIONS: Bactericidal; inhibits cell wall synthesis

DOSAGE: *Adults.* 250–500 mg qid. *Peds <40 kg.* 12.5–25 mg/kg/d ÷ qid

SUPPLIED: Caps 125, 250, 500 mg; soln 62.5 mg/5 mL

NOTES: Take on an empty stomach

Dicyclomine (Bentyl)

COMMON USES: Functional irritable bowel syndromes

ACTIONS: Smooth muscle relaxant

DOSAGE: *Adults.* 20 mg PO qid; ↑ to a max dose of 160 mg/d or 20 mg IM q6h. *Peds.* Infants >6 mo: 5 mg/dose tid–qid. *Children:* 10 mg/dose tid–qid

SUPPLIED: Caps 10, 20 mg; tabs 20 mg; syrup 10 mg/5 mL; inj 10 mg/mL

NOTES: Anticholinergic side effects may limit dose

Didanosine [DDI] (Videx)

COMMON USES: HIV infection in zidovudine-intolerant patients

ACTIONS: Nucleoside antiretroviral agent

DOSAGE: *Adults.* >60 kg: 400 mg/d PO or 200 mg PO bid. *<60 kg:* 250 mg/d PO or 125 mg PO bid. *Peds.* Dose by following table

BSA (m²)	Tablets (mg)	Powder (mg)
1.1–1.4	100 mg bid	125 mg bid
0.8–1	75 mg bid	94 mg bid
0.5–0.7	50 mg bid	62 mg bid
<0.4	25 mg bid	31 mg bid

SUPPLIED: Chewable tabs 25, 50, 100, 150, 200 mg; powder packets 100, 167, 250, 375 mg; powder for soln 2, 4 g
NOTES: Reconstitute powder with water; side effects include pancreatitis, peripheral neuropathy, diarrhea, and headache; adults should take 2 tabs/administration. Dose adjust in renal impairment; do not mix powder with fruit juice or other acidic beverages

Diflunisal (Dolobid)

COMMON USES: Mild to moderate pain; osteoarthritis
ACTIONS: NSAID
DOSAGE: *Pain:* 500 mg PO bid. *Osteoarthritis:* 500–1500 mg PO in 2–3 ÷ doses
SUPPLIED: Tabs 250, 500 mg
NOTES: May prolong bleeding time

Digoxin (Lanoxin, Lanoxicaps)

Used for emergency cardiac care (see Chapter 21)
COMMON USES: CHF, AF and flutter, and PAT
ACTIONS: Positive inotrope; increases the refractory period of the AV node
DOSAGE: *Adults.* PO digitalization: 0.50–0.75 mg PO, then 0.25 mg PO q6–8h to total 1.0–1.5 mg. *IV or IM digitalization:* 0.25–0.50 mg IM or IV, then 0.25 mg q4–6h to total ≅1 mg. *Daily maintenance:* 0.125–0.500 mg/d PO, IM, or IV (average daily dose 0.125–0.250 mg). *Peds.* Preterm infants: *Digitalization:* 30 µg/kg PO or 25 µg/kg IV; give ½ of dose initially, then ¼ at 8–12-h intervals for 2 doses. *Maintenance:* 5–7.5 µg/kg/24h PO or 4–6 µg/kg/24h IV ÷ q12h. *Term infants: Digitalization:* 25–35 µg/kg PO or 20–30 µg/kg IV; give ½ the dose initially, then ¼ of the dose at 8–12 h. *Maintenance:* 6–10 µg/kg/24h PO or 5–8 µg/kg/24h ÷ q12h. *1 mo–2 y: Digitalization:* 35–60 µg/kg PO or 30–50 µg/kg IV; give ½ the dose initially, then ¼ of the dose at 8–12 intervals for 2 doses. *Maintenance:* 10–15 µg/kg/24h PO or 7.5–15 µg/kg/24h IV ÷ q12h. *2–10 y: Digitalization:* 30–40 µg/kg PO or 25 µg/kg IV; give ½ dose initially, then ¼ of the dose at 8–12-h intervals for 2 doses. *Maintenance:* 8–10 µg/kg/24h PO or 6–8 µg/kg/24h IV ÷ q12h. *>10 y:* Same as for adults
SUPPLIED: Caps 0.05, 0.1, 0.2 mg; tabs 0.125, 0.25, 0.5 mg; elixir 0.05 mg/mL; inj 0.1, 0.25 mg/mL
NOTES: Can cause heart block; low potassium can potentiate toxicity; ↓ in renal failure. *Toxicity symptoms:* Nausea and vomiting, headache, fatigue, visual disturbances (yellow-green halos around lights), and cardiac arrhythmias; IM inj can be painful and has erratic absorption (See Drug Levels, Table 22–7, pages 631–634)

Digoxin Immune Fab (Digibind)

Used for emergency cardiac care (see Chapter 21)
COMMON USES: Life-threatening digoxin intoxication
ACTIONS: Antigen-binding fragments bind digoxin, rendering it inactive
DOSAGE: *Adults & Peds.* Based on serum level and patient's weight. See dosing charts provided with the drug
SUPPLIED: Inj 38 mg/vial
NOTES: Each vial binds ≅0.6 mg of digoxin; in renal failure, may require redosing in several days because of breakdown of the immune complex

Diltiazem (Cardizem, Dilacor, Tiazac)

Used for emergency cardiac care (see Chapter 21)
COMMON USES: Angina pectoris, prevention of reinfarction, HTN, AF or flutter, and PAT
ACTIONS: Calcium channel-blocker
DOSAGE: *Oral:* Initially, 30 mg PO qid; ↑ to 180–360 mg/d in 3–4 ÷ doses PRN. *SR:* 60–120 mg PO bid; ↑ to effect to max dose 360 mg/d. *CD:* 120–360 mg/d (max 480 mg/d). *IV:* 0.25 mg/kg IV bolus over 2 min; may repeat the dose in 15 min at 0.35 mg/kg. May begin cont inf of 5–15 mg/h
SUPPLIED: Tabs 30, 60, 90, 120 mg; SR caps 60, 90, 120 mg; CD caps 120, 180, 240, 300, 360 mg, 420 mg; inj 5 mg/mL
NOTES: Contra in sick sinus syndrome, AV block, and hypotension; Cardizem CD, Dilacor XR, and Tiazac not interchangeable

Dimenhydrinate (Dramamine, other)

COMMON USES: Prevention and Rx of nausea, vomiting, dizziness, or vertigo of motion sickness
ACTIONS: Antiemetic
DOSAGE: *Adults.* 50–100 mg PO q4–6h to a max of 400 mg/d; 50 mg IM/IV PRN. *Peds.* 5 mg/kg/24h PO or IV ÷ qid (max 300 mg/d)
SUPPLIED: Tabs 50 mg; chewable tabs 50 mg; liq 12.5 mg/4 mL, 12.5 mg/5 mL, 15.62 mg/5 mL; inj 50 mg/mL
NOTES: Anticholinergic side effects

Dimethyl Sulfoxide [DMSO] (Rimso-50)

COMMON USES: Interstitial cystitis
ACTIONS: Unknown
DOSAGE: Intravesical, 50 mL, retain for 15 min; repeat q 2 wk until relief
SUPPLIED: 50 % soln in 50 mL

Diphenhydramine (Benadryl, others)

COMMON USES: Allergic reactions, motion sickness, potentiate narcotics, sedation, cough suppression, and treatment of extrapyramidal reactions
ACTIONS: Antihistamine, antiemetic
DOSAGE: *Adults.* 25–50 mg PO, IV, or IM bid–tid. *Peds.* 5 mg/kg/24h PO or IM ÷ q6h (max 300 mg/d)
SUPPLIED: Tabs and caps 25, 50 mg; chewable tabs 12.5 mg; elixir 12.5 mg/5 mL; syrup 12.5 mg/5 mL; liq 6.25 mg/5 mL, 12.5 mg/5 mL; inj 50 mg/mL
NOTES: Anticholinergic side effects, including dry mouth and urinary retention; causes sedation; ↑ interval in moderate to severe renal failure

Diphenoxylate + Atropine (Lomotil) [C]

COMMON USES: Diarrhea
ACTIONS: Constipating meperidine congener
DOSAGE: *Adults.* Initially, 5 mg PO tid–qid until under control, then 2.5–5.0 mg PO bid. *Peds >2 y:* 0.3–0.4 mg/kg/24h (of diphenoxylate) ÷ bid–qid
SUPPLIED: Tabs 2.5 mg of diphenoxylate/0.025 mg of atropine; liq 2.5 mg diphenoxylate/0.025 mg atropine/5 mL
NOTES: Atropine-type side effects

Dipivefrin (Propine)

COMMON USES: Open-angle glaucoma
ACTIONS: α-Adrenergic agonist
DOSAGE: 1 gtt into eye q12h
SUPPLIED: 0.1% soln

Dirithromycin (Dynabac)

COMMON USES: Bronchitis, community-acquired pneumonia, and skin and skin structure infections

ACTIONS: Macrolide antibiotic

DOSAGE: 500 mg/d PO

SUPPLIED: Tabs 250 mg

NOTES: Absorption enhanced when taken with food

Disopyramide (Norpace, Napamide)

COMMON USES: Suppression and prevention PVC

ACTIONS: Class 1A antiarrhythmic

DOSAGE: *Adults.* 400–800 mg/d ÷ q6h for regular-release products and q12h for SR products. *Peds.* <1 y: 10–30 mg/kg/24h PO (÷ qid). *1–4 y:* 10–20 mg/kg/24h PO (÷ qid). *4–12 y:* 10–15 mg/kg/24h PO (÷ qid). *12–18 y:* 6–15 mg/kg/24h PO (÷ qid)

SUPPLIED: Caps 100, 150 mg; SR caps 100, 150 mg

NOTES: Anticholinergic side effects (urinary retention); negative inotropic properties may induce CHF; ↓ in impaired hepatic function and renal dysfunction. (See Table 22–7, pages 631–634, for levels.)

Dobutamine (Dobutrex)

Used for emergency cardiac care (see Chapter 21)

COMMON USES: Short-term use in cardiac decompensation secondary to depressed contractility

ACTIONS: Positive inotropic agent

DOSAGE: *Adults & Peds.* Cont IV inf of 2.5–15 µg/kg/min; rarely, 40 µg/kg/min may be required; titrate according to response

SUPPLIED: Inj 250 mg/20 mL

NOTES: Monitor ECG for ↑ heart rate, BP, and ectopic activity; monitor PWP and cardiac output if possible. (See also Table 20–10, page 637.)

Docetaxel (Taxotere)

COMMON USES: Breast (anthracycline-resistant), ovarian, and lung cancers

ACTIONS: Antimitotic agent; promotes microtubular aggregation; semisynthetic taxoid

DOSAGE: 100 mg/m² by 1-h IV infusion q 3 wk. Start dexamethasone 8 mg bid prior to docetaxel and continue for 3–4 d. (Refer to specific protocols.)

SUPPLIED: Inj 20, 40, 80 mg/mL

NOTES: *Toxicity symptoms:* Myelosuppression, neuropathy, and nausea and vomiting; fluid retention syndrome cumulative doses of 300–400 mg/m² without corticosteroid preparation and post-treatment and 600–800 mg/m² with corticosteroid preparation. Hypersensitivity reactions possible, but only rarely with corticosteroid preparation. ↓ Dose with ↑ bilirubin levels

Docusate Calcium (Surfak, others)/Docusate Potassium (Dialose)/Docusate Sodium (Doss, Colace, others)

COMMON USES: Constipation; adjunct to painful anorectal conditions (hemorrhoids)

ACTIONS: Stool softener

DOSAGE: *Adults.* 50–500 mg PO ÷ qd–qid. *Peds.* Infants–3 y: 10–40 mg/24h ÷ qd–qid. *3–6 y:* 20–60 mg/24h ÷ qd–qid. *6–12 y:* 40–150 mg/24h ÷ qd–qid

SUPPLIED: *Ca:* Caps 50, 240 mg. *K:* Caps 100, 240 mg. *Na:* Caps 50, 100 mg; syrup 50, 60 mg/15 mL; liq 150 mg/15 mL; soln 50 mg/mL

NOTES: No significant side effects; no laxative action

Dolasetron (Anzemet)

COMMON USES: Prevention of nausea and vomiting associated with chemotherapy

ACTIONS: 5-HT₃ receptor antagonists

DOSAGE: *Adults & Peds.* 1.8 mg/kg IV as a single dose 30 min prior to chemotherapy. *Adults.* 100 mg PO as a single dose. 1 h prior to chemotherapy. *Peds.* 1.8 mg/kg PO to max 100 mg as a single dose
SUPPLIED: Tabs 50, 100 mg; Inj 20 mg/mL
NOTES: May prolong QT interval

Dopamine (Intropin, Dopastat)

Used for emergency cardiac care (see Chapter 21)
COMMON USES: Short-term use in cardiac decompensation secondary to decreased contractility; increases organ perfusion
ACTIONS: Positive inotropic agent with dose-related response. 2–10 μg/kg/min β-effects (increases cardiac output and renal perfusion). 10–20 μg/kg/min α-effects (peripheral vasoconstriction, pressor). >20 μg/kg/min peripheral and renal vasoconstriction
DOSAGE: *Adults & Peds.* 5 μg/kg/min by cont inf, ↑ increments of 5 μg/kg/min to a max of 50 μg/kg/min based on effect
SUPPLIED: Inj 40, 80, 160 mg/mL
NOTES: Dosage >10 μg/kg/min may ↓ renal perfusion; monitor urinary output; monitor ECG for ↑ in heart rate, BP, and ectopic activity; monitor PCWP and cardiac output if possible. (See also Table 20–10, page 637.)

Dornase Alfa (Pulmozyme)

COMMON USES: ↓ Frequency of respiratory infections in patients with CF
ACTIONS: Enzyme that selectively cleaves DNA
DOSAGE: Inhal 2.5 mg/d
SUPPLIED: Soln for inhalation 1 mg/mL
NOTES: Use with recommended nebulizer

Dorzolamide (Trusopt)

COMMON USES: Glaucoma
ACTIONS: Carbonic anhydrase inhibitor
DOSAGE: 1 gtt in eye(s) tid
SUPPLIED: 2% soln

Dorzolamide and Timolol (Cosopt)

COMMON USES: Glaucoma
ACTIONS: Carbonic anhydrase inhibitor with β-adrenergic blocker
DOSAGE: 1 gtt in eye(s) bid
SUPPLIED: Soln dorzolamide 2% and timolol 0.5%

Doxazosin (Cardura)

COMMON USES: HTN and BPH
ACTIONS: α_1-Adrenergic blocker; relaxation of bladder neck smooth muscle fibers
DOSAGE: *HTN:* Initially 1 mg/d PO; may be ↑ to 16 mg/d PO. *BPH:* Initially 1 mg/d PO, may be ↑ to 8 mg/d PO
SUPPLIED: Tabs 1, 2, 4, 8 mg
NOTES: Doses >4 mg ↑ likelihood of excessive postural hypotension, asthenia, retrograde ejaculation

Doxepin (Sinequan, Adapin)

COMMON USES: Depression, anxiety, and chronic pain
ACTIONS: Tricyclic antidepressant; increases the synaptic concentrations of serotonin or norepinephrine in CNS
DOSAGE: 25–150 mg/d PO, usually hs, but can be in ÷ doses
SUPPLIED: Caps 10, 25, 50, 75, 100, 150 mg; oral conc 10 mg/mL
NOTES: Anticholinergic, CNS, and cardiovascular side effects

Doxepin Topical (Zonalon)

COMMON USES: Short-term Rx pruritus (atopic dermatitis or lichen simplex chronicus)
ACTIONS: Tricyclic antidepressant; increases synaptic concentrations of serotonin or norepinephrine
DOSAGE: Apply thin coating qid for max 8 d
SUPPLIED: 5% cream
NOTES: Apply to limited areas to avoid systemic toxicity (anticholinergic, CNS, and cardiovascular side effects)

Doxorubicin (Adriamycin, Rubex)

COMMON USES: Acute leukemias; Hodgkin's and non-Hodgkin's lymphomas; breast cancer; soft tissue and osteosarcomas; Ewing's sarcoma; Wilms' tumor; neuroblastoma; bladder, ovarian, gastric, thyroid, and lung cancers
ACTIONS: DNA intercalating agent; inhibitor of DNA topoisomerases I and II
DOSAGE: $60–75$ mg/m^2 q 3 wk; reduced cardiotoxicity with weekly (20 mg/m^2/wk) or cont inf ($60–90$ mg/m^2 over 96 h) schedules. (Refer to specific protocols)
SUPPLIED: Inj 10, 20, 50, 75, 200 mg
NOTES: *Toxicity symptoms:* Myelosuppression; extravasation leads to tissue damage; venous streaking and phlebitis, nausea and vomiting, diarrhea, mucositis, and radiation recall phenomenon. Cardiomyopathy rare but dose-related; limit of 550 mg/m^2 cumulative dose (400 mg/m^2 if prior history of mediastinal irradiation)

Doxycycline (Vibramycin)

COMMON USES: Broad-spectrum antibiotic, including activity against *Rickettsia* spp., *Chlamydia*, and *M. pneumoniae*
ACTIONS: Tetracycline; interferes with protein synthesis
DOSAGE: *Adults.* 100 mg PO q12h on 1st day, then 100 mg PO qd–bid or 100 mg IV q12h. *Peds >8 y.* 5 mg/kg/24h PO, to a max of 200 mg/d ÷ qd–bid
SUPPLIED: Tabs 50, 100 mg; caps 20, 50, 100 mg; syrup 50 mg/5 mL; susp 25 mg/5 mL; inj 100, 200 mg/vial
NOTES: Useful for chronic bronchitis; tetracycline of choice for patients with renal impairment

Dronabinol (Marinol) [C]

COMMON USES: Nausea and vomiting; appetite stimulation
ACTIONS: Antiemetic; inhibits the vomiting center in the medulla
DOSAGE: *Adults & Peds.* Antiemetic: 5–15 mg/m^2/dose q4–6h PRN. *Adults.* Appetite: 2.5 mg PO before lunch and dinner
SUPPLIED: Caps 2.5, 5, 10 mg
NOTES: Principal psychoactive substance present in marijuana; many CNS side effects

Droperidol (Inapsine)

COMMON USES: Nausea and vomiting; premedication for anesthesia
ACTIONS: Tranquilization, sedation, and antiemetic
DOSAGE: *Adults.* Nausea: 2.5–5 mg IV or IM q3–4h PRN. *Premed:* 2.5–10 mg IV, 30–60 min preop. *Peds.* Premed: 0.1–0.15 mg/kg/dose
SUPPLIED: Inj 2.5 mg/mL
NOTES: Drowsiness, moderate hypotension, and occasional tachycardia

Econazole (Spectazole)

COMMON USES: Most tinea, cutaneous *Candida*, and tinea versicolor infections
ACTIONS: Topical antifungal
DOSAGE: Apply to affected areas bid (qd for tinea versicolor) for 2–4 wk
SUPPLIED: Topical cream 1%

NOTES: Relief of symptoms and clinical improvement may be seen early in treatment, but carry out course of therapy to avoid recurrence

Echothiophate Iodine (Phospholine Ophthalmic)

COMMON USES: Glaucoma
ACTIONS: Cholinesterase inhibitor
DOSAGE: 1 gtt eye(s) bid with one dose hs
SUPPLIED: Powder to reconstitute 1.5 mg/0.03%; 3 mg/0.06%; 6.25 mg/0.125%; 12.5 mg/0.25%

Edrophonium (Tensilon)

COMMON USES: Diagnosis of MyG; acute myasthenic crisis; curare antagonist
ACTIONS: Anticholinesterase
DOSAGE: *Adults.* Test for MyG: 2 mg IV in 1 min; if tolerated, give 8 mg IV; a positive test is a brief increase in strength. *Peds.* Test for MyG: Total dose of 0.2 mg/kg. Give 0.04 mg/kg as a test dose. If no reaction occurs, give the remainder of the dose in 1-mg increments to max of 10 mg
SUPPLIED: Inj 10 mg/mL
NOTES: Can cause severe cholinergic effects; keep atropine available

Efavirenz (Sustiva)

COMMON USES: HIV infections
ACTIONS: Antiretroviral agent, nonnucleoside reverse transcriptase inhibitor
DOSAGE: *Adults.* 600 mg/d PO. *Peds.* Refer to product information for dosing chart
SUPPLIED: Caps 50, 100, 200 mg
NOTES: Take hs, may cause somnolence, vivid dreams, dizziness; may cause rash

Enalapril (Vasotec)

COMMON USES: HTN, CHF, and asymptomatic LVD
ACTIONS: ACE inhibitor
DOSAGE: *Adults.* 2.5–5 mg/d PO ↑ by effect to 10–40 mg/d as 1–2 ÷ doses, or 1.25 mg IV q6h. *Peds.* 0.05–0.08 mg/kg/dose PO q12–24h
SUPPLIED: Tabs 2.5, 5, 10, 20 mg; inj 1.25 mg/mL
NOTES: Initial dose can produce symptomatic hypotension, especially with concomitant diuretics; discontinue diuretic for 2–3 d prior to initiation if possible; monitor closely for ↑ in serum potassium; may cause a nonproductive cough

Enoxaparin (Lovenox)

COMMON USES: Prevention and Rx of DVT; Rx PE; unstable angina and non-Q-wave MI
ACTIONS: Low-molecular-weight heparin
DOSAGE: *Prevention:* 30 mg bid SC or 40 mg SC q24h. *DVT/PE:* 1 mg/kg SC q12h or 1.5 mg/kg SC q24h. *Angina:* 1 mg/kg SC q12h
SUPPLIED: Inj 10 mg/0.1 mL (30-, 40-, 60-, 80-, 100-mg syringes)
NOTES: Does not significantly affect bleeding time, platelet function, PT, or APTT

Entacapone (Comtan)

COMMON USES: Parkinson's disease
ACTION: Selective and reversible inhibitor of COMT
DOSAGE: 200 mg administered concurrently with each levodopa/carbidopa dose to a max of 8×/d
SUPPLIED: Tabs 200 mg

Ephedrine

COMMON USES: Acute bronchospasm, nasal congestion, hypotension, narcolepsy, enuresis, and MyG
ACTIONS: Sympathomimetic that stimulates both α- and β-receptors

DOSAGE: *Adults.* 25–50 mg IM or IV q 10 min to a max of 150 mg/d or 25–50 mg PO q3–4h PRN.
Peds. 0.2–0.3 mg/kg/dose IM or IV q4–6h PRN
SUPPLIED: Inj 25, 50 mg/mL; caps 25, 50 mg; syrup 11, 20 mg/5 mL

Epinephrine (Adrenalin, Sus-Phrine, others)

Used for emergency cardiac care (see Chapter 21)
COMMON USES: Cardiac arrest, anaphylactic reactions, and acute asthma
ACTIONS: β-Adrenergic agonist with some α-effects
DOSAGE: *Adults.* Emergency cardiac care: 0.5–1.0 mg (5–10 mL of 1:10,000) IV q 5 min to response. *Anaphylaxis:* 0.3–0.5 mL of 1:1000 dilution SC; may repeat q 10–15 min to a max of 1 mg/dose and 5 mg/d. *Asthma:* 0.3–0.5 mL of 1:1000 dilution SC. repeated at 20-min–4-h intervals or 1 inhal (met-dose) repeated in 1–2 min or susp 0.1–0.3 mL SC for extended effect. *Peds.* Emergency cardiac care: 0.1 mL/kg of 1:10,000 dilution IV q 3–5 min to response
SUPPLIED: Inj 1:1000, 1:2000, 1:10,000, 1:100,000; susp for inj 1:200; aerosol; soln for inhal
NOTES: Sus-Phrine offers sustained action. In acute cardiac settings, can be given via endotracheal tube if central line not available

Epoetin Alfa [Erythropoietin] (Epogen, Procrit)

COMMON USES: Anemia associated with CRF, zidovudine treatment in HIV-infected patients, and patients receiving cancer chemotherapy; reduction in transfusions associated with surgery
ACTIONS: Erythropoietin supplementation
DOSAGE: *Adults & Peds.* 50–150 U/kg 3×/wk; adjust the dose q 4–6 wk as needed. *Surgery:* 300 U/kg/d for 10 d prior to surgery
SUPPLIED: Inj 2000, 3000, 4000, 10,000, 20,000 U/mL
NOTES: May cause HTN, headache, tachycardia, nausea, and vomiting; store in refrigerator

Epoprostenol (Flolan)

COMMON USES: Pulmonary HTN
ACTIONS: Dilates the pulmonary and systemic arterial vascular beds; inhibits platelet aggregation
DOSAGE: 4 ng/kg/min IV cont inf; make dosage adjustments based on clinical status and package insert guidelines
SUPPLIED: Inj 0.5, 1.5 mg
NOTES: Availability through PBM

Eprosartan (Teveten)

COMMON USES: HTN
ACTIONS: Angiotensin II receptor antagonist
DOSAGE: 400–800 mg/d as single dose or bid
SUPPLIED: Tabs 400, 600 mg
NOTES: Avoid use during PRG

Eptifibatide (Integrilin)

COMMON USES: Acute coronary syndrome
ACTIONS: Glycoprotein IIb/IIIa inhibitor
DOSAGE: 180 µg/kg IV bolus, followed by 2 µg/kg/min cont inf
SUPPLIED: Inj 0.75, 2 mg/mL

Erythromycin (E-mycin, Ilosone, Erythrocin, others)

COMMON USES: Infections caused by group A streptococci (*S. pyrogenes*), α-hemolytic streptococci, and *Neisseria gonorrhoeae* infections in penicillin-allergic patients, *S. pneumoniae*, *M. pneumoniae*, and *Legionella* infections
ACTIONS: Bacteriostatic; interferes with protein synthesis
DOSAGE: *Adults.* 250–500 mg PO qid or 500 mg–1 g IV qid. *Peds.* 30–50 mg/kg/24h PO or IV ÷ q6h, to a max of 2 g/d

SUPPLIED: *Powder for inj as lactobionate and gluceptate salts:* 500 mg, 1 g; *Base:* Tabs 250, 333, 500 mg; caps 250 mg; *Estolate:* Tabs 500 mg; caps 250 mg; susp 125, 250 mg per 5 mL; *Stearate:* Tabs 250, 500 mg; *Ethylsuccinate:* Chewable tabs 200 mg; tabs 400 mg; susp 200, 400 mg/5 mL
NOTES: Frequent mild GI disturbances; estolate salt associated with cholestatic jaundice; erythromycin base not well absorbed from the GI tract; some forms better tolerated with respect to GI irritation; lactobionate salt contains benzyl alcohol, so use with caution in neonates; used as part of the Condon bowel prep

Erythromycin and Benzoyl Peroxide (Benzamycin)

COMMON USES: Topical control of acne vulgaris
ACTIONS: Macrolide antibiotic with keratolytic
DOSAGE: Apply bid (AM & PM)
SUPPLIED: Gel erythromycin 30 mg/benzoyl peroxide 50 mg/g

Erythromycin and Sulfisoxazole (Eryzole, Pediazole)

COMMON USES: Bacterial infections of the upper and lower respiratory tract; otitis media in children due to *H. influenzae;* other infections in penicillin-allergic patients
ACTIONS: Macrolide antibiotic with sulfonamide
DOSAGE: Based on erythromycin content. *Adults.* 400 mg erythromycin/1200 mg sulfisoxazole PO q6h. *Peds >2 mo.* 40–50 mg/kg/d of erythromycin PO ÷ tid–qid; max 2 g erythromycin or 6 g sulfisoxazole/d or estimated dose of 1.25 mL/kg/d ÷ tid–qid
SUPPLIED: Susp erythromycin ethylsuccinate 200 mg/sulfisoxazole 600 mg/5 mL

Erythromycin, Ophthalmic (Ilotycin Ophthalmic)

COMMON USES: Conjunctival infections
ACTIONS: Macrolide antibiotic
DOSAGE: Apply q6h
SUPPLIED: 0.5% Oint

Erythromycin, Topical (Akne-Mycin Topical, Del-Mycin Topical, Emgel Topical, Staticin Topical, others)

COMMON USES: Acne
ACTIONS: Macrolide antibiotic
DOSAGE: Wash and dry area, apply 2% product over area bid
SUPPLIED: Soln 1.5, 2%;gel; impregnated pads and swabs 2%

Esmolol (Brevibloc)

Used for emergency cardiac care (see Chapter 21)
COMMON USES: SVT and noncompensatory sinus tachycardia
ACTIONS: β-Adrenergic blocking agent; class II antiarrhythmic
DOSAGE: *Adults & Peds.* Initiate treatment with 500 μg/kg load over 1 min, then 50 μg/kg/min for 4 min; if inadequate response, repeat the loading dose and follow with maintenance infusion of 100 μg/kg/min for 4 min; continue the titration process by repeating the loading dose followed by incremental ↑ in the maintenance dose of 50 μg/kg/min for 4 min until the desired heart rate is reached or BP decreases ; average dose 100 μg/kg/min
SUPPLIED: Inj 10, 250 mg/mL
NOTES: Monitor closely for hypotension; ↓ or discontinuing infusion reverses hypotension in ≅30 min

Estazolam (Prosom) [C]

COMMON USES: Insomnia
ACTIONS: Benzodiazepine
DOSAGE: 1–2 mg PO hs PRN
SUPPLIED: Tabs 1, 2 mg

Esterified Estrogens (Estratab, Menest)

COMMON USES: Vasomotor symptoms, atrophic vaginitis, or kraurosis vulvae associated with menopause; female hypogonadism
ACTIONS: Estrogen supplementation
DOSAGE: *Menopause:* 0.3–1.25 mg/d, administered cyclically 3 wk on and 1 wk off. *Hypogonadism:* 2.5 mg PO qd–tid
SUPPLIED: Tabs 0.3, 0.625, 1.25, 2.5 mg

Esterified Estrogens + Methyltestosterone (Estratest)

COMMON USES: Moderate to severe vasomotor symptoms associated with menopause; postpartum breast engorgement
ACTIONS: Estrogen and androgen supplementation
DOSAGE: 1 tab/d for 3 wk, then 1 wk off
SUPPLIED: Tabs (estrogen/methyltestosterone) 0.625 mg/1.25 mg, 1.25 mg/2.5 mg

Estradiol, (Estrace)

COMMON USES: Atrophic vaginitis and kraurosis vulvae associated with menopause, vasomotor symptoms
ACTIONS: Estrogen supplementation
DOSAGE: *Oral:* 1–2 mg/d, adjust dose as necessary to control symptoms. *Vaginal cream:* 2–4 g/d for 2 wk, then 1 g 1–3×/wk
SUPPLIED: Tabs 0.5, 1, 2 mg; vaginal cream

Estradiol, Transdermal (Estraderm, others)

COMMON USES: Severe vasomotor symptoms associated with menopause; female hypogonadism
ACTIONS: Estrogen supplementation
DOSAGE: 0.1 mg/d patch 1–2×/wk depending on product; adjust dose as necessary to control symptoms
SUPPLIED: TD patches (delivers mg/24h) 0.025, 0.0375, 0.05, 0.075, 0.1

Estramustine Phosphate (Estracyte, Emcyt)

COMMON USES: Advanced prostate cancer
ACTIONS: Antimicrotubule agent; weak estrogenic and antiandrogenic activity
DOSAGE: 14 mg/kg/d in 3–4 ÷ doses
SUPPLIED: Caps 140 mg
NOTES: *Toxicity symptoms:* Nausea and vomiting, exacerbation of preexisting CHF, gynecomastia in 20–100%

Estrogen, Conjugated (Premarin)

COMMON USES: Moderate to severe vasomotor symptoms associated with menopause; atrophic vaginitis; palliative therapy of advanced prostatic carcinoma; prevention of estrogen deficiency-induced osteoporosis
ACTIONS: Hormonal replacement
DOSAGE: 0.3–1.25 mg/d PO cyclically; prostatic carcinoma requires 1.25–2.5 mg PO tid
SUPPLIED: Tabs 0.3, 0.625, 0.9, 1.25, 2.5 mg; inj 25 mg/mL
NOTES: Do NOT use in PRG; associated with an increased risk of endometrial carcinoma, gallbladder disease, thromboembolism, and possibly breast cancer; generic products not equivalent

Estrogen, Conjugated + Methylprogesterone (Premarin + Methylprogesterone)

COMMON USES: Vasomotor symptoms associated with menopause
ACTIONS: Estrogen and androgen combination
DOSAGE: 1 tab/d
SUPPLIED: Tabs containing 0.625 mg of estrogen, conjugated, and 5 mg of methylprogesterone

Estrogen, Conjugated + Methyltestosterone (Premarin + Methyltestosterone)

COMMON USES: Moderate to severe vasomotor symptoms associated with menopause; postpartum breast engorgement
ACTIONS: Estrogen and androgen combination
DOSAGE: 1 tab/d for 3 wk, then 1 wk off
SUPPLIED: Tabs (estrogen/methyltestosterone) 0.625 mg/5 mg, 1.25 mg/10 mg

Ethacrynic Acid (Edecrin)

COMMON USES: Edema, CHF, and ascites; any time rapid diuresis is desired
ACTIONS: Loop diuretic; inhibits reabsorption of sodium and chlorine in the ascending loop of Henle and the distal renal tubule
DOSAGE: *Adults.* 50–200 mg PO qd or 50 mg IV PRN. *Peds.* 1 mg/kg/dose IV. Repeated doses NOT recommended
SUPPLIED: Tabs 25, 50 mg; powder for inj 50 mg
NOTES: Contra in anuria; severe side effects reported

Ethambutol (Myambutol)

COMMON USES: Pulmonary TB and other mycobacterial infections
ACTIONS: Inhibits cellular metabolism
DOSAGE: *Adults & Peds >12 y.* 15–25 mg/kg/d PO as a single dose
SUPPLIED: Tabs 100, 400 mg
NOTES: May cause vision changes and GI upset

Ethinyl Estradiol (Estinyl, Feminone)

COMMON USES: Vasomotor symptoms associated with menopause; female hypogonadism
ACTIONS: Estrogen supplementation
DOSAGE: 0.02–1.5 mg/d ÷ qd–tid
SUPPLIED: Tabs 0.02, 0.05, 0.5 mg

Ethosuximide (Zarontin)

COMMON USES: Seizures
ACTIONS: Anticonvulsant; increases the seizure threshold
DOSAGE: *Adults.* Initially, 500 mg PO ÷ bid; ↑ by 250 mg/d q 4–7 d PRN (max 1500 mg/d) *Peds.* 20–40 mg/kg/24h PO ÷ bid to a max of 1500 mg/d
SUPPLIED: Caps 250 mg; syrup 250 mg/5 mL
NOTES: Blood dyscrasias as well as CNS and GI side effects may occur; use caution in renal or hepatic impairment. (See Table 27–7, pages 631–634, for levels.)

Etidronate Disodium (Didronel)

COMMON USES: Hypercalcemia of malignancy and hypertropic ossification
ACTIONS: Inhibition of normal and abnormal bone resorption
DOSAGE: 5–20 mg/kg/d, may be given in ÷ doses. (Duration of therapy 3–6 mo) 7.5 mg/kg/d IV infusion over 2 h
SUPPLIED: Tabs 200, 400 mg; inj 50 mg/mL
NOTES: GI intolerance may be ↓ by ÷ oral daily doses

Etodolac (Lodine)

COMMON USES: Arthritis and pain
ACTIONS: NSAID
DOSAGE: 200–400 mg PO bid–qid (max 1200 mg/d)
SUPPLIED: Tabs 400, 500 mg; ER tabs 400, 500, 600 mg; caps 200, 300 mg

22

Etoposide [VP-16] (Vepesid)

COMMON USES: Testicular cancer, non-small-cell lung cancers, Hodgkin's and non-Hodgkin's lymphomas, pediatric ALL, and allogeneic and autologous BMT in high doses
ACTIONS: Topoisomerase II inhibitor
DOSAGE: 50 mg/m^2/d IV for 3–5 d; 50 mg/m^2/d PO for 21 d (bioavailability of the oral formulation ≈50% of the IV form); 2–6 g/m^2 or 25–70 mg/kg used in BMT. (Refer to specific protocols)
SUPPLIED: Caps 50 mg; inj 20 mg/mL
NOTES: *Toxicity symptoms:* Myelosuppression, nausea and vomiting, and alopecia; hypotension may occur if infused too rapidly; anaphylaxis or lesser hypersensitivity reactions (wheezing) rare; potential for secondary leukemias

Famciclovir (Famvir)

COMMON USES: Acute herpes zoster (shingles) and genital herpes infections
ACTIONS: Inhibits viral DNA synthesis
DOSAGE: *Zoster:* 500 mg PO q8h. *Simplex:* 125–250 mg PO bid
SUPPLIED: Tabs 125, 250, 500 mg

Famotidine (Pepcid)

COMMON USES: Short-term Rx of active duodenal ulcer and benign gastric ulcer; maintenance therapy for duodenal ulcer, hypersecretory conditions, GERD, and heartburn
ACTIONS: H$_2$-antagonist; inhibits gastric acid secretion
DOSAGE: *Adults.* Ulcer: 20–40 mg PO hs or 20 mg IV q12h. *Hypersecretion:* 20–160 mg PO q6h. *GERD:* 20 mg PO bid; maintenance 20 mg PO hs. *Heartburn:* 10 mg PO PRN heartburn; *Peds.* 1–2 mg/kg/d
SUPPLIED: Tabs 10, 20, 40 mg; chewable tabs 10 mg; susp 40 mg/5 mL; inj 10 mg/mL
NOTES: ↓ Dose in severe renal insufficiency

Felodipine (Plendil)

COMMON USES: HTN and CHF
ACTIONS: Ca channel-blocker
DOSAGE: 5–20 mg PO qd
SUPPLIED: ER tabs 2.5, 5, 10 mg
NOTES: Closely monitor BP in elderly and in impaired hepatic function; do NOT use doses >10 mg in these patients; bioavailability is ↑ when administered with grapefruit juice

Fenofibrate (Tricor)

COMMON USES: Hypertriglyceridemia
ACTIONS: Inhibits triglyceride synthesis
DOSAGE: Initially 67 mg/d, ↑ to 67 mg tid or 200 mg/d
SUPPLIED: Caps 67, 200 mg
NOTES: Take with meals to increase bioavailability; May cause cholecystitis; monitor LFTs

Fenoldopam (Corlopam)

COMMON USES: Hypertensive emergency
ACTIONS: Rapid acting vasodilator
DOSAGE: Initial dose 0.03–0.1 µg/kg/min IV cont inf, titrate to effect q 15 min with 0.05–0.1 µg/kg/min increments
SUPPLIED: Inj 10 mg/mL
NOTES: Avoid concurrent use with β-blockers

Fenoprofen (Nalfon)

COMMON USES: Arthritis and pain
ACTIONS: NSAID

DOSAGE: 200–600 mg q4–8h, to a max of 3200 mg/d
SUPPLIED: Caps 200, 300 mg; tabs 600 mg

Fentanyl (Sublimaze) [C-II]

COMMON USES: Short-acting analgesic used in conjunction with anesthesia
ACTIONS: Narcotic
DOSAGE: *Adults & Peds.* 0.025–0.15 mg/kg IV/IM titrated to effect
SUPPLIED: Inj 0.05 mg/mL
NOTES: Causes significant sedation; 0.1 mg of fentanyl = 10 mg of morphine IM

Fentanyl, Transdermal (Duragesic) [C-II]

COMMON USES: Chronic pain
ACTIONS: Narcotic
DOSAGE: Apply a patch to the upper torso q72h. Dose calculated from the narcotic requirements for the previous 24 h
SUPPLIED: TD patches deliver 25, 50, 75, 100 µg/h
NOTES: 0.1 mg of fentanyl = 10 mg of morphine IM

Fentanyl, Transmucosal System (Actiq, Fentanyl Oralet) [C-II]

COMMON USES: Induction of anesthesia and breakthrough cancer pain
ACTIONS: Narcotic
DOSAGE: *Adults & Peds.* Anesthesia: 5–15 µg/kg. *Pain:* 200 µg consumed over 15 min, titrate to appropriate effect
SUPPLIED: Lozenges 100, 200, 300, 400 µg; lozenges on stick 200, 400, 600, 800, 1200, 1600 µg

Ferric Gluconate Complex (Ferrlecit)

COMMON USES: Iron deficiency in patients receiving supplemental erythropoietin therapy
ACTIONS: Supplemental iron
DOSAGE: Give test dose of 2 mL (25 mg Fe) infused over 1 h. If no reaction, 125 mg (10 mL) IV over 1 h until favorable hematocrit achieved. Usual cumulative dose 1 g Fe administered over 8 sessions
SUPPLIED: Inj 12.5 mg/mL Fe
NOTES: Dosage is expressed as mg Fe; may be infused during dialysis

Ferrous Gluconate (Fergon, others)

COMMON USES: Fe deficiency anemia and Fe supplementation
ACTIONS: Dietary supplementation
DOSAGE: *Adults.* 100–200 mg Fe/d
SUPPLIED: Tabs 240 (27 mg Fe), 325 mg (36 mg Fe)
NOTES: 12% Fe; may turn stool and urine dark

Ferrous Sulfate

COMMON USES: Fe deficiency anemia and Fe supplementation
ACTIONS: Dietary supplementation
DOSAGE: *Adults.* 300 mg PO bid–tid. *Peds.* 1–4 mg/kg/24h ÷ qd–bid
SUPPLIED: Tabs 187, 200, 324 mg; SR caplets and tabs 160 mg; gtt 75 mg/0.6 mL; elixir 220 mg/5 mL; syrup 90 mg/5 mL
NOTES: May turn stools and urine dark; can cause GI upset and constipation; vitamin C taken with ferrous sulfate ↑ absorption of Fe, especially in patients with atrophic gastritis

Fexofenadine (Allegra)

COMMON USES: Relief of allergic rhinitis
ACTIONS: Antihistamine

DOSAGE: *Adults & Peds >12 y.* 60 mg bid or 180 mg/d
SUPPLIED: Caps 60 mg, 180 mg tabs; also available in combination with pseudoephedrine (60 mg fexoferadine/120 mg pseudoephedrine)

Filgrastim [G-CSF] (Neupogen)

COMMON USES: Decrease incidence of infection in febrile neutropenic patients, and Rx chronic neutropenia
ACTIONS: Recombinant G-CSF
DOSAGE: *Adults & Peds.* 5 µg/kg/d SC or IV as a single daily dose
SUPPLIED: Inj 300 µg/mL
NOTES: May cause bone pain. Discontinue therapy when ANC >10,000

Finasteride (Proscar, Propecia)

COMMON USES: BPH and androgenetic alopecia
ACTIONS: Inhibits 5α reductase
DOSAGE: *BPH:* 5 mg/d PO [Proscar]. *Alopecia:* 1 mg/d PO [Propecia]
SUPPLIED: Tabs 1, 5 mg
NOTES: Decreases PSA levels; may take 3–6 mo to see effect on urinary symptoms

Flavoxate (Urispas)

COMMON USES: Symptomatic relief of dysuria, urgency, nocturia, suprapubic pain, urinary frequency, and incontinence
ACTIONS: Counteracts smooth muscle spasm of the urinary tract
DOSAGE: 100–200 mg PO tid–qid
SUPPLIED: Tabs 100 mg
NOTES: May cause drowsiness, blurred vision, and dry mouth

Flecainide (Tambocor)

COMMON USES: Prevention of PAF/flutter and PSVT, Rx life-threatening ventricular arrhythmias
ACTIONS: Class 1C antiarrhythmic
DOSAGE: *Adults.* 100 mg PO q12h; ↑ in increments of 50 mg q12h q 4 d to a max of 400 mg/d. *Peds.* 3–6 mg/kg/d in 3 ÷ doses
SUPPLIED: Tabs 50, 100, 150 mg
NOTES: May cause new or worsened arrhythmias; therapy should be initiated in the hospital; may dose q8h if the patient is intolerant or uncontrolled at 12-h intervals; drug interactions with propranolol, digoxin, verapamil, and disopyramide; may cause CHF

Floxuridine (FUDR)

COMMON USES: Colon carcinoma, pancreatic carcinoma, liver cancer, biliary tract cancers, and adenocarcinoma of the GI tract metastatic to the liver
ACTIONS: Inhibitor of thymidylate synthase; interferes with DNA synthesis (S phase-specific)
DOSAGE: 0.1–0.6 mg/kg/d for 1–6 wk
SUPPLIED: Inj 500 mg
NOTES: *Toxicity symptoms:* Myelosuppression, nausea and vomiting, anorexia, abdominal cramps, diarrhea, mucositis, alopecia, skin rash, and hyperpigmentation; rare neurotoxicity (blurred vision, depression, nystagmus, vertigo, and lethargy). Intraarterial catheter-related problems (ischemia, thrombosis, bleeding, and infection)

Fluconazole (Diflucan)

COMMON USES: Oropharyngeal and esophageal candidiasis; cryptococcal meningitis; *Candida* infections of the lungs, peritoneum, and urinary tract; prevention of candidiasis in BMT patients on chemotherapy or radiation; and candidal vaginitis
ACTIONS: Antifungal; inhibits fungal cytochrome P-450 sterol demethylation

DOSAGE: *Adults.* 100–400 mg/d PO or IV. *Vaginitis:* 150 mg PO as a single dose. *Peds.* 3–6 mg/kg/d PO or IV
SUPPLIED: Tabs 50, 100, 150, 200 mg; susp 10, 40 mg/mL; inj 2 mg/mL
NOTES: Adjust dose in renal insufficiency; oral dosing produces the same blood levels as IV dosing, so use oral route whenever possible

Fludarabine Phosphate (Fludara)

COMMON USES: CLL, low-grade lymphoma, and mycosis fungoides
ACTIONS: Inhibits ribonucleotide reductase; blocks DNA polymerase-induced DNA repair
DOSAGE: 18–30 mg/m^2/d for 5 d, given as a 30-min inf (Refer to specific protocols)
SUPPLIED: Inj 50 mg
NOTES: *Toxicity symptoms:* Myelosuppression, nausea and vomiting, diarrhea, and hepatic transaminase elevations; severe CNS toxicity rare in leukemic patients and pulmonary toxicity

Fludrocortisone Acetate (Florinef)

COMMON USES: Partial treatment for adrenocortical insufficiency
ACTIONS: Mineralocorticoid replacement
DOSAGE: *Adults.* 0.05–0.2 mg/d PO. *Peds.* 0.05–0.1 mg/d PO
SUPPLIED: Tabs 0.1 mg
NOTES: For adrenal insufficiency, must be used in conjunction with a glucocorticoid supplement; dosage changes based on plasma renin activity

Flumazenil (Romazicon)

Used for emergency (see Chapter 21)
COMMON USES: For complete or partial reversal of the sedative effects of benzodiazepines (diazepam, etc)
ACTIONS: Benzodiazepine receptor antagonist
DOSAGE: *Adults.* 0.2 mg IV over 15 s; dose may be repeated if the desired level of consciousness is not obtained, to a max dose of 1 mg. *Peds.* 0.01 mg/kg to a max of 0.2 mg IV over 15 s. Repeat doses 0.005 mg/kg at 1-min intervals
SUPPLIED: Inj 0.1 mg/mL
NOTES: Does NOT reverse narcotics

Flunisolide (Aerobid, Nasalide)

COMMON USES: Control of bronchial asthma in patients requiring chronic corticosteroid therapy; relief of seasonal or perennial allergic rhinitis
ACTIONS: Topical steroid
DOSAGE: *Adults.* 2–4 inhal bid. *Nasal:* 2 sprays/nostril bid. *Peds >6 y.* 2 inhal bid. *Nasal:* 1–2 sprays/nostril bid
SUPPLIED: Met-dose aerosol 250 mg; nasal spray 0.025%
NOTES: May cause oral candidiasis; NOT for acute asthma attack

Fluorouracil [5-FU] (Adrucil)

COMMON USES: Colorectal, bladder, gastric, pancreatic, anal, head and neck, and breast cancers; topical application for basal cell carcinoma of the skin
ACTIONS: Inhibitor of thymidylate synthetase (interferes with DNA synthesis, S phase-specific)
DOSAGE: 370–1000 mg/m^2/d for 1–5 d; intravenously as IV push to 24-h cont inf; protracted venous infusion of 200–300 mg/m^2/d. (See specific protocols.)
SUPPLIED: Inj 50 mg/mL
NOTES: *Toxicity symptoms:* Stomatitis, esophagopharyngitis, diarrhea, anorexia, and nausea and vomiting. Myelosuppression (leukocytopenia, thrombocytopenia, and anemia); rash, dry skin, and photosensitivity frequent. Tingling in the hands and feet followed by pain (palmar-plantar erythrodysesthesia); phlebitis and discoloration at inj sites

Fluorouracil, Topical [5-FU] (Efudex)

COMMON USES: Basal cell carcinoma of the skin, actinic and solar keratosis
ACTIONS: Inhibitor of thymidylate synthetase (interferes with DNA synthesis, S phase-specific)
DOSAGE: Apply 5% cream bid for 4–6 wk
SUPPLIED: Cream 1, 5%; soln 1, 2, 5%
NOTES: Toxicity symptoms: Rash, dry skin, and photosensitivity

Fluoxetine (Prozac, Sarafem)

COMMON USES: Depression, OCD, bulimia, PMDD
ACTIONS: SSRI
DOSAGE: Initially, 20 mg/d PO; ↑to a max of 80 mg/24h; ÷ doses of >20 mg/d. *Bulimia:* 60 mg/d in AM. *PMDD:* 20 mg/d
SUPPLIED: Caps 10, 20 mg; tabs 10 mg; soln 20 mg/5 mL
NOTES: May cause nausea, nervousness, and weight loss; hepatic failure dosage adjustment

Fluoxymesterone (Halotestin)

COMMON USES: Androgen-responsive metastatic breast cancer
ACTIONS: Inhibition of secretion of LH and FSH by feedback inhibition
DOSAGE: 10–40 mg/d
SUPPLIED: Tabs 2, 5, 10 mg
NOTES: *Toxicity symptoms:* Virilization, amenorrhea and menstrual irregularities, hirsutism, alopecia and acne, nausea, and cholestasis. *Hematologic toxicity symptoms:* Suppression of clotting factors II, V, VII, and X and polycythemia. ↑ libido, headache, and anxiety

Fluphenazine (Prolixin, Permitil)

COMMON USES: Psychotic disorders
ACTIONS: Phenothiazine antipsychotic; blocks postsynaptic mesolimbic dopaminergic receptors in the brain
DOSAGE: 0.5–10 mg/d in ÷ doses PO q6–8h; average maintenance 5.0 mg/d or 1.25 mg IM initially, then 2.5–10 mg/d in ÷ doses q6–8h PRN
SUPPLIED: Tabs 1, 2.5, 5, 10; conc 5 mg/mL; elixir 2.5 mg/5 mL; inj 2.5 mg/mL; depot inj 25 mg/mL
NOTES: ↓ Dose in elderly; monitor LFT; may cause drowsiness; do NOT administer conc with caffeine, tannic acid, or pectin-containing products

Flurazepam (Dalmane) [C]

COMMON USES: Insomnia
ACTIONS: Benzodiazepine
DOSAGE: *Adults & Peds >15 y.* 15–30 mg PO hs PRN
SUPPLIED: Caps 15, 30 mg
NOTES: ↓ Dose in elderly

Flurbiprofen (Ansaid)

COMMON USES: Arthritis
ACTIONS: NSAID
DOSAGE: 50–100 mg bid–qid, to a max of 300 mg/d
SUPPLIED: Tabs 50, 100 mg

Flutamide (Eulexin)

COMMON USES: Advanced prostate cancer (in combination with GnRH agonists, eg, leuprolide or goserelin) with or without radiation for localized prostate cancer
ACTIONS: Nonsteroidal antiandrogen
DOSAGE: 250 mg PO tid (750 mg total)
SUPPLIED: Caps 125 mg

NOTES: *Toxicity symptoms:* Hot flashes, loss of libido, impotence, diarrhea, nausea and vomiting, and gynecomastia; follow LFT

Fluticasone Nasal (Flonase)

COMMON USES: Seasonal allergic rhinitis
ACTIONS: Topical steroid
DOSAGE: *Adults & adolescents.* 100–250 µg bid. *Nasal:* 1–2 sprays/nostril/d. *Peds 4–11 y.* 50 µg bid. *Nasal:* 1–2 sprays/nostril/d
SUPPLIED: Nasal spray 50 µg/actuation

Fluticasone Oral (Flovent, Flovent Rotadisk)

COMMON USES: Chronic treatment of asthma
ACTIONS: Topical steroid
DOSAGE: *Adults & adolescents.* 2–4 puffs bid. *Peds 4–11 y.* 50 µg bid
SUPPLIED: Multidose inhaler 44, 110, or 220 µg/activation; Rotadisk dry powder 50, 100, and 250 µg/activation; risk of thrush
NOTES: Counsel patients carefully on use of device

Fluvastatin (Lescol)

COMMON USES: Adjunct to diet in the treatment of elevated total cholesterol
ACTIONS: HMG-CoA reductase inhibitor
DOSAGE: 20–40 mg PO hs, may be ↑ to 80 mg/d
SUPPLIED: Caps 20, 40 mg
NOTES: Avoid concurrent use with gemfibrozil

Fluvoxamine (Luvox)

COMMON USES: OCD
ACTIONS: SSRI
DOSAGE: Initial 50 mg as single hs dose, may be ↑ to 300 mg/d in ÷ doses
SUPPLIED: Tabs 25, 50, 100 mg
NOTES: ÷ doses of >100 mg; numerous drug interactions

Folic Acid

COMMON USES: Megaloblastic anemia
ACTIONS: Dietary supplementation
DOSAGE: *Adults.* Supplement: 0.4 mg/d PO. *PRG:* 0.8 mg/d PO. *Folate deficiency:* 1.0 mg PO qd–tid. *Peds.* Supplement: 0.04–0.4 mg/24h PO, IM, IV, or SC. *Folate deficiency:* 0.5–1.0 mg/24h PO, IM, IV, or SC
SUPPLIED: Tabs 0.1, 0.4, 0.8, 1.0 mg; inj 5 mg/mL
NOTES: Recommended for all women of childbearing age; ↓ incidence of fetal neural tube defects by 50%

Foscarnet (Foscavir)

COMMON USES: CMV; acyclovir-resistant herpes infections
ACTIONS: Inhibits viral DNA polymerase and reverse transcriptase
DOSAGE: *Induction:* 60 mg/kg IV q8h for 14–21 d. *Maintenance:* 90–120 mg/kg/d IV (Monday–Friday)
SUPPLIED: Inj 24 mg/mL
NOTES: Dosage must be adjusted for renal function; nephrotoxic; monitor ionized calcium closely (causes electrolyte abnormalities); administer through a central line

Fosfomycin (Monurol)

COMMON USES: Uncomplicated UTI
ACTIONS: Inhibits bacterial cell wall synthesis

DOSAGE: 3 g PO dissolved in 90–120 mL of water as single dose
SUPPLIED: Granule packets 3 g
NOTES: May take 2–3 d for symptoms to improve

Fosinopril (Monopril)

COMMON USES: HTN and heart failure
ACTIONS: ACE inhibitor
DOSAGE: Initially, 10 mg/d PO; may be ↑ to a max of 80 mg/d PO ÷ qd–bid
SUPPLIED: Tabs 10, 20, 40 mg
NOTES: ↓ Dose in elderly; may cause nonproductive cough and dizziness

Fosphenytoin (Cerebyx)

COMMON USES: Status epilepticus
ACTION: Inhibits seizure spread in the motor cortex
DOSAGE: Dosed as phenytoin equivalents (PE) Loading 15–20 mg PE/kg, maintenance 4–6 mg PE/kg/d
SUPPLIED: Inj; 150 mg (= phenytoin 100 mg); 750 mg (= phenytoin 500 mg)
NOTES: Requires 15 min to convert the prodrug fosphenytoin to phenytoin; administer at <150 mg PE/min to prevent hypotension; administer with BP monitoring; dosage adjustment/plasma monitoring may be necessary in hepatic impairment

Furosemide (Lasix)

Used for emergency cardiac care (see Chapter 21)
COMMON USES: Edema, HTN, and CHF
ACTIONS: Loop diuretic; inhibits Na and Cl reabsorption in the ascending loop of Henle and the distal renal tubule
DOSAGE: *Adults.* 20–80 mg PO or IV qd–bid. *Peds.* 1 mg/kg/dose IV q6–12h; 2 mg/kg/dose PO q12h–24h
SUPPLIED: Tabs 20, 40, 80 mg; soln 10 mg/mL, 40 mg/5 mL; inj 10 mg/mL
NOTES: Monitor for hypokalemia; use with caution in hepatic disease; high doses of the IV form may cause ototoxicity

Gabapentin (Neurontin)

COMMON USES: Adjunctive therapy in the treatment of partial seizures
ACTIONS: Anticonvulsant
DOSAGE: 900–1800 mg/d PO in 3 ÷ doses
SUPPLIED: Caps 100, 300, 400 mg
NOTES: Not necessary to monitor serum gabapentin levels; dosage adjustment in renal impairment

Gallium Nitrate (Ganite)

COMMON USES: Hypercalcemia of malignancy; bladder cancer
ACTIONS: Inhibits resorption of Ca from the bones
DOSAGE: *Hypercalcemia:* 10–200 mg/m^2/d for 5 d. *Cancer:* 350 mg/m^2 cont inf for 5 d to 700 mg/m^2 rapid IV inf q 2 wk in antineoplastic settings
SUPPLIED: Inj 25 mg/mL
NOTES: Can cause renal insufficiency; may cause hypocalcemia, hypophosphatemia, and decreased bicarbonate; <1% of patients developed acute optic neuritis; for bladder cancer, use in combination with vinblastine and ifosfamide

Ganciclovir (Cytovene, Vitrasert)

COMMON USES: Rx and prevention of CMV retinitis and prevention of CMV disease in transplant recipients
ACTIONS: Inhibits viral DNA synthesis

DOSAGE: *Adults & Peds.* IV: 5 mg/kg IV q12h for 14–21 d, then maintenance of 5 mg/kg/d IV for 7 d/wk or 6 mg/kg/d IV for 5 d/wk. *Ocular implant:* One implant q 5–8 mo. *Adults.* PO: Following induction, 1000 mg PO tid. *Prevention:* 1000 mg PO tid
SUPPLIED: Caps 250, 500 mg; inj 500 mg; ocular implant 4.5 mg
NOTES: NOT a cure for CMV; granulocytopenia and thrombocytopenia are major toxicities; injection should be handled with cytotoxic precautions; take caps with food; implant confers no systemic benefit; dosage adjustment in renal impairment

Gatifloxacin (Tequin)

COMMON USES: Acute exacerbation of chronic bronchitis, sinusitis, community acquired pneumonia, UTI
ACTIONS: Quinolone antibiotic, inhibits DNA-gyrase
DOSAGE: 400 mg/d PO or IV
SUPPLIED: Tabs 200, 400 mg; inj
NOTES: Avoid use with antacids; do NOT use in children <18 y, pregnant or lactating women; reliable activity against *S. pneumoniae;* dosage adjustment in renal impairment

Gemcitabine (Gemzar)

COMMON USES: Pancreatic cancer, gastric cancer, and lung cancer
ACTIONS: Antimetabolite; inhibits ribonucleotide reductase; produces false nucleotide base-inhibiting DNA synthesis
DOSAGE: 1000 mg/m^2 as a 1-h IV inf weekly for 3–4 wk or 6–8 wk
SUPPLIED: Inj 20 mg/mL
NOTES: *Toxicity symptoms:* Myelosuppression, nausea and vomiting, diarrhea, drug fever, and skin rash

Gemfibrozil (Lopid)

COMMON USES: Hypertriglyceridemia, and reduction of CHD risk
ACTIONS: Lipid-regulating agent
DOSAGE: 1200 mg/d PO in 2 ÷ doses 30 min ac AM and PM
SUPPLIED: Tabs 600 mg; caps 300 mg
NOTES: Monitor AST, ALT, LDH, alkaline phosphatase, and serum lipids during therapy; cholelithiasis may occur secondary to treatment; may enhance the effect of warfarin; avoid concurrent use with the HMG-CoA reductase inhibitors

Gentamicin (Garamycin, others)

COMMON USES: Serious infections caused by susceptible *Pseudomonas, Proteus, E. coli, Klebsiella, Enterobacter,* and *Serratia,* and for initial treatment of gram (−) sepsis
ACTIONS: Bactericidal; inhibits protein synthesis
DOSAGE: See also Aminoglycoside dosing (page 620). *Adults.* 3–5 mg/kg/24h IV ÷ q8–24h. *Peds. Infants <7 d <1200 g:* 2.5 mg/kg/dose q18–24h. *>1200 g:* 2.5 mg/kg/dose q12–18h. *Infants >7 d:* 2.5 mg/kg/dose IV q8–12h. *Children:* 2.5 mg/kg/d IV q8h
SUPPLIED: Inj 10, 40 mg/mL, IT preservative-free 2 mg/mL
NOTES: Nephrotoxic and ototoxic; ↓ dose with renal insufficiency; monitor CrCl and serum concentration for dosage adjustments (see Table 22–7, pages 631–634). Daily dosing becoming popular

Gentamicin, Ophthalmic (Garamycin, Genoptic, Gentacidin, others)

COMMON USES: Conjunctival infections
ACTIONS: Bactericidal; inhibits protein synthesis
DOSAGE: Oint apply bid or tid; soln: 1–2 gtt q2–4h, up to 2 gtt/h for severe infections
SUPPLIED: Soln and oint 0.3%

22

Gentamicin, Topical (Garamycin, G-Myticin)

COMMON USES: Skin infections caused by susceptible organisms
ACTIONS: Bactericidal; inhibits protein synthesis
DOSAGE: *Adult and Peds >1 y.* Apply tid–qid
SUPPLIED: Cream; oint; soln 0.3%

Gentamicin and Prednisolone, Ophthalmic (Pred-G Ophthalmic)

COMMON USES: Steroid-responsive ocular and conjunctival infections sensitive to gentamicin (eg, *Staphylococcus, E. coli, H. influenzae, Klebsiella, Neisseria, Pseudomonas, Proteus,* and *Serratia* spp)
ACTIONS: Bactericidal; inhibits protein synthesis
DOSAGE: Oint apply bid or tid; Soln: 1–2 gtt q2–4h, up to 2 gtt/h for severe infections
SUPPLIED: Oint, ophth: Prednisolone acetate 0.6% and gentamicin sulfate 0.3% (3.5 g); Susp, ophth: Prednisolone acetate 1% and gentamicin sulfate 0.3% (2 mL, 5 mL, 10 mL); Soln and oint 0.3%

Glimepiride (Amaryl)

COMMON USES: Type 2 DM
ACTION: Sulfonylurea. Stimulates the release of insulin from the pancreas; increases insulin sensitivity at peripheral sites; reduces glucose output from the liver
DOSAGE: 1–4 mg/d, up to max of 8 mg
SUPPLIED: Tabs 1, 2, 4 mg

Glipizide (Glucotrol)

COMMON USES: Type 2 DM
ACTION: Sulfonylurea. Stimulates the release of insulin from the pancreas; increases insulin sensitivity at peripheral sites; reduces glucose output from the liver
DOSAGE: 5–15 mg qd–bid
SUPPLIED: Tabs 5, 10 mg; ER tabs 5, 10 mg

Glucagon

Emergency care (see Chapter 21)
COMMON USES: Severe hypoglycemic reactions in diabetic patients with sufficient liver glycogen stores or β-blocker overdose
ACTIONS: Accelerates liver gluconeogenesis
DOSAGE: *Adults.* 0.5–1.0 mg SC, IM, or IV; repeat after 20 min PRN. β-*Blocker overdose:* 3–10 mg IV; repeat in 10 min PRN; may be given as cont inf. *Peds.* Neonates: 0.3 mg/kg/dose SC, IM, or IV q4h PRN. *Children:* 0.025–0.1 mg/kg/dose SC, IM, or IV; repeat after 20 min PRN
SUPPLIED: Inj 1 mg
NOTES: Administration of glucose IV necessary; ineffective in states of starvation, adrenal insufficiency, or chronic hypoglycemia

Glyburide (Diaβeta, Micronase Glynase Prestab)

COMMON USES: Type 2 DM
ACTION: Sulfonylurea. Stimulates the release of insulin from the pancreas; increases insulin sensitivity at peripheral sites; reduces glucose output from the liver
DOSAGE: *Nonmicronized:* 1.25–10 mg qd–bid. *Micronized:* 1.5–6 mg qd–bid
SUPPLIED: Tabs 1.25, 2.5, 5 mg; micronized tabs [Glynase] 1.5, 3, 4.5, 6 mg
NOTES: NOT recommended in renal impairment

Glycerin Suppository

COMMON USES: Constipation
ACTIONS: Hyperosmolar laxative
DOSAGE: *Adults.* 1 adult supp PR PRN. *Peds.* 1 infant supp PR qd–bid PRN

22

SUPPLIED: Supp (adult, infant); liq 4 mL/applicatorful

Gonadorelin (Lutrepulse)

COMMON USES: Primary hypothalamic amenorrhea
ACTIONS: Stimulates the pituitary to release the gonadotropins LH and FSH
DOSAGE: 5–20 μg IV q 90 min for 21 d using a reservoir and pump
SUPPLIED: Inj 0.8 mg, 3.2 mg
NOTES: Risk of multiple pregnancies

Goserelin (Zoladex)

COMMON USES: Advanced prostate cancer and with radiation for localized prostate cancer; endometriosis
ACTIONS: Slow-release form of LHRH agonist, thereby inhibiting the release of gonadotropin, decreasing testosterone levels
DOSAGE: 3.6 mg SC (implant) q 28 d or 10.8 mg SC q 3 mo
SUPPLIED: Subcutaneous implant 3.6, 10.8 mg
NOTES: *Toxicity symptoms:* Hot flashes, ↓ libido, gynecomastia, and transient exacerbation of cancer-related bone pain ("flare reaction" 7–10 d after 1st dose)

Granisetron (Kytril)

COMMON USES: Prevention of nausea and vomiting
ACTIONS: Serotonin receptor antagonist
DOSAGE: *Adults & Peds.* 10 mg/kg IV 30 min prior to initiation of chemotherapy. *Adults.* 1 mg PO 1 h prior to chemotherapy, then 12 h later
SUPPLIED: Tabs 1 mg; inj 1 mg/mL

Guaifenesin (Robitussin, others)

COMMON USES: Symptomatic relief of dry, nonproductive cough
ACTIONS: Expectorant
DOSAGE: *Adults.* 200–400 mg (10–20 mL) PO q4h. *Peds.* <2 y: 12 mg/kg/d in 6 ÷ doses. *2–5 y:* 50–100 mg (2.5–5 mL) PO q4h. *6–11 y:* 100–200 mg (5–10 mL) PO q4h
SUPPLIED: Tabs 100, 200, 1200 mg; SR tabs 600 mg; caps 200 mg; SR caps 300 mg; liq 100, 200 mg/5 mL

Guaifenesin and Codeine (Robitussin A-C, Brontex, others) [C]

COMMON USES: Symptomatic relief of dry, nonproductive cough
ACTIONS: Antitussive with expectorant
DOSAGE: *Adults.* 10 mL or 1 tab PO q6–8h. *Peds.* 2–6 y: 1–1.5 kg/kg codeine/d ÷ dose q4–6h; *6–12 y:* 5 mL q4h; *>12 y:* 10 mL q4h, max 60 mL/24h
SUPPLIED: Brontex tab contains 10 mg codeine; Brontex liq 2.5 mg codeine/5 mL; others 10 mg codeine/5 mL

Guaifenesin and Dextromethorphan (Many OTC Brands)

COMMON USES: Cough due to upper respiratory irritation
ACTIONS: Antitussive with expectorant
DOSAGE: *Adults & Peds >12 y.* 10 mL PO q6h. *Peds.* 2–6 y: 2.5 mL q6–8h, 10 mL/d max; *6–12 y:* 5 mL q6–8h, 20 mL max/d

Guanabenz (Wytensin)

COMMON USES: HTN
ACTIONS: Central α-adrenergic agonist
DOSAGE: *Adults.* Initially, 4 mg PO bid; ↑ by 4 mg/d increments at 1–2-wk intervals up to 32 mg bid. *Peds >12 y.* Initially, 0.5–4 mg/d; ↑ by increments of 0.5–2 mg/d at 1-wk intervals up to 24 mg/d ÷ bid

SUPPLIED: Tabs 4, 8 mg
NOTES: Sedation, dry mouth, dizziness, and headache common

Guanadrel (Hylorel)

COMMON USES: HTN
ACTIONS: Inhibits norepinephrine release from peripheral storage sites
DOSAGE: Initially, 5 mg PO bid; ↑ by 10 mg/d increments at 1-wk intervals up to 75 mg PO bid
SUPPLIED: Tabs 10, 25 mg
NOTES: Interactions with tricyclic antidepressants; lower incidence of orthostatic changes and impotence than guanethidine; dosage adjustment in renal impairment

Guanethidine (Ismelin)

COMMON USES: Moderate to severe HTN or renal HTN
ACTIONS: Inhibits release of norepinephrine from peripheral storage sites
DOSAGE: *Adults.* Initially, 10–25 mg PO qd. *Peds.* Initially, 0.2 mg/kg/24h PO; ↑ by 0.2 mg/kg/24h increments q 7–10 d to a max of 3 mg/kg/24h
SUPPLIED: Tabs 10, 25 mg
NOTES: May produce profound orthostatic hypotension, especially with diuretic use; may potentiate the effects of vasopressor agents; increased bowel movements and explosive diarrhea possible; interaction with tricyclic antidepressants reduces effectiveness

Guanfacine (Tenex)

COMMON USES: HTN
ACTIONS: Centrally acting α-adrenergic agonist
DOSAGE: Initially, 1 mg hs; ↑ by 1 mg/24h increments to a max of 3 mg/24h; split the dose bid if BP increases at the end of the dosing interval
SUPPLIED: Tabs 1, 2 mg
NOTES: Use with a thiazide diuretic recommended; sedation and drowsiness common; rebound HTN possible with abrupt cessation of therapy

Haemophilus B Conjugate Vaccine (Prohibit, Comvax, others)

COMMON USES: Routine immunization of children against diseases caused by *H. influenzae* type B
ACTIONS: Active immunization against *Haemophilus B*
DOSAGE: *Peds.* 0.5 mL (25 mg) IM in deltoid or vastus lateralis
SUPPLIED: Inj 7.5, 10, 15, 25 µg/0.5 mL
NOTES: Booster NOT required; observe for anaphylaxis. (See Table 22–9, page 636.)

Haloperidol (Haldol)

COMMON USES: Psychotic disorders, agitation, Tourette's disorders, and hyperactivity in children
ACTIONS: Antipsychotic, neuroleptic
DOSAGE: *Adults.* Moderate symptoms: 0.5–2.0 mg PO bid–tid. *Severe symptoms or agitation:* 3–5 mg PO bid–tid or 1–5 mg IM q4h PRN (max 100 mg/d). *Peds.* 3–6 y: 0.01–0.03 mg/kg/24h PO qd. *6–12 y:* Initially, 0.5–1.5 mg/24h PO; ↑ by increments of 0.5 mg/24h to maintenance of 2–4 mg/24h (0.05–0.1 mg/kg/24h) or 1–3 mg/dose IM q4–8h to a max of 0.1 mg/kg/24h; Tourette's syndrome may require up to 15 mg/24h PO
SUPPLIED: Tabs 0.5, 1, 2, 5, 10, 20 mg; conc liq 2 mg/mL; inj 5 mg/mL; decanoate inj 50, 100 mg/mL
NOTES: Can cause extrapyramidal symptoms and hypotension; ↓ dose in elderly

Haloprogin (Halotex)

COMMON USES: Topical treatment of tinea pedis, tinea cruris, tinea corporis, tinea manus
ACTIONS: Topical antifungal
DOSAGE: *Adults.* Apply bid for up to 2 wk; intertriginous may require up to 4 wk
SUPPLIED: 1% Cream; soln

Heparin

Used for emergency cardiac care (see Chapter 21)
COMMON USES: Rx and prevention of DVT and PE, AF with emboli formation, and acute arterial occlusion
ACTIONS: Acts with antithrombin III to inactivate thrombin and inhibit thromboplastin formation
DOSAGE: *Adults.* Prophylaxis: 3000–5000 U SC q8–12h. *Thrombosis Rx:* Loading dose of 50–75 U/kg IV, then 10–20 U/kg IV qh (adjust based on PTT). *Peds.* Infants: Loading dose 50 U/kg IV bolus, then 20 U/kg/h IV by cont inf. *Children:* Loading dose 50 U/kg IV, then 15–25 U/kg cont inf or 100 U/kg/dose q4h IV intermittent bolus
SUPPLIED: Inj 10, 100, 1000, 2000, 2500, 5000, 7500, 10,000, 20,000, 40,000 U/mL
NOTES: Follow PTT, thrombin time, or activated clotting time to assess effectiveness; heparin has little effect on the prothrombin time; with proper dose, PTT is about 1.5–2 × the control; can cause thrombocytopenia; follow platelet counts

Hepatitis A Vaccine (Havrix, Vaqta)

COMMON USES: Prevention of hepatitis A in individuals at high risk, eg, travelers, those in certain professions, or those practicing high-risk behavior
ACTIONS: Provides active immunity
DOSAGE: (Expressed as ELISA units [EL.U]) *Havrix: Adults.* 1440 EL.U. as a single IM dose. *Peds >2 y.* 720 EL.U. as a single IM dose. *Vaqta: Adults.* 50 U as a single IM dose. *Peds.* 25 U as a single IM dose
SUPPLIED: Inj 720 EL.U./0.5 mL, 1440 EL.U./1 mL.; 50 U/mL
NOTES: Booster is recommended 6–12 mo after primary vaccination

Hepatitis B Immune Globulin [HBIG] (BayhepB, NAbi-HB)

COMMON USES: Exposure to HBsAg-positive materials, eg, blood, plasma, or serum (accidental needle-stick, mucous membrane contact, or oral ingestion)
ACTIONS: Passive immunization
DOSAGE: *Adults & Peds.* 0.06 mL/kg IM to a max of 5 mL; within 24 h of needle-stick or percutaneous exposure; within 14 d of sexual contact; repeat 1 and 6 mo after exposure
SUPPLIED: Inj
NOTES: Administered in gluteal or deltoid muscle; if exposure continues, the patient should also receive the hepatitis B vaccine

Hepatitis B Vaccine (Engerix-B, Recombivax HB)

COMMON USES: Prevention of hepatitis B
ACTIONS: Active immunization
DOSAGE: *Adults.* 3 IM doses of 1 mL each, the first 2 doses given 1 mo apart, the 3rd 6 mo after the first. *Peds.* 0.5 mL IM given on the same schedule as for adults (see Table 22–9, page 636)
SUPPLIED: *Engerix-B:* Inj 20 μg/mL; Ped inj 10 μg/0.5 mL. *Recombivax HB:* Inj 10 and 40 μg/mL; Ped inj 5 μg/0.5 mL
NOTES: Administer IM injections for adults and older Peds in the deltoid; in other Peds, administer in the anterolateral thigh; may cause fever, inj site soreness; derived from recombinant DNA technology

Hetastarch (Hespan)

COMMON USES: Plasma volume expansion as an adjunct in the treatment of shock and leukapheresis
ACTIONS: Synthetic colloid with actions similar to those of albumin
DOSAGE: 500–1000 mL (do not exceed 1500 mL/d) IV at a rate not to exceed 20 mL/kg/h. *Leukapheresis:* 250–700 mL
SUPPLIED: Inj 6 g/100 mL
NOTES: NOT a substitute for blood or plasma; contra in patients with severe bleeding disorders, severe CHF, or renal failure with oliguria or anuria

Hydralazine (Apresoline, others)

COMMON USES: Moderate to severe HTN
ACTIONS: Peripheral vasodilator
DOSAGE: *Adults.* Begin at 10 mg PO qid, then ↑ to 25 mg qid to max of 300 mg/d. *Peds.* 0.75–3 mg/kg/24h PO ÷ q12–6h
SUPPLIED: Tabs 10, 25, 50, 100 mg; inj 20 mg/mL
NOTES: Use caution with impaired hepatic function and CAD; compensatory sinus tachycardia can be eliminated with the addition of propranolol; chronically high doses can cause SLE-like syndrome and Vitamin B_6 deficiency; SVT can occur following IM administration; dosage adjustment in renal impairment

Hydrochlorothiazide (Hydrodiuril, Esidrix, others)

COMMON USES: Edema, HTN, and CHF
ACTIONS: Thiazide diuretic; inhibits Na reabsorption in the distal tubule
DOSAGE: *Adults.* 25–100 mg/d PO in single or ÷ doses. *Peds.* <6 mo: 2–3 mg/kg/d in 2 ÷ doses. >6 mo: 2 mg/kg/d in 2 ÷ doses
SUPPLIED: Tabs 25, 50, 100 mg; caps 12.5 mg; oral soln 50 mg/5 mL
NOTES: Hypokalemia frequent; hyperglycemia, hyperuricemia, hyperlipidemia, and hyponatremia common

Hydrochlorothiazide and Amiloride (Moduretic)

COMMON USES: HTN; adjunctive therapy for CHF
ACTIONS: Combined effects of a thiazide diuretic and a potassium-sparing diuretic
DOSAGE: 1–2 tabs/d PO
SUPPLIED: Tabs (amiloride/hydrochlorothiazide) 5 mg/50 mg
NOTES: Do NOT give to diabetics or patients with renal failure

Hydrochlorothiazide and Spironolactone (Aldactazide)

COMMON USES: Edema (CHF, cirrhosis) and HTN
ACTIONS: Combined effects of a thiazide diuretic and a K-sparing diuretic
DOSAGE: 25–200 mg each component/d in ÷ doses
SUPPLIED: Tabs (hydrochlorothiazide/spironolactone) 25 mg/25 mg, 50 mg/50 mg

Hydrochlorothiazide and Triamterene (Dyazide, Maxzide)

COMMON USES: Edema and HTN
ACTIONS: Combined effects of a thiazide diuretic and a K-sparing diuretic
DOSAGE: *Dyazide:* 1–2 caps PO qd–bid. *Maxzide:* 1 tab/d PO
SUPPLIED: (triamterene/HCTZ) 37.5 mg/25 mg, 50 mg/25 mg, 75 mg/50 mg
NOTES: HCTZ component in Maxzide more bioavailable than Dyazide; can cause hyperkalemia as well as hypokalemia; follow serum K levels

Hydrocodone and Acetaminophen (Lorcet, Vicodin, others) [C-III]

COMMON USES: Moderate to severe pain; hydrocodone has antitussive properties
ACTIONS: Narcotic analgesic with nonnarcotic analgesic
DOSAGE: 1–2 caps or tabs PO q4–6h PRN
SUPPLIED: Many different combinations; specify hydrocodone/acetaminophen dose. Caps 5/500; tabs 2.5/500, 5/400, 5/500, 7.5/400, 7.5/650, 7.5/750, 10/325, 10/400, 10/500, 10/650; elixir and soln (fruit punch flavor) 2.5 mg hydrocodone/167 mg acetaminophen/5 mL

Hydrocodone and Aspirin (Lortab ASA, others) [C-III]

COMMON USES: Moderate-to-severe pain
ACTIONS: Narcotic analgesic with NSAID
DOSAGE: 1–2 PO q4–6h PRN
SUPPLIED: 5 mg hydrocodone/500 mg aspirin/tab

Hydrocodone and Guaifenesin (Hycotuss Expectorant, others) [C-III]

COMMON USES: Nonproductive cough associated with respiratory infection
ACTIONS: Expectorant plus cough suppressant
DOSAGE: *Adults & Peds.* >12 y: 5 mL q4h, pc and hs. *Peds.* <2 y: 0.3 mg/kg/d ÷ qid; *2–12 y:* 2.5 mL q4h pc and hs
SUPPLIED: Hydrocodone 5 mg/guaifenesin 100 mg/5 mL

Hydrocodone and Homatropine (Hycodan, others) [C-III]

COMMON USES: Relief of cough
ACTIONS: Combination antitussive
DOSAGE: Dose based on hydrocodone. *Adults.* 5–10 mg q4–6h. *Peds.* 0.6 mg/kg/d ÷ tid–qid
SUPPLIED: Syrup 5-mg hydrocodone/5 mL; tabs 5-mg hydrocodone

Hydrocodone and Ibuprofen (Vicoprofen) [C-III]

COMMON USES: Moderate to severe pain (<10 d)
ACTIONS: Narcotic with NSAID
DOSAGE: 1–2 tabs q4–6h PRN
SUPPLIED Tabs 7.5 mg hydrocodone/200 mg ibuprofen

Hydrocodone and Pseudoephedrine (Entuss-D, Histussin-D, others) [C-III]

COMMON USES: Cough and nasal congestion
ACTIONS: Narcotic cough suppressant with decongestant
DOSAGE: 5 mL qid, PRN
SUPPLIED: Entuss-D 5-mg hydrocodone/30 mg pseudoephedrine/5 mL; Histussin-D 5-mg hydrocodone/60 mg pseudoephedrine/5 mL

Hydrocodone, Chlorpheniramine, Phenylephrine, Acetaminophen, and Caffeine (Hycomine Compound) [C-III]

COMMON USES: Cough and symptoms of upper respiratory infections
ACTIONS: Narcotic cough suppressant with decongestants and analgesic
DOSAGE: 1 PO, q4h, PRN
SUPPLIED: Hydrocodone 5 mg/chlorpheniramine/2 mg/phenylephrine/10 mg/acetaminophen 250 mg/caffeine 30 mg/tab

Hydrocortisone

See Steroids (topical Table 22–6, pages 628–630, systemic, Table 22–5, page 627)

Hydrocortisone, Rectal (Anusol-HC Suppository, C Ortifoam Rectal, Proctocort others)

COMMON USES: Adjunct to painful anorectal conditions; radiation proctitis, management of ulcerative colitis
ACTIONS: Antiinflammatory steroid
DOSAGE: *Adults.* Ulcerative colitis 10–100 mg rectally qd–bid 2–3 wk 1–2×/d for 2–3 wk
SUPPLIED: *Hydrocortisone acetate:* Rectal aerosol 90 mg/applicator; supp 25 mg; *Hydrocortisone base:* Rectal 1%; rectal susp: 100 mg/60 mL

Hydrocortisone, Topical (see also Table 22–6, pages 628–630)

Hydromorphone (Dilaudid) [C-II]

COMMON USES: Moderate to severe pain
ACTIONS: Narcotic analgesic
DOSAGE: 1–4 mg PO, IM, IV, or PR q4–6h PRN; 3 mg PR q6–8h PRN
SUPPLIED: Tabs 1, 2, 3, 4, 8 mg; liq 5 mg/mL; inj 1, 2, 4, 10 mg/mL; supp 3 mg
NOTES: 1.5 mg IM = 10 mg of morphine IM

22

Hydroxyurea (Hydrea, Droxia)

COMMON USES: CML, head and neck cancer, ovarian cancer, melanoma, colon cancer, acute leukemia, and sickle cell anemia, HIV
ACTIONS: Probable inhibitor of the ribonucleotide reductase system
DOSAGE: 50–75 mg/kg for WBC counts of >100,000 cells/mL; 20–30 mg/kg in refractory CML. *HIV:* 1000–1500 mg/d in single or ÷ doses
SUPPLIED: Caps 200, 300, 400, 500 mg
NOTES: *Toxicity symptoms:* Myelosuppression (primarily leukopenia), nausea and vomiting, rashes, facial erythema, radiation recall reactions, and renal dysfunction; dosage adjustment in renal dysfunction

Hydroxyzine (Atarax, Vistaril)

COMMON USES: Anxiety, tension, sedation, itching
ACTIONS: Antihistamine, anxiety
DOSAGE: *Adults.* Anxiety or sedation: 50–100 mg PO or IM qid or PRN (max 600 mg/d). *Itching:* 25–50 mg PO or IM tid–qid. *Peds.* 0.5–1.0 mg/kg/24h PO or IM q6h
SUPPLIED: Tabs 10, 25, 50, 100 mg; caps 25, 50, 100 mg; syrup 10 mg/5 mL; susp 25 mg/5 mL; inj 25, 50 mg/mL
NOTES: Useful in potentiating effects of narcotics; NOT for IV use; drowsiness and anticholinergic effects common

Hyoscyamine (Anaspaz, Cystospaz, Levsin, others)

COMMON USES: Spasm associated with GI and bladder disorders
DOSAGE: *Adults.* 0.125–0.25 mg (1–2 tabs) SL 3–4/×/d, pc and hs; 1 SR caps q12h
SUPPLIED: Caps SR [Cystospaz-M, Levsinex])

Hyoscyamine, Atropine, Scopolamine, and Phenobarbital (Donnatal, others)

COMMON USES: Irritable bowel, spastic colitis, peptic ulcer, spastic bladder
DOSAGE: 0.125–0.25 mg (1–2 tabs) 3–4×/d, 1 cap q12h (SR), 5–10 mL elixir 3–4×/d or q8h

Ibuprofen (Motrin, Rufen, Advil, others)

COMMON USES: Arthritis and pain
ACTIONS: NSAID
DOSAGE: *Adults.* 200–800 mg PO bid–qid. *Peds.* 30–40 mg/kg/d in 3–4 ÷ doses
SUPPLIED: Tabs 100, 200, 400, 600, 800 mg; chewable tabs 50, 100 mg; caps 200 mg; susp 100 mg/2.5 mL, 100 mg/5 mL, 40 mg/mL

Ibutilide (Corvert)

COMMON USES: Rapid conversion of Afib or flutter
ACTIONS: Class III antiarrhythmic agent
DOSAGE: 0.01 mg/kg (max 1 mg) IV inf over 10 min. May be repeated once
SUPPLIED: Inj 0.1 mg/mL
NOTES: Do NOT administer Class I or III antiarrhythmics concurrently or within 4 h of ibutilide inf

Idarubicin (Idamycin)

COMMON USES: AML (in combination with cytarabine), CML in blast crisis, and ALL
ACTIONS: DNA intercalating agent; inhibits of DNA topoisomerases I and II
DOSAGE: 10–12 mg/m^2/d for 3–4 d
SUPPLIED: Inj 1 mg/mL (5-, 10-, 20-mg vials
NOTES: *Toxicity symptoms:* Myelosuppression, cardiotoxicity, nausea and vomiting, mucositis, alopecia, and irritation at sites of IV administration; rare changes in renal and hepatic function; dosage adjustment in renal or hepatic dysfunction

Ifosfamide (Ifex, Holoxan)

COMMON USES: Lung cancer (small-cell and non-small-cell), soft tissue sarcoma, testicular cancer, and non-Hodgkin's lymphoma
ACTIONS: Alkylating agent
DOSAGE: 1.2 g/m²/d for 5 d by bolus or cont inf; 2.4 g/m²/d for 3 d; with MESNA uroprotection (see MESNA)
SUPPLIED: Inj 1, 3 g
NOTES: *Toxicity symptoms:* Hemorrhagic cystitis, nephrotoxicity, nausea and vomiting, mild to moderate leukopenia, lethargy and confusion, alopecia, and hepatic enzyme elevations; dosage adjustment in renal impairment

Imipenem-Cilastatin (Primaxin)

COMMON USES: Serious infections caused by a wide variety of susceptible bacteria; inactive against *S. aureus,* group A and B streptococci, etc
ACTIONS: Bactericidal; interferes with cell wall synthesis
DOSAGE: *Adults.* 250–500 mg (imipenem) IV q6h. *Peds.* 60–100 mg/kg/24h IV ÷ q6h
SUPPLIED: Inj (imipenem/cilastatin) 250 mg/250 mg, 500 mg/500 mg
NOTES: Seizures may occur if drug accumulates; ↓ dosage for renal insufficiency to avoid drug accumulation if calculated CrCl is <70 mL/min

Imipramine (Tofranil)

COMMON USES: Depression, enuresis, and chronic pain
ACTIONS: Tricyclic antidepressant; ↑ synaptic conc of serotonin or norepinephrine in the CNS
DOSAGE: *Adults.* Hospitalized: Start at 100 mg/24h PO in ÷ doses; can ↑ over several weeks to 250–300 mg/24h. *Outpatient:* Maintenance of 50–150 mg PO hs, not to exceed 200 mg/24h. *Peds.* Antidepressant: 1.5–5.0 mg/kg/24h ÷ 1–4×/d. *Enuresis:* >6 y: 10–25 mg PO hs; ↑ by 10–25 mg at 1–2-wk intervals; treat for 2–3 mo, then taper
SUPPLIED: Tabs 10, 25, 50 mg; caps 75, 100, 125, 150 mg
NOTES: Do NOT use with MAO inhibitors; less sedation than with amitriptyline

Imiquimod Cream, 5% (Aldara)

COMMON USES: External genital warts
ACTIONS: Exact mechanism unknown; may induce cytokines
DOSAGE: Applied 3×/wk; leave on skin for 6–10 h, continue therapy for a max of 16 wk
SUPPLIED: Single-dose packets (250 mg of the cream)
NOTES: Local skin reactions common

Immune Globulin, Intravenous (Gamimmune N, Sandoglobulin, Gammar IV)

COMMON USES: IgG antibody deficiency disease states (eg, congenital agammaglobulinemia), CVH, and BMT; and ITP
ACTIONS: IgG supplementation
DOSAGE: *Adults & Peds.* Immunodeficiency: 100–200 mg/kg/mo IV at a rate of 0.01–0.04 mL/kg/min to a max of 400 mg/kg/dose. *ITP:* 400 mg/kg/dose IV qd for 5 d. *BMT:* 500 mg/kg/wk
SUPPLIED: Inj
NOTES: Adverse effects associated mostly with rate of infusion

Indapamide (Lozol)

COMMON USES: HTN and CHF
ACTIONS: Thiazide diuretic; enhances Na, Cl, and water excretion in the proximal segment of the distal tubule
DOSAGE: 1.25–5.0 mg/d PO
SUPPLIED: Tabs 1.25, 2.5 mg
NOTES: Doses >5 mg do NOT have additional effects on lowering BP

Indinavir (Crixivan)

COMMON USES: HIV infection when antiretroviral therapy is indicated
ACTIONS: Protease inhibitor; inhibits maturation of immature noninfectious virions to mature infectious virus
DOSAGE: 800 mg PO q8h
SUPPLIED: Caps 200, 400 mg
NOTES: Use in combination with other antiretroviral agents; take on an empty stomach; may cause nephrolithiasis; drink six 8-oz glasses of water/d; numerous drug interactions; dosage adjustment in hepatic impairment

Indomethacin (Indocin)

COMMON USES: Arthritis and closure of the ductus arteriosus; tocolytic
ACTIONS: Inhibits prostaglandin synthesis
DOSAGE: *Adults.* 25–50 mg PO bid–tid, to a max of 200 mg/d. SR dosed 1–2 × day *Tocolysis:* 50–100 10 PR, then 25 mg PO/PR q4–6h/× 48h. *Infants:* 0.2–0.25 mg/kg/dose IV; may be repeated in 12–24 h for up to 3 doses
SUPPLIED: Inj 1 mg/vial; caps 25, 50 mg; SR caps 75 mg; supp 50 mg; susp 25 mg/5 mL
NOTES: Monitor renal function carefully

Infliximab (Remicade)

COMMON USES: Moderate to severe Crohn's disease; RA (in combination with methotrexate)
ACTIONS: IgG1κ neutralizes biologic activity of TNFα
DOSAGE: *Crohn's disease:* 5 mg/kg IV inf, may follow with subsequent doses given at 2 and 6 wk after initial inf. *RA:* 3 mg/kg IV inf at 0, 2, 6 wk, followed by q 8 wk
SUPPLIED: Inj
NOTES: May cause hypersensitivity reaction, made up of human constant and murine variable regions; patients are predisposed to infection

Influenza Vaccine (Fluzone, Fluogen, Flushield, Flu-immune)

COMMON USES: Prevention of influenza in high-risk populations (chronic medical conditions, eg, heart disease, lung disease, or diabetes; children with asthma; residents of chronic care facilities; and any person >50 y). Health care workers or members of households who may come into contact with these patients also encouraged to be immunized
ACTIONS: Active immunization to inactivated virus grown in eggs
DOSAGE: 0.5 mL/dose IM in adults. Optimal time for vaccination in the U.S. is October–November because protection begins 1–2 wk after vaccination and lasts up to 6 mo
SUPPLIED: Each year, specific vaccines manufactured based on predictions of the strains likely to be active in the influenza season. The flu season generally December–Spring in the U.S. (Flu-immune = surface antigen, Fluogen = split virus, Flurone = whole virus)
NOTES: Soreness at the inj site and fever or malaise common after inj; severe reactions rare. Whole or split virus usually given to adults; give children <13 y split virus or purified surface antigen form to decrease febrile reactions

Insulin

COMMON USES: DM refractory to diet change or oral hypoglycemic agents; adjunct to the management of acute life-threatening hyperkalemia
ACTIONS: Insulin supplementation
DOSAGE: Based on serum glucose levels; usually given SC but can also be given IV or IM (only regular insulin can be given IV)
SUPPLIED: See Table 22–2 (page 622)
NOTES: Highly purified insulins ↑ free insulin; monitor patients closely for several weeks when changing doses

22

Interferon Alfa (Roferon-A, Intron A)

COMMON USES: HCL, Kaposi's sarcoma, multiple myeloma, CML, renal cell carcinoma, bladder cancer, melanoma, and chronic hepatitis C
ACTIONS: Direct antiproliferative action against tumor cells; modulation of the host immune response
DOSAGE: Dictated by treatment protocol. *Alfa-2a (Roferon)*: 3 million IU/d for 16–24 wk SC or IM. *Alfa-2b (Intron A)*: 2 million IU/m^2 IM or SC 3×/wk for 2–6 mo; intravesical 50–100 million IU in 50 mL/wk NS × 6
SUPPLIED: Injectable forms
NOTES: May cause flu-like symptoms; fatigue common; anorexia occurs in 20–30% of patients; neurotoxicity may occur at high doses; neutralizing antibodies can occur in up to 40% of patients receiving prolonged therapy

Interferon Alfa-2B and Ribavirin Combination (Rebetron)

COMMON USES: Chronic hepatitis C in patients with compensated liver disease who have relapsed following α-interferon therapy
ACTIONS: Combination antiviral agents
DOSAGE: 3 million U Intron A SC 3×/wk with 1000–1200 mg of Rebtrol PO ÷ bid dose for 24 wk; *Patients <75 kg:* 1000 mg of Rebetrol/d
SUPPLIED: *Patients <75 kg:* Combination pack; 6 vials Intron A (3 million U/0.5 mL) with 6 syringes and alcohol swabs; 70 Rebtrol caps. One 18-million-U multidose vial of Intron A inj (22.8 million U/3.8 mL; 3 million U/0.5 mL) and 6 syringes and alcohol swabs; 70 Rebetrol caps. One 18 million IU Intron A inj multidose pen (22.5 million IU/1.5 mL; 3 million IU/0.2 mL) and 6 disposable needles and alcohol swabs 70 Rebetrol caps. *Patients >75 kg:* Identical except for 84 Rebetrol caps/pack
NOTES: Instruct patients in self-administration of SC Intron A

Interferon Alfacon-1 (Infergen)

COMMON USES: Management of chronic hepatitis C
ACTIONS: Biologic response modifier
DOSAGE: 9 μg SC 3×/wk
SUPPLIED: Inj 9, 15 μg
NOTES: At least 48 h between inj

Interferon β-1B (Betaseron)

COMMON USES: Management of MS
ACTIONS: Biologic response modifier
DOSAGE: 0.25 mg SC qod
SUPPLIED: Powder for inj 0.3 mg
NOTES: May cause flu-like syndrome

Interferon Gamma-1B (Actimmune)

COMMON USES: Chronic granulomatous disease
ACTIONS: Biologic response modifier
DOSAGE: 50 mg/m^2 SC 3×/wk
SUPPLIED: Inj 100 mg
NOTES: 100 mg = 3 million U; may cause flu-like syndrome

Ipecac Syrup

See also Chapter 21
COMMON USES: Drug overdose and certain cases of poisoning
ACTIONS: Irritation of the GI mucosa; stimulation of the chemoreceptor trigger zone
DOSAGE: *Adults.* 15–30 mL PO, followed by 200–300 mL of water; if no emesis occurs in 20 min, may repeat once. *Peds.* Children 6–12 mo: 5–10 mL PO, followed by 10–20 mL/kg of water; if no

emesis occurs in 20 min, may repeat once. *Children 1–12 y:* 15 mL PO followed by 10–20 mL/kg of water; if no emesis occurs in 20 min, may repeat once
SUPPLIED: Syrup 15, 30 mL
NOTES: Do NOT use for ingestion of petroleum distillates or strong acid, base, or other corrosive or caustic agents; NOT for use in comatose or unconscious patients; caution in CNS depressant overdose

Ipratropium (Atrovent)

COMMON USES: Bronchospasm associated with COPD, bronchitis, and emphysema; rhinorrhea
ACTIONS: Synthetic anticholinergic agent similar to atropine
DOSAGE: *Adults & Peds >12 y.* 2–4 puffs qid. Nasal: 2 sprays/nostril bid–tid
SUPPLIED: Met-dose inhaler 18 µg/dose; soln for inhal 0.02%; nasal spray 0.03%, 0.06%
NOTES: Not for initial treatment of acute episodes of bronchospasm

Irbesartan (Avapro)

COMMON USES: HTN
ACTIONS: Angiotensin II receptor antagonists
DOSAGE: 150 mg/d PO, may be $\uparrow$ to 300 mg/d
SUPPLIED: Tabs 75, 150, 300 mg

Irinotecan (Camptosar)

COMMON USES: Advanced colorectal cancer; lung cancer
ACTIONS: Topoisomerase I inhibitor; interferes with DNA synthesis
   Dose: 125–250 mg/m^2 weekly to every other week
SUPPLIED: Inj 20 mg/mL
NOTES: *Toxicity symptoms:* Myelosuppression, diarrhea (acute or subacute), nausea and vomiting, abdominal cramping, and alopecia. Diarrhea dose-limiting in many studies; acute diarrhea associated with crampy abdominal pain successfully treated with atropine; subacute diarrhea treated with Imodium or loperamide. Diarrhea correlated to levels of metabolite SN-38

Iron Dextran (Dexferrum, InFeD)

COMMON USES: Iron deficiency when oral supplementation not possible
ACTIONS: Parenteral iron supplementation
DOSAGE: Based on estimate of iron deficiency, given IM/IV. A 0.5-mL test dose (0.25 mL in infants) prior to starting iron dextran. Total replacement dose (mL) = 0.0476 × weight (kg) × [desired hemoglobin (g/dL) − measured hemoglobin (g/dL)] + 1 mL/5 kg weight (max 14 mL). *Max daily dose: Adults >50 kg.* 100 mg Fe. *Peds <5 kg.* 25 mg Fe, 5–10 kg: 50 mg Fe, 0–50 kg: 100 mg Fe
SUPPLIED: Inj 50 mg (Fe)/mL
NOTES: Use test dose because anaphylaxis common; may be given deep IM using the "Z-track" technique, although IV route preferred

Isoetharine (Bronkosol, Bronkometer)

COMMON USES: Bronchial asthma and reversible bronchospasm
ACTIONS: Sympathomimetic bronchodilator
DOSAGE: *Adults.* 0.25–1.0 mL diluted 1:3 with saline q4–6h. *Peds.* 0.01 mL/kg; min dose 0.1 mL; max dose 0.5 mL; dilute with saline q4–6h
SUPPLIED: Soln for inhal; aerosol

Isoniazid (INH)

COMMON USES: Treatment and prophylaxis of *Mycobacterium* spp infections
ACTIONS: Bactericidal; interferes with mycolic acid synthesis, thus disrupting the bacterial cell wall

DOSAGE: *Adults.* Active TB: 5 mg/kg/24h PO or IM (usually 300 mg/d). *Prophylaxis:* 300 mg/d PO for 6–12 mo. *Peds.* Active TB: 10–20 mg/kg/24h PO or IM to a max of 300 mg/d. *Prophylaxis:* 10 mg/kg/24h PO
SUPPLIED: Tabs 50, 100, 300 mg; syrup 50 mg/5 mL; inj 100 mg/mL
NOTES: Can cause severe hepatitis; given with other antituberculous drugs for active TB; consult *MMWR* for the latest recommendations on the treatment and prophylaxis of TB; IM route rarely used; to prevent peripheral neuropathy, give pyridoxine 50–100 mg/d; dosage adjustment in hepatic impairment

Isoproterenol (Isuprel, Medihaler-Iso)

Used for emergency cardiac care (see Chapter 21)
COMMON USES: Shock, cardiac arrest, and AV nodal block; antiasthmatic
ACTIONS: β_1- and β_2-receptor stimulant
DOSAGE: *Adults.* For emergency cardiac care, also see Chapter 21. *Shock:* 1–4 mg/min IV inf; titrate to effect. *AV nodal block:* 20–60 mg IV push; may repeat q 3–5 min; maintenance 1–5 mg/min IV inf. *Inhalation:* 1–2 inhal 4–6×/d. *Peds.* For emergency cardiac care, also see Chapter 21. *Inhal:* 1–2 inhal 4–6×/d
SUPPLIED: Metered inhaler; soln for neb 0.5%, 1%; inj 0.02 mg/mL, 0.2 mg/mL
NOTES: Contra in tachycardia; pulse >130 may induce ventricular arrhythmias. (See Table 20–10, page 637.)

Isosorbide Dinitrate (Isordil, Sorbitrate)

COMMON USES: Rx and prevention of angina pectoris
ACTIONS: Relaxation of vascular smooth muscle
DOSAGE: *Acute angina:* 5–10 mg PO (chewable tabs) q2–3h or 2.5–10 mg SL PRN q 5–10 min; >3 doses should not be given in a 15–30-min period. *Angina prophylaxis:* 5–60 mg PO tid
SUPPLIED: Tabs 5, 10, 20, 30, 40 mg; SR tabs 40 mg; SL tabs 2.5, 5, 10 mg; chewable tabs 5, 10 mg; SR caps 40 mg
NOTES: Do NOT give nitrates on a chronic q6h or qid basis because of development of tolerance; can cause headaches; higher oral dose usually needed to achieve same results as SL forms

Isosorbide Mononitrate (Ismo, Imdur)

COMMON USES: Prevention of angina pectoris
ACTIONS: Causes relaxation of the vascular smooth muscle
DOSAGE: 20 mg PO bid, with the 2 doses given 7 h apart or ER (Imdur) 30–120 mg/d PO
SUPPLIED: Tabs 10, 20 mg; ER 30, 60, 120 mg

Isotretinoin [13-cis Retinoic Acid] (Accutane)

COMMON USES: Refractory severe acne
ACTIONS: Retinoic acid derivative
DOSAGE: 0.5–2 mg/kg/d PO ÷ bid
SUPPLIED: Caps 10, 20, 40 mg
NOTES: Contra in PRG and lactation; isolated reports of depression, psychosis, suicidal thoughts; dosage adjustment in hepatic impairment

Isradipine (Dyna-Circ)

COMMON USES: HTN and CHF
ACTIONS: Ca channel-blocker
DOSAGE: 2.5–10 mg PO bid
SUPPLIED: Caps 2.5, 5.0 mg; tabs CR 5, 10 mg

Itraconazole (Sporanox)

COMMON USES: Systemic fungal infections caused by *Aspergillus, Blastomycosis,* and *Histoplasma*
ACTIONS: Inhibits synthesis of ergosterol

22

DOSAGE: 200 mg PO or IV qd–bid
SUPPLIED: Caps 100 mg; soln 10 mg/mL; inj 10 mg/mL
NOTES: Administer with meals or cola; do NOT use concurrently with H_2-antagonist, omeprazole, antacids, terfenadine, astemizole, or cisapride; numerous other interactions

Kaolin-Pectin (Kaodene, Kao-Spen, Kapectolin)

COMMON USES: Diarrhea
ACTIONS: Adsorbent demulcent
DOSAGE: *Adults.* 60–120 mL PO after each loose stool or q3–4h PRN. *Peds.* 3–6 y: 15–30 mL/dose PO PRN. *6–12 y:* 30–60 mL/dose PO PRN
SUPPLIED: Multiple OTC forms
NOTES: Also available with opium (Parepectolin [C-V])

Ketoconazole (Nizoral)

COMMON USES: Systemic fungal infections (candidiasis, chronic mucocutaneous candidiasis, blastomycosis, coccidioidomycosis, histoplasmosis, and paracoccidioidomycosis); topical cream for localized fungal infections due to dermatophytes and yeast; short-term treatment of prostate cancer when rapid reduction of testosterone needed (ie, spinal cord compression)
ACTIONS: Inhibits fungal cell wall synthesis
DOSAGE: *Adults.* Oral: 200 mg PO qd; ↑ to 400 mg PO qd for serious infections; prostate cancer 400 mg PO tid (short term). *Topical:* Apply to the affected area qd (cream or shampoo). *Peds >2 y.* 5–10 mg/kg/24h PO ÷ q12–24h
SUPPLIED: Tabs 200 mg; topical cream 2%; shampoo 2%
NOTES: Systemic use associated with hepatotoxicity; monitor LFT; drug interaction with any agent ↑ gastric pH prevents absorption of ketoconazole; avoid concurrent use with cisapride; may enhance oral anticoagulants; may react with alcohol to produce a disulfiram-like reaction; numerous other drug interactions

Ketoprofen (Orudis, Oruvail)

COMMON USES: Arthritis and pain
ACTIONS: NSAID; inhibits prostaglandin synthesis
DOSAGE: 25–75 mg PO tid–qid, to a max of 300 mg/d
SUPPLIED: Tabs 12.5 mg; caps 50, 75 mg; caps, SR 100, 150, 200 mg

Ketorolac (Toradol)

COMMON USES: Arthritis and pain
ACTIONS: NSAID; inhibits prostaglandin synthesis
DOSAGE: 15–30 mg IV/IM q6h or 10 mg PO qid
SUPPLIED: Tabs 10 mg; inj 15 mg/mL, 30 mg/mL
NOTES: Do NOT use for longer than 5 d; adjust dose for age and renal dysfunction

Ketorolac Ophthalmic (Acular)

COMMON USES: Relief of ocular itching caused by seasonal allergic conjunctivitis
ACTIONS: NSAID
DOSAGE: 1 gt qid
SUPPLIED: Soln 0.5%

Labetalol (Trandate, Normodyne)

COMMON USES: HTN and hypertensive emergencies
ACTIONS: α- and β-Adrenergic blocking agent
DOSAGE: *Adults.* HTN: Initially, 100 mg PO bid; then 200–400 mg PO bid. *Hypertensive emergency:* 20–80 mg IV bolus, then 2 mg/min IV infusion, titrated to effect. *Peds.* Oral: 3–20 mg/kg/d in ÷ doses. *Hypertensive emergency:* 0.4–3 mg/kg/h IV cont inf
SUPPLIED: Tabs 100, 200, 300 mg; inj 5 mg/mL. (See Table 22–10, page 637.)

22

Lactic Acid and Ammonium Hydroxide [Ammonium Lactate] (Lac-Hydrin)

COMMON USES: Severe xerosis and ichthyosis
ACTIONS: Emollient moisturizer
DOSAGE: Apply bid
SUPPLIED: Lactic acid 12% with ammonium hydroxide

Lactobacillus (Lactinex Granules)

COMMON USES: Control of diarrhea, especially after antibiotic therapy
ACTIONS: Replaces normal intestinal flora
DOSAGE: *Adult and Peds >3 y.* 1 packet, 2 caps, or 4 tabs with meals or liqs tid–qid
SUPPLIED: Tabs; caps; EC caps; powder in packets

Lactulose (Chronulac, Cephulac)

COMMON USES: Hepatic encephalopathy; laxative
ACTIONS: Acidifies the colon, allowing ammonia to diffuse into the colon
DOSAGE: *Adults.* Acute hepatic encephalopathy: 30–45 mL PO q1h until soft stools are observed, then tid–qid. *Chronic laxative therapy:* 30–45 mL PO tid–qid; adjust the dosage q 1–2 d to produce 2–3 soft stools/d. *Rectally:* 200 g diluted with 700 mL of water instilled PR. *Peds.* Infants: 2.5–10 mL/24h ÷ tid–qid. *Children:* 40–90 mL/24h ÷ tid–qid
SUPPLIED: Syrup 10 g/15 mL
NOTES: Can cause severe diarrhea

Lamivudine (Epivir, Epivir-HBV)

COMMON USES: HIV infection when therapy warranted based on clinical or immunologic evidence of disease progression, and chronic hepatitis B
ACTIONS: Inhibits HIV reverse transcriptase, resulting in viral DNA chain termination
DOSAGE: *HIV: Adults & Peds >12 y.* 150 mg PO bid. *Peds <12 y.* 4 mg/kg bid. *HBV:* 100 mg/d
SUPPLIED: Tabs 100, 150 mg; soln 5 mg/mL, 10 mg/mL
NOTES: Use in combination with zidovudine; use with caution in pediatric patients because of an increased incidence of pancreatitis; adjust dose for renal dysfunction

Lamotrigine (Lamictal)

COMMON USES: Partial seizures
ACTIONS: Phenyltriazine antiepileptic
DOSAGE: *Adults.* Initial dose 50 mg/d PO, followed by 50 mg PO bid for 2 wk, then maintenance dose of 300–500 mg/d in 2 ÷ doses. *Peds.* 0.15 mg/kg in 1–2 ÷ doses for weeks 1 and 2, then 0.3 mg/kg for weeks 3 and 4, then maintenance dose of 1 mg/kg/d in 1–2 ÷ doses
SUPPLIED: Tabs 25, 100, 150, 200 mg; chewable tabs 5, 25 mg
NOTES: May cause rash and photosensitivity; value of therapeutic monitoring not established; interacts with other antiepileptics

Lansoprazole (Prevacid)

COMMON USES: Duodenal ulcers, *H. pylori* infection, erosive esophagitis, and hypersecretory conditions
ACTIONS: Proton pump inhibitor
DOSAGE: 15–30 mg/d PO
SUPPLIED: Caps 15, 30 mg

Latanoprost (Xalatan)

COMMON USES: Refractory glaucoma
ACTIONS: Prostaglandin
DOSAGE: 1 gtt
SUPPLIED: 0.005% Soln
NOTES: May darken light irides

22

Leflunomide (Arava)

COMMON USES: Active RA
ACTIONS: Inhibits pyrimidine synthesis
DOSAGE: Initial 100 mg/d for 3 d, followed by 10–20 mg/d
SUPPLIED: Tabs 10, 20, 100 mg
NOTES: PRG category X **DO NOT USE;** monitor serum transaminase levels during initial therapy

Lepirudin (Refludan)

COMMON USES: Heparin-induced thrombocytopenia
ACTIONS: Direct inhibitor of thrombin
DOSAGE: Bolus 0.4 mg/kg IV, followed by 0.15 mg/kg cont inf
SUPPLIED: Inj 50 mg
NOTES: Adjust dose based on aPTT ratio; maintain aPTT ratio of 1.5–2.0

Letrozole (Femara)

COMMON USES: Advanced breast cancer
ACTIONS: Nonsteroidal inhibitor of the aromatase enzyme system
DOSAGE: 2.5 mg/d
SUPPLIED: Tabs 2.5 mg
NOTES: Requires periodic CBC, thyroid function, electrolyte, LFT, and renal monitoring

Leucovorin (Wellcovorin)

COMMON USES: Overdose of folic acid antagonist; augmentation of 5-FU
ACTIONS: Reduced folate source; circumvents the action of folate reductase inhibitors (ie, methotrexate)
DOSAGE: *Adults & Peds.* MTX rescue: 10 mg/m^2/dose IV or PO q6h for 72 h until MTX level <10^{-8}. *5-FU:* 200 mg/m^2/d IV 1–5 d during daily 5-FU treatment or 500 mg/m^2/wk with weekly 5-FU therapy. *Adjunct to antimicrobials:* 5–15 mg/d PO
SUPPLIED: Tabs 5, 15, 25 mg; inj
NOTES: Many different dosing schedules for leucovorin rescue following MTX therapy

Leuprolide (Lupron, Viadur)

COMMON USES: Prostate cancer, endometriosis, and CPP
ACTIONS: LHRH agonist; paradoxically inhibits release of gonadotropin, resulting in decreased LH and testosterone levels
DOSAGE: *Adults.* Prostate: 7.5 mg IM q 28 d or 22.5 mg IM q 3 mo of depot. *Endometriosis (depot only)*: 3.75 mg IM as a single monthly dose. Viadur: SQ implant 1 × year *Peds.* CPP: 50 mg/kg/d as a daily SC inj. ↑ by 10 mg/kg/d until total down-regulation achieved. *Depot: <25 kg:* 7.5 mg IM q 4 wk. *>25–37.5 kg:* 11.25 mg IM q 4 wk. *>37.5 kg:* 15 mg IM q 4 wk
SUPPLIED: Inj 5 mg/mL; depot forms 3.75, 7.5, 11.25, 15, 22.5, 30 mg; Viadur 12 mo implant
NOTES: *Toxicity symptoms:* Hot flashes, gynecomastia, nausea and vomiting, constipation, anorexia, dizziness, headache, insomnia, paresthesias, peripheral edema, and bone pain (transient "flare reaction" at 7–14 d after the first dose due to testosterone surge)

Levalbuterol (Xopenex)

COMMON USES: Rx and prevention of bronchospasm
ACTIONS: Sympathomimetic bronchodilator
DOSAGE: 0.63 mg neb q6–8h
SUPPLIED: Soln for inhal 0.63, 1.25 mg/3mL
NOTES: Therapeutically active *R*-isomer of albuterol

Levamisole (Ergamisol)

COMMON USES: Adjuvant therapy of Dukes C colon cancer (in combination with 5-FU)
ACTIONS: Multiple poorly understood immunostimulatory effects
DOSAGE: 50 mg PO q8h for 3 d q 14 d during 5-FU therapy
SUPPLIED: Tabs 50 mg
NOTES: *Toxicity symptoms:* Nausea and vomiting, diarrhea, abdominal pain, taste disturbance, anorexia, hyperbilirubinemia, disulfiram-like reaction on alcohol ingestion, minimal bone marrow depression, fatigue, fever, and conjunctivitis

Levetiracetam (Keppra)

COMMON USES: Partial onset seizures
ACTIONS: Unknown
DOSAGE: 500 mg PO bid, may be ↑ to a max of 3000 mg/d
SUPPLIED: Tabs 250, 500, 750 mg
NOTES: May cause dizziness and somnolence; may impair coordination; adjust dosage in renal impairment

Levobunolol (Betagan, Liquidfilm Ophthalmic)

COMMON USES: Glaucoma
ACTIONS: β-Adrenergic blocker
DOSAGE: 1–2 gtt/d 0.5% or 1–2 gtt 0.25% bid
SUPPLIED: Soln 0.25, 0.5%

Levocabastine (Livostin)

COMMON USES: Allergic seasonal conjunctivitis
ACTIONS: Antihistamine
DOSAGE: 1 gtt in eye(s) qid up to 4 wk
SUPPLIED: 0.05% soln

Levofloxacin (Levaquin)

COMMON USES: Lower respiratory tract infections, sinusitis, and UTI
ACTIONS: Quinolone antibiotic, inhibits DNA gyrase
DOSAGE: 250–500 mg/d PO or IV
SUPPLIED: Tabs 250, 500 mg; inj 5, 25 mg/mL
NOTES: Reliable activity against *S. pneumoniae,* drug interactions with cation-containing products; renal dosage adjustment

Levonorgestrel Implant (Norplant)

COMMON USES: Contraceptive (Progestin)
DOSAGE: Implant 6 caps in the midforearm during first 7 days of menses
SUPPLIED: Kits containing 6 implantable caps, each containing 36 mg
NOTES: Prevents pregnancy for up to 5 y; caps may be removed if pregnancy desired

Levorphanol (Levo-Dromoran) [C-II]

COMMON USES: Moderate to severe pain
ACTIONS: Narcotic analgesic
DOSAGE: 2 mg PO or SC PRN q6–8h
SUPPLIED: Tabs 2 mg; inj 2 mg/mL

Levothyroxine (Synthroid)

COMMON USES: Hypothyroidism
ACTIONS: Supplementation of L-thyroxine

22

DOSAGE: *Adults.* Initially, 25–50 μg/d PO or IV; ↑ by 25–50 μg/d every month; usual dose 100–200 μg/d. *Peds.* 0–1 y: 8–10 μg/kg/24h PO or IV. *1–5 y:* 4–6 μg/kg/24h PO or IV. *>5 y:* 3–4 μg/kg/24h PO or IV
SUPPLIED: Tabs 25, 50, 75, 88, 100, 112, 125, 150, 175, 200, 300 μg; inj 200, 500 μg
NOTES: Titrate dosage based on clinical response and thyroid function tests; can ↑ dosage more rapidly in young to middle-aged patients

Lidocaine (Anestacon Topical, Xylocaine, others)

Used for emergency cardiac care (see Chapter 21)
COMMON USES: Local anesthetic; treatment of cardiac arrhythmias
ACTIONS: Anesthetic; class IB antiarrhythmic
DOSAGE: *Adults.* Antiarrhythmic, endotracheal: 5 mg/kg; follow with 0.5 mg/kg in 10 min if effective. *IV Load:* 1 mg/kg/dose bolus over 2–3 min; repeat in 5–10 min up to 200–300 mg/h; cont inf of 20–50 μg/kg/min or 1–4 mg/min. *Peds.* Antiarrhythmic, endotracheal, Loading dose: 1 mg/kg; repeat in 10–15 min max total dose of 5 mg/kg; then IV inf 20–50 μg/kg/min. *Topical:* Apply max 3 mg/kg/dose. *Local inj anesthetic:* Max 4.5 mg/kg; See Chapter 17.
SUPPLIED: Inj (*Local*) 0.5, 1, 1.5, 2, 4, 10, 20%; (*Inj IV*) 1% (10 mg/mL, 2% 20 mg/mL); admixture 4, 10, 20%; (*IV inf*) 0.2%, 0.4%; cream 2%; gel 2, 2.5%; oint 2.5, 5%; liq 2.5%; soln 2, 4%; viscous 2%. (For infusion, see Table 20–10, page 637.)
NOTES: Endotracheal doses should be diluted to 1–2 mL with NS; epinephrine may be added for local anesthesia to prolong effect and help decrease bleeding; do NOT use lidocaine with epinephrine on the digits, ears, or nose because vasoconstriction may cause necrosis; for IV forms, ↓ dose with liver disease or CHF; dizziness, paresthesias, and convulsions associated with toxicity; see Table 22–7 (pages 631–634) for drug levels

Lidocaine/Prilocaine (EMLA)

COMMON USES: Topical anesthetic; adjunct to phlebotomy or invasive dermal procedures
ACTIONS: Topical anesthetic
DOSAGE: *Adults.* EMLA cream and anesthetic disc (1 g/10 cm²): Apply thick layer of cream 2–2.5 g to intact skin and cover with an occlusive dressing (eg, Tegaderm) for at least 1 h. *Anesthetic disc:* 1 g/10 cm² for at least 1 h. *Peds.* Max dose: ≤3 mo or <5 kg: 1 g/10 cm² for 1 h. *3–12 mo and >5 kg:* 2 g/20 cm² for 4 h. *1–6 y and »10 kg:* 10 g/100 cm² for 4 h. *7–12 y and >20 kg:* 20 g/200 cm² for 4 h
SUPPLIED: Cream 2.5% lidocaine/2.5% prilocaine; anesthetic disc (1 g)
NOTES: Not for ophth use; use with caution when risk of methemoglobinemia; longer contact time gives greater effect

Lindane (Kwell)

COMMON USES: Head lice, crab lice, scabies
ACTIONS: Ectoparasiticide and ovicide
DOSAGE: *Adults & Peds.* Cream or lotion: Apply thin layer after bathing and leave in place for 8–12h (6–8 h for children, 6 h for infants), pour on laundry. *Shampoo:* Apply 30 mL and develop a lather with warm water for 4 min; comb out nits
SUPPLIED: Lotion 1%; shampoo 1%
NOTES: Caution with overuse; may be absorbed into blood; repeat in 7 d if necessary

Linezolid (Zyvox)

COMMON USES: Infections caused by gram+ bacteria, including vancomycin-resistant and methicillin-resistant strains
ACTIONS: Unique action, binds ribosomal bacterial RNA; bacteriocidal for strep, bacteriostatic for enterococci and staph
DOSAGE: 400–600 mg IV or PO q12h
SUPPLIED: Inj 2 mg/mL; tabs 400, 600 mg; susp 100 mg/5 mL
NOTES: Reversible MAO inhibitor; avoid foods containing tyramine; avoid cough and cold products containing pseudoephedrine

Liothyronine (Cytomel)

COMMON USES: Hypothyroidism
ACTIONS: T_3 replacement
DOSAGE: *Adults.* Initial dose of 25 μg/24h, then titrate q 1–2 wk according to clinical response and TFT to maintenance of 25–100 μg/d PO. *Myxedema coma:* 25–50 μg IV. *Peds.* Initial dose of 5 μg/24h, then titrate by 5 μg/24h increments at 1–2-wk intervals; maintenance 25–75 μg/24h PO qd
SUPPLIED: Tabs 5, 25, 50 μg; inj 10 μg/mL
NOTES: ↓ Dose in elderly; monitor TFT

Lisinopril (Prinivil, Zestril)

COMMON USES: HTN, heart failure, and AMI
ACTIONS: ACE inhibitor
DOSAGE: 5–40 mg/24h PO qd–bid. *AMI:* 5 mg within 24h of MI, followed by 5 mg after 24h, 10 mg after 48 h, then 10 mg/d
SUPPLIED: Tabs 2.5, 5, 10, 20, 30, 40 mg
NOTES: Dizziness, headache, and cough common side effects; Do NOT use in PRG

Lithium Carbonate (Eskalith, others)

COMMON USES: Manic episodes of bipolar illness; maintenance therapy in recurrent disease
ACTIONS: Effects shift toward intraneuronal metabolism of catecholamines
DOSAGE: *Adults.* Acute mania: 600 mg PO tid or 900 mg SR bid. *Maintenance:* 300 mg PO tid–qid. *Peds 6–12 y.* 15–60 mg/kg/d in 3–4 ÷ doses
SUPPLIED: Caps 150, 300, 600 mg; tabs 300 mg; SR tabs 300, 450 mg; syrup 300 mg/5 mL
NOTES: Dosage must be titrated; follow serum levels (Table 22–7, pages 631–634); common side effects polyuria and tremor; contra in patients with severe renal impairment; Na retention or diuretic use may potentiate toxicity

Lodoxamide (Alomide Ophthalmic)

COMMON USES: Seasonal allergic conjunctivitis
ACTIONS: Stabilizes mast cells
DOSAGE: *Adults & Peds >2 y.* 1–2 gtt in eye(s) qid up to 3 mo
SUPPLIED: Soln 0.1%

Lomefloxacin (Maxaquin)

COMMON USES: UTI and lower respiratory tract infections caused by gram– bacteria; prophylaxis in transurethral procedures
ACTIONS: Quinolone antibiotic; inhibits DNA gyrase
DOSAGE: 400 mg/d PO
SUPPLIED: Tabs 400 mg
NOTES: May cause photosensitivity; renal dosage adjustment

Lomustine (CCNU, CeeNu)

COMMON USES: Hodgkin's lymphoma and primary brain tumors
ACTIONS: Nitrosourea alkylating agent
DOSAGE: 130 mg/m^2 single dose repeated q 6 wk
SUPPLIED: Caps 10, 40, 100 mg; dose pack
NOTES: *Toxicity symptoms:* Myelosuppression, renal injury, anorexia, nausea and vomiting, stomatitis, pulmonary fibrosis, and hepatotoxicity. High lipid solubility translates into excellent penetration into the CNS

Loperamide (Imodium)

COMMON USES: Diarrhea
ACTIONS: Slows intestinal motility

DOSAGE: *Adults.* Initially, 4 mg PO; then 2 mg after each loose stool, up to 16 mg/d. *Peds.* 0.4–0.8 mg/kg/24h PO ÷ q6–12h until diarrhea resolves or for 7 d max
SUPPLIED: Caps 2 mg; tabs 2 mg; liq 1 mg/5 mL, 1 mg/mL
NOTES: Do NOT use in acute diarrhea caused by *Salmonella, Shigella,* or *C. difficile*

Loracarbef (Lorabid)

COMMON USES: Infections caused by susceptible bacteria involving the upper and lower respiratory tract, skin, bone, urinary tract, abdomen, and gynecologic system
ACTIONS: 2nd-generation cephalosporin; inhibits cell wall synthesis
DOSAGE: *Adults.* 200–400 mg PO bid. *Peds.* 7.5–15 mg/kg/d PO ÷ bid
SUPPLIED: Caps 200, 400 mg; susp 125, 250 mg/5 mL
NOTES: More gram (−) activity than 1st-generation cephalosporins

Loratadine (Claritin)

COMMON USES: Allergic rhinitis
ACTIONS: Nonsedating antihistamine
DOSAGE: 10 mg/d PO
SUPPLIED: Tabs 10 mg; syrup 1 mg/mL
NOTES: Take on an empty stomach

Lorazepam (Ativan, others) [C-IV]

COMMON USES: Anxiety and anxiety mixed with depression; preop sedation; control of status epilepticus; antiemetic
ACTIONS: Benzodiazepine; antianxiety agent
DOSAGE: *Adults.* Anxiety: 1–10 mg/d PO in 2–3 ÷ doses. *Preop sedation:* 0.05 mg/kg to a max of 4 mg IM 2 h before surgery. *Insomnia:* 2–4 mg PO hs. *Status epilepticus:* 4 mg/dose IV may be repeated at 10–15-min intervals; usual total dose 8 mg. *Antiemetic:* 0.5–2 mg IV or PO q4–6h PRN. *Peds.* Status epilepticus: 0.05 mg/kg/dose IV repeated at 1–20-min intervals × 2 PRN. *Antiemetic, 2–15 y old:* 0.05 mg/kg (to 2 mg/dose) prior to chemotherapy
SUPPLIED: Tabs 0.5, 1, 2 mg; soln, oral conc 2 mg/mL; inj 2, 4 mg/mL
NOTES: ↓ Dose in elderly; do NOT administer IV faster than 2 mg/min or 0.05 mg/kg/min; may take up to 10 min to see effect when given IV

Losartan (Cozaar)

COMMON USES: HTN
ACTIONS: Angiotensin II antagonist
DOSAGE: 25–50 mg PO qd–bid
SUPPLIED: Tabs 25, 50, 100 mg
NOTES: Do NOT use in PRG; symptomatic hypotension may occur in patients on diuretics; dosage adjustment in elderly or hepatic impairment

Lovastatin (Mevacor)

COMMON USES: Hypercholesterolemia; to slow the progression of atherosclerosis
ACTIONS: HMG-CoA reductase inhibitor
DOSAGE: 20 mg/d PO with PM meal; may ↑ at 4-wk intervals to a max of 80 mg/d taken with meals
SUPPLIED: Tabs 10, 20, 40 mg
NOTES: Patient must maintain standard cholesterol-lowering diet throughout treatment; monitor LFT q 6 wk during the 1st year of therapy; headache and GI intolerance common; patient should promptly report any unexplained muscle pain, tenderness, or weakness; avoid concurrent use with gemfibrozil

Lyme Disease Vaccine (Lymerix)

COMMON USE: Prevention of Lyme disease
ACTION: Provides active immunity against *Borrelia burgdorferi*

DOSAGE: 30 μg/0.5 mL IM administered at 0, 1, and 12 mo
SUPPLIED: Vaccine 0.3 μg/0.5 mL

Magaldrate (Riopan, Lowsium)

COMMON USES: Hyperacidity associated with peptic ulcer, gastritis, and hiatal hernia
ACTIONS: Low-Na antacid
DOSAGE: 5–10 mL PO between meals and hs
SUPPLIED: Susp
NOTES: <0.3 mg Na/tab or tsp; do NOT use in renal insufficiency due to Mg content

Magnesium Citrate

COMMON USES: Vigorous bowel preparation; constipation
ACTIONS: Cathartic laxative
DOSAGE: *Adults.* 120–240 mL PO PRN. *Peds.* 0.5 mL/kg/dose, to a max of 200 mL PO
SUPPLIED: Effervescent soln
NOTES: Do NOT use in renal insufficiency or intestinal obstruction

Magnesium Hydroxide (Milk of Magnesia)

COMMON USES: Constipation
ACTIONS: Saline laxative
DOSAGE: *Adults.* 15–30 mL PO PRN. *Peds.* 0.5 mL/kg/dose PO PRN
SUPPLIED: Tabs 311 mg, liq 400 mg/5 mL, 800 mg/5 mL
NOTES: Do NOT use in renal insufficiency or intestinal obstruction

Magnesium Oxide (Mag-Ox 400, others)

COMMON USES: Replacement for low plasma levels
ACTIONS: Mg supplementation
DOSAGE: 400–800 mg/d ÷ qd–qid. (See Chapter 9)
SUPPLIED: Caps 140 mg; tabs 400 mg
NOTES: May cause diarrhea

Magnesium Sulfate

Used for emergency cardiac care (see Chapter 21)
COMMON USES: Replacement for low plasma levels; refractory hypokalemia and hypocalcemia; preeclampsia and premature labor
ACTIONS: Mg supplement
DOSAGE: *Adults.* Supplement: 1–2 g IM or IV; repeat dosing based on response and continued hypomagnesemia. (See also Chapter 9.) *Preeclampsia, premature labor:* 4 g load then 1–4 g/h IV infusion. *Peds.* 25–50 mg/kg/dose IM or IV q4–6h for 3–4 doses; may repeat if hypomagnesemia persists
SUPPLIED: Inj 100, 125, 250, 500 mg/mL; oral soln 500 mg/mL; granules 40 meq/5 g
NOTES: ↓ Dose with low urine output or renal insufficiency

Mannitol

Used for emergency care (see Chapter 21)
COMMON USES: Cerebral edema, oliguria, anuria, myoglobinuria
ACTIONS: Osmotic diuretic
DOSAGE: *Adults.* Diuresis: 0.2 g/kg/dose IV over 3–5 min; if no diuresis within 2 h, discontinue. *Peds.* Diuresis: 0.75 g/kg/dose IV over 3–5 min; if no diuresis within 2 h, discontinue. *Adults & Peds.* Cerebral edema: 0.25 g/kg/dose IV push, repeated at 5-min intervals PRN; ↑ incrementally to 1 g/kg/dose PRN for increased intracranial pressure
SUPPLIED: Inj 5%, 10%, 15%, 20%, 25%
NOTES: Caution with CHF or volume overload

Maprotiline (Ludiomil)

COMMON USES: Depressive neurosis, bipolar illness, major depressive disorder, and anxiety associated with depression
ACTIONS: Tetracyclic antidepressant
DOSAGE: 75–150 mg/d hs, to a max of 300 mg/d
SUPPLIED: Tabs 25, 50, 75 mg
NOTES: Contra with MAO inhibitors or seizure history; patients >60 y, give only 50–75 mg/d; anticholinergic side effects

Mechlorethamine (Mustargen)

COMMON USES: Hodgkin's and non-Hodgkin's lymphoma, cutaneous T-cell lymphoma (mycosis fungoides), lung cancer, CLL, CML, and malignant pleural effusions
ACTIONS: Alkylating agent (bifunctional)
DOSAGE: 0.4 mg/kg single dose or 0.1 mg/kg/d for 4 d; 6 mg/m^2 1–2 ×/mo
SUPPLIED: Inj 10 mg
NOTES: *Toxicity symptoms:* Myelosuppression, thrombosis, or thrombophlebitis at inj site; tissue damage with extravasation (Na thiosulfate may be used topically to treat); nausea and vomiting; skin rash; amenorrhea; and sterility. High rates of sterility (especially in men) and secondary leukemia in patients treated for Hodgkin's disease. Highly volatile; must be administered within 30–60 min of preparation

Meclizine (Antivert)

COMMON USES: Motion sickness; vertigo associated with diseases of the vestibular system
ACTIONS: Antiemetic, anticholinergic, and antihistaminic properties
DOSAGE: *Adults & Peds >12 y.* 25 mg PO tid–qid PRN
SUPPLIED: Tabs 12.5, 25, 50 mg; chewable tabs 25 mg; caps 25, 30 mg
NOTES: Drowsiness, dry mouth, and blurred vision common

Medroxyprogesterone (Provera, Depot Provera, Cycrin)

COMMON USES: Secondary amenorrhea and abnormal uterine bleeding caused by hormonal imbalance; endometrial cancer
ACTIONS: Progestin supplement
DOSAGE: *Secondary amenorrhea:* 5–10 mg/d PO for 5–10 d. *Abnormal uterine bleeding:* 5–10 mg/d PO for 5–10 d beginning on the 16th or 21st d of the menstrual cycle. *Endometrial cancer:* 400–1000 mg/wk IM
SUPPLIED: Tabs 2.5, 5, 10 mg; depot inj 100, 150, 400 mg/mL
NOTES: Contra with past thromboembolic disorders or with hepatic disease

Megestrol Acetate (Megace)

COMMON USES: Breast and endometrial cancers; appetite stimulant in cancer and HIV-related cachexia
ACTIONS: Hormone; progesterone analogue
DOSAGE: *Cancer:* 40–320 mg/d PO in ÷ doses. *Appetite:* 800 mg/d PO
SUPPLIED: Tabs 20, 40 mg; soln 40 mg/mL
NOTES: May induce DVT; do NOT abruptly discontinue therapy

Meloxicam (Mobic)

COMMON USES: Osteoarthritis
ACTIONS: NSAID agent
DOSAGE: 7.5–15 mg/d PO
SUPPLIED: Tabs 7.5 mg
NOTES: ↓ Dose in renal impairment

Melphalan [ʟ-PAM] (Alkeran)

COMMON USES: Multiple myeloma, breast cancer, testicular cancer, ovarian cancer, melanoma, and allogenic and ABMT in high doses
ACTIONS: Alkylating agent (bifunctional)
DOSAGE: (Per protocol) 9 mg/m^2 or 0.25 mg/kg/d for 4–7 d, repeated at 4–6-wk intervals, or 1 mg/kg single dose once q 4–6 wk; 0.15 mg/kg/d for 5 d q 6 wk. *High dose for high-risk multiple myeloma:* Single dose 140 mg/m^2..*ABMT:* 140–240 mg/m^2 IV
SUPPLIED: Tabs 2 mg; inj 50 mg
NOTES: *Toxicity symptoms:* Myelosuppression (leukopenia and thrombocytopenia), secondary leukemia, alopecia, dermatitis, stomatitis, and pulmonary fibrosis; very rare hypersensitivity reactions

Meperidine (Demerol) [C-II]

COMMON USES: Relief of moderate to severe pain
ACTIONS: Narcotic analgesic
DOSAGE: *Adults.* 50–150 mg PO or IM q3–4h PRN. *Peds.* 1–1.5 mg/kg/dose PO or IM q3–4h PRN, up to 100 mg/dose
SUPPLIED: Tabs 50, 100 mg; syrup 50 mg/mL; inj 10, 25, 50, 75, 100 mg/mL
NOTES: 75 mg IM = 10 mg of morphine IM; beware of respiratory depression; do NOT use in renal failure; ↓ dose in elderly and renal impairment

Meprobamate (Equanil, Miltown) [C-IV]

COMMON USES: Short-term relief of anxiety
ACTIONS: Mild tranquilizer; antianxiety
DOSAGE: *Adults.* 400 mg PO tid–qid up to 2400 mg/d; SR 400–800 mg PO bid. *Peds 6–12 y.* 100–200 mg bid–tid; SR 200 mg bid
SUPPLIED: Tabs 200, 400, 600 mg; SR caps 200, 400 mg
NOTES: May cause drowsiness; adjust dose for renal impairment

Mercaptopurine [6-MP] (Purinethol)

COMMON USES: Acute leukemias of children and adults, 2nd-line Rx of CML and non-Hodgkin's lymphoma, maintenance therapy of ALL in children, and immunosuppressant therapy for autoimmune diseases (Crohn's disease)
ACTIONS: Antimetabolite; mimics hypoxanthine
DOSAGE: 80–100 mg/m^2/d or 2.5–5 mg/kg/d; maintenance 1.5–2.5 mg/kg/d
SUPPLIED: Tabs 50 mg
NOTES: *Toxicity symptoms:* Mild hematologic toxicity; uncommon GI toxicity, except mucositis, stomatitis, and diarrhea. Rash, fever, eosinophilia, jaundice, and hepatitis. Concurrent allopurinol therapy requires a 67–75% ↓ of 6-MP because of interference with metabolism by xanthine oxidase

Meropenem (Merrem)

COMMON USES: Serious infections caused by a wide variety of bacteria including intraabdominal and polymicrobial; bacterial meningitis
ACTIONS: Carbapenem; inhibition of cell wall synthesis, a β-lactam
DOSAGE: *Adults.* 1 g IV q8h. *Peds.* 20–40 mg/kg IV q8h
SUPPLIED: Inj
NOTES: Adjust dose for renal function; less seizure potential than imipenem; beware of possible anaphylaxis

Mesalamine [5-Amino salicylic acid] (Rowasa, Asacol, Pentasa)

COMMON USES: Mild to moderate distal ulcerative colitis, proctosigmoiditis, or proctitis
ACTIONS: Unknown; may topically inhibit prostaglandins
DOSAGE: Retention enema qd hs or insert 1 supp bid. *Oral:* 800–1000 mg PO 3–4×/d
SUPPLIED: Tabs 400 mg; caps 250 mg; supp 500 mg; rectal susp 4 g/60 mL

Mesna (Mesnex)

COMMON USES: ↓ Incidence of ifosfamide and cyclophosphamide-induced hemorrhagic cystitis
ACTIONS: Antidote
DOSAGE: 20% of the ifosfamide dose (+/–) or cyclophosphamide dose IV at 15 min prior to and 4 and 8 h after chemotherapy
SUPPLIED: Inj 100 mg/mL

Mesoridazine (Serentil)

COMMON USES: Schizophrenia, acute and chronic alcoholism, and chronic brain syndrome
ACTIONS: Phenothiazine antipsychotic
DOSAGE: Initially, 25–50 mg PO or IV tid; ↑ to a max of 300–400 mg/d
SUPPLIED: Tabs 10, 25, 50, 100 mg; oral conc 25 mg/mL; inj 25 mg/mL
NOTES: Low incidence of extrapyramidal side effects

Metaproterenol (Alupent, Metaprel)

COMMON USES: Bronchodilator for asthma and reversible bronchospasm
ACTIONS: Sympathomimetic bronchodilator
DOSAGE: *Adults.* Inhal: 1–3 inhal q3–4h to a max of 12 inhal/24h; allow at least 2 min between inhal. *Oral:* 20 mg q6–8h. *Peds.* Inhal: 0.5 mg/kg/dose to a max of 15 mg/dose inhaled q4–6h by neb or 1–2 puffs q4–6h. *Oral:* 0.3–0.5 mg/kg/dose q6–8h
SUPPLIED: Aerosol 75, 150 mg; soln for inhal 0.4%, 0.6% 5%; tabs 10, 20 mg; syrup 10 mg/5 mL
NOTES: Fewer β_1-effects than isoproterenol and longer acting

Metaraminol (Aramine)

COMMON USES: Prevention and Rx of hypotension due to spinal anesthesia
ACTIONS: α-Adrenergic agent
DOSAGE: *Adults.* Prevention: 2–10 mg IM q10–15min PRN. *Rx:* 0.5–5 mg IV bolus followed by IV inf of 1–4 mg/kg/min titrated to effect. *Peds.* Prevention: 0.1 mg/kg/dose IM PRN. *Rx:* 0.01 mg/kg IV bolus followed by IV inf of 5 mg/kg/min titrated to effect
SUPPLIED: Injectable forms
NOTES: Allow 10 min for max effect; employ other shock management techniques, eg, fluid resuscitation as needed; may cause cardiac arrhythmias

Metaxalone (Skelaxin)

COMMON USES: Relief of painful musculoskeletal conditions
ACTIONS: Centrally acting skeletal muscle relaxant
DOSAGE: 800 mg PO 3–4×/d
SUPPLIED: Tabs 400 mg

Metformin (Glucophage)

COMMON USES: Type 2 DM
ACTIONS: Decreases hepatic glucose production; ↓ intestinal absorption of glucose; improves insulin sensitivity
DOSAGE: Initial dose of 500 mg PO bid; may ↑ to max dose 2500 mg/d
SUPPLIED: Tabs 500, 850 mg
NOTES: Administer with the AM and PM meals; may cause lactic acidosis; do NOT use if SCr >1.3 in females or >1.4 in males; withhold prior to and following IV contrast studies; contra in hypoxemic conditions, including acute CHF and sepsis

Methadone (Dolophine) [C-II]

COMMON USES: Severe pain; detoxification and maintenance of narcotic addiction
ACTIONS: Narcotic analgesic

DOSAGE: *Adults.* 2.5–10 mg IM q 3–8h or 5–15 mg PO q8h; titrate as needed. *Peds.* 0.7 mg/kg/24h PO or IM ÷ q8h
SUPPLIED: Tabs 5, 10, 40 mg; oral soln 5, 10 mg/5 mL; oral conc 10 mg/mL; inj 10 mg/mL
NOTES: Equianalgesic with parenteral morphine; long half-life; ↑ slowly to avoid respiratory depression

Methenamine (Hiprex, Urex, others)

COMMON USES: Suppression or elimination of bacteriuria associated with chronic and recurrent UTI
DOSAGE: *Adults.* Hippurate: 1 g bid, mandelate: 1 g qid pc and hs. *Peds 6–12 y.* Hippurate: 25–50 mg/kg/d ÷ bid. *Mandelate:* 50–75 mg/kg/d ÷ qid
SUPPLIED: *Methenamine hippurate (Hiprex, Urex):* 1-g tabs. *Methenamine mandelate:* 500 mg/1 g EC tabs
NOTES: Contra in patients with renal insufficiency, severe hepatic disease, and severe dehydration

Methimazole (Tapazole)

COMMON USES: Hyperthyroidism and preparation for thyroid surgery or radiation
ACTIONS: Blocks the formation of T_3 and T_4
DOSAGE: *Adults.* Initial: 15–60 mg/d PO ÷ tid. *Maintenance:* 5–15 mg PO qd. *Peds.* Initial: 0.4–0.7 mg/kg/24h PO ÷ tid. *Maintenance:* ⅓–⅔ of the initial dose PO qd
SUPPLIED: Tabs 5, 10 mg
NOTES: Follow patient clinically and with TFT

Methocarbamol (Robaxin)

COMMON USES: Relief of discomfort associated with painful musculoskeletal conditions
ACTIONS: Centrally acting skeletal muscle relaxant
DOSAGE: *Adults.* 1.5 g PO qid for 2–3 d, then 1 g PO qid maintenance therapy; IV form rarely indicated. *Peds.* 15 mg/kg/dose may be repeated if necessary. (Recommended for tetanus only)
SUPPLIED: Tabs 500, 750 mg; inj 100 mg/mL
NOTES: Can discolor urine; may cause drowsiness or GI upset; contra with MyG

Methotrexate (Folex, Rheumatrex)

COMMON USES: ALL and AML, leukemic meningitis, trophoblastic tumors (chorioepithelioma, choriocarcinoma, chorioadenoma destruens, hydatidiform mole), breast cancer, Burkitt's lymphoma, mycosis fungoides, osteosarcoma, head and neck cancer, Hodgkin's and non-Hodgkin's lymphoma, lung cancer; psoriasis; and RA
ACTIONS: Inhibits dihydrofolate reductase-mediated generation of tetrahydrofolate
DOSAGE: *Cancer, "conventional dose":* 15–30 mg PO or IV 1–2×/wk q 1–3 wk. *"Intermediate dose":* 50–240 mg or 0.5–1 g/m² IV once q 4 d to 3 wk. *"High dose":* 1–12 g/m² IV once q 1–3 wk; 12 mg/m² (max 15 mg) IT, weekly until the CSF cell count returns to normal. *RA:* 7.5 mg/wk PO as a single dose or 2.5 mg q12h PO for 3 doses/wk
SUPPLIED: Tabs 2.5 mg; inj 2.5, 25 mg/mL; preservative-free inj 25 mg/mL
NOTES: *Toxicity symptoms:* Myelosuppression, nausea and vomiting, anorexia, mucositis, diarrhea, hepatotoxicity (transient and reversible; may progress to atrophy, necrosis, fibrosis, cirrhosis), rashes, dizziness, malaise, blurred vision, renal failure, pneumonitis, and, rarely, pulmonary fibrosis. Chemical arachnoiditis and headache with IT delivery. High-dose therapy requires leucovorin rescue to prevent severe hematologic and mucosal toxicity (see page 559); monitor blood counts and MTX levels carefully

Methoxamine (Vasoxyl)

COMMON USES: Support, restoration, or maintenance of blood pressure during anesthesia; for termination of some episodes of PSVT
ACTIONS: α-Adrenergic
DOSAGE: *Adults.* Anesthesia: 10–15 mg IM; if emergency, 3–5 mg slow IV push. *PSVT:* 10 mg by slow IV push. *Peds.* 0.25 mg/kg/dose IM or 0.08 mg/kg/dose slow IV push

SUPPLIED: Injectable forms
NOTES: IM dose requires 15 min to act; use 5–10 mg phentolamine locally in case of extravasation; interaction with MAO inhibitors and tricyclic antidepressants to potentiate methoxamine effect

Methyldopa (Aldomet)

COMMON USES: Essential HTN
ACTIONS: Centrally acting antihypertensive
DOSAGE: *Adults.* 250–500 mg PO bid–tid (max 2–3 g/d) or 250 mg–1 g IV q6–8h. *Peds.* 10 mg/kg/24h PO in 2–3 ÷ doses (max 40 mg/kg/24h ÷ q6–12h) or 5–10 mg/kg/dose IV q6–8h to total dose of 20–40 mg/kg/24h
SUPPLIED: Tabs 125, 250, 500 mg; oral susp 50 mg/mL; inj 50 mg/mL
NOTES: Do NOT use in the presence of liver disease; can discolor urine; initial transient sedation or drowsiness frequent

Methylergonovine (Methergine)

COMMON USES: Prevention and Rx postpartum hemorrhage caused by uterine atony
ACTIONS: Ergotamine derivative
DOSAGE: 0.2 mg IM after delivery of placenta, may repeat at 2–4-h intervals or 0.2–0.4 mg PO q6–12h for 2–7 d
SUPPLIED: Injectable forms, 0.2 mg tabs
NOTES: IV doses should be given over a period of not less than 1 min with frequent BP monitoring

Methylprednisolone (Solu-Medrol)

See Steroids (Table 22–5, see page 627).

Metoclopramide (Reglan, Clopra, Octamide)

COMMON USES: Relief of diabetic gastroparesis; symptomatic GERD; relief of cancer chemotherapy-induced nausea and vomiting
ACTIONS: Stimulates motility of the upper GI tract and blocks dopamine in the chemoreceptor trigger zone
DOSAGE: *Adults.* Diabetic gastroparesis: 10 mg PO 30 min ac and hs for 2–8 wk PRN; or same dose given IV for 10 d, then switch to PO. *Reflux:* 10–15 mg PO 30 min ac and hs. *Antiemetic:* 1–3 mg/kg/dose IV 30 min prior to antineoplastic agent, then q2h for 2 doses, then q3h for 3 doses. *Peds.* Reflux: 0.1 mg/kg/dose PO qid. *Antiemetic:* 1–2 mg/kg/dose IV on the same schedule as for adults
SUPPLIED: Tabs 5, 10 mg; syrup 5 mg/5 mL; soln 10 mg/mL; inj 5 mg/mL
NOTES: Dystonic reactions common with high doses; can be treated with IV diphenhydramine; can also be used to facilitate small bowel intubation and radiologic evaluation of the upper GI tract

Metolazone (Mykrox, Zaroxolyn)

COMMON USES: Mild to moderate essential HTN and edema of renal disease or cardiac failure
ACTIONS: Thiazide-like diuretic; inhibits reabsorption of sodium in the distal tubules
DOSAGE: *Adults.* HTN: 2.5–5 mg/d PO. *Edema:* 5–20 mg/d PO. *Peds.* 0.2–0.4 mg/kg/d PO ÷ q12h–qd
SUPPLIED: Tabs 0.5, 2.5, 5, 10 mg
NOTES: Monitor fluid and electrolyte status during treatment

Metoprolol (Lopressor, Toprol XL)

Used for emergency cardiac care (see also Chapter 21)
COMMON USES: HTN, angina, and AMI
ACTIONS: Competitively blocks β-adrenergic receptors, $β_1$.
DOSAGE: *Angina:* 50–100 mg PO bid. *HTN:* 100–450 mg/d PO. *AMI:* 5 mg IV × 3 doses, then 50 mg PO q6h × 48 h, then 100 mg PO bid
SUPPLIED: Tabs 50, 100 mg; ER tabs 50, 100, 200 mg; inj 1 mg/mL

Metronidazole (Flagyl, Metrogel)

COMMON USES: Amebiasis, trichomoniasis, *C. difficile, H. pylori,* anaerobic infections, and bacterial vaginosis

ACTIONS: Interferes with DNA synthesis

DOSAGE: *Adults.* Anaerobic infections: 500 mg IV q6–8h. *Amebic dysentery:* 750 mg/d PO for 5–10 d. *Trichomoniasis:* 250 mg PO tid for 7 d or 2 g PO in a single dose. *C. difficile infection:* 500 mg PO or IV q8h for 7–10 d. *Vaginosis:* 1 applicatorful intravaginally bid or 500 mg PO bid for 7 d. *Acne rosacea and skin:* Apply bid. *Peds.* Anaerobic infections: 15 mg/kg/24h PO or IV ÷ q6h. *Amebic dysentery:* 35–50 mg/kg/24h PO in 3 ÷ doses for 5–10 d

SUPPLIED: Tabs 250, 500 mg; ER tabs 750 mg; caps 375 mg; topical lotion and gel 0.75%; gel, vaginal 0.75% (5 g/applicator 37.5 mg in 70 g tube)

NOTES: For *Trichomonas* infections, also treat patient's partner; ↓ in hepatic failure; no activity against aerobic bacteria; use in combination in serious mixed infections; may cause a disulfiram-like reaction; adjust dose in renal failure

Metyrapone (Metopirone)

COMMON USES: Diagnostic test for hypothalamic-pituitary ACTH function

ACTIONS: Inhibits adrenocortical synthesis by blocking 11b-hydroxylase

DOSAGE: *Metyrapone test: Day 1:* Control period, collect 24 h urine to measure 17-OHCS or 17-KSG. *Day 2:* ACTH test, administer 50 U of ACTH infused over 8 h and measure 24-h urinary steroids. *Days 3–4:* Rest period. *Day 5:* Administer metyrapone with milk or a snack. *Adults.* 750 mg PO q4h for 6 doses. *Peds.* 15 mg/kg q4h for 6 doses (min 250-mg dose). *Day 6:* Determine 24-h urinary steroids

SUPPLIED: Tabs 250 mg (Limited availability in U.S.)

NOTES: Normal 24-h urine 17-OHCS is 3–12 mg; following ACTH, it ↑ to 15–45 mg/24h; normal response to metyrapone is 2-fold to 4-fold increase in 17-OHCS excretion; drug interactions with phenytoin, cyproheptadine, and estrogens may lead to subnormal response

Metyrosine (Demser)

COMMON USES: Pheochromocytoma; short-term preop and long-term when surgery contraindicated

ACTIONS: Tyrosine hydroxylase inhibitor

DOSAGE: *Adults & Peds >12 y.* 250 mg PO qid, ↑ by 250–500 mg/d up to 4 g/d. *Maintenance dose:* 2–3 g/d ÷ qid

SUPPLIED: 250 mg caps

NOTES: Administer at least 5–7 d preop

Mexiletine (Mexitil)

COMMON USES: Suppression of symptomatic ventricular arrhythmias; diabetic neuropathy

ACTIONS: Class IB antiarrhythmic

DOSAGE: Administer with food or antacids; 200–300 mg PO q8h; do not exceed 1200 mg/d

SUPPLIED: Caps 150, 200, 250 mg

NOTES: Do NOT use in cardiogenic shock or 2nd- or 3rd-degree AV block if no pacemaker; may worsen severe arrhythmias; monitor LFT during therapy; drug interactions with hepatic enzyme inducers and suppressors requiring dosage changes

Mezlocillin (Mezlin)

COMMON USES: Infections caused by susceptible strains of gram (−) bacteria (including *Klebsiella, Proteus, E. coli, Enterobacter, P. aeruginosa,* and *Serratia*) involving the skin, bone, respiratory tract, urinary tract, abdomen, and septicemia

ACTIONS: Bactericidal; inhibits cell wall synthesis

DOSAGE: *Adults.* 3 mg IV q4–6h. *Peds.* 200–300 mg/kg/d ÷ q4–6h

SUPPLIED: Inj

NOTES: Often used in combination with aminoglycoside; adjust dosage for renal impairment

Miconazole (Monistat, others)

COMMON USES: Severe systemic fungal infections, including coccidioidomycosis, candidiasis, *Cryptococcus*, etc; various tinea forms; cutaneous candidiasis; vulvovaginal candidiasis; tinea versicolor
ACTIONS: Fungicidal; alters permeability of the fungal cell membrane
DOSAGE: *Adults.* Apply to affected area bid for 2–4 wk. *Candidiasis:* 600–1800 mg/day ÷ Q8h *Intravaginally:* Insert 1 applicatorful or supp hs for 7 d
SUPPLIED: Topical cream 2%; lotion 2%; powder 2%; spray 2%; vaginal supp 100, 200 mg; vaginal cream 2%, IU forms
NOTES: Antagonistic to amphotericin B *in vivo;* rapid IV infusion may cause tachycardia or arrhythmias; may potentiate warfarin drug activity

Midazolam (Versed) [C-IV]

COMMON USES: Preoperative sedation, conscious sedation for short procedures, and induction of general anesthesia
ACTIONS: Short-acting benzodiazepine
DOSAGE: *Adults.* 1–5 mg IV or IM; titrate dose to effect. *Peds.* Conscious sedation: 0.08 mg/kg IM in a single dose. *General anesthesia:* 0.15 mg/kg IV followed by 0.05 mg/kg/dose q 2 min for 1–3 doses as needed to induce anesthesia
SUPPLIED: Inj 1, 5 mg/mL; syrup 2 mg/mL
NOTES: Monitor for respiratory depression; may produce hypotension in conscious sedation

Mifepristone [RU 486] (Mifeprex)

COMMON USES: Termination of intrauterine pregnancies of <49 d
ACTIONS: Antiprogestin; increases prostaglandins, resulting in uterine contraction
DOSAGE: Must be administered with 3 office visits: Day 1, three 200-mg tablets, PO; Day 3 if no abortion has occurred, give two 200-µg misoprostol PO; on or about day 14, verify termination of pregnancy
SUPPLIED: Tabs 200 mg
NOTES: Must be administered under physician supervision; can cause abdominal pain and 1–2 wk of uterine bleeding

Miglitol (Glyset)

COMMON USES: Type 2 DM
ACTIONS: α-Glucosidase inhibitor; delays digestion of ingested carbohydrates
DOSAGE: Initial 25 mg PO tid taken at the first bite of each meal; maintenance 50–100 mg tid with meals
SUPPLIED: Tabs 25, 50, 100 mg
NOTES: May be used alone or in combination with sulfonylureas

Milrinone (Primacor)

COMMON USES: CHF
ACTIONS: Positive inotrope and vasodilator, with little chronotropic activity
DOSAGE: Loading dose of 50 µg/kg, followed by cont inf of 0.375–0.75 µg/kg/min
SUPPLIED: Inj 1 µg/mL
NOTES: Carefully monitor fluid and electrolyte status; dosage adjustment in renal impairment

Mineral Oil

COMMON USES: Constipation
ACTIONS: Emollient laxative
DOSAGE: *Adults.* 5–45 mL PO PRN. *Peds >6 y.* 5–20 mL PO bid
SUPPLIED: Liq

Minoxidil (Loniten, Rogaine)

COMMON USES: Severe HTN; male and female pattern baldness
ACTIONS: Peripheral vasodilator; stimulates vertex hair growth
DOSAGE: *Adults.* Oral: 2.5–10 mg PO bid–qid. *Topical:* [Rogaine] Apply bid to the affected area. *Peds.* 0.2–1 mg/kg/24h ÷ PO q12–24h
SUPPLIED: Tabs 2.5, 10 mg; topical soln (Rogaine) 2%
NOTES: Pericardial effusion and volume overload may occur with oral use; hypertrichosis after chronic use

Mirtazapine (Remeron)

COMMON USES: Depression
ACTIONS: Tetracyclic antidepressant, unrelated to tricyclics or MAOIs.
DOSAGE: 15 mg PO hs, up to 45 mg/d hs
SUPPLIED: Tabs 15, 30, 45 mg
NOTES: Do NOT ↑ dose at intervals of less than 1–2 wk; may cause agranulocytosis

Misoprostol (Cytotec)

COMMON USES: Prevention of NSAID-induced gastric ulcers
ACTIONS: Synthetic prostaglandin with both antisecretory and mucosal protective properties
DOSAGE: 200 μg PO qid with meals
SUPPLIED: Tabs 100, 200 μg
NOTES: Do NOT take during PRG; can cause miscarriage with potentially dangerous bleeding; GI side effects common

Mitomycin C (Mutamycin)

COMMON USES: Adenocarcinomas of the stomach, pancreas, colon, and breast; non-small-cell lung cancer; head and neck cancer; cervical cancer; squamous cell carcinoma of the anus; and bladder cancer (intravesically)
ACTIONS: Alkylating agent; may also generate oxygen free radicals, which induce DNA strand breaks
DOSAGE: 20 mg/m^2 q 6–8 wk or 10 mg/m^2 in combination with other myelosuppressive drugs; bladder cancer 20–40 mg in 40 mL of NS via a urethral catheter once/wk for 8 wk, followed by monthly treatments for 1 y
SUPPLIED: Inj
NOTES: *Toxicity symptoms:* Myelosuppression, which may persist up to 3–8 wk after a dose and may be cumulative (minimized by a lifetime dose <50–60 mg/m^2), nausea and vomiting, anorexia, stomatitis, and renal toxicity. Microangiopathic hemolytic anemia (similar to hemolytic-uremic syndrome) with progressive renal failure. Venoocclusive disease of the liver, interstitial pneumonia, and alopecia (rare); extravasation reactions can be severe. Adjust dose in renal impairment

Mitotane (Lysodren)

COMMON USES: Palliative treatment of inoperable adrenal cortex carcinoma
ACTIONS: Exact action unclear; induces mitochondrial injury in adrenocortical cells
DOSAGE: 8–10 g/d in 3–4 ÷ doses (begin at 2 g/d with full glucocorticoid replacement therapy)
SUPPLIED: Tabs 500 mg
NOTES: *Toxicity symptoms:* Anorexia, nausea and vomiting, and diarrhea. Acute adrenal insufficiency may be precipitated by physical stresses (shock, trauma, infection), in which case corticosteroid replacement necessary. Allergic reactions (rare), visual disturbances, hemorrhagic cystitis, albuminuria, hematuria, HTN or hypotension, minor aches, and fever

Mitoxantrone (Novantrone)

COMMON USES: AML (with cytarabine), ALL, CML, breast and prostate cancer, non-Hodgkin's lymphoma
ACTIONS: DNA-intercalating agent; inhibitor of DNA topoisomerase II

DOSAGE: 12 mg/m^2/d for 3 d (ANLL induction), 12–14 mg/m^2 q 3 wk (advanced solid tumors)
SUPPLIED: Inj 20, 25, 30 mg
NOTES: *Toxicity symptoms:* Myelosuppression, nausea and vomiting, stomatitis, alopecia (infrequent), cardiotoxicity; cumulative dose not to exceed 160 mg/m^2 in patients receiving mediastinal radiation therapy or 120 mg/m^2 in patients receiving prior anthracycline therapy; dosage adjustment for hepatic failure may be warranted

Mivacurium (Mivacron)

COMMON USES: Adjunct to general anesthesia or mechanical ventilation
ACTIONS: Nondepolarizing neuromuscular blocker
DOSAGE: *Adults.* 0.15 mg/kg/dose IV; may need to repeat at 15-min intervals. *Peds.* 0.2 mg/kg/dose IV; may need to repeat at 10-min interval
SUPPLIED: Inj 0.5, 2 mg/mL
NOTES: Dosage adjustment in renal impairment

Moexipril (Univasc)

COMMON USES: HTN
ACTIONS: ACE inhibitor
DOSAGE: 7.5–30 mg in 1–2 ÷ doses administered 1 h ac
SUPPLIED: Tabs 7.5, 15 mg; adjust dose in renal impairment

Molindone (Moban)

COMMON USES: Psychotic disorders
ACTIONS: Piperazine phenothiazine
DOSAGE: *Adults.* 50-75 mg/d, ↑ to 225 mg/d if necessary. *Peds.* 3–5 y: 1–2.5 mg/d in 4 ÷ doses. *5–12 y:* 0.5–1.0 mg/kg/d in 4 ÷ doses
SUPPLIED: Tabs 5, 10, 25, 50, 100 mg; conc 20 mg/mL

Montelukast (Singulair)

COMMON USES: Prophylaxis and Rx of chronic asthma
ACTIONS: Leukotriene receptor antagonist
DOSAGE: *Adults >15 y.* 10 mg/d PO taken in PM. *Peds.* 6–14 y: 5 mg/d PO taken in PM. *2–5 y:* 4 mg/d PO taken in PM
SUPPLIED: Tabs 10 mg; chewable tabs 4, 5 mg
NOTES: NOT for acute asthma attacks

Moricizine (Ethmozine)

COMMON USES: Ventricular arrhythmias
ACTIONS: Class I antiarrhythmic
DOSAGE: 200–300 mg PO tid
SUPPLIED: Tabs 200, 250, 300 mg

Morphine (Roxanol, Duramorph, MS Contin, others) [C-II]

Used for emergency cardiac care (see Chapter 21)
COMMON USES: Relief of severe pain
ACTIONS: Narcotic analgesic
DOSAGE: *Adults.* Oral: 10–30 mg q4h PRN; SR tabs 30–60 mg q8–12h. *IV/IM:* 2.5–15 mg q2-6h. *Peds.* 0.1–0.2 mg/kg/dose IM/IV q2–4h PRN, to a max of 15 mg/dose
SUPPLIED: Tabs 10, 15, 30 mg; SR tabs 15, 30, 60 mg; soln 10, 20, 100 mg; supp 5, 10, 20 mg; inj 2, 4, 5, 8, 10, 15 mg/mL; preservative-free inj 0.5, 1 mg/mL
NOTES: Large number of narcotic side effects; may require scheduled dosing to relieve severe chronic pain. Duramorph and MS Contin commonly used SR forms

Moxifloxacin (Avelox)

COMMON USES: Acute sinusitis, acute bronchitis, and community acquired pneumonia
ACTIONS: Quinolone; inhibits DNA gyrase
DOSAGE: 400 mg/d once
SUPPLIED: Tabs 400 mg
NOTES: Active against gram (−) bacteria and *S. pneumoniae;* interactions with Mg, Ca, Al and Fe containing products and Class IA and III antiarrhythmic agents

Mupirocin (Bactroban)

COMMON USES: Impetigo; eradication of MRSA nasal carrier state
ACTIONS: Inhibits bacterial protein synthesis
DOSAGE: *Topical:* Apply small amount to affected area. *Nasal:* Apply bid in the nostrils
SUPPLIED: Oint 2%; cream 2%
NOTES: Do NOT use concurrently with other nasal products

Muromonab-CD3 [OKT3] (Orthoclone OKT3)

COMMON USES: Acute rejection following organ transplantation
ACTIONS: Blocks T-cell function
DOSAGE: *Adults.* 5 mg/d IV for 10–14 d. *Peds.* 0.1 mg/kg/d for 10–14 d
SUPPLIED: Inj 5 mg/5 mL
NOTES: Murine antibody; may cause significant fever and chills after the first dose; requires close patient monitoring for anaphylaxis B or pulmonary edema

Mycophenolate (CellCept)

COMMON USES: Prevention of organ rejection following transplantation
ACTIONS: Inhibits immunologically mediated inflammatory responses
DOSAGE: 1 g PO bid
SUPPLIED: Caps (as Mofetil) 250, 500 mg, inj 500 mg
NOTES: Used in conjunction with corticosteroids and cyclosporine

Nabumetone (Relafen)

COMMON USES: Arthritis and pain
ACTIONS: NSAID; inhibits prostaglandin synthesis
DOSAGE: 1000–2000 mg/d ÷ qd–bid
SUPPLIED: Tabs 500, 750 mg

Nadolol (Corgard)

COMMON USES: HTN and angina
ACTIONS: Competitively blocks β-adrenergic receptors (β_1 and β_2)
DOSAGE: 40–80 mg/d; up to 240 mg/d (angina) or 320 mg/d (HTN) may be needed
SUPPLIED: Tabs 20, 40, 80, 120, 160 mg

Nafcillin (Nallpen)

COMMON USES: Infections caused by susceptible strains of *Staphylococcus* and *Streptococcus*
ACTIONS: Bactericidal; inhibits cell wall synthesis
DOSAGE: *Adults.* 1–2 g IV q4–6h. *Peds.* 50–200 mg/kg/d ÷ q4–6h
SUPPLIED: Inj
NOTES: No adjustments for renal function

Naftifine (Naftin)

COMMON USES: Tinea cruris and tinea corporis
ACTIONS: Antifungal antibiotic
DOSAGE: Apply bid
SUPPLIED: 1% cream; gel

Nalbuphine (Nubain)

COMMON USES: Moderate to severe pain; preop and obstetrical analgesia
ACTIONS: Narcotic agonist–antagonist; inhibits ascending pain pathways
DOSAGE: *Adults.* 10–20 mg IM or IV q4–6h PRN; max of 160 mg per d; single max dose, 20 mg. *Peds.* 0.2 mg/kg IV or IM to a max dose of 20 mg
SUPPLIED: Inj 10, 20 mg/mL
NOTES: Causes CNS depression and drowsiness; use with caution in patients receiving opiates

Nalidixic Acid (NegGram)

COMMON USES: UTI caused by susceptible strains of *Proteus, Klebsiella, Enterobacter,* and *E. coli,* but not *Pseudomonas*
ACTIONS: Inhibits bacterial RNA and DNA synthesis
DOSAGE: *Adults.* 1 g PO qid. *Suppressive:* 500 mg PO qid. *Peds.* 55 mg/kg/24h in 4 ÷ doses. *Suppressive:* 33 mg/kg/d in 4 ÷ doses
SUPPLIED: Tabs 250 mg, 500 mg, 1 g; oral susp 250 mg/5 mL
NOTES: Resistance emerges within 48 h in a significant percentage of trials; may enhance the effect of oral anticoagulants; may cause CNS adverse effects that reverse on discontinuation; decreased effect with concurrent use of antacids

Naloxone (Narcan)

Used for emergency care (see also Chapter 21)
COMMON USES: Reversal of narcotic effect
ACTIONS: Competitive narcotic antagonist
DOSAGE: *Adults.* 0.4–2.0 mg IV, IM, or SC q 5 min; max total dose of 10 mg. *Peds.* 0.01–1.0 mg/kg/dose IV, IM, or SC; may repeat IV q 3 min for 3 doses PRN
SUPPLIED: Inj 0.4, 1.0 mg/mL; neonatal inj 0.02 mg/mL
NOTES: May precipitate acute withdrawal in addicts; if no response after 10 mg, suspect nonnarcotic cause

Naltrexone (Revia)

COMMON USES: Alcoholism and narcotic addiction
ACTIONS: Competitively binds to opioid receptors
DOSAGE: 50 mg/d PO
SUPPLIED: Tabs 50 mg
NOTES: May cause hepatotoxicity; do NOT give until opioid-free for 7–10 d

Naphazoline and Antazoline (Albalon-A Ophthalmic, others)
Naphazoline and Pheniramine Acetate (Naphcon A)

COMMON USES: Temporary relief from ocular redness and itching caused by allergy
ACTIONS: Vasoconstrictor and antihistamine
DOSAGE: 1–2 gtt up to 4×/d
SUPPLIED: Soln 15 mL
NOTES: Contra in those with glaucoma, children <6 y, and with contact lens use

Naproxen (Aleve [OTC], Naprosyn, Anaprox)

COMMON USES: Arthritis and pain
ACTIONS: NSAID; inhibits prostaglandin synthesis
DOSAGE: *Adults & Peds >12 y.* 200–500 mg bid–tid, to a max of 1500 mg/d
SUPPLIED: Tabs 200 [OTC], 250, 375, 500 mg; DR tabs 375, 500 mg; susp 125 mg/5 mL
NOTES: ↓ Dose in hepatic impairment

Naratriptan (Amerge)

COMMON USES: Acute migraine attacks
ACTIONS: Serotonin 5-HT$_1$ receptor antagonist

DOSAGE: 1–2.5 mg PO once; may be repeated once in 4 h
SUPPLIED: Tabs 1, 2.5 mg
NOTES: Contra in persons with severe renal impairment; adjust dose in renal dysfunction; avoid in angina, ischemic heart disease, uncontrolled HTN, and ergot administration

Nedocromil (Tilade)

COMMON USES: Mild to moderate asthma
ACTIONS: Antiinflammatory agent
DOSAGE: 2 inhal 4×/d
SUPPLIED: Met-dose inhaler

Nefazodone (Serzone)

COMMON USES: Depression
ACTIONS: Inhibits neuronal uptake of serotonin and norepinephrine
DOSAGE: Initially, 100 mg PO bid; usual effective range is 300–600 mg/d in 2 ÷ doses
SUPPLIED: Tabs 100, 150, 200, 250 mg
NOTES: May cause postural hypotension and allergic reactions

Nelfinavir (Viracept)

COMMON USES: HIV infection
ACTIONS: Protease inhibitor; results in formation of immature, noninfectious virion
DOSAGE: *Adults.* 750 mg PO tid or 1250 mg PO bid. *Peds.* 20–30 mg/kg PO tid
SUPPLIED: Tabs 250 mg; oral powder
NOTES: Food necessary to increase absorption; interacts with St. John's wort

Neomycin, Bacitracin and Polymyxin B (Neosporin Ointment) (see Bacitracin, Neomycin and Polymyxin, page 502)

Neomycin, Colistin, and Hydrocortisone (Cortisporin-TC Otic Drops)
Neomycin, Colistin, Hydrocortisone, and Thonzonium (Cortisporin-TC Otic Suspension)

COMMON USES: External otitis, infections of mastoidectomy and fenestration cavities
ACTIONS: Antibiotic and antiinflammatory
DOSAGE: *Adults.* 4–5 gtt in the ear(s) tid–qid. *Peds.* 3–4 gtt in ear(s) tid–qid
SUPPLIED: Otic gtt and susp

Neomycin and Dexamethasone (Neo-Dexameth Ophthalmic, NeoDecadron Ophthalmic)

COMMON USES: Steroid responsive inflammatory conditions of the cornea, conjunctiva, lid, and anterior segment
ACTIONS: Antibiotic with antiinflammatory corticosteroid
DOSAGE: 1–2 gtt in eye(s) q3–4h or thin coat tid–qid until response observed, then reduce dose to qd
SUPPLIED: Cream neomycin 0.5%/dexamethasone 0.1%; oint neomycin 0.35%/dexamethasone 0.05%; soln neomycin 0.35%/dexamethasone 0.1%

Neomycin, Polymyxin B (Neosporin Cream)

COMMON USES: Infection in minor cuts, scrapes, and burns
ACTIONS: Bactericidal antibiotic
DOSAGE: Apply bid–qid
SUPPLIED: Cream neomycin 3.5 mg/polymyxin B 10,000 U/g
NOTES: Different from Neosporin oint (See page 502)

Neomycin, Polymyxin-B and Dexamethasone, (Maxitrol)

COMMON USES: Steroid-responsive ocular conditions with bacterial infection
ACTIONS: Antibiotic with antiinflammatory corticosteroid
DOSAGE: 1–2 gtt in eye(s) q4–6h; apply oint in eye(s) 3–4×/d
SUPPLIED: Oint neomycin sulfate 3.5 mg/ polymyxin B sulfate 10,000 U/dexamethasone 0.1%/g; susp identical/5 mL
NOTES: Should be used under supervision of ophthalmologist

Neomycin, Polymyxin Bladder Irrigant

COMMON USES: Continuous irrigant for prophylaxis against bacteriuria and gram– bacteremia associated with indwelling catheter use
ACTIONS: Bactericidal antibiotic
DOSAGE: 1-mL irrigant added to 1 L of 0.9% NaCl; continuous irrigation of the bladder with 1–2 L of soln/24h
SUPPLIED: Ampules 1, 20 mL
NOTES: Potential for bacterial or fungal superinfection; slight possibility for neomycin-induced ototoxicity or nephrotoxicity

Neomycin, Polymyxin, and Hydrocortisone (Cortisporin Ophthalmic and Otic)

COMMON USES: Ocular and otic bacterial infections
ACTIONS: Antibiotic and antiinflammatory
DOSAGE: *Otic:* 3–4 gtt in the ear(s) 3–4×/d. *Ophth:* Apply a thin layer to the eye(s) or 1 gt 1–4×/d
SUPPLIED: Otic susp; ophth soln; ophth oint

Neomycin, Polymyxin-B and Prednisolone (Poly-Pred Opthalmic)

COMMON USES: Steroid-responsive ocular conditions with bacterial infection
ACTIONS: Antibiotic and antiinflammatory
DOSAGE: 1–2 gtt in eye(s) q4–6h; apply oint in eye(s) 3–4×/d
SUPPLIED: Susp, neomycin 0.35%/polymyxin B 10,000 U/prednisolone 0.5%/mL
NOTES: Should be used under supervision of ophthalmologist

Neomycin Sulfate

COMMON USES: Hepatic coma and preoperative bowel preparation
ACTIONS: Aminoglycoside; suppresses GI bacterial flora
DOSAGE: *Adults.* 3–12 g/24h PO in 3–4 ÷ doses. *Peds.* 50–100 mg/kg/24h PO in 3–4 ÷ dose
SUPPLIED: Tabs 500 mg; oral soln 125 mg/5 mL
NOTES: Part of the Condon bowel prep

Nevirapine (Viramune)

COMMON USES: HIV infection
ACTIONS: Nonnucleoside reverse transcriptase inhibitor
DOSAGE: *Adults.* Initially 200 mg/d for 14 d; then 200 mg bid. *Peds.* <8 y: 4 mg/kg/d for 14 d; then 7 mg/kg bid. >8 y: 4 mg/kg/d for 14 d; then 4 mg/kg bid
SUPPLIED: Tabs 200 mg; susp 50 mg/5 mL
NOTES: May cause life-threatening rash; give without regard to food

Niacin (Nicolar)

COMMON USES: Adjunctive therapy in patients with significant refractory hyperlipidemia
ACTIONS: Inhibits lipolysis; decreases esterification of triglycerides; increases lipoprotein lipase activity
DOSAGE: 1–6 g tid; max of 9 g/d
SUPPLIED: SR caps 125, 250, 300, 400, 500 mg; tabs 25, 50, 100, 250, 500 mg; SR tabs 150, 250, 500, 750 mg; elixir 50 mg/5 mL
NOTES: Upper body and facial flushing and warmth following dose; may cause GI upset

22

Nicardipine (Cardene)

COMMON USES: Chronic stable angina and HTN; prophylaxis of migraine
ACTIONS: Ca channel-blocker
DOSAGE: *Oral:* 20–40 mg PO tid. *SR:* 30–60 mg PO bid. *IV:* 5 mg/h IV cont inf; ↑ by 2.5 mg/h q 15 min to max 15 mg/h
SUPPLIED: Caps 20, 30 mg; SR caps 30, 45, 60 mg; inj 2.5 mg/mL
NOTES: *Oral-to-IV conversion:* 20 mg tid = 0.5 mg/h, 30 mg tid = 1.2 mg/h, 40 mg tid = 2.2 mg/h; adjust dose in renal or hepatic impairment

Nicotine Gum (Nicorette, Nicorette DS)

COMMON USES AND ACTIONS: See Nicotine, Transdermal
DOSAGE: 9–12 pieces/d PRN. Max 30 pieces/d
SUPPLIED: 2 mg (96 pieces/box); Nicorette DS has 4 mg/piece
NOTES: Patients must stop smoking and perform behavior modification for max effect

Nicotine Nasal Spray (Nicotrol NS)

COMMON USES: Aid to smoking cessation for the relief of nicotine withdrawal
ACTIONS: Provides systemic delivery of nicotine
DOSAGE: 0.5 mg/actuation; 1–2 sprays/h, not to exceed 10 sprays/h.
SUPPLIED: Nasal inhaler 10 mg/mL
NOTES: Patients must stop smoking and perform behavior modification for max effect

Nicotine, Transdermal (Habitrol, Nicoderm, Nicotrol, Prostep)

COMMON USES: Aid to smoking cessation for the relief of nicotine withdrawal
ACTIONS: Provides systemic delivery of nicotine
DOSAGE: Individualized to the patient's needs; apply 1 patch (14–22 mg/d), and taper over 6 wk
SUPPLIED: Habitrol and Nicoderm 7, 14, 21 mg of nicotine/24h; Nicotrol 5, 10, 15 mg/24h; ProStep 11, 22 mg/24h
NOTES: Nicotrol to be worn for 16 h to mimic smoking patterns; others worn for 24 h; patients must stop smoking and perform behavior modification for max effect

Nifedipine (Procardia, Procardia Xl, Adalat, Adalat CC)

COMMON USES: Vasospastic or chronic stable angina and HTN; tocolytic
ACTIONS: Ca channel-blocker
DOSAGE: *Adults.* SR tabs 30–90 mg/d. *Tocolysis:* 10–20 mg PO q4–6h. *Peds.* 0.6–0.9 mg/kg/24h ÷ tid–qid
SUPPLIED: Caps 10, 20 mg; SR tabs 30, 60, 90 mg
NOTES: Headaches common on initial treatment; reflex tachycardia may occur with regular release dosage forms; Adalat CC and Procardia XL are NOT interchangeable; SL administration NOT advisable

Nilutamide (Nilandron)

COMMON USES: Combination with surgical castration for the treatment of metastatic prostate cancer
ACTIONS: Nonsteroidal antiandrogen
DOSAGE: 300 mg/d in ÷ doses for the first 30 d, then 150 mg/d
SUPPLIED: 50-, 150-mg tabs
NOTES: *Toxicity symptoms:* Hot flashes, loss of libido, impotence, diarrhea, nausea, vomiting, gynecomastia, hepatic dysfunction (follow LFTs), and interstitial pneumonitis

Nimodipine (Nimotop)

COMMON USES: Prevention of vasospasm following subarachnoid hemorrhage
ACTIONS: Ca channel-blocker
DOSAGE: 60 mg PO q4h for 21 d

SUPPLIED: Caps 30 mg
NOTES: Contents of caps may be extracted and administered down a NG tube if caps cannot be swallowed whole; dosage adjustment in hepatic failure

Nisoldipine (Sular)

COMMON USES: HTN
ACTIONS: Ca channel-blocker
DOSAGE: 10–60 mg/d PO
SUPPLIED: ER tabs 10, 20, 30, 40 mg
NOTES: Do NOT take with grapefruit juice or high-fat meal; ↓ starting doses in elderly or hepatic impairment

Nitrofurantoin (Macrodantin, Furadantin, Macrobid)

COMMON USES: Prevention and Rx UTI
ACTIONS: Bacteriostatic; interferes with carbohydrate metabolism
DOSAGE: *Adults.* Suppression: 50–100 mg/d PO. *Rx:* 50–100 mg PO qid. *Peds.* 5–7 mg/kg/24h in 4 ÷ doses
SUPPLIED: Caps and tabs 50, 100 mg; SR caps [Macrobid] 100 mg; susp 25 mg/5 mL
NOTES: GI side effects common; should be taken with food, milk, or antacid; macrocrystals (Macrodantin) cause less nausea than other forms of the drug; avoid if CrCl <50 mL/min

Nitroglycerin (Nitrostat, Nitrolingual, Nitro-Bid Ointment, Nitro-Bid IV, Nitrodisc, Transderm-Nitro, others)

Used for emergency cardiac care (see Chapter 21)
COMMON USES: Angina pectoris, acute and prophylactic therapy, CHF, BP control
ACTIONS: Relaxation of vascular smooth muscle
DOSAGE: *Adults.* SL: 1 tab q 5 min SL PRN for 3 doses. *Translingual:* 1–2 met-doses sprayed onto the oral mucosa q3–5 min, max 3 doses. *Oral:* 2.5–9 mg tid. *IV:* 5–20 µg/min, titrated to effect. *Topical:* Apply 1–2 in. of oint to the chest wall q6h, then wipe off at night. *TD:* 5–20-cm patch qd. *Peds.* 1 µg/kg/min IV, titrated to effect
SUPPLIED: SL tabs 0.3, 0.4, 0.6 mg; translingual spray 0.4 mg/dose; SR caps 2.5, 6.5, 9, 13 mg; SR tabs 2.6, 6.5, 9.0 mg; inj 0.5, 5, 10 mg/mL; oint 2%; TD patches 2.5, 5, 7.5, 10, 15 mg/24h; buccal CR 1, 2, 3 mg
NOTES: Tolerance to nitrates develops with chronic use after 1–2 wk; can be avoided by providing a nitrate-free period each day; use shorter-acting nitrates tid, and remove long-acting patches and oint before hs to prevent development of tolerance. (See Table 20–10, page 637.)

Nitroprusside (Nitropress)

COMMON USES: Hypertensive emergency, aortic dissection, and pulmonary edema
ACTIONS: Reduces systemic vascular resistance
DOSAGE: *Adults & Peds.* 0.5–10 µg/kg/min IV inf, titrated to desired effect; usual dose 3 µg/kg/min
SUPPLIED: Inj 10 mg/mL, 25 mg/mL
NOTES: Thiocyanate, the metabolite, excreted by the kidney; thiocyanate toxicity occurs at plasma levels of 5–10 mg/dL; if used to treat aortic dissection; use β-blocker concomitantly. (See Table 20–10, page 637.)

Nizatidine (Axid)

COMMON USES: Duodenal ulcers, GERD, and heartburn
ACTIONS: H_2-receptor antagonist
DOSAGE: *Active ulcer:* 150 mg PO bid or 300 mg PO hs; maintenance 150 mg PO hs. *GERD:* 150 mg PO bid; maintenance PO hs. *Heartburn:* 75 mg PO bid
SUPPLIED: Caps 75, 150, 300 mg
NOTES: Dosage adjustment in renal impairment

Norepinephrine (Levophed)

Used for emergency cardiac care (see Chapter 21)
COMMON USES: Acute hypotensive states
ACTIONS: Peripheral vasoconstrictor acting on both the arterial and venous beds
DOSAGE: *Adults.* 8–12 µg/min IV, titrated to desired effect. *Peds.* 0.05–0.1 mg/kg/min IV, titrated to desired effect
SUPPLIED: Inj 1 mg/mL
NOTES: Correct blood volume depletion as much as possible prior to initiation of vasopressor therapy; drug interaction with tricyclic antidepressants leading to severe profound HTN; infuse into large vein to avoid extravasation; phentolamine 5–10 mg/10 mL NS injected locally as an antidote to extravasation. (See Table 20–10, page 637.)

Norfloxacin (Noroxin)

COMMON USES: Complicated and uncomplicated UTI caused by a wide variety of gram (−) bacteria, prostatitis, and infectious diarrhea
ACTIONS: Quinolone, inhibits DNA gyrase
DOSAGE: *Adults.* 400 mg PO bid. *Gonorrhea:* 800 mg as single dose. *Conjunctivitis:* 1–2 gtt qid
SUPPLIED: Tabs 400 mg; ophth soln 0.3%
NOTES: Do NOT use in PRG; drug interactions with antacids, theophylline, and caffeine; good concentrations in the kidney and urine, poor blood levels; do NOT use for urosepsis; dosage adjustment in renal impairment

Norgestrel (Ovrette)

COMMON USES: Contraceptive
ACTIONS: Prevent follicular maturation and ovulation
DOSAGE: 1 tab/d; begin day 1 of menses
SUPPLIED: Tabs 0.075 mg
NOTES: Progestin-only products have higher risk of failure in prevention of pregnancy

Nortriptyline (Aventyl, Pamelor)

COMMON USES: Endogenous depression
ACTIONS: Tricyclic antidepressant; increases the synaptic concentrations of serotonin and/or norepinephrine in the CNS
DOSAGE: *Adults.* 25 mg PO tid–qid; doses >150 mg/d NOT recommended. *Elderly:* 10–25 mg hs. *Peds.* 6–7 y: 10 mg/d. *8–11 y:* 10–20 mg/d. *>11 y:* 25–35 mg/d
SUPPLIED: Caps 10, 25, 50, 75 mg; soln 10 mg/5 mL
NOTES: Many anticholinergic side effects, including blurred vision, urinary retention, and dry mouth; max effect seen after 2 wk of therapy

Nystatin (Mycostatin, Nilstat, others)

COMMON USES: Mucocutaneous *Candida* infections (thrush, vaginitis)
ACTIONS: Alters membrane permeability
DOSAGE: *Adults.* Oral: 400,000–600,000 U PO "swish and swallow" qid. *Vaginal:* 1 tab vaginally hs for 2 wk. *Topical:* Apply bid–tid to the affected area. *Peds.* Infants: 200,000 U PO q6h. *Children:* See Adult dosage
SUPPLIED: Oral susp 100,000 U/mL; oral tabs 500,000 U; troches 200,000 U; vaginal tabs 100,000 U; topical cream and oint 100,000 U/g
NOTES: Not absorbed orally; therefore, NOT effective for systemic infections

Octreotide (Sandostatin)

COMMON USES: Suppresses or inhibits severe diarrhea associated with carcinoid and neuroendocrine tumors of the intestinal tract; bleeding esophageal varices
ACTIONS: Long-acting peptide that mimics the natural hormone somatostatin

DOSAGE: *Adults.* 100–600 µg/d SC in 2–4 ÷ doses; initiate at 50 µg qd–bid. *Peds.* 1–10 µg/kg/24h SC in 2–4 ÷ doses
SUPPLIED: Inj 0.05, 0.1, 0.2, 0.5, 1 mg/mL
NOTES: May cause nausea, vomiting, and abdominal discomfort

Ofloxacin (Floxin, Ocuflox Ophthalmic)

COMMON USES: Infections of the lower respiratory tract, skin and skin structure, and urinary tract, prostatitis, uncomplicated gonorrhea, and *Chlamydia* infections; topical for bacterial conjunctivitis; acute otitis media in children >1 y tympanostomy tubes; otitis externa in adults and children >1 y; if perforated ear drum >12 y
ACTIONS: Bactericidal: inhibits DNA gyrase
DOSAGE: *Adults.* 200–400 mg PO bid or IV q12h. *Adults & Peds.* >1 y: Ophth 1–2 gtt in eye(s) q2–4h for 2 d, then qid for 5 more d. *Peds.* Do NOT administer systemically in children <18 y. *Peds 1–12 y:* Otic 5 gtt in ear(s) bid for 10 d. *Adults & Peds >12 y:* Otic 10 gtt in ear(s) bid for 10 d
SUPPLIED: Tabs 200, 300, 400 mg; inj 20, 40 mg/mL; ophth 0.3%
NOTES: May cause nausea and vomiting, diarrhea, insomnia, and headache; drug interactions with antacids, sucralfate, and aluminum-, calcium-, magnesium-, iron-, or zinc-containing products decrease absorption; may increase theophylline levels; dosage adjustment in renal impairment; ophth form used for ears

Olanzapine (Zyprexa)

COMMON USES: Psychotic disorders
ACTIONS: Dopamine and serotonin antagonist
DOSAGE: ↑ to max of 20 mg/d
SUPPLIED: Tabs 5, 7.5, 10 mg
NOTES: May take many weeks to titrate to therapeutic dose; cigarette smoking will decrease levels

Olsalazine (Dipentum)

COMMON USES: Maintenance of remission of ulcerative colitis
ACTIONS: Topical antiinflammatory activity
DOSAGE: 500 mg PO bid
SUPPLIED: Caps 250 mg
NOTES: Take with food; may cause diarrhea

Omeprazole (Prilosec)

COMMON USES: Duodenal and gastric ulcers, Zollinger–Ellison syndrome, GERD, and *H. pylori* infections
ACTIONS: Proton-pump inhibitor
DOSAGE: 20–40 mg PO qd–bid
SUPPLIED: Caps 10, 20, 40 mg
NOTES: Combination (ie, antibiotic) therapy necessary for *H. pylori* infection

Ondansetron (Zofran)

COMMON USES: Prevention of nausea and vomiting associated with cancer chemotherapy and postoperative nausea and vomiting
ACTIONS: Serotonin receptor antagonist
DOSAGE: *Adults & Peds.* Chemotherapy: 0.15 mg/kg/dose IV prior to chemotherapy, then repeated 4 and 8 h after the first dose or 4–8 mg PO tid; administer the first dose 30 min prior to chemotherapy. *Adults.* Postop: 4 mg IV immediately before induction of anesthesia or postop
SUPPLIED: Tabs 4, 8 mg; inj 2 mg/mL
NOTES: May cause diarrhea and headache; administer on a schedule, NOT PRN

Oprelvekin (Neumega)

COMMON USES: Prevention of severe thrombocytopenia due to chemotherapy
ACTIONS: Promotes proliferation and maturation of megakaryocytes
DOSAGE: *Adults.* 50 µg/kg/d SC for 10–21 d. *Peds.* 75–100 µg/kg/d SC for 10–21 d
SUPPLIED: Inj
NOTES: Interleukin-11

Oral Contraceptives, Biphasic, Monophasic, Triphasic, Progestin Only (see Table 22–3, pages 623–625)

COMMON USES: Birth control and regulation of anovulatory bleeding
ACTIONS: *Birth Control:* Suppresses LH surge, prevents ovulation, progestins thicken cervical mucous, inhibits fallopian tubule cilia, ↓ endometrial thickness and hence ↓ chances of fertilization. *Anovulatory bleeding:* Cyclic hormones mimic the body's natural cycle and help regulate the endometrial lining, resulting in regular bleeding q 28 d; may also reduce uterine bleeding and dysmenorrhea
DOSAGE: 28-d cycle pills taken qd. 21-d cycle pills taken qd, no pills taken during the last 7 d of the cycle (during the menstrual period)
SUPPLIED: 28-d cycle pills (21 hormonally active pills + 7 placebo/Fe supplementation). 21-d cycle pills (21 hormonally active pills). See Table 22–3, page 000
NOTES: Taken correctly, 99.9% effective for preventing pregnancy, but do not protect against STD; encourage use of additional barrier contraceptive. Over long periods can ↓ risk of ectopic pregnancy, benign breast disease, and future development of ovarian, and uterine cancer. *Absolute contra:* Undiagnosed abnormal vaginal bleeding, pregnancy, estrogen-dependent malignancy, hypercoagulation disorders, liver disease, and smokers >35 y. *Relative contra:* Migraine headaches, HTN, diabetes, sickle cell disease, and gallbladder disease. *Rx for menstrual cycle control:* Start with a monophasic pill. Pill must be taken for 3 mo before switching to another brand. Abnormal bleeding continues, changed to higher estrogen dose pill.

   Rx for birth control: Choose pill with the most beneficial side effect profile for particular patient. Side effects numerous and due to symptoms of estrogen excess or progesterone deficiency. Because each pill's side effect profile is unique (found in package insert), Rx may be tailored to specific patient. *Common side effects:* Intramenstrual bleeding, oligomenorrhea, amenorrhea, increased appetite/weight gain, loss of libido, fatigue, depression, mood swings, mastalgia, headaches, melasma, increase vaginal discharge, acne/greasy skin, corneal edema, nausea

Orphenadrine (Norflex)

COMMON USES: Muscle spasms
ACTIONS: Central atropine-like effects cause indirect skeletal muscle relaxation, euphoria, and analgesia
DOSAGE: 100 mg PO bid, 60 mg IM/IV q12h
SUPPLIED: Tabs 100 mg; SR tabs 100 mg; inj 30 mg/mL

Oseltamivir (Tamiflu)

COMMON USES: Influenza A and B
ACTIONS: Inhibition of viral neuraminidase
DOSAGE: 75 mg bid for 5 d
SUPPLIED: Caps 75 mg
NOTES: Initiate within 48 h of symptom onset; ↓ dose in renal impairment

Oxacillin (Bactocill, Prostaphlin)

COMMON USES: Infections caused by susceptible strains of *S. aureus* and *Streptococcus*
ACTIONS: Bactericidal; inhibits cell wall synthesis

DOSAGE: *Adults.* 1–2 mg IV q4–6h. *Peds.* 150–200 mg/kg/d IV q4–6h
SUPPLIED: Inj; caps 250, 500 mg; soln 250 mg/5 mL

Oxaprozin (Daypro)

COMMON USES: Arthritis and pain
ACTIONS: NSAID; inhibits prostaglandin synthesis
DOSAGE: 600–1200 mg/d
SUPPLIED: Caplets 600 mg

Oxazepam (Serax) [C]

COMMON USES: Anxiety, acute alcohol withdrawal, and anxiety with depressive symptoms
ACTIONS: Benzodiazepine
DOSAGE: *Adults.* 10–15 mg PO tid–qid; severe anxiety and alcohol withdrawal may require up to 30 mg qid. *Peds.* 1 mg/kg/d in ÷ doses
SUPPLIED: Caps 10, 15, 30 mg; tabs 15 mg
NOTES: One of the metabolites of diazepam (Valium); avoid abrupt discontinuation

Oxcarbazepine (Trileptal)

COMMON USES: Partial seizures
ACTIONS: Produce blockage of voltage-sensitive Na channels, resulting in stabilization of hyperexcited neural membranes
DOSAGE: *Adults.* 300 mg bid, ↑ dose weekly to a usual dose of 1200–2400 mg/d. *Peds.* 8–10 mg/kg bid, NOT to exceed 600 mg/d; ↑ dose weekly to target maintenance dose
SUPPLIED: Tabs 150, 300, 600 mg
NOTES: May cause clinically significant hyponatremia; possible cross-sensitivity to carbamazepine

Oxiconazole (Oxistat)

COMMON USES: Tinea pedis, tinea cruris, and tinea corporis
ACTIONS: Antifungal antibiotic
DOSAGE: Apply bid
SUPPLIED: 1% Cream; lotion

Oxybutynin (Ditropan, Ditropan XL)

COMMON USES: Symptomatic relief of urgency, nocturia, and incontinence associated with neurogenic or reflex neurogenic bladder
ACTIONS: Direct antispasmodic effect on smooth muscle; increases bladder capacity
DOSAGE: *Adults & Peds > 5 y.* 5 mg PO tid–qid. *Adults.* ER 5 mg PO qd; ↑ to 30 mg/d PO, (5 and 10 mg/tab). *Peds 1–5 y.* 0.02 mg/kg/dose bid–qid (syrup 5 mg/5 mL)
SUPPLIED: Tabs 5 mg; ER tabs 5, 10, 15 mg; syrup 5 mg/5 mL
NOTES: Anticholinergic side effects

Oxycodone [Dihydrohydroxycodeinone] (OxyContin, OxyIR, Roxicodone) [C-II]

COMMON USES: Moderate to severe pain, normally used in combination with nonnarcotic analgesics
ACTIONS: Narcotic analgesic
DOSAGE: *Adults.* 5 mg PO q6h PRN. *Peds.* 6–12 y: 1.25 mg PO q6h PRN. >*12 y:* 2.5 mg q6h PRN
SUPPLIED: Immediate release caps (OxyIR) 5 mg; tabs (Percolone) 5 mg tabs; CR (OxyContin) 10, 20, 40, 80 mg; liq 5 mg/5 mL; soln conc 20 mg/mL
NOTES: Usually prescribed in combination with acetaminophen or aspirin; OxyContin useful for chronic cancer pain

Oxycodone and Acetaminophen (Percocet, Tylox) [C-II]

COMMON USES: Moderate to severe pain

ACTIONS: Narcotic analgesic
DOSAGE: *Adults.* 1–2 tabs/caps PO q4–6h PRN. *Peds.* Oxycodone 0.05–0.15 mg/kg/dose q4–6h PRN; up to 5 mg/dose
SUPPLIED: Percocet tabs 5 mg of oxycodone, 325 mg of acetaminophen; Tylox caps 5 mg of oxycodone, 500 mg of acetaminophen. Soln 5 mg of oxycodone and 325 mg of acetaminophen/5 mL
NOTES: Acetaminophen max dose of 4 g/d

Oxycodone and Aspirin (Percodan, Percodan-Demi) [C-II]

COMMON USES: Moderate to moderately severe pain
ACTIONS: Narcotic analgesic with NSAID
DOSAGE: *Adults.* 1–2 tabs/caps PO q4–6h PRN. *Peds.* 0.05–0.15 mg/kg/dose q4–6h, max 5 mg/dose (based on oxycodone)
SUPPLIED: Percodan 4.5 mg oxycodone hydrochloride 0.38 mg oxycodone terephthalate, 325 mg aspirin; Percodan-Demi 2.25 mg oxycodone hydrochloride, 0.19 mg oxycodone terephthalate, 325 mg aspirin

Oxymorphone (Numorphan) [C-II]

COMMON USES: Moderate to severe pain, sedative
ACTIONS: Narcotic analgesic
DOSAGE: 0.5 mg IM, SC, IV initially, 1–1.5 mg q4–6h PRN. *PR:* 5 mg q4–6h PRN
SUPPLIED: Inj 1, 1.5 mg/mL; supp 5 mg
NOTES: Chemically related to hydromorphone

Oxytocin (Pitocin, Syntocinon)

COMMON USES: Induction of labor and control of postpartum hemorrhage; promote milk let down in lactating woman
ACTIONS: Stimulate muscular contractions of the uterus, stimulate milk flow during nursing
DOSAGE: 0.001–0.002 U/min IV inf; titrate to desired effect, to a max of 0.02 U/min. *Breast feeding:* 1 spray in both nostrils 2–3 min before feeding
SUPPLIED: Inj 10 U/mL; nasal soln 40 U/mL
NOTES: Can cause uterine rupture and fetal death; monitor vital signs closely; nasal form for breast feeding only

Paclitaxel (Taxol)

COMMON USES: Ovarian and breast cancer
ACTIONS: Mitotic spindle poison promotes microtubule assembly and stabilization against depolymerization (a taxrane)
DOSAGE: 135–250 mg/m^2 as a 3–24-h IV inf
SUPPLIED: Inj 6 mg/mL
NOTES: *Toxicity symptoms:* Hypersensitivity reactions (dyspnea, hypotension, urticaria, rash) usually within 10 min of starting infusion; minimize with corticosteroid, antihistamine (H$_1$ and H$_2$ antagonist) pretreatment. Myelosuppression, peripheral neuropathy, transient ileus, myalgia, bradycardia, hypotension, mucositis, diarrhea, nausea and vomiting, fever, rash, headache, and phlebitis. Hematologic toxicity schedule-dependent; leukopenia dose-limiting by 24-h inf; neurotoxicity dose-limiting by short (1–3-h) inf. Infuse this agent in glass or polyolefin containers using polyethylene-lined nitroglycerin tubing sets. PVC inf sets result in leaching of plasticizer

Pamidronate (Aredia)

COMMON USES: Hypercalcemia of malignancy and Paget's disease; palliation of symptomatic bone metastases
ACTIONS: Inhibition of normal and abnormal bone resorption
DOSAGE: *Hypercalcemia:* 60 mg IV over 4 h or 90 mg IV over 24 h. *Paget's disease:* 30 mg/d IV for 3 d
SUPPLIED: Powder for inj 30, 60, 90 mg

NOTES: *Toxicity symptoms:* Fever, tissue irritation at inj site, uveitis, fluid overload, HTN, abdominal pain, nausea and vomiting, constipation, UTI, bone pain, hypokalemia, hypocalcemia, hypomagnesemia, and hypophosphatemia; slow inf rate necessary

Pancreatin/Pancrelipase (Pancrease, Cotazyme, Creon, Ultrase)

COMMON USES: Exocrine pancreatic secretion deficiency (CF, chronic pancreatitis, other pancreatic insufficiency) and for steatorrhea of malabsorption syndrome
ACTIONS: Pancreatic enzyme supplementation
DOSAGE: *Adults & Peds.* 1–3 caps (tabs) with meals and snacks; dosage ↑ to 8 caps (tabs)
SUPPLIED: Caps, tabs
NOTES: Avoid antacids; may cause nausea, abdominal cramps, or diarrhea; do not crush or chew EC products; dosage dependent on patient's digestive requirements

Pancuronium (Pavulon)

COMMON USES: Rx of patients on mechanical ventilation
ACTIONS: Nondepolarizing neuromuscular blocker
DOSAGE: *Adults.* 2–4 mg IV q2–4h PRN. *Peds.* 0.02–0.10 mg/kg/dose q2–4h PRN
SUPPLIED: Inj 1, 2 mg/mL
NOTES: Intubate patient and keep on controlled ventilation; use an adequate amount of sedation or analgesia; adjust dose for renal or hepatic impairment

Pantoprazole (Protonix)

COMMON USES: GERD
ACTION: Proton pump inhibitor
DOSAGE: 40 mg/d PO
SUPPLIED: Tabs 40 mg
NOTES: DR tabs, therefore do NOT crush or chew tabs

Paregoric [C]

COMMON USES: Diarrhea, pain and neonatal opiate withdrawal syndrome
ACTIONS: Narcotic
DOSAGE: *Adults.* 5–10 mL PO qd–qid PRN. *Peds.* 0.25–0.5 mL/kg qd–qid. *Neonatal withdrawal syndrome:* 3–6 gtt PO q3–6h PRN to relieve symptoms for 3–5 d, then taper over 2–4 wk
NOTES: Contains opium; short-term use only. (See also Kaolin-Pectin.)

Paroxetine (Paxil)

COMMON USES: Depression, OCD, panic disorder, and social anxiety disorder
ACTIONS: Serotonin reuptake inhibitor
DOSAGE: 10–60 mg PO as a single daily dose
SUPPLIED: Tabs 10, 20, 30,40 mg; susp 10 mg/5 mL
NOTES: Should be administered in AM; may cause sexual dysfunction

Penbutolol (Levatol)

COMMON USES: HTN
ACTIONS: Competitively blocks β-adrenergic receptors, β_1, β_2
DOSAGE: 20–40 mg/d
SUPPLIED: Tabs 20 mg

Penciclovir (Denavir)

COMMON USES: Herpes simplex
ACTIONS: Competitive inhibitor of DNA polymerase
DOSAGE: Apply topically at first sign of lesions, then q2h for 4 d
SUPPLIED: Cream 1%

Penicillin G, Aqueous (Potassium or Sodium) (Pfizerpen)

COMMON USES: Most gram (+) infections (except penicillin-resistant staphylococci), including streptococci, *N. meningitidis,* syphilis, clostridia, and some coliforms
ACTIONS: Bactericidal; inhibits cell wall synthesis
DOSAGE: *Adults.* 400,000–800,000 U PO qid; IV doses vary greatly depending on indications; range from 1.2–24 million U/d in ÷ doses q4h. *Peds.* Newborns <1 wk: 25,000–50,000 U/kg/dose IV q12h. *Infants 1 wk < 1 mo:* 25,000–50,000 U/kg/dose IV q8h. *Children:* 100,000–300,000 U/kg/24h IV ÷ q4h
SUPPLIED: Powder for inj
NOTES: Beware of hypersensitivity reactions. Dosage adjustment in renal impairment

Penicillin G Benzathine (Bicillin)

COMMON USES: Useful as a single-dose treatment regimen for streptococcal pharyngitis, rheumatic fever and glomerulonephritis prophylaxis, and syphilis
ACTIONS: Bactericidal; inhibits cell wall synthesis
DOSAGE: *Adults.* 1.2–2.4 million U deep IM inj q 2–4 wk. *Peds.* 50,000 U/kg/dose to a max of 2.4 million U/dose deep IM inj q 2–4 wk
SUPPLIED: Inj 300,000, 600,000 U/mL
NOTES: Sustained action with detectable levels up to 4 wk; considered the drug of choice for treatment of noncongenital syphilis; Bicillin L-A contains the benzathine salt only; Bicillin C-R contains a combination of the benzathine and procaine (300,000 U of procaine with 300,000 U of benzathine/mL or 900,000 U of benzathine with 300,000 U of procaine/2 mL)

Penicillin G Procaine (Wycillin, others)

COMMON USES: Moderately severe infections caused by penicillin G-sensitive organisms that respond to low, persistent serum levels
ACTIONS: Bactericidal; inhibits cell wall synthesis
DOSAGE: *Adults.*0.6–4.8 million U/d in ÷ doses q12–24h. *Peds.* 25,000–50,000 U/kg/d IM ÷ qd–bid
SUPPLIED: Inj 300,000, 500,000, 600,000 U/mL
NOTES: Long-acting parenteral penicillin; blood levels up to 15 h; give probenecid at least 30 min prior to administration of penicillin to prolong action

Penicillin V (Pen-Vee K, Veetids, others)

COMMON USES: Most gram (+) infections, including streptococci, *N. meningitidis,* syphilis, clostridia, and some coliforms
ACTIONS: Bactericidal; inhibits cell wall synthesis
DOSAGE: *Adults.* 250–500 mg PO q6h. *Peds.* 25–50 mg/kg/24h PO in 4 ÷ doses
SUPPLIED: Tabs 125, 250, 500 mg; susp 125, 250 mg/5 mL
NOTES: Well-tolerated oral penicillin; 250 mg = 400,000 U of penicillin G

Pentamidine (Pentam 300, Nebupent)

COMMON USES: Rx and prevention of PCP
ACTIONS: Inhibits DNA, RNA, phospholipid, and protein synthesis
DOSAGE: *Adults & Peds.* 4 mg/kg/24h IV qd for 14–21 d. *Adults & Peds >5 y.* Prevention: 300 mg once q 4 wk, administered via Respigard II neb
SUPPLIED: Inj 300 mg/vial; aerosol 300 mg
NOTES: Monitor for severe hypotension following IV administration; associated with pancreatic islet cell necrosis leading to hypoglycemia and hyperglycemia; monitor hematology lab results for leukopenia and thrombocytopenia; IV requires dosage adjustment in renal impairment

Pentazocine (Talwin) [C-IV]

COMMON USES: Moderate to severe pain

ACTIONS: Partial narcotic agonist–antagonist
DOSAGE: *Adults.* 30 mg IM or IV; 50–100 mg PO q3–4h PRN. *Peds.* 5–8 y: 15 mg IM q4h PRN. *8–14 y:* 30 mg IM q4h PRN
SUPPLIED: Tabs 50 mg (+ naloxone 0.5 mg); inj 30 mg/mL
NOTES: 30–60 mg IM equianalgesic to 10 mg of morphine IM; associated with considerable dysphoria; dosage adjustment in renal impairment

Pentobarbital (Nembutal, others) [C-II]

COMMON USES: Insomnia, convulsions, and induced coma following severe head injury
ACTIONS: Barbiturate
DOSAGE: *Adults.* Sedative: 20–40 mg PO or PR q6–12h. *Hypnotic:* 100–200 mg PO or PR hs PRN. *Induced coma:* Load 5–10 mg/kg IV, then maintenance 1–3 mg/kg/h IV cont inf to keep the serum level between 20 and 50 mg/mL. *Peds.* Hypnotic: 2–6 mg/kg/dose PO hs PRN. *Induced coma:* See adult dosage
SUPPLIED: Caps 50, 100 mg; elixir 18.5 mg/5 mL; supp 30, 60, 120, 200 mg; inj 50 mg/mL
NOTES: Can cause respiratory depression; may produce profound hypotension when used aggressively IV for cerebral edema; tolerance to sedative–hypnotic effect acquired within 1–2 wk; reduce dose in severe hepatic impairment

Pentosan Polysulfate Sodium (Elmiron)

COMMON USES: Relief of pain/discomfort associated with interstitial cystitis
ACTIONS: Acts as buffer on bladder wall
DOSAGE: 100 mg PO tid on empty stomach with water 1 h ac or 2 h pc
SUPPLIED: Caps 100 mg
NOTES: *Toxicity symptoms:* Alopecia, diarrhea, nausea, and headaches

Pentostatin (Nipent)

COMMON USES: Hairy cell leukemia, CLL, mycosis fungoides, ALL, and adult T-cell leukemia
ACTIONS: Irreversible inhibitor of adenosine deaminase
DOSAGE: 4–5 mg/m^2/wk for 3 consecutive weeks
SUPPLIED: Inj 10 mg
NOTES: *Toxicity symptoms:* Renal dysfunction; myelosuppression (especially leukopenia), lymphocytopenia, fever, and infection possible; neurologic toxicity symptoms (lethargy and fatigue, dry skin, keratoconjunctivitis, and nausea and vomiting); dosage adjustment in renal impairment

Pentoxifylline (Trental)

COMMON USES: Symptomatic management of peripheral vascular disease
ACTIONS: Lowers blood cell viscosity by restoring erythrocyte flexibility
DOSAGE: 400 mg PO tid pc
SUPPLIED: Tabs 400 mg
NOTES: Treat for at least 8 wk to see full effect; ↓ to bid if GI or CNS effects occur

Pergolide (Permax)

COMMON USES: Parkinson's disease
ACTIONS: Centrally active dopamine receptor agonist
DOSAGE: Initially, 0.05 mg PO tid, titrated q 2–3 d to desired effect, usual maintenance dose 2–3 mg/d in ÷ doses
SUPPLIED: Tabs 0.05, 0.25, 1.0 mg
NOTES: May cause hypotension during initiation of therapy

Perindopril Erbumine (Aceon)

COMMON USES: HTN and CHF
ACTIONS: ACE inhibitor
DOSAGE: 4–8 mg/d

SUPPLIED: Tabs 2, 4, 8 mg
NOTES: Avoid taking with food; dosage adjustment in renal impairment; contra in PRG

Permethrin (Nix, Elimite)

COMMON USES: Eradication of lice and scabies
ACTIONS: Pediculicide
DOSAGE: *Adults & Peds.* Saturate the hair and scalp; allow to remain in the hair for 10 min before rinsing out
SUPPLIED: Topical liq 1%; cream 5%

Perphenazine (Trilafon)

COMMON USES: Psychotic disorders, intractable hiccups, and severe nausea
ACTIONS: Phenothiazine; blocks postsynaptic mesolimbic dopaminergic receptors in the brain
DOSAGE: *Adults.* Antipsychotic: 4–16 mg PO tid; max 64 mg/d. *Hiccups:* 5 mg IM q6h PRN or 1 mg IV at not less than 1–2 mg/min intervals to a max of 5 mg. *Peds.* 1–6 y: 4–6 mg/d in ÷ doses. *6–12 y:* 6 mg/d in ÷ doses. *>12 y:* 4–16 mg 2–4×/d
SUPPLIED: Tabs 2, 4, 8, 16 mg; oral conc 16 mg/5 mL; inj 5 mg/mL

Phenazopyridine (Pyridium, others)

COMMON USES: Lower urinary tract irritation
ACTIONS: Local anesthetic on urinary tract mucosa
DOSAGE: *Adults.* 100–200 mg PO tid. *Peds 6–12 y.* 12 mg/kg/24h PO in 3 ÷ doses
SUPPLIED: Tabs 95, 100, 200 mg
NOTES: GI disturbances; causes red-orange urine color, which can stain clothing; dosage adjustment in renal impairment

Phenelzine (Nardil)

COMMON USES: Depression
ACTIONS: MAO inhibitor
DOSAGE: *Adults.* 15 mg tid. *Elderly:* 15–60 mg/d in ÷ doses
SUPPLIED: Tabs 15 mg
NOTES: May cause postural hypotension; may take 2–4 wk to see therapeutic effect; avoid tyramine-containing foods

Phenobarbital [C-IV]

COMMON USES: Seizure disorders, insomnia, and anxiety
ACTIONS: Barbiturate
DOSAGE: *Adults.* Sedative–hypnotic: 30–120 mg/f PO or IM PRN. *Anticonvulsant:* Loading dose of 10–12 mg/kg in 3 ÷ doses, then 1–3 mg/kg/24h PO, IM, or IV. *Peds.* Sedative–hypnotic: 2–3 mg/kg/24h PO or IM hs PRN. *Anticonvulsant:* Loading dose of 15–20 mg/kg ÷ into 2 equal doses 4 h apart, then 3–5 mg/kg/24h PO ÷ in 2–3 doses
SUPPLIED: Tabs 8, 15, 16, 30, 32, 60, 65, 100 mg; elixir 15, 20 mg/5 mL; inj 30, 60, 65, 130 mg/mL
NOTES: Tolerance develops to sedation; paradoxic hyperactivity seen in pediatric patients; long half-life allows single daily dosing. (See Table 22–7, pages 631–634.)

Phenylephrine (Neo-Synephrine)

COMMON USES: Vascular failure in shock, hypersensitivity, or drug-induced hypotension; nasal congestion; mydriatic
ACTIONS: α-Adrenergic agonist
DOSAGE: *Adults.* Mild to moderate hypotension: 2–5 mg IM or SC elevates BP for 2 h; 0.1–0.5 mg IV elevates BP for 15 min. *Severe hypotension or shock:* Initiate cont inf at 100–180 mg/min; after BP is stabilized, maintenance rate of 40–60 mg/min. *Nasal congestion:* 1–2 sprays/nostril PRN. *Ophth:* 1 gtt 15–30 min before examination. *Peds.* Hypotension: 5–20 µg/kg/dose IV q 10–15 min

or 0.1–0.5 mg/kg/min IV infusion, titrated to desired effect. *Nasal congestion:* 1 spray/nostril q3–4h PRN
SUPPLIED: Inj 10 mg/mL; nasal soln 0.125, 0.16, 0.25, 0.5, 1%; ophth soln 0.12, 2.5, 10%
NOTES: Promptly restore blood volume if loss has occurred; use with extreme caution in patients with hyperthyroidism, bradycardia, partial heart block, myocardial disease, or severe arteriosclerosis; use large veins for infusion to avoid extravasation; phentolamine 10 mg in 10–15 mL of NS for local inj as antidote for extravasation; activity potentiated by oxytocin, MAO inhibitors, and tricyclic antidepressants. (See Table 20–10, page 637.)

Phenytoin (Dilantin)

COMMON USES: Seizure disorders
ACTIONS: Inhibits seizure spread in the motor cortex
DOSAGE: *Adults & Peds.* Load: 15–20 mg/kg IV at a max inf rate of 25 mg/min or orally in 400-mg doses at 4-h intervals. *Adults.* Maintenance: Initially, 200 mg PO or IV bid or 300 mg hs; then follow serum concentrations. *Peds.* Maintenance: 4–7 mg/kg/24h PO or IV ÷ qd–bid
SUPPLIED: Caps 30, 100 mg; chewable tabs 50 mg; oral susp 30, 125 mg/5 mL; inj 50 mg/mL
NOTES: Use caution with cardiac depressant side effects, especially with IV administration; follow levels as needed (see Table 22–7, pages 631–634); nystagmus and ataxia early signs of toxicity; gum hyperplasia occurs with long-term use; avoid use of oral susp if possible because of erratic absorption; avoid use in pregnancy

Physostigmine (Antilirium)

COMMON USES: Antidote for tricyclic antidepressant, atropine, and scopolamine overdose; glaucoma
ACTIONS: Reversible cholinesterase inhibitor
DOSAGE: *Adults.* 2 mg IV or IM q 20 min. *Peds.* 0.01–0.03 mg/kg/dose IV q 15–30 min, to total of 2 mg if necessary
SUPPLIED: Inj 1 mg/mL; ophth oint 0.25%
NOTES: Rapid IV administration associated with convulsions; cholinergic side effects; may cause asystole. (See also Chapter 21.)

Phytonadione [Vitamin K] (AquaMEPHYTON, others)

COMMON USES: Coagulation disorders caused by faulty formation of factors II, VII, IX, and X; hyperalimentation
ACTIONS: Supplementation; needed for the production of factors II, VII, IX, and X
DOSAGE: *Children and Adults.* Anticoagulant-induced prothrombin deficiency: 2.5–10.0 mg PO or IV slowly. *Hyperalimentation:* 10 mg IM or IV q wk. *Infants.* 0.5–1.0 mg/dose IM, SC, or PO
SUPPLIED: Tabs 5 mg; inj 2, 10 mg/mL
NOTES: With parenteral treatment, the first change in prothrombin usually seen in 12–24 h; anaphylaxis can result from IV dosage; administer IV slowly

Pindolol (Visken)

COMMON USES: HTN
ACTIONS: Competitively blocks β-adrenergic receptors, β_1, β_2, ISA
DOSAGE: 5–10 mg bid, to max dose of 60 mg/d
SUPPLIED: Tabs 5, 10 mg

Pioglitazone (Actos)

COMMON USES: Type 2 DM in combination with diet or other agents
ACTIONS: Increases insulin sensitivity
DOSAGE: 15–45 mg/d
SUPPLIED: Tabs 15, 30, 45 mg
NOTES: Do NOT use in hepatic impairment

Pipecuronium (Arduan)

COMMON USES: Adjunct to general anesthesia
ACTIONS: Nondepolarizing neuromuscular blocker
DOSAGE: *Adults & Peds.* 0.05–0.085 mg/kg initially, followed by 0.5–2 µg/kg/min (ICU)
SUPPLIED: Inj 10 mg
NOTES: Dosage adjustment in renal failure

Piperacillin (Pipracil)

COMMON USES: Infections caused by susceptible strains of gram– bacteria (including *Klebsiella, Proteus, E. coli, Enterobacter, P. aeruginosa,* and *Serratia*) involving the skin, bone, respiratory tract, urinary tract, abdomen, and septicemia
ACTIONS: Bactericidal; inhibits cell wall synthesis
DOSAGE: *Adults.* 3 gm IV q4–6h. *Peds.* 200–300 mg/kg/d IV ÷ q4–6h
SUPPLIED: Inj
NOTES: Often used in combination with aminoglycosides; dosage adjustment in renal failure

Piperacillin-Tazobactam (Zosyn)

COMMON USES: Infections caused by susceptible strains of gram (–) bacteria (including *Klebsiella, Proteus, E. coli, Enterobacter, P. aeruginosa,* and *Serratia*) involving the skin, bone, respiratory tract, urinary tract, abdomen, and septicemia
ACTIONS: Bactericidal; inhibits cell wall synthesis
DOSAGE: *Adults.* 3.375–4.5 g IV q6h
SUPPLIED: Inj
NOTES: Often used in combination with aminoglycoside; dosage adjustment in renal failure

Pirbuterol (Maxair)

COMMON USES: Prevention and Rx of reversible bronchospasm
ACTIONS: β_2-Adrenergic agonist
DOSAGE: *Adults & Peds >12 y.* 2 inhal q4–6h; max 12 inhal/d
SUPPLIED: Aerosol 0.2 mg/actuation
NOTES: Mouth rinsed with water after each use

Piroxicam (Feldene)

COMMON USES: Arthritis and pain
ACTIONS: NSAID; inhibits prostaglandin synthesis
DOSAGE: 10–20 mg/d
SUPPLIED: Caps 10, 20 mg

Plasma Protein Fraction (Plasmanate, others)

COMMON USES: Shock and hypotension
ACTIONS: Plasma volume expansion
DOSAGE: *Adults.* Initially, 250–500 mL IV (NOT >10 mL/min); subsequent inf depend on clinical response. *Peds.* 10–15 mL/kg/dose IV; subsequent inf depend on clinical response
SUPPLIED: Inj 5%
NOTES: Hypotension associated with rapid inf; 130–160 meq Na/L; NOT substitute for RBC

Plicamycin (Mithracin)

COMMON USES: Hypercalcemia of malignancy; disseminated embryonal cell carcinoma or germ cell tumors of the testis
ACTIONS: Antibiotic; binds to the outside of the DNA molecule, interrupting DNA-directed RNA synthesis, DNA intercalation
DOSAGE: *Hypercalcemia:* 25 mg/kg/d IV qod for 3–8 doses. *Cancer:* 25–30 mg/kg/d for 8–10 d
SUPPLIED: Inj

22

NOTES: *Toxicity symptoms:* Thrombocytopenia; drug-induced deficiency of clotting factors II, V, VII, and X, resulting in bleeding and bruising; dosage adjustment in renal or hepatic impairment

Pneumococcal Vaccine, Polyvalent (Pneumovax-23)

COMMON USES: Immunization against pneumococcal infections in patients predisposed to or at high risk. (See Table 22–9, page 636.)
ACTIONS: Active immunization
DOSAGE: *Adults & Peds >2 y.* 0.5 mL IM
SUPPLIED: Inj 25 mg each of polysaccharide isolates/0.5-mL dose
NOTES: Do NOT vaccinate during immunosuppressive therapy

Pneumococcal 7-valent Conjugate Vaccine (Prevnar)

COMMON USES: Immunization against pneumococcal infections in infants and children. (See Table 22–9, page 636.)
ACTIONS: Active immunization
DOSAGE: 0.5 mL IM/dose; series consists of 3 doses; 1st dose at 2 mo of age with subsequent doses q 2 mo
SUPPLIED: Inj

Podophyllin (Podocon-25, Condylox Gel 0.5%, Condylox)

COMMON USES: Topical therapy of benign growths (genital and perianal warts [condylomata acuminata], papillomas, fibroids
ACTIONS: Direct antimitotic effect. Exact mechanism unknown
DOSAGE: Condylox gel and Condylox are applied 3 consecutive d/wk for 4 wk. Use Podocon-25 sparingly on the lesion, leave on for 1–4 h, then thoroughly wash off
SUPPLIED: Podocon-25 contains benzoin 15 mL bottles; Condylox gel 0.5% 35 g clear gel; Condylox soln 0.5% 35 g clear
NOTES: Podocon-25 applied only by the clinician; NOT to be dispensed to patient. Contra in PRG, diabetics, bleeding lesions, immunocompromised

Polyethylene Glycol [PEG] Electrolyte Solution (GoLYTELY, CoLyte)

COMMON USES: Bowel cleansing prior to examination or surgery
ACTIONS: Osmotic cathartic
DOSAGE: *Adults.* Following 3–4-h fast, drink 240 mL of soln q 10 min until 4 L is consumed. *Peds.* 25–40 mL/kg/h for 4–10 h
SUPPLIED: Powder for reconstitution to 4 L in container
NOTES: 1st bowel movement should occur in approximately 1 h; may cause some cramping or nausea

Polymyxin B and Hydrocortisone (Otobiotic Otic)

COMMON USES Superficial bacterial infections of external ear canal
ACTIONS: Antibiotic antiinflammatory combination
DOSAGE: 4 gtt in ear(s) tid–qid
SUPPLIED: Soln polymyxin B 10,000 U/ hydrocortisone 0.5%/ mL
NOTES: Useful in neomycin allergy

Potassium Citrate (Urocit-K)

COMMON USES: Alkalinize urine, prevention of urinary stones (uric acid, calcium stones if hypocitraturic)
ACTIONS: Urinary alkalinizer
DOSAGE: 10–20 mEq PO tid with meals, max 100 mEq/d
NOTES: Tabs 540 mg = 5 mEq, 1080 mg = 10 mEq

Potassium Citrate and Citric Acid (Polycitra-K)

COMMON USES: Alkalinize urine, prevention of urinary stones (uric acid, calcium stones if hypocitraturic)
ACTIONS: Urinary alkalinizer
DOSAGE: 10–20 mEq PO tid with meals, max 100 mEq/d
NOTES: Soln 10 mEq/5 mL; powder 30 mEq/packet

Potassium Idodide [Lugol's Solution] (SSKI, Thyro-Block)

COMMON USES: Thyroid crisis, reduction of vascularity before thyroid surgery, block thyroid uptake of radioactive isotopes of iodine, thin bronchial secretions
ACTIONS: Iodine supplement
DOSAGE: *Adults & Peds.* Preop thyroidectomy: 50–250 mg PO tid (2–6 gtt strong iodine soln); administer 10 d preop. *Thyroid crisis: Adults & Peds >1 y.* 300 mg (6 gtt SSKI q8h). *Infants <1 y.* ½ dose)
SUPPLIED: Tabs 130 mg; soln SSKI 1 g/mL; Lugol's soln, strong iodine 100 mg/mL ; syrup 325 mg/5 mL

Potassium Supplements (Kaon, Kaochlor, K-Lor, Slow-K, Micro-K, Klorvess, others). (See Table 22–4, page 626.)

COMMON USES: Prevention or Rx of hypokalemia (often related to diuretic use)
ACTIONS: Supplementation of potassium
DOSAGE: Adult: 20–100 mEq/d PO ÷ qd–bid; IV 10–20 mEq/h, max 40 mEq/h and 150 mEq/d (monitor frequent potassium levels when using high-dose IV infusions). *Peds.* Calculate potassium deficit; 1–3 mEq/kg/d PO ÷ qd–qid; IV max dose 0.5–1 mEq/kg/h
SUPPLIED: Oral forms (see Table 22–4, page 626); injectable forms
NOTES: Can cause GI irritation; mix powder and liquid with beverage (unsalted tomato juice, etc); use cautiously in renal insufficiency as well as with NSAIDs and ACE inhibitors. Cl salt recommended in coexisting alkalosis, for coexisting acidosis use acetate, bicarbonate, citrate or gluconate salt. (See also Chapter 9.)

Pramipexole (Mirapex)

COMMON USES: Parkinson's disease
ACTION: Dopamine agonist
DOSAGE: 1.5–4.5 mg/d, beginning with 0.375 mg/d in 3 ÷ doses
SUPPLIED: Tabs 0.125, 0.25, 1, 1.5 mg
NOTES: Titrate dosage slowly

Pramoxine (Anusol Ointment, Proctofoam-NS, others)

COMMON USES: Relief of pain and itching from external and internal hemorrhoids and anorectal surgery; topical for burns and dermatosis
ACTIONS: Topical anesthetic
DOSAGE: Apply cream, oint, gel or spray, freely to anal area q3–h
SUPPLIED: [OTC] all 1%; foam (Proctofoam NS), cream, oint, lotion, gel, pads, spray

Pramoxine + Hydrocortisone (Enzone, Proctofoam-HC)

COMMON USES: Relief of pain and itching from hemorrhoids
ACTIONS: Topical anesthetic
DOSAGE: Apply freely to anal area tid–qid
SUPPLIED: Cream pramoxine hydrochloride 1% hydrocortisone acetate 0.5/1%; foam pramoxine 1% hydrocortisone 1%; lotion pramoxine 1% hydrocortisone 0.25/1/2.5%, pramoxine 2.5% and hydrocortisone 1%

Pravastatin (Pravachol)

COMMON USES: Reduction of elevated cholesterol levels
ACTIONS: HMG-CoA reductase inhibitor

22

DOSAGE: 10–40 mg PO hs
SUPPLIED: Tabs 10, 20, 40 mg
NOTES: Avoid concurrent use with gemfibrozil. Follow LFT's

Prazepam (Centrax) [C]

COMMON USES: Anxiety disorders and alcohol withdrawal
ACTIONS: Benzodiazepine
DOSAGE: 5–10 mg PO tid–qid, or 20–50 mg PO as a single dose hs to minimize daytime drowsiness
SUPPLIED: Discontinued

Prazosin (Minipress)

COMMON USES: HTN and CHF
ACTIONS: Peripherally acting α-adrenergic blocker
DOSAGE: 1 mg PO tid; can ↑ to max daily dose of up to 20 mg/d. *Peds.* 5–25 µg/kg/dose q6h, up to 25 µg/kg/dose
SUPPLIED: Caps 1, 2, 5 mg
NOTES: Can cause orthostatic hypotension, so the patient should take the first dose hs; tolerance develops to this effect; tachyphylaxis may result

Prednisolone

See Steroids, systemic (Table 22–5, page 627)

Prednisone

See Steroids, systemic (Table 22–5, page 627)

Probenecid (Benemid, others)

COMMON USES: Prevention of gout and hyperuricemia; prolong serum levels of penicillins or cephalosporins
ACTIONS: Renal tubular blocking agent
DOSAGE: *Adults.* Gout: 250 mg bid for 1 wk, then 0.5 g PO bid. Can ↑ by 500 mg/mo up to 2–3 g/d. *Antibiotic effect:* 1–2 g PO 30 min prior to dose of antibiotic. *Peds >2 y.* 25 mg/kg, then 40 mg/kg/d PO ÷ qid
SUPPLIED: Tabs 500 mg

Procainamide (Pronestyl, Procan)

Used for emergency cardiac care (see Chapter 21)
COMMON USES: Supraventricular and ventricular arrhythmias
ACTIONS: Class 1A antiarrhythmic
DOSAGE: *Adults.* For emergency cardiac care, see Chapter 21. *Chronic dosing:* 50 mg/kg/d PO in ÷ doses q4–6h. *Peds.* For emergency cardiac care, see Chapter 21. *Maintenance:* 15–50 mg/kg/24h PO ÷ q3–6h
SUPPLIED: Tabs and caps 250, 375, 500 mg; SR tabs 250, 500, 750, 1000 mg; inj 100, 500 mg/mL
NOTES: Can cause hypotension and a lupus-like syndrome; dosage adjustment required with renal or hepatic impairment (see Table 22–7, pages 631–634. See also Table 20–10, p. 637.)

Procarbazine (Matulane)

COMMON USES: Hodgkin's disease, non-Hodgkin's lymphoma, and brain tumors
ACTIONS: Alkylating agent; inhibition of DNA and RNA synthesis
DOSAGE: 2–4 mg/kg/d × 7 d, then 4–6 mg/kg/d until response. Maintenance 1–2 mg/kg/d/ in combination, 60–100 mg/m²/d × 10–14 d
SUPPLIED: Caps 50 mg
NOTES: *Toxicity symptoms:* Myelosuppression, hemolytic reactions (with G6PD deficiency), nausea, vomiting, and diarrhea; disulfiram-like reaction. Cutaneous reactions. Constitutional symp-

22

toms, myalgia, and arthralgia. CNS effects may be related to the high concentrations of drug reached in CSF or because of MAO inhibitor effects. Azoospermia and cessation of menses common

Prochlorperazine (Compazine)

COMMON USES: Nausea and vomiting, agitation, and psychotic disorders
ACTIONS: Phenothiazine; blocks postsynaptic mesolimbic dopaminergic receptors in the brain
DOSAGE: *Adults.* Antiemetic: 5–10 mg PO tid–qid or 25 mg PR bid or 5–10 mg deep IM q4–6h. *Antipsychotic:* 10–20 mg IM acutely or 5–10 mg PO tid–qid for maintenance. **Peds.** 0.1–0.15 mg/kg/dose IM q4–6h or 0.4 mg/kg/24h PO ÷ tid–qid
SUPPLIED: Tabs 5, 10, 25 mg; SR caps 10, 15, 30 mg; syrup 5 mg/5 mL; supp 2.5, 5, 25 mg; inj 5 mg/mL
NOTES: A much larger dose may be required for antipsychotic effect; extrapyramidal side effects common; treat acute extrapyramidal reactions with diphenhydramine

Procyclidine (Kemadrin)

COMMON USES: Parkinson's syndrome
ACTIONS: Blocking excess acetylcholine
DOSAGE: 2.5 mg PO tid, up to 20 mg/d
SUPPLIED: Tabs 5 mg
NOTES: Contra in glaucoma

Promethazine (Phenergan)

COMMON USES: Nausea and vomiting, motion sickness, sedation
ACTIONS: Phenothiazine; blocks postsynaptic mesolimbic dopaminergic receptors in the brain
DOSAGE: *Adults.* 12.5–50 mg PO, PR, or IM bid–qid PRN. **Peds.** 0.1–0.5 mg/kg/dose PO or IM q12–6h PRN
SUPPLIED: Tabs 12.5, 25, 50 mg; syrup 6.25 mg/5 mL, 25 mg/5 mL; supp 12.5, 25, 50 mg; inj 25, 50 mg/mL
NOTES: High incidence of drowsiness

Propafenone (Rythmol)

COMMON USES: Life-threatening ventricular arrhythmias
ACTIONS: Class IC antiarrhythmic
DOSAGE: 150–300 mg PO q8h
SUPPLIED: Tabs 150, 225, 300 mg
NOTES: May cause dizziness, unusual taste, 1st-degree heart block, and prolongation of QRS and QT intervals

Propantheline (Pro-Banthine)

COMMON USES: Symptomatic treatment of small intestine hypermotility, spastic colon, ureteral spasm, bladder spasm, pylorospasm
ACTIONS: Antimuscarinic agent
DOSAGE: *Adults.* 15 mg PO ac and 30 mg PO hs. **Peds.** 1–3 mg/kg/24h PO ÷ tid–qid
SUPPLIED: Tabs 7.5, 15 mg
NOTES: Anticholinergic side effects, eg, dry mouth and blurred vision common

Propofol (Diprivan)

COMMON USES: Induction or maintenance of anesthesia; continuous sedation in intubated patients
ACTIONS: Sedative hypnotic; mechanism unknown
DOSAGE: *Anesthesia:* 2–2.5 mg/kg induction then 0.1–0.2 mg/kg/min cont inf. *ICU sedation:* 5–50 μg/kg/min cont inf
SUPPLIED: Inj 10 mg/mL
NOTES: 1 mL of propofol contains 0.1 g of fat; may increase serum triglycerides when administered for extended periods

Propoxyphene (Darvon) [C-IV]

Propoxyphene and Acetaminophen (Darvocet) [C-IV]

Propoxyphene and Aspirin (Darvon Compound-65, Darvon-N + Aspirin) [C-IV]

COMMON USES: Mild to moderate pain
ACTIONS: Narcotic analgesic
DOSAGE: 1–2 PO q4h PRN
SUPPLIED: Darvon: propoxyphene HCl caps 65 mg; Darvon-N: propoxyphene napsylate 100-mg tabs; Darvocet-N: propoxyphene napsylate 50 mg/acetaminophen 325 mg; Darvocet-N 100: propoxyphene napsylate 100 mg/acetaminophen 650 mg; Darvon Compound-65: propoxyphene HCl 65-mg/aspirin 389-mg/caffeine 32-mg caps; Darvon-N with aspirin: propoxyphene napsylate 100 mg/aspirin 325 mg
NOTES: Intentional overdose can be **lethal**

Propranolol (Inderal)

Used for emergency cardiac care (see also Chapter 21)
COMMON USES: HTN, angina, MI
ACTIONS: Competitively blocks β-adrenergic receptors, β_1, β_2
DOSAGE: *Adults.* Angina: 80–320 mg/d PO ÷ bid–qid or 80–160 mg/d SR. *Arrhythmia:* 10–80 mg PO tid–qid or 1 mg IV slowly, repeat q 5 min up to 5 mg. *HTN:* 40 mg PO bid or 60–80 mg/d SR, ↑ weekly to max 640 mg/d. *Hypertrophic subaortic stenosis:* 20–40 mg PO tid–qid. *MI:* 180–240 mg PO ÷ tid–qid. *Migraine prophylaxis:* 80 mg/d ÷ qid–tid, ↑ weekly to max 160–240 mg/d ÷ tid–qid; wean off if no response in 6 wk. *Pheochromocytoma:* 30–60 mg/d ÷ tid–qid. *Thyrotoxicosis:* 1–3 mg IV single dose; 10–40 mg PO q6h. *Tremor:* 40 mg PO bid, ↑ as needed to max 320 mg/d. *Peds.* Arrhythmia: 0.5–1.0 mg/kg/d ÷ tid–qid, ↑ as needed q3–7d to max 60 mg/d; 0.01–0.1 mg/kg IV over 10 min, max dose 1 mg. *HTN:* 0.5–1.0 mg/kg ÷ bid–qid, ↑ as needed q 3–7 d to 2 mg/kg/d max
SUPPLIED: Tabs 10, 20, 40, 60, 80, 90 mg; caps SR 60, 80, 120, 160 mg; oral soln 4 mg/mL, 8 mg/mL, 80 mg/mL; inj 1 mg/mL
NOTES: Dosage adjustment in renal impairment

Propylthiouracil [PTU]

COMMON USES: Hyperthyroidism
ACTIONS: Inhibits production of T_3 and T_4 and conversion of T_4 to T_3
DOSAGE: *Adults.* Initial: 100 mg PO q8h (may need up to 1200 mg/d for control); after the patient is euthyroid (6–8 wk), taper the dose by ½ q 4–6 wk to *Maintenance:* 50–150 mg/24h; can usually be discontinued in 2–3 y. *Peds.* Initial: 5–7 mg/kg/24h PO ÷ q8h. *Maintenance:* ⅓–⅔ of the initial dose
SUPPLIED: Tabs 50 mg
NOTES: Follow the patient clinically; monitor TFT

Protamine Sulfate

COMMON USES: Reversal of heparin effect
ACTIONS: Neutralizes heparin by forming a stable complex
DOSAGE: *Adults & Peds.* Based on amount of heparin reversal desired; give IV slowly; 1 mg reverses approximately 100 U of heparin given in the preceding 3–4 h, to a max dose of 50 mg
SUPPLIED: Inj 10 mg/mL
NOTES: Follow coagulation studies; may have anticoagulant effect if given without heparin

Pseudoephedrine (Sudafed, Novafed, Afrinol, others)

COMMON USES: Decongestant
ACTIONS: Stimulates α-adrenergic receptors, resulting in vasoconstriction
DOSAGE: *Adults.* 30–60 mg PO q6–8h; SR caps 120 mg PO q12h. *Peds.* 4 mg/kg/24h PO ÷ qid

22

SUPPLIED: Tabs 30, 60 mg; caps 60 mg; SR tabs 120, 240 mg; SR caps 120 mg; liq 7.5 mg/0.8 mL, 15, 30 mg/5 mL
NOTES: Contra in patients with poorly controlled HTN or CAD and in patients taking MAO inhibitors; ingredient in many cough and cold preparations

Psyllium (Metamucil, Serutan, Effer-Syllium)

COMMON USES: Constipation and diverticular disease of the colon
ACTIONS: Bulk laxative
DOSAGE: 1 tsp (7 g) in a glass of water qd–tid
SUPPLIED: Granules 4, 25 g/tsp; powder 3.5 g/packet
NOTES: Do NOT use if suspected bowel obstruction; one of the safest laxatives; psyllium in effervescent (Effer-Syllium) form usually contains potassium and should be used with caution in renal failure

Pyrazinamide

COMMON USES: Active TB
ACTIONS: Bacteriostatic; mechanism unknown
DOSAGE: *Adults.* 15–30 mg/kg/24h PO ÷ tid–qid; max 2 g/d. *Peds.* 15–30 mg/kg/d PO ÷ qd–bid
SUPPLIED: Tabs 500 mg
NOTES: May cause hepatotoxicity; use in combination with other antituberculosis drugs; consult *MMWR* for the latest recommendations on the treatment of tuberculosis; dosage regimen differs for directly observed therapy; adjust dose for renal or hepatic impairment

Pyridoxine [Vitamin B$_6$] (Nestrex)

COMMON USES: Rx and prevention of vitamin B$_6$ deficiency, including drug-induced (ie INH, hydralazine)
ACTIONS: Supplementation of vitamin B$_6$
DOSAGE: *Adults.* Deficiency: 10–20 mg/d. PO *Drug-induced neuritis:* 100–200 mg/d; 25–100 mg/d prophylaxis. *Peds.* 5–25 mg/d × 3 wk
SUPPLIED: Tabs 25, 50, 100 mg; inj 100 mg/mL

Quazepam (Doral) [CIV]

COMMON USES: Insomnia
ACTIONS: Benzodiazepine
DOSAGE: 7.5–15 mg PO hs PRN
SUPPLIED: Tabs 7.5, 15 mg
NOTES: ↓ Dose in the elderly; do NOT discontinue abruptly

Quetiapine (Seroquel)

COMMON USES: Acute exacerbations of schizophrenia
ACTIONS: Serotonin and dopamine antagonism
DOSAGE: 150–750; mg/d; initiate at 25–100 mg bid–tid
SUPPLIED: Tabs 25, 100, 200 mg
NOTES: ↑ Dose slowly; adjust dose for hepatic and geriatric patients

Quinapril (Accupril)

COMMON USES: HTN and heart failure
ACTIONS: ACE inhibitor
DOSAGE: 10–80 mg PO qd in a single dose
SUPPLIED: Tabs 5, 10, 20, 40 mg
NOTES: Dosage adjustment in renal impairment

Quinidine (Quinidex, Quinaglute)

22

COMMON USES: Prevention of tachydysrhythmias

ACTIONS: Class 1A antiarrhythmic
DOSAGE: *Adults.* PAC, PVCs: 200–300 mg PO tid–qid. *Conversion of AF or flutter:* Use after digitalization, 200 mg q2–3h for 8 doses; then ↑ daily dose to a max of 3–4 g or until normal rhythm. *Peds.* 15–60 mg/kg/24h PO in 4–5 ÷ dose
SUPPLIED: *Sulfate:* Tabs 200, 300 mg; SR tabs 300 mg; *Gluconate:* SR tabs 324 mg; inj 80 mg/mL
NOTES: Contra in digitalis toxicity and AV block; follow serum levels if available (see Table 22–7, pages 631–634); extreme hypotension seen with IV administration. Sulfate salt contains 83% quinidine; gluconate salt contains 62% quinidine; dosage adjustment in renal impairment

Quinupristin/Dalfopristin (Synercid)

COMMON USES: Infections caused by vancomycin-resistant *Entercoccus faecium,* and other gram+ organisms
ACTIONS: Inhibits both the early and late phase of protein synthesis at the ribosomes
DOSAGE: *Adults & Peds.* 7.5 mg/kg IV q8–12h
SUPPLIED: Inj 500 mg (150 mg quinupristin/350 mg dalfopristin)
NOTES: Administer through central line if possible; NOT compatible with saline or heparin, therefore flush IV lines with dextrose

Rabeprazole (Aciphex)

COMMON USES: Peptic ulcers, GERD, and hypersecretory conditions
ACTIONS: Proton pump inhibitor
DOSAGE: 20 mg/d; may be ↑ to 60 mg/d
SUPPLIED: Tabs 60 mg
NOTES: Do NOT crush tabs

Raloxifene (Evista)

COMMON USES: Prevention of osteoporosis
ACTIONS: Partial antagonist of estrogen that behaves like estrogen
DOSAGE: 60 mg/d
SUPPLIED: Tabs 60 mg

Ramipril (Altace)

COMMON USES: HTN and heart failure
ACTIONS: ACE inhibitor
DOSAGE: 2.5–20 mg/d PO ÷ qd–bid
SUPPLIED: Caps 1.25, 2.5, 5, 10 mg
NOTES: May use in combination with diuretics; may cause a nonproductive cough; dosage adjustment in renal impairment

Ranitidine (Zantac)

COMMON USES: Duodenal ulcer, active benign ulcers, hypersecretory conditions, and GERD
ACTIONS: H_2-receptor antagonist
DOSAGE: *Adults.* Ulcer: 150 mg PO bid, 300 mg PO hs, or 50 mg IV q6–8h; or 400 mg IV/d cont inf, then maintenance of 150 mg PO hs. *Hypersecretion:* 150 mg PO bid, up to 600 mg/d. *GERD:* 300 mg PO bid; maintenance 300 mg PO hs. *Peds.* 0.75–1.5 mg/kg/dose IV q6–8h or 1.25–2.5 mg/kg/dose PO q12
SUPPLIED: Tabs 75, 150, 300 mg; syrup 15 mg/mL; inj 25 mg/mL
NOTES: ↓ Dose with renal failure; oral and parenteral doses are different

Repaglinide (Prandin)

COMMON USES: Type 2 DM
ACTIONS: Stimulates insulin release from pancreas
DOSAGE: 0.5–4 mg ac
SUPPLIED: Tabs 0.5, 1, 2 mg

Reteplase (Retavase)

COMMON USES: Post-AMI
ACTIONS: Thrombolytic agent
DOSAGE: 10 U IV over 2 min, 2nd dose 30 min later of 10 U IV over 2 min
SUPPLIED: Inj 10.8 U/2 mL

Ribavirin (Virazole)

COMMON USES: RSV infection in infants and; hepatitis C, (in combination with interferon alfa-2b)
ACTIONS: Unknown
DOSAGE: *RSV:* 6 g in 300 mL of sterile water inhaled over 12–18 h. *Hep C:* 600 mg PO bid in combination with interferon alfa-2b (See Rebetron, page 000)
SUPPLIED: Powder for aerosol 6 g; caps 200 mg
NOTES: Aerosolized by a SPAG ; may accumulate on soft contact lenses; monitor H/H frequently; PRG test monthly

Rifabutin (Mycobutin)

COMMON USES: Prevention of *M. avium* complex infection in AIDS patients with a CD4 count <100
ACTIONS: Inhibits DNA-dependent RNA polymerase activity
DOSAGE: 150–300 mg/d PO
SUPPLIED: Caps 150 mg
NOTES: Adverse effects and drug interactions similar to rifampin

Rifampin (Rifadin)

COMMON USES: TB and Rx and prophylaxis of *N. meningitidis, H. influenzae,* or *S. aureus* carriers
ACTIONS: Inhibits DNA-dependent RNA polymerase activity
DOSAGE: *Adults.* N. meningitidis and *H. influenzae* carrier: 600 mg/d PO for 4 d. *TB:* 600 mg PO or IV qd or 2×/wk with combination-therapy regimen. *Peds.* 10–20 mg/kg/dose PO or IV qd–bid
SUPPLIED: Caps 150, 300 mg; inj 600 mg
NOTES: Multiple drug interactions; causes orange-red discoloration of bodily secretions, including tears; never used as a single agent to treat active TB

Rifapentine (Priftin)

COMMON USES: TB
ACTIONS: Inhibits DNA-dependent RNA polymerase activity
DOSAGE: *Intensive phase:* 600 mg PO 2×/wk for 2 mo; separate doses by 3 or more days. *Continuation phase:* 600 mg/wk
SUPPLIED: Tabs 150 mg
NOTES: Adverse effects and drug interactions similar to rifampin

Rimantadine (Flumadine)

COMMON USES: Prophylaxis and Rx of influenza A virus infections
ACTIONS: Antiviral agent
DOSAGE: *Adults.* 100 mg PO bid. *Peds.* 5 mg/kg/d PO, NOT to exceed 150 mg/d
SUPPLIED: Tabs 100 mg; syrup 50 mg/5 mL
NOTES: Dosage adjustment in severe renal or hepatic impairment; initiate within 48 h of symptom onset

Rimexolone (Vexol Ophthalmic)

COMMON USES: Postop inflammation and uveitis
ACTIONS: Steroid
DOSAGE: *Adults & Peds > 2 y.* Uveitis: 1–2 gtt/h daytime and q2h at night, taper to 1 gtt q4h; postop 1–2 gtt qid up to 2 wk

SUPPLIED: 1% susp
NOTES: Taper dose to zero

Risedronate (Actonel)

COMMON USES: Prevention and Rx of postmenopausal osteoporosis; Paget's disease
ACTIONS: Bisphosphonate; inhibits osteoclast-mediated bone resorption
DOSAGE: 5 mg/d PO with 6–8 oz water; 30 mg/d for 2 mo for Paget's disease
SUPPLIED: Tabs 5, 30 mg
NOTES: Take 30 min before first food or drink of the day; maintain upright position for at least 30 min after administration, interaction with calcium supplements; may cause GI distress and arthralgia; NOT recommended in moderate to severe renal impairment

Risperidone (Risperdal)

COMMON USES: Psychotic disorders
ACTIONS: Benzisoxazole antipsychotic agent
DOSAGE: 1–6 mg PO bid
SUPPLIED: Tabs 1, 2, 3, 4 mg
NOTES: ↓ Starting doses in elderly, renal or hepatic impairment; orthostatic hypotension; extrapyramidal reactions with higher doses

Ritonavir (Norvir)

COMMON USES: HIV infection when therapy is warranted
ACTIONS: Protease inhibitor; inhibits maturation of immature noninfectious virions to mature infectious virus
DOSAGE: 600 mg PO bid or 400 mg PO bid in combination with Saquinavir
SUPPLIED: Caps 100 mg; soln 80 mg/mL
NOTES: Titrate dose over 1 wk to avoid GI complications; take with food; has many drug interactions; may cause perioral and peripheral paresthesias; store in refrigerator

Rivastigmine (Exelon)

COMMON USES: Mild to moderate dementia associated with Alzheimer's disease
ACTIONS: Enhances cholinergic activity
DOSAGE: 1.5 mg bid; ↑ to 6 mg bid, with dosage increases at 2-wk intervals
SUPPLIED: Caps 1.5, 3, 4.5, 6 mg; soln 2 mg/mL
NOTES: Associated with significant dose-related GI adverse effects

Rizatriptan (Maxalt)

COMMON USES: Acute migraine attacks
ACTIONS: Serotonin 5-HT$_1$ receptor antagonist
DOSAGE: 5–10 mg PO; may repeat once in 2 h
SUPPLIED: Tabs 5, 10 mg; disintegrating tabs 5, 10 mg

Rofecoxib (Vioxx)

COMMON USES: Osteoarthritis, acute pain, and primary dysmenorrhea
ACTIONS: NSAID; COX-2 inhibitor
DOSAGE: 12.5–50 mg/d
SUPPLIED: Tabs 12.5, 25 mg; susp 12.5 mg/5 mL, 25 mg/5 mL
NOTES: Alert patients to be aware of GI ulceration or bleeding; use with caution in renal impairment; ↓ dose in elderly

Rosiglitazone (Avandia)

COMMON USES: Type 2 DM
ACTIONS: ↑ Insulin sensitivity
DOSAGE: 4–8 mg/d PO or in 2 ÷ doses

22

SUPPLIED: Tabs 2, 4, 8 mg
NOTES: May be taken without regard to meals; do NOT use in active liver disease

Salmeterol (Serevent)

COMMON USES: Asthma and exercise-induced bronchospasm
ACTIONS: Sympathomimetic bronchodilator
DOSAGE: 2 inhal bid
SUPPLIED: Met-dose inhaler; NOT for relief of acute attacks

Saquinavir (Fortovase)

COMMON USES: HIV infection
ACTIONS: HIV protease inhibitor
DOSAGE: 1200 mg PO tid within 2 h pc
SUPPLIED: Caps 200 mg

Sargramostim [GM-CSF] (Leukine)

COMMON USES: Myeloid recovery following BMT or cancer chemotherapy
ACTIONS: Activates mature granulocytes and macrophages
DOSAGE: *Adults & Peds.* 250 mg/m^2/d IV for 21 d (BMT)
SUPPLIED: Inj 250, 500 mg
NOTES: May cause bone pain

Scopolamine, Transdermal (Transderm-Scop)

COMMON USES: Prevention of nausea and vomiting associated with motion sickness
ACTIONS: Anticholinergic, antiemetic
DOSAGE: Apply 1 TD patch behind the ear q 3 d; 0.3–0.65 IM/IV/SC, repeat PRN q4–6h
SUPPLIED: Patch 1.5 mg, injectable forms
NOTES: May cause dry mouth, drowsiness, and blurred vision. Apply at least 4 h before exposure

Secobarbital (Seconal) [C-II]

COMMON USES: Insomnia
ACTIONS: Rapid-acting barbiturate
DOSAGE: *Adults.* 100–200 mg IM hs PRN. *Peds.* 3–5 mg/kg/dose IM hs PRN, up to 100 mg
SUPPLIED: Inj 50 mg/mL
NOTES: Beware of respiratory depression; tolerance acquired within 1–2 wk

Selegiline (Eldepryl)

COMMON USES: Parkinson's disease
ACTIONS: Inhibits MAO activity
DOSAGE: 5 mg PO bid
SUPPLIED: Tabs 5 mg
NOTES: May cause nausea and dizziness

Selenium Sulfide (Exsel Shampoo, Selsun Blue Shampoo, Selsun Shampoo)

COMMON USES: Scalp seborrheic dermatitis, itching and flaking of the scalp due to dandruff; treatment of tinea versicolor
ACTIONS: Antiseborrheic
DOSAGE: *Dandruff, seborrhea:* Massage 5–10 mL into wet scalp, leave on 2–3 min, rinse and repeat; use 2×/wk, then once q 1–4 wk PRN. *Tinea versicolor:* Apply qd for 7 d, 2.5% on area and lather with small amounts of water; leave on skin for 10 min, then rinse
SUPPLIED: Shampoo 1, 2.5%

Sertraline (Zoloft)

COMMON USES: Depression
ACTIONS: Inhibits neuronal uptake of serotonin
DOSAGE: 50–200 mg/d PO
SUPPLIED: Tabs 25, 50, 100 mg
NOTES: Can activate manic/hypomanic state; has caused weight loss in clinical trials; caution in hepatic impairment

Sibutramine (Meridia)

COMMON USES: Obesity
ACTIONS: Blocks uptake of norepinephrine, serotonin, and dopamine
DOSAGE: 10 mg/d, may ↓ to 5 mg after 4 wk
SUPPLIED: Caps 5, 10, 15 mg
NOTES: Use with low-calorie diet, monitor BP

Sildenafil (Viagra)

COMMON USES: Erectile dysfunction
ACTIONS: Smooth muscle relaxation and increased inflow of blood to the corpus cavernosum; inhibits phosphodiesterase type 5 responsible for cGMP breakdown resulting in increased cGMP activity
DOSAGE: 25–100 mg 1 h prior to attempted sexual activity, max dosing is once daily
SUPPLIED: Tabs 25, 50, 100 mg
NOTES: Contra with nitrates of any form; adjust dose in persons >65 y, hepatic/severe renal impairment, potent CYP3A4 inhibitors (ie, protease inhibitors); may cause headache, blue haze visual disturbance, usually reversible; cardiac events in the absence of nitrate use debatable

Silver Nitrate (Dey-Drop)

COMMON USES: Prevention of ophthalmia neonatorium due to GC; removal of granulation tissue, warts and cauterization of wounds
ACTIONS: Caustic antiseptic and astringent
DOSAGE: *Adults & Peds.* Apply to moist surface 2–3×/wk for several weeks or until desired effect. *Peds.* Newborns: Apply 2 gtt into conjunctival sac immediately after birth
SUPPLIED: Topical impregnated applicator sticks, 10% oint, 10, 25, 50% soln; ophth 1% amp
NOTES: May stain tissue black, usually resolves

Silver Sulfadiazine (Silvadene)

COMMON USES: Prevention of sepsis in 2nd- and 3rd-degree burns
ACTIONS: Bactericidal
DOSAGE: *Adults & Peds.* Aseptically cover the affected area with ⅟₁₆-in. coating bid
SUPPLIED: Cream 1%
NOTES: Can have systemic absorption with extensive application

Simethicone (Mylicon)

COMMON USES: Flatulence
ACTIONS: Defoaming action
DOSAGE: *Adults & Peds.* 40–125 mg PO pc and hs PRN
SUPPLIED: Tabs 40, 80, 125 mg; caps 125 mg; gtt 40 mg/0.6 mL

Simvastatin (Zocor)

COMMON USES: Reduction of elevated cholesterol levels
ACTIONS: HMG-CoA reductase inhibitor
DOSAGE: 5–80 mg PO hs
SUPPLIED: Tabs 5, 10, 20, 40 mg
NOTES: Avoid concurrent use of gemfibrozil

Sirolimus [Rapamycin] (Rapamune)

COMMON USES: Prophylaxis of organ rejection
ACTIONS: Inhibits T-lymphocyte activation
DOSAGE: 2 mg/d PO
SUPPLIED: Soln 1 mg/mL
NOTES: Dilute in water or orange juice; do NOT drink grapefruit juice while on sirolimus; take 4 h after cyclosporin; dosage adjustment in hepatic impairment. Routine blood levels not needed except in Peds or liver failure (trough 9–17 ng/mL)

Sodium Bicarbonate

Used for emergency cardiac care (see Chapter 21)
COMMON USES: Alkalinization of urine, RTA, metabolic acidosis
DOSAGE: *Adults.* Emergency cardiac care: Initiate adequate ventilation, 1 mEq/kg/dose IV ; can repeat 0.5 mEq/kg in 10 min once or based on acid–base status. *Metabolic acidosis:* 2–5 mEq/kg IV over 8 h and PRN based on acid–base status. *Alkalinize urine:* 4 g (48 mEq) PO, then 1–2 g q4h; adjust based on urine pH. *Chronic renal failure:* 1–3 mEq/kg/d. *Distal RTA:* 1 mEq/kg/d PO. *Peds.* >1 y: Emergency cardiac care: See Adult. *<1 y: Emergency cardiac care:* Initiate adequate ventilation, 1:1 dilution 1 mEq/mL dosed 1 mEq/kg IV; can repeat with 0.5 mEq/kg in 10 min once or based on acid–base status. *Chronic renal failure:* See Adult. *Distal RTA:* 2–3 mEq/kg/d PO. *Proximal RTA:* 5–10 mEq/kg/d titrate based on serum bicarbonate levels. *Urine alkalinization:* 84–840 mg/kg/d (1–10 mEq/kg/d) ÷ doses; adjust based on urine pH
SUPPLIED: IV inf, powder, and tabs. 300 mg = 3.6 mEq; 325 mg = 3.8 mEq; 520 mg = 6.3 mEq; 600 mg = 7.3 mEq; 650 mg = 7.6 mEq
NOTES: 1 g neutralizes 12 mEq of acid; in infants, do NOT exceed 10 mEq/min inf

Sodium Citrate (Bicitra)

COMMON USES: Alkalinization of urine; dissolve uric acid and cysteine stones
ACTIONS: Urinary alkalinizer
DOSAGE: *Adults:* 2–6 tsp (10–30 mL) diluted in 1–3 oz water pc and hs. *Peds.* 1–3 tsp (5–15 mL) diluted in 1–3 oz water pc and hs
SUPPLIED: 15- or 30-mL unit dose: 16 (473 mL) or 4 (118 mL) fl oz
NOTES: Do NOT give to patients on aluminum-based antacids. Contra in patients with severe renal impairment of sodium-restricted diets

Sodium Polystyrene Sulfonate (Kayexalate)

COMMON USES: Hyperkalemia
ACTIONS: Sodium and potassium ion-exchange resin
DOSAGE: *Adults.* 15–60 g PO or 30–60 g PR q6h based on serum K^+. *Peds.* 1 g/kg/dose PO or PR q6h based on serum K^+
SUPPLIED: Powder; susp 15 g/60 mL sorbitol
NOTES: Can cause hypernatremia; given with an agent, eg, sorbitol to promote movement through the bowel

Sorbitol

COMMON USES: Constipation
ACTIONS: Laxative
DOSAGE: 30–60 mL of a 20–70% soln PRN
SUPPLIED: Liq 70%

Sotalol (Betapace)

COMMON USES: Ventricular arrhythmias
ACTIONS: β-Adrenergic-blocking agent
DOSAGE: 80 mg PO bid; may be ↑ to 240–320 mg/d

SUPPLIED: Tabs 80, 120, 160, 240 mg
NOTES: Adjust dosage for renal insufficiency

Spironolactone (Aldactone)

COMMON USES: Hyperaldosteronism, essential HTN, and edematous states (CHF, cirrhosis)
ACTIONS: Aldosterone antagonist; K-sparing diuretic
DOSAGE: *Adults.* 25–100 mg PO qid. *Peds.* 1–3.3 mg/kg/24h PO ÷ bid–qid. *Neonates:* 0.5–1 mg/kg/dose q8h
SUPPLIED: Tabs 25, 50, 100 mg
NOTES: Can cause hyperkalemia and gynecomastia; avoid prolonged use; diuretic of choice for cirrhotic edema and ascites

Stavudine (Zerit)

COMMON USES: Advanced HIV disease
ACTIONS: Reverse-transcriptase inhibitor
DOSAGE: *Adults.* >60 kg: 40 mg bid. *<60 kg:* 30 mg bid
SUPPLIED: Caps 15, 20, 30, 40 mg; soln 1 mg/mL
NOTES: May cause peripheral neuropathy; not a cure for HIV; dosage adjustment in renal impairment

Steroids, Systemic (see also Table 22–5, page 627)

The following relates only to the commonly used systemic glucocorticoids.
COMMON USES: Endocrine disorders (adrenal insufficiency), rheumatoid disorders, collagen-vascular diseases, dermatologic diseases, allergic states, edematous states (cerebral, nephrotic syndrome), immunosuppression for transplantation, hypercalcemia, malignancies (breast, lymphomas), preoperatively (in any patient who has been on steroids in the previous year, known hypoadrenalism, preop for adrenalectomy); injection into joints/tissue
ACTIONS: Glucocorticoid
DOSAGE: Varies with use and institutional protocols. *Adrenal insufficiency, acute (Addisonian crisis): Adult.* Hydrocortisone: 100 mg IV q8h; then 300 mg/d ÷ q8h; convert to 50 mg PO q8h × 6 doses, taper to 30–50 mg/d ÷ bid. *Peds.* Hydrocortisone: 1–2 mg/kg IV; then 150–250 mg/d ÷ tid. *Adrenal insufficiency, chronic (physiologic replacement):* May need mineralocorticoid supplementation such as Florinef *Adults.* Hydrocortisone 20 mg PO qAM, 10 mg PO qPM; cortisone 0.5–0.75 mg/kg/d ÷ bid; cortisone 0.25–0.35 mg/kg/d IM; dexamethasone 0.03–0.15 mg/kg/d or 0.6–0.75 mg/m^2/d in ÷ q6–12h PO, IM, IV. *Peds.* Hydrocortisone 0.5–0.75 mg/kg/d PO tid; hydrocortisone succinate 0.25–0.35 mg/kg/d IM. *Asthma, acute: Peds.* Prednisolone 1–2 mg/kg/d or prednisone 1–2 mg/kg/d ÷ qd–bid for up to 5 d; prednisolone 2–4 mg/kg/d IV ÷ tid. *Congenital adrenal hyperplasia: Peds.* Initially hydrocortisone 30–36 mg/m^2/d PO ÷ ⅓ dose q AM, ⅔ dose q PM; maintenance: 20–25 mg/m^2/d ÷ bid. *Extubation/airway edema:* Dexamethasone 0.5–1 mg/kg/d IM/IV ÷ q6h, start beginning 24 h prior to extubation; continue for 4 additional doses. *Immunosuppressive/antiinflammatory: Adults & Older Peds.* Hydrocortisone 15–240 mg PO, IM, IV q12h; methylprednisolone: 4–48 mg/d PO, taper to lowest effective dose; methylprednisolone sodium succinate 10–80 mg/d IM. *Adults.* Prednisone or prednisolone 5–60 mg/d PO, ÷ qd–qid. *Infants and Younger Children.* 2.5–10 mg/kg/d hydrocortisone PO ÷ q6–8h; 1–5 mg/kg/d IM/IV ÷ bid. *Nephrotic syndrome: Peds.* Prednisolone or prednisone 2 mg/kg/d PO ÷ tid–qid until urine is protein-free for 5 d, use up to 28 d; for persistent proteinuria, 4 mg/kg/dose PO qod max 120 mg/d for an additional 28 d; maintenance: 2 mg/kg/dose qod for 28 d; taper over 4–6 wk (max 80 mg/d). *Septic shock: Adults.* Hydrocortisone 500 mg–1 g IM/IV q2–6h. *Peds.* Hydrocortisone 50 mg/kg IM/IV, repeat q4–24h PRN. *Status asthmaticus: Adult and Peds.* Hydrocortisone 1–2 mg/kg/dose IV q6h; then by 0.5–1 mg/kg q6h. *Rheumatic disease: Adults.* Intraarticular: Hydrocortisone acetate 25–37.5 mg large joint; 10–25 mg small joint; methylprednisolone acetate 20–80 mg large joint, 4–10 mg small joint. *Intrabursal:* Hydrocortisone acetate 25–37.5 mg. *Intraganglial:* Hydrocortisone acetate 25–37.5 mg. *Tendon sheath:* Hydrocortisone acetate 5–12.5 mg. *Perioperative steroid coverage:* Hydrocortisone 100 mg IV night before surgery, 1 h preop, intraop, and 4, 8, and

22

12 h postop; pod #1 100 mg IV q6h; pod #2 100 mg IV q8h; pod #3 100 mg IV q12h; pod #4 50 mg IV q12h; pod #5 25 mg IV q12h; then resume prior oral dosing if chronic use or discontinue if only perioperative coverage required. *Cerebral edema:* Dexamethasone 10 mg IV; then 4 mg IV q4–6h
NOTES: See Table 22–5, page 627. All can cause hyperglycemia, "steroid psychosis," adrenal suppression; never acutely stop steroids, especially if chronic treatment; taper dose. Hydrocortisone succinate administered systemically, acetate form intraarticular

Steroids, Topical

See Table 22–6 (pages 628–630)
COMMON USES: Relief of inflammatory and pruritic manifestations of corticosteroid-response dermatoses
ACTIONS: Corticosteroid, antiinflammatory
DOSAGE: Varies with indication and formulation (See Table 22–6 (pages 628–630) for frequency of application)
SUPPLIED: See Table 22–6, pages 628–630

Streptokinase (Streptase, Kabikinase)

Used for emergency cardiac care (see Chapter 21)
COMMON USES: Coronary artery thrombosis, acute massive PE, DVT, and some occluded vascular grafts
ACTIONS: Activates plasminogen to plasmin that degrades fibrin; fibrinolytic
DOSAGE: *Adults.* PE. Loading dose of 250,000 IU IV through a peripheral vein over 30 min, then 100,000 IU/h IV for 24–72 h. *Coronary artery thrombosis:* 1.5 million U IV over 60 min. *DVT or arterial embolism:* Load as with PE, then 100,000 IU/h for 72 h. *Peds.* 3500–4000 U/kg over 30 min, followed by 1000–1500 U/kg/h
SUPPLIED: Powder for inj 250,000, 600,000, 750,000, 1,500,000 IU
NOTES: If maintenance inf inadequate to maintain thrombin clotting time 2–5 × control, refer to the package insert, or the *American Hospital Formulary* Service for adjustments. Antibodies remain 3–6 mo following dose

Streptomycin

COMMON USES: TB or serious *Enterococcus* infections
ACTIONS: Aminoglycoside; interferes with protein synthesis
DOSAGE: 1–4 g/d IM in 1–2 ÷ doses (endocarditis); TB 15 mg/kg/d
SUPPLIED: Inj 400 mg/mL
NOTES: Increased incidence of vestibular toxicity; adjust dose in renal impairment

Streptozocin (Zanosar)

COMMON USES: Pancreatic islet cell tumors and carcinoid tumors
ACTIONS: DNA–DNA (interstrand) cross-linking; DNA, RNA, and protein synthesis inhibitor
DOSAGE: 1–1.5 g/m^2 q 4 wk (single agent); 500 mg –1 g/m^2/d for 5 d q 4–6 wk (combination regimens)
SUPPLIED: Inj 1 g
NOTES: *Toxicity symptoms:* Nausea and vomiting and duodenal ulcers; myelosuppression rare (20%) and mild; nephrotoxicity (proteinuria and azotemia often heralded by hypophosphatemia) can be dose-limiting. Hypo- or hyperglycemia may occur; phlebitis and pain at the site of inj may also occur. Use with caution; adjust dose in renal impairment

Succimer (Chemet)

COMMON USES: Lead poisoning
ACTIONS: Heavy metal-chelating agent
DOSAGE: *Adults & Peds.* 8–15 kg: 100 mg PO; *16–23 kg:* 200 mg PO; *24–34 kg:* 300 mg PO; *35–44 kg:* 400 mg PO; *>45 kg:* 500 mg PO. Give dose noted q8h for 5 d, q12h for 14 d

SUPPLIED: Caps 100 mg

NOTES: May cause a rash; patients should drink a lot of fluids

Succinylcholine (Anectine, Quelicin, Sucostrin)

COMMON USES: Adjunct to general anesthesia to facilitate endotracheal intubation and to induce skeletal muscle relaxation during surgery or mechanically supported ventilation

ACTIONS: Depolarizing neuromuscular blocking agent

DOSAGE: *Adults.* 0.6 mg/kg IV over 10–30 s, followed by 0.04–0.07 mg/kg as needed to maintain muscle relaxation. *Peds.* 1–2 mg/kg/dose IV, followed by 0.3–0.6 mg/kg/dose at intervals of 10–20 min

SUPPLIED: Inj 20, 50, 100 mg/mL; powder for inj 100 mg, 500 mg, 1 g/vial

NOTES: May precipitate malignant hyperthermia; respiratory depression or prolonged apnea may occur; many drug interactions potentiating activity of succinylcholine; observe for cardiovascular effects; use only freshly prepared solutions; ↓ in severe liver disease

Sucralfate (Carafate)

COMMON USES: Duodenal and gastric ulcers

ACTIONS: Forms ulcer-adherent complex that protects against acid, pepsin, and bile acid

DOSAGE: *Adults.* 1 g PO qid, 1 h prior to meals and hs. *Peds.* 40–80 mg/kg/d ÷ q6h

SUPPLIED: Tabs 1 g; susp 1 g/10 mL

NOTES: Continue treatment for 4–8 wk unless healing is demonstrated by x-ray or endoscopy; constipation most frequent side effect

Sufentanil (Sufenta) [C-II]

COMMON USES: Analgesic adjunct to maintain balanced general anesthesia

ACTIONS: Potent synthetic opioid

DOSAGE: Adjunctive: 1–8 µg/kg with nitrous oxide/oxygen; maintenance of 10–50 µg PRN. *General anesthesia:* 8–30 µg/kg with oxygen and a skeletal muscle relaxant. *Maintenance:* 25–50 µg PRN.

SUPPLIED: Inj 50 µg/mL

NOTES: Respiratory depressant effects persisting longer than the analgesic effects; 80 times more potent than morphine

Sulfacetamide (Bleph-10, Cetamide, Sodium Sulamyd)

COMMON USES: Conjunctival infections

ACTIONS: Sulfonamide antibiotic

DOSAGE: 10% Oint apply qid and hs; soln for keratitis apply q2–3h depending on severity

SUPPLIED: Oint 10%; soln 10, 15, 30%

Sulfacetamide Prednisolone (Blephamide, others)

COMMON USES: Steroid-responsive inflammatory ocular conditions with infection or a risk of infection

ACTIONS: Antibiotic and antiinflammatory

DOSAGE: *Adult and Peds > 2 y.* Apply oint to lower conjunctival sac qd–qid; soln 1–3 gtt 2–3 h while awake

SUPPLIED: Oint: Sulfacetamide 10%/prednisolone 0.5%, sulfacetamide 10%/prednisolone 0.2%, sulfacetamide 10%/prednisolone 0.25%; susp: sulfacetamide 10%/prednisolone/0.25%, sulfacetamide 10%/prednisolone 0.5%, sulfacetamide sodium 10%/prednisolone 0.2%, sulfacetamide 10% and prednisolone 0.25%

NOTES: Ophth susp can be used as an otic agent

Sulfasalazine (Azulfidine)

COMMON USES: Ulcerative colitis

ACTIONS: Sulfonamide; actions not clear

DOSAGE: *Adults.* Initially, 1 g tid–qid; ↑ to a max of 8 g/d in 3–4 ÷ doses; maintenance 500 mg PO qid. *Peds.* Initially, 40–60 mg/kg/24h PO ÷ q4–6h; maintenance 20–30 mg/kg/24h PO ÷ q6h
SUPPLIED: Tabs 500 mg; EC tabs 500 mg; oral susp 250 mg/5 mL
NOTES: Can cause severe GI upset; discolors urine

Sulfinpyrazone (Anturane)

COMMON USES: Acute and chronic gout
ACTIONS: Inhibits renal tubular absorption of uric acid
DOSAGE: 100–200 mg PO bid for 1 wk, then ↑ as needed to maintenance of 200–400 mg bid
SUPPLIED: Tabs 100 mg; caps 200 mg
NOTES: Avoid in renal impairment; take with food or antacids, take with plenty of fluids; avoid salicylates

Sulindac (Clinoril)

COMMON USES: Arthritis and pain
ACTIONS: NSAID; inhibits prostaglandin synthesis
DOSAGE: 150–200 mg bid
SUPPLIED: Tabs 150, 200 mg

Sumatriptan (Imitrex)

COMMON USES: Acute treatment of migraine attacks
ACTIONS: Vascular serotonin receptor agonist
DOSAGE: *SC:* 6 mg SC as a single dose, PRN, to a max of 12 mg/24h; *Oral:* 25 mg, repeat in 2 h, PRN, 100 mg/d max oral dose; max 300 mg/d. *Nasal spray:* 1 single spray into 1 nostril, may repeat in 2 h, max 40 mg/24hh
SUPPLIED: Inj 12 mg/mL; tabs 25, 50 mg; nasal spray 5, 20 mg
NOTES: May cause pain and bruising at the injection site; avoid in angina, ischemic heart disease, uncontrolled HTN, and ergot administration

Tacrine (Cognex)

COMMON USES: Mild to moderate dementia
ACTIONS: Cholinesterase inhibitor
DOSAGE: 10–40 mg PO qid, up to 160 mg/d
SUPPLIED: Caps 10, 20, 30, 40 mg
NOTES: May cause elevations in transaminases; monitor LFT regularly; separate doses from food

Tacrolimus [FK 506] (Prograf)

COMMON USES: Prophylaxis of organ rejection
ACTIONS: Macrolide immunosuppressant
DOSAGE: *IV:* 0.05–0.1 mg/kg/d as cont inf. *PO:* 0.15–0.3 mg/kg/d ÷ into 2 doses
SUPPLIED: Caps 1, 5 mg; inj 5 mg/mL
NOTES: May cause neurotoxicity and nephrotoxicity; ↓ in renal impairment; may need to ↓ in hepatic impairment

Tamoxifen (Nolvadex)

COMMON USES: Breast cancer (postmenopausal, estrogen receptor-positive), endometrial cancer, melanoma, reduction of breast cancer in high-risk women
ACTIONS: Nonsteroidal antiestrogen; mixed agonist–antagonist effect
DOSAGE: 20–40 mg/d (typically 10 mg bid or 20 mg/d)
SUPPLIED: Tabs 10, 20 mg
NOTES: *Toxicity symptoms:* Menopausal symptoms (hot flashes, nausea, and vomiting) in premenopausal patients. Vaginal bleeding and menstrual irregularities. Skin rash, pruritus vulvae, dizziness, headache, and peripheral edema. Acute flare of bone metastasis pain and hypercalcemia.

With high doses, retinopathy. Increased risk of pregnancy in sexually active premenopausal women by inducing ovulation

Tamsulosin (Flomax)

COMMON USES: Benign prostatic hyperplasia
ACTIONS: Antagonist of α-receptors on the prostate
DOSAGE: 0.4 mg/d
SUPPLIED: Caps 0.4 mg; do NOT crush, chew, or open caps

Tazarotene (Tazorac)

COMMON USES: Facial acne vulgaris; stable plaque psoriasis up to 20% body surface area
ACTIONS: Keratolytic
DOSAGE: *Adults & Peds > 12 y.* Acne: Cleanse face, dry, and apply thin film qd hs on acne lesions. *Psoriasis:* Apply hs
SUPPLIED: Gel 0.05, 0.1%

Telmisartan (Micardis)

COMMON USES: HTN
ACTIONS: Angiotensin II receptor antagonists
DOSAGE: 40–80 mg/d
SUPPLIED: Tabs 40, 80 mg
NOTES: Avoid use during PRG

Temazepam (Restoril) [C-IV]

COMMON USES: Insomnia
ACTIONS: Benzodiazepine
DOSAGE: 15–30 mg PO hs PRN
SUPPLIED: Caps 7.5, 15, 30 mg
NOTES: ↓ Dose in elderly

Tenecteplase (TNKase)

COMMON USES: Reduction of mortality associated with AMI
ACTIONS: Thrombolytic; TPA
DOSAGE: 30–50 mg; see following table

Weight (kg)	TNKase Volume (mg)	TNKase[a] (mL)
<60	30	6
≥60–<70	35	7
≥70–<80	40	8
≥80–<90	45	9
≥90	50	10

[a]From one vial of reconstituted TNKase.

SUPPLIED: Inj 50 mg, reconstituted with 10 mL sterile water

Teniposide [VM-26] (Vumon)

COMMON USES: ALL (refractory pediatric), small-cell lung cancer, Kaposi's sarcoma, non-Hodgkin's lymphoma

ACTIONS: Topoisomerase II inhibitor, interfering with strand passage and DNA ligase activities of topoisomerase II. Cell cycle-specific activity late S, early G_2 phase
DOSAGE: 45–60 mg/m^2/d × 5 d q 21 d; 120–160 mg/m^2 on d 1, 3, and 5 q 21 d; 100 mg/m^2 on d 1 and 2 q 3 wk; 100 mg/m^2/wk
SUPPLIED: Inj 10 mg/mL
NOTES: *Toxicity symptoms:* Myelosuppression (especially leukopenia and thrombocytopenia), hypotension, chemical phlebitis, skin rashes, HTN, hypersensitivity reactions (urticaria, flushing, rashes, or hypotension), and secondary leukemia. Adjust dose in significant renal impairment; consider adjustment in hepatic impairment

Terazosin (Hytrin)

COMMON USES: BPH and HTN
ACTIONS: α-1 Blocker (blood vessel and bladder neck/prostate)
DOSAGE: Initially, 1 mg PO hs; ↑ to a max of 20 mg/d PO
SUPPLIED: Tabs 1, 2, 5, 10 mg; caps 1, 2, 5, 10 mg
NOTES: Hypotension and syncope following first dose; dizziness, weakness, nasal congestion, peripheral edema common; should be used with thiazide diuretic for HTN

Terbinafine (Lamisil)

COMMON USES: Onychomycosis, athlete's foot
ACTIONS: Inhibits squalene epoxidase resulting in fungal death
DOSAGE: *Oral:* 250 mg/d PO for 6–12 wk. *Topical:* Apply to affected area
SUPPLIED: Tabs 250 mg; cream 1%
NOTES: Full clinical effect may take months due to need for new nail growth; NO occlusive dressings; dosage adjustment in renal impairment

Terbutaline (Brethine, Bricanyl)

COMMON USES: Reversible bronchospasm (asthma, COPD); inhibition of labor
ACTIONS: Sympathomimetic
DOSAGE: *Adults.* Bronchodilator: 2.5–5 mg PO qid or 0.25 mg SC; may repeat in 15 min (max 0.5 mg in 4 h). *Met-dose inhaler:* 2 inhal q4–6h. *Premature labor:* Acutely 2.5–10 mg/min/IV, gradually ↑ as tolerated q 10–20 min; maintenance 2.5 – 10 mg PO q 4–6h until term; or 0.25 mg SC q 30 min. *Peds.* Oral: 0.05–0.15 mg/kg/dose PO tid; max 5 mg/24h
SUPPLIED: Tabs 2.5, 5 mg; inj 1 mg/mL; met-dose inhaler
NOTES: Caution with diabetes, HTN, hyperthyroidism; high doses may precipitate β-1-adrenergic effects

Terconazole (Terazol [vaginal])

COMMON USES: Vaginal fungal infections
ACTIONS: Topical antifungal
DOSAGE: 1 applicatorful or 1 supp intravaginally hs for 7 d
SUPPLIED: Vaginal cream 0.4%, vaginal supp 80 mg

Tetanus Immune Globulin [TIG]

COMMON USES: Passive immunization against tetanus for any person with a suspected contaminated wound and unknown immunization status (Chapter 17)
ACTIONS: Passive immunization
DOSAGE: *Adults & Peds.* 250–500 U IM (higher doses if delay in initiation of therapy)
SUPPLIED: Inj 250-U vial or syringe
NOTES: May begin active immunization series at different inj site if required

Tetanus Toxoid

COMMON USES: Protection against tetanus
ACTIONS: Active immunization

DOSAGE: See Chapter 17 and Table 22–9, page 636 for tetanus prophylaxis
SUPPLIED: Inj tetanus toxoid, fluid, measured in limes flocculation (Lf) units of toxoid: 4–5 Lf units/0.5 mL; tetanus toxoid, adsorbed, 5, 10 Lf units/0.5 mL

Tetracycline (Achromycin V, Sumycin)

COMMON USES: Broad-spectrum antibiotic treatment against *Staphylococcus, Streptococcus, Chlamydia, Rickettsia,* and *Mycoplasma*
ACTIONS: Bacteriostatic; inhibits protein synthesis
DOSAGE: *Adults.* 250–500 mg PO bid–qid. *Peds >8 y.* 25–50 mg/kg/24h PO q6–12h. Do NOT use in children <8 y old
SUPPLIED: Caps 100, 250, 500 mg; tabs 250, 500 mg; oral susp 250 mg/5 mL
NOTES: Can stain enamel and depress bone formation in children; caution with use in pregnancy; do NOT use in the presence of impaired renal function (see Doxycycline page 531)

Theophylline (Theolair, Theo-Dur, Somophyllin, others)

COMMON USES: Asthma, bronchospasm
ACTIONS: Relaxes smooth muscle of the bronchi and pulmonary blood vessels
DOSAGE: *Adults.* 900 mg PO ÷ q6h; SR products may be ÷ q8–12h × (maintenance). *Peds.* 16–22 mg/kg/24h PO ÷ q6h; SR products may be ÷ q8–12h × (maintenance)
SUPPLIED: Elixir 80, 150 mg/15 mL; liq 80, 160 mg/15 mL; caps 100, 200, 250 mg; tabs 100, 125, 200, 225, 250, 300 mg; SR caps 50, 75, 100, 125, 200, 250, 260, 300 mg; SR tabs 100, 200, 250, 300, 400, 450, 500 mg
NOTES: See drug levels in Table 22–7 (pages 631–634); many drug interactions; side effects include nausea, vomiting, tachycardia, and seizures

Thiamine [Vitamin B₁]

COMMON USES: Thiamine deficiency (beriberi); alcoholic neuritis; Wernicke's encephalopathy
ACTIONS: Dietary supplementation
DOSAGE: *Adults.* Deficiency: 100 mg/d IM for 2 wk, then 5–10 mg/d PO for 1 mo. *Wernicke's encephalopathy:* 100 mg IV in single dose, then 100 mg/d IM for 2 wk. *Peds.* 10–25 mg/d IM for 2 wk, then 5–10 mg/24h PO for 1 mo
SUPPLIED: Tabs 5, 10, 25, 50, 100, 500 mg; inj 100, 200 mg/mL
NOTES: IV thiamine administration associated with anaphylactic reaction; give IV slowly

Thiethylperazine (Torecan)

COMMON USES: Nausea and vomiting
ACTIONS: Antidopaminergic antiemetic
DOSAGE: 10 mg PO, PR, or IM qd–tid
SUPPLIED: Tabs 10 mg; supp 10 mg; inj 5 mg/mL
NOTES: Extrapyramidal reactions may occur

6-Thioguanine [6-TG] (Tabloid)

COMMON USES: AML, ALL, CML
ACTIONS: Purine-based antimetabolite (substitutes for natural purines interfering with nucleotide synthesis)
DOSAGE: 2–3 mg/kg/d
SUPPLIED: Tabs 40 mg
NOTES: *Toxicity symptoms:* Myelosuppression (especially leukopenia and thrombocytopenia), nausea and vomiting, anorexia, stomatitis, and diarrhea. Hepatotoxicity rare; dosage adjustment in renal or hepatic impairment

Thioridazine (Mellaril)

COMMON USES: Psychotic disorders; short-term treatment of depression, agitation, organic brain syndrome

22

ACTIONS: Phenothiazine antipsychotic
DOSAGE: *Adults.* Initially, 50–100 mg PO tid; maintenance 200–800 mg/24h PO in 2–4 ÷ doses. *Peds >2 y.* 0.5–3 mg/kg/24h PO in 2–3 ÷ doses
SUPPLIED: Tabs 10, 15, 25, 50, 100, 150, 200 mg; oral conc 30, 100 mg/mL; oral susp 25, 100 mg/5 mL
NOTES: Low incidence of extrapyramidal effects; may cause ventricular arrhythmias

Thiothixene (Navane)

COMMON USES: Psychotic disorders
ACTIONS: Antipsychotic
DOSAGE: *Adults & Peds >12 y.* Mild to moderate psychosis: 2 mg PO tid, up to 20–30 mg/d. *Severe psychosis:* 5 mg PO bid; ↑ to a max of 60 mg/24h PRN. *IM use:* 16–20 mg/24h ÷ bid–qid; max 30 mg/d. *Peds <12 y.* 0.25 mg/kg/24h PO ÷ q6–12h
SUPPLIED: Caps 1, 2, 5, 10, 20 mg; oral conc 5 mg/mL; inj 2, 5 mg/mL
NOTES: Drowsiness and extrapyramidal side effects most common

Tiagabine (Gabitril)

COMMON USES: Adjunctive therapy in treatment of partial seizures
ACTIONS: Inhibition of GABA
DOSAGE: Initial 4 mg/d, ↑ by 4 mg during 2nd wk; may keep increasing by 4–8 mg/d until clinical response achieved; max dose 56 mg/d
SUPPLIED: Tabs 4, 12, 16, 20 mg
NOTE: Use gradual withdrawal; used in combination with other anticonvulsants

Ticarcillin (Ticar)

COMMON USES: Infections caused by susceptible strains of gram (−) bacteria (including *Klebsiella, Proteus, E. coli, Enterobacter, P. aeruginosa,* and *Serratia*) involving the skin, bone, respiratory tract, urinary tract, abdomen, and septicemia
ACTIONS: Bacteriocidal; inhibits cell wall synthesis
DOSAGE: *Adults.* 3 g IV q4–6h. *Peds.* 200–300 mg/kg/d IV ÷ q4–6h
SUPPLIED: Inj
NOTES: Often used in combination with aminoglycoside; dosage adjustment in renal impairment

Ticarcillin/Potassium Clavulanate (Timentin)

COMMON USES: Infections caused by susceptible strains of gram (−) bacteria (including *Klebsiella, Proteus, E. coli, Enterobacter, P. aeruginosa,* and *Serratia*) involving the skin, bone, respiratory tract, urinary tract, abdomen, and septicemia
ACTIONS: Bactericidal; inhibits cell wall synthesis
DOSAGE: *Adults.* 3.1 g IV q4–6h. *Peds.* 200–300 mg/kg/d IV ÷ q4–6h
SUPPLIED: Inj
NOTES: Often used in combination with aminoglycosides; dosage adjustment in renal impairment

Ticlopidine (Ticlid)

COMMON USES: Reduces the risk of thrombotic stroke
ACTIONS: Platelet aggregation inhibitor
DOSAGE: 250 mg PO bid
SUPPLIED: Tabs 250 mg
NOTES: Administer with food; may cause neutropenia, monitor WBC and LFTs

Timolol (Blocadren)

COMMON USES: HTN and MI
ACTIONS: Competitively blocks β-adrenergic receptors, β_1, β_2
DOSAGE: *HTN:* 10–20 mg bid, up to 60 mg/d. *MI:* 10 mg bid
SUPPLIED: Tabs 5, 10, 20 mg

Timolol, Ophthalmic (Timoptic)

COMMON USES: Glaucoma
ACTIONS: β-Blocker
DOSAGE: 0.25% 1 gt bid; ↓ to qd when controlled; use 0.5% if needed; 1 gt gel qd
SUPPLIED: Soln 0.25/0.5%; Timoptic XE (0.25, 0.5%) gel-forming soln

Tioconazole (Vagistat)

COMMON USES: Vaginal fungal infections
ACTIONS: Topical antifungal
DOSAGE: 1 applicatorful intravaginally hs (single dose)
SUPPLIED: Vaginal oint 6.5%

Tirofiban (Aggrastat)

COMMON USES: Acute coronary syndrome
ACTIONS: Glycoprotein IIb/IIIa inhibitor
DOSAGE: Initial 0.4 μg/kg/min for 30 min, followed by 0.1 μg/kg/min
SUPPLIED: Inj 50 μg/mL, 250 μg/mL
NOTES: Adjust dose in renal insufficiency; use in combination with heparin

Tobramycin (Nebcin)

COMMON USES: Serious gram– infections, especially *Pseudomonas*
ACTIONS: Aminoglycoside; inhibits protein synthesis
DOSAGE: *Adults.* 1–2.5 mg/kg/dose IV q8–24h (see page 620). *Peds.* 2.5 mg/kg/dose IV q8h
SUPPLIED: Inj 10, 40 mg/mL
NOTES: Nephrotoxic and ototoxic; ↓ with renal insufficiency; monitor creatinine clearance and serum concentrations for dosage adjustments (see Table 22–7, pages 631–634, and page 620).

Tobramycin Ophthalmic (AK Tob, Tobrex)

COMMON USES: Ocular bacterial infections
ACTIONS: Aminoglycoside antibiotic
DOSAGE: 1–2 gtt q4h; oint bid–tid; if severe infections, use oint q3–4h, or 2 gtt q 30–60 min, then less frequently
SUPPLIED: Oint and soln tobramycin 0.3%

Tobramycin and Dexamethasone Ophthalmic (TobraDex)

COMMON USES: Ocular bacterial infections associated with significant inflammation
ACTIONS: Antibiotic with antiinflammatory
DOSAGE: 0.3% oint apply q3–8h or soln 0.3% apply 1–2 gtt q1–4h
SUPPLIED: Oint and soln tobramycin 0.3% and dexamethasone 0.1%

Tocainide (Tonocard)

COMMON USES: Suppression of ventricular arrhythmias, including PVCs, and ventricular tachycardia
ACTIONS: Class IB antiarrhythmic
DOSAGE: 400–600 mg PO q8h, up to 2400 mg/d
SUPPLIED: Tabs 400, 600 mg
NOTES: Properties similar to those of lidocaine; ↓ dose in renal failure; CNS and GI side effects common

Tolazamide (Tolinase)

COMMON USES: Type 2 DM
ACTION: Sulfonylurea. Stimulates the release of insulin from the pancreas; increases insulin sensitivity at peripheral sites; reduces glucose output from the liver
DOSAGE: 100–500 mg/d
SUPPLIED: Tabs 100, 250, 500 mg

22

Tolazoline (Priscoline)

COMMON USES: Persistent pulmonary vasoconstriction and HTN of the newborn, peripheral vasospastic disorders
ACTIONS: Competitively blocks α-adrenergic receptors
DOSAGE: *Adults.* 10–50 mg IM/IV/SC qid
   Neonates. 1–2 mg/kg IV over 10–15 min, followed by 1–2 mg/kg/h
SUPPLIED: Inj 25 mg/mL

Tolbutamide (Orinase)

COMMON USES: Type 2 DM
ACTION: Sulfonylurea. Stimulates the release of insulin from the pancreas; increases insulin sensitivity at peripheral sites; reduces glucose output from the liver
DOSAGE: 500–1000 mg bid
SUPPLIED: Tabs 500 mg
NOTES: May require dosage adjustment in hepatic impairment

Tolmetin (Tolectin)

COMMON USES: Arthritis and pain
ACTIONS: NSAID; inhibits prostaglandin synthesis
DOSAGE: 200–600 mg tid, to a max of 2000 mg/d
SUPPLIED: Tabs 200, 600 mg; caps 400 mg

Tolnaftate [OTC] (Tinactin)

COMMON USES: Tinea pedis, tinea cruris, tinea corporis, tinea manus, tinea versicolor
ACTIONS: Topical antifungal
DOSAGE: Apply to area bid for 2–4 wk
SUPPLIED: OTC 1% liq; gel; powder; cream; soln

Tolterodine (Detrol, Detrol LA)

COMMON USES: Management of overactive bladder (frequency, urgency, urge incontinence)
ACTIONS: Anticholinergic
DOSAGE: Detrol 1–2 mg PO bid; Detrol LA 2–4 mg/d
SUPPLIED: Detrol tabs 1, 2 mg; Detrol LA tabs 2, 4 mg
NOTES: Do not administer to patients with urinary retention, gastric retention, or uncontrolled narrow-angle glaucoma; dry mouth common side effect

Topiramate (Topamax)

COMMON USES: Partial onset seizures
ACTIONS: Anticonvulsant
DOSAGE: Total dose 400 mg/d. See product information for 8-wk titration schedule
SUPPLIED: Tabs 25, 100, 200 mg; caps sprinkles 15, 25, 50 mg
NOTES: May precipitate kidney stones; dosage adjustment in renal impairment

Topotecan (Hycamtin)

COMMON USES: Ovarian cancer (cisplatin-refractory), small-cell lung cancer, and non-Hodgkin's lymphoma
ACTIONS: Topoisomerase I inhibitor; interferes with DNA synthesis
DOSAGE: 1.5 mg/m^2/d as an 1-h IV inf for 5 consecutive days, repeated q 3 wk
SUPPLIED: Vials containing 4 mg of lyophilized drug reconstituted in sterile water and diluted in NS or 5% dextrose
NOTES: *Toxicity symptoms:* Myelosuppression, nausea and vomiting, diarrhea, drug fever, and skin rash. ↓ Dose for renal dysfunction

Torsemide (Demadex)

COMMON USES: Edema, HTN, CHF, and hepatic cirrhosis
ACTIONS: Loop diuretic; inhibits reabsorption of sodium and chloride in the ascending loop of Henle and distal tubule
DOSAGE: 5–20 mg/d PO or IV
SUPPLIED: Tabs 5, 10, 20, 100 mg; inj 10 mg/mL

Tramadol (Ultram)

COMMON USES: Moderate to severe pain
ACTIONS: Centrally acting analgesic
DOSAGE: 50–100 mg PO q4–6h PRN, not to exceed 400 mg/d
SUPPLIED: Tabs 50 mg
NOTES: Lowers seizure threshold, tolerance or dependence may develop

Trandolapril (Mavik)

COMMON USES: HTN, CHF, LVD, post-AMI
ACTIONS: ACE inhibitor
DOSAGE: *HTN:* 2–4 mg/d. *CHF/LVD:* 4 mg/d
SUPPLIED: Tabs 1, 2, 4 mg
NOTES: Dosage adjustment in renal or hepatic impairment

Trazodone (Desyrel)

COMMON USES: Depression
ACTIONS: Antidepressant; inhibits reuptake of serotonin and norepinephrine
DOSAGE: *Adults & Adolescents.* 50–150 mg PO qd–qid; max 600 mg/d
SUPPLIED: Tabs 50, 100, 150, 300 mg
NOTES: May take 1–2 wk for symptomatic improvement; anticholinergic side effects

Tretinoin, Systemic [Tretinoic Acid] (Vesanoid)

COMMON USES: APL induction therapy
ACTIONS: Differentiating agent; all *trans* retinoic acid
DOSAGE: 45 mg/m^2/d in ÷ doses for approximately 40 d
SUPPLIED: Caps 10 mg
NOTES: *Toxicity symptoms:* Cutaneous (dryness, chafing), neurologic (headache), hypertriglyceridemia, and treatment-related leukocytosis reported in APL, as well as "retinoic acid syndrome"

Tretinoin, Topical [Retinoic Acid] (Retin-A, Avita)

COMMON USES: Acne vulgaris, sun-damaged skin, some skin cancers
ACTIONS: Exfoliant retinoic acid derivative
DOSAGE: *Adults & Peds> 12.* Apply qd hs; if irritation develops, ↓ frequency
SUPPLIED: Cream 0.025, 0.05, 0.1%; gel 0.01, 0.025, 0.1%; liq 0.05%
NOTES: Avoid sunlight

Triamcinolone and Nystatin (Mycolog-II)

COMMON USES: Cutaneous candidiasis
ACTIONS: Antifungal and antiinflammatory
DOSAGE: Apply lightly to area bid; max 25 d
SUPPLIED: Cream and oint 15, 30, 60, 120 mg
NOTES: Contra in varicella

Triamterene (Dyrenium)

COMMON USES: Edema associated with CHF, cirrhosis
ACTIONS: Potassium-sparing diuretic
DOSAGE: *Adults.* 100–300 mg/24h PO ÷ qd–bid. *Peds.* 2–4 mg/kg/d in 1–2 ÷ doses

SUPPLIED: Caps 50, 100 mg
NOTES: Can cause hyperkalemia, blood dyscrasias, liver damage, and other reactions; dosage adjustment in renal or hepatic impairment

Triazolam (Halcion) [C-IV]

COMMON USES: Short-term management of insomnia
ACTIONS: Benzodiazepine
DOSAGE: 0.125–0.25 mg/d PO hs PRN
SUPPLIED: Tabs 0.125, 0.25 mg
NOTES: Additive CNS depression with alcohol and other CNS depressants; ↓ dose; avoid in cirrhosis

Triethanolamine (Cerumenex)

COMMON USES: Cerumen removal
ACTIONS: Ceruminolytic agent
DOSAGE: Fill the ear canal and insert the cotton plug; irrigate with water after 15 min; repeat as needed
SUPPLIED: Soln 6, 12 mL

Triethylene-Triphosphoramide [Thiotepa, TESPA, TSPA] (Thioplex)

COMMON USES: Hodgkin's and non-Hodgkin's lymphomas; leukemia; breast, ovarian, and bladder cancers (IV and intravesical therapy), preparative regimens for allogeneic and autologous BMT in high doses
ACTIONS: Polyfunctional alkylating agent
DOSAGE: 0.5 mg/kg q 1–4 wk, 6 mg/m^2 IM or IV × 4 d q 2–4 wk, 15–35 mg/m^2 by cont IV inf over 48 h; 60 mg instilled into the bladder and retained 2 h q 1–4 wk; 900–125 mg/m^2 in ABMT regimens (the highest dose that can be administered without ABMT is 180 mg/m^2); 1–10 mg/m^2 (typically 15 mg) IT once or twice a week; 0.8 mg/kg in 1–2 L of soln may be instilled intraperitoneally
SUPPLIED: Inj 15 mg
NOTES: *Toxicity symptoms:* Myelosuppression, nausea, vomiting, dizziness, headache, allergy, and paresthesias

Trifluoperazine (Stelazine)

COMMON USES: Psychotic disorders
ACTIONS: Phenothiazine; blocks postsynaptic mesolimbic dopaminergic receptors in the brain
DOSAGE: *Adults.* 2–10 mg PO bid. *Peds 6–12 y.* 1 mg PO qd–bid initially, then gradually ↑ up to 15 mg/d
SUPPLIED: Tabs 1, 2, 5, 10 mg; oral conc 10 mg/mL; inj 2 mg/mL
NOTES: ↓ Dose in elderly and debilitated patients; oral conc must be diluted to 60 mL or more prior to administration; requires several weeks for onset of effects

Trifluridine (Viroptic)

COMMON USES: Herpes simplex keratitis and conjunctivitis
ACTIONS: Antiviral
DOSAGE: 1 gt q2h (max 9 gtt/d); ↓ to 1 gt q4h after healing begins; treat up to 14 d
SUPPLIED: 1% soln

Trihexyphenidyl (Artane)

COMMON USES: Parkinson's disease
ACTIONS: Blocks excess acetylcholine at cerebral synapses
DOSAGE: 2–5 mg PO qd–qid
SUPPLIED: Tabs 2, 5 mg; SR caps 5 mg; elixir 2 mg/5 mL
NOTES: Contra in narrow-angle glaucoma

Trimethobenzamide (Tigan)

COMMON USES: Nausea and vomiting
ACTIONS: Inhibits medullary chemoreceptor trigger zone
DOSAGE: *Adults.* 250 mg PO or 200 mg PR or IM tid–qid PRN. *Peds.* 20 mg/kg/24h PO or 15 mg/kg/24h PR or IM in 3–4 ÷ doses (NOT recommended for infants)
SUPPLIED: Caps 100, 250 mg; supp 100, 200 mg; inj 100 mg/mL
NOTES: In the presence of viral infections, may mask emesis or mimic CNS effects of Reye's syndrome; may cause parkinsonian-like syndrome

Trimethoprim (Trimpex, Proloprim)

COMMON USES: UTI due to susceptible gram+ and gram– organisms; often used for suppression of UTI
ACTIONS: Inhibits dihydrofolate reductase
DOSAGE: *Adults.* 100 mg/d PO bid or 200 mg/d PO. *Peds.* 4 mg/kg/d in 2 ÷ doses
SUPPLIED: Tabs 100, 200 mg; oral soln 50 mg/5 mL
NOTES: ↓ Dose in renal failure

Trimethoprim-Sulfamethoxazole [Co-trimoxazole] (Bactrim, Septra)

COMMON USES: UTI, otitis media, sinusitis, bronchitis, and *Shigella, P. carinii,* and *Nocardia* infections
ACTIONS: Dual effect of SMX-inhibiting synthesis of dihydrofolic acid and TMP-inhibiting dihydrofolate reductase to impair protein synthesis
DOSAGE: *Adults.* 1 DS tab PO bid or 5–20 mg/kg/24h (based on TMP component) IV in 3–4 ÷ doses. *P. carinii:* 15–20 mg/kg/d IV or PO (TMP component) in 4 ÷ doses. *Nocardia:* 10–15 mg/kg/d IV or PO (TMP component) in 4 ÷ doses. *Peds.* 8–10 mg/kg/24h (TMP) PO ÷ into 2 doses or 3–4 doses IV; do NOT use in newborns
SUPPLIED: Regular tabs 80 mg of TMP and 400 mg of SMX; DS tabs 160 mg of TMP and 800 mg of SMX; oral susp 40 mg of TMP and 200 mg of SMX/ 5 mL; inj 80 mg of TMP and 400 mg of SMX/5 mL
NOTES: Synergistic combination; reduce dosage in renal failure; maintain adequate hydration

Trimetrexate (Neutrexin)

COMMON USES: Moderate to severe PCP
ACTIONS: Inhibits dihydrofolate reductase
DOSAGE: 45 mg/m^2 IV q24h for 21 d
SUPPLIED: Inj
NOTES: Administer with leucovorin 20 mg/m^2 IV q6h for 24 d; use cytotoxic precautions; infuse over 60 min; ↓ in hepatic impairment

Trimipramine (Surmontil)

COMMON USES: Depression
ACTIONS: Tricyclic antidepressant; increases synaptic concentration of serotonin and/or norepinephrine in CNS
DOSAGE: 50–300 mg/d PO hs
SUPPLIED: Caps 25, 50, 100 mg

Urokinase (Abbokinase)

COMMON USES: PE, DVT, restore patency to IV catheters
ACTIONS: Converts plasminogen to plasmin that causes clot lysis
DOSAGE: *Adults & Peds.* Systemic effect: 4400 IU/kg IV over 10 min, followed by 4400–6000 IU/kg/h for 12 h. *Restore catheter patency:* Inject 5000 IU into catheter and gently aspirate
SUPPLIED: Powder for inj 5000 IU/mL, 250,000 IU vial
NOTES: Do NOT use systemically within 10 d of surgery, delivery, or organ biopsy

22

Valacyclovir (Valtrex)

COMMON USES: Herpes zoster; genital herpes
ACTIONS: Prodrug of acyclovir, inhibits viral DNA replication
DOSAGE: 1 g PO tid; genital herpes treatment 500 mg bid × 7 d, prophylaxis 500–1000 mg/d
SUPPLIED: Caplets 500 mg
NOTES: Dosage adjustment in renal impairment

Valproic Acid and Divalproex (Depakene, Depakote)

COMMON USES: Rx epilepsy, mania; prophylaxis of migraines
ACTIONS: Anticonvulsant; increases the availability of GABA
DOSAGE: *Adults & Peds.* Seizures: 30–60 mg/kg/24h PO ÷ tid (after initiation of 10–15 mg/dh/24h). *Mania:* 750 mg in 3 ÷ doses, ↑ to a max of 60 mg/kg/d. *Migraines:* 250 mg bid, ↑ to 1000 mg/d
SUPPLIED: *Valproic acid:* caps 250 mg; syrup 250 mg/5 mL. *Divalproex:* EC tabs 125, 250, 500; caps 125 mg
NOTES: Monitor LFT and follow serum levels (see Table 22–7, pages 631–634); concurrent use of phenobarbital and phenytoin may alter serum levels of these agents; ↓ dose in hepatic impairment

Valrubicin (Valstar)

COMMON USES: Intravesical treatment of BCG-refractory CIS when immediate cystectomy would be associated with unacceptable morbidity or mortality
ACTIONS: Semisynthetic doxorubicin analogue; cytotoxic
DOSAGE: 800 mg intravesically weekly for 6 wk
SUPPLIED: Liq 200 mg/5 mL
NOTES: Dilute 800 mg in approximately 75 mL NS; minimal systemic absorption with intact bladder. Do NOT use within 1–2 wk of biopsy as systemic absorption can cause myelosuppression; can cause local bladder symptoms; contra with bladder capacity of < 75 mL or active UTI

Valsartan (Diovan)

COMMON USES: HTN
ACTIONS: Angiotensin II receptor antagonist
DOSAGE: 80 –160 mg/d
SUPPLIED: Caps 80, 160 mg
NOTES: Use with caution with K-sparing diuretics or K supplements

Vancomycin (Vancocin, Vancoled)

COMMON USES: Serious MRSA infections and in enterococcal endocarditis in combination with aminoglycosides in penicillin-allergic patients; oral treatment of *C. difficile* pseudomembranous colitis
ACTIONS: Inhibits cell wall synthesis
DOSAGE: *Adults.* 1 g IV q12h; for colitis 125–500 mg PO q6h. *Peds (NOT neonates).* 40 mg/kg/24h IV in ÷ doses q6–12h
SUPPLIED: Caps 125, 250 mg; powder for oral soln; powder for inj 500 mg, 1000 mg, 10 g/vial
NOTES: Ototoxic and nephrotoxic; NOT absorbed orally, provides local effect in gut only; IV dose must be given slowly over 1 h to prevent "red-man syndrome"; adjust dose in renal failure (for drug levels, see Table 22–7, pages 631–634)

Varicella Virus Vaccine (Varivax)

COMMON USES: Prevention of varicella (chicken pox) infection
ACTIONS: Active immunization
DOSAGE: *Adults & Peds.* 0.5 mL SC, repeated in 4–8 wk
SUPPLIED: Powder for inj
NOTES: Live virus; do NOT administer to immunocompromised

Vasopressin [Antidiuretic Hormone (ADH)] (Pitressin)

COMMON USES: Diabetes insipidus; relief of gaseous GI tract distention; severe GI bleeding
ACTIONS: Posterior pituitary hormone, potent GI vasoconstrictor
DOSAGE: *Adults & Peds.* Diabetes insipidus: 2.5–10 U SC or IM tid–qid or 1.5–5.0 U IM q 1–3 d of the tannate. *GI hemorrhage:* 0.2–0.4 U/min
SUPPLIED: Inj 20 U/mL
NOTES: Use with caution with any vascular disease

Vecuronium (Norcuron)

COMMON USES: Skeletal muscle relaxation during surgery or mechanical ventilation
ACTIONS: Nondepolarizing neuromuscular blocker
DOSAGE: *Adults & Peds.* 0.08–0.1 mg/kg IV bolus; maintenance of 0.010–0.015 mg/kg after 25–40 min followed with additional doses q 12–15 min
SUPPLIED: Powder for inj 10 mg
NOTES: Drug interactions leading to an increased effect of vecuronium include aminoglycosides, tetracycline, and succinylcholine; fewer cardiac effects than with pancuronium

Venlafaxine (Effexor)

COMMON USES: Depression
ACTIONS: Potentiation of neurotransmitter activity in the CNS
DOSAGE: 75–375 mg/d ÷ into 2–3 equal doses
SUPPLIED: Tabs 25, 37.5, 50, 75, 100 mg; ER caps 37.5, 75, 150 mg
NOTES: Dosage adjustment in renal or hepatic impairment

Verapamil (Calan, Isoptin)

Used for emergency cardiac care (see Chapter 21)
COMMON USES: Angina, essential HTN, and arrhythmias
ACTIONS: Ca channel-blocker
DOSAGE: *Adults.* Arrhythmias: See Chapter 21. *Angina:* 80–120 mg PO tid, up to 480 mg/24h. *HTN:* 80–180 mg PO tid or SR tabs 120–240 mg PO qd to 240 mg bid. **Peds.** <1 y: 0.1–0.2 mg/kg IV over 2 min (may repeat in 30 min). *1–16 y:* 0.1–0.3 mg/kg IV over 2 min (may repeat in 30 min); do NOT exceed 5 mg. *Oral: 1–5 y:* 4–8 mg/kg/d in 3 ÷ doses. *>5 y:* 80 mg q6–8h
SUPPLIED: Tabs 40, 80, 120 mg; SR tabs 120, 180, 240 mg; SR caps 120, 180, 240, 360 mg; inj 5 mg/2 mL
NOTES: Use caution with elderly patients; ↓ dose in renal or hepatic failure; constipation common

Vinblastine (Velban, Velbe)

COMMON USES: Hodgkin's and non-Hodgkin's lymphomas, mycosis fungoides, testicular cancer, choriocarcinoma, breast cancer, histiocytosis X, non-small-cell lung cancer, AIDS-related Kaposi's sarcoma, renal cell carcinoma
ACTIONS: Inhibits microtubule assembly through binding to tubulin
DOSAGE: 0.1–0.5 mg/kg/wk (4–20 mg/m^2)
SUPPLIED: Inj 1 mg/mL
NOTES: *Toxicity symptoms:* Myelosuppression (especially leukopenia), nausea and vomiting (rare), constipation, neurotoxicity (similar to that listed for vincristine but less frequent), alopecia, rash; myalgia and tumor pain common; dosage adjustment in hepatic impairment

Vincristine (Oncovin, Vincasar PFS)

COMMON USES: ALL, breast carcinoma, sarcoma (including Ewing's and rhabdomyosarcoma), Wilms' tumor, Hodgkin's and non-Hodgkin's lymphomas, neuroblastoma, small-cell lung cancer, multiple myeloma
ACTIONS: Promotes disassembly of mitotic spindle, causing metaphase arrest
DOSAGE: 0.4–1.4 mg/m^2 (single doses do NOT usually exceed 2 mg)
SUPPLIED: Inj 1 mg/mL

NOTES: *Toxicity symptoms:* Neurotoxicity commonly dose-limiting, jaw pain (trigeminal neuralgia), fever, fatigue and anorexia, constipation and paralytic ileus, bladder atony, no significant myelosuppression observed with standard doses. Soft tissue necrosis possible with extravasation; dosage adjustment in hepatic impairment

Vinorelbine (Navelbine)

COMMON USES: Non-small-cell lung cancer (single agent or with cisplatin), breast cancer
ACTIONS: Inhibits polymerization of microtubules, impairing mitotic spindle formation, semisynthetic vinca alkaloid
DOSAGE: 30 mg/m^2/wk
SUPPLIED: Inj 10 mg
NOTES: *Toxicity symptoms:* Myelosuppression (especially leukopenia), mild GI effects and infrequent neurotoxicity (6– 29%), constipation and paresthesias (rare). Tissue damage can result from extravasation. Dosage adjustment in hepatic impairment

Vitamin B₁

See Thiamine (page 609)

Vitamin B₆

See Pyridoxine (page 596)

Vitamin B₁₂

See Cyanocobalamin (page 521)

Vitamin K

See Phytonadione (page 589)

Warfarin (Coumadin)

COMMON USES: Prophylaxis and Rx of PE and DVT, AF with embolization, other postoperative indications
ACTIONS: Inhibits vitamin K-dependent production of clotting factors in the order VII-IX-X-II
DOSAGE: See Table 22–10 (page 637) for anticoagulation guidelines. *Adults.* Individualize dose to keep INR 2.0–3.0 for most indications, for mechanical heart valves desired INR is 2.5–3.5. ACCP guidelines recommend initiation with 5 mg, unless rapid attainment of therapeutic INR is necessary (use 7.5–10 mg) if patient elderly or has other bleeding risk factors (↓). others recommend 10–15 mg PO, IM, or IV qd for 1–3 d; then maintenance, 2–10 mg/d PO, IV, or IM; follow daily INR during initial phase to guide dosage. *Peds.* 0.05–0.34 mg/kg/24h PO, IM, or IV. Follow PT/INR closely to adjust dosage
SUPPLIED: Tabs 1, 2, 2.5, 3, 4, 5, 6, 7.5, 10 mg; inj
NOTES: INR now the preferred test rather than PT; Check INR periodically on maintenance dose; beware of bleeding caused by over anticoagulation (PT >3 × control or INR >5.0– 6.0); to rapidly correct over coumadinization, use vitamin K or FFP or both; highly teratogenic; do NOT use in pregnancy. Caution patient on taking Coumadin with other medications, especially aspirin. *Common warfarin interactions:* Potentiates acetaminophen, alcohol (with liver disease), amiodarone, cimetidine, ciprofloxacin, co-trimoxazole, erythromycin, fluconazole, flu vaccine, isoniazid, itraconazole, metronidazole, omeprazole, phenytoin, propranolol, quinidine, tetracycline. Inhibits barbiturates, carbamazepine, chlordiazepoxide, cholestyramine, dicloxacillin, nafcillin, rifampin, sucralfate, high vitamin K foods

Witch Hazel (Tucks Pads, others)

COMMON USES: After bowel movement cleansing to decrease local irritation or relieve hemorrhoids; after anorectal surgery and episiotomy
DOSAGE: Apply PRN
SUPPLIED: Presoaked pads, liq

Zafirlukast (Accolate)

COMMON USES: Prophylaxis and chronic Rx of asthma
ACTIONS: Selective and competitive inhibitor of leukotriene D4 and E4
DOSAGE: 20 mg bid
SUPPLIED: Tabs 20 mg
NOTES: NOT for acute exacerbations of asthma, contra in nursing women; associated with hepatic dysfunction, which has been reversible on discontinuation

Zalcitabine [DdC] (Hivid)

COMMON USES: HIV patients intolerant of zidovudine and didanosine
ACTIONS: Antiretroviral agent
DOSAGE: 0.75 mg PO tid
SUPPLIED: Tabs 0.375, 0.75 mg
NOTES: May be used in combination with zidovudine; may cause peripheral neuropathy; dosage adjustment in renal impairment

Zaleplon (Sonata)

COMMON USES: Insomnia
ACTION: A nonbenzodiazepine sedative hypnotic, a pyrazolopyrimidine
DOSAGE: 5–20 mg hs PRN
SUPPLIED: Caps 5, 10 mg

Zanamivir (Relenza)

COMMON USES: Influenza
ACTIONS: Inhibits viral neuraminidase
DOSAGE: 2 inhal (10 mg) bid for 5 d
SUPPLIED: Powder for inhal 5 mg
NOTES: Uses a Diskhaler for administration; initiate within 48 h of symptom onset; do NOT use in pulmonary disease

Zidovudine (Retrovir)

COMMON USES: HIV infections
ACTIONS: Inhibits reverse transcriptase
DOSAGE: *Adults.* 200 mg PO tid or 300 mg PO bid or 1–2 mg/kg/dose IV q4h. *Pregnancy:* 100 mg PO 5×/d until the start of labor, then during labor 2 mg/kg over 1 h followed by 1 mg/kg/h until clamping of the umbilical cord. *Peds.* 160 mg/m^2/dose q8h
SUPPLIED: Caps 100 mg; tabs 300 mg; syrup 50 mg/5 mL; inj 10 mg/mL
NOTES: Not a cure for HIV infections; hematologic toxicity; dosage adjustment in renal impairment

Zidovudine and Lamivudine (Combivir)

COMMON USES: HIV infections
ACTIONS: Combination inhibitors of reverse transcriptase
DOSAGE: *Adults & Peds 12 y.* 1 tab bid
SUPPLIED: Caps zidovudine 300 mg/lamivudine 150 mg
NOTES: An alternative to ↓ number of caps for combination therapy with the two agents

Zileuton (Zyflo)

COMMON USES: Prophylaxis and chronic treatment of asthma
ACTIONS: Inhibitor of 5-lipoxygenase
DOSAGE: 600 mg qid
SUPPLIED: Tabs 600 mg
NOTES: MUST take on a regular basis; does NOT treat acute exacerbation; hepatotoxic/do NOT use in hepatic impairment

22

Zolmitriptan (Zomig)

COMMON USES: Acute treatment of migraine

Action: Selective agonist of serotonin to cause vasoconstriction

DOSAGE: Initial 2.5 mg, may repeat after 2 h to a max of 10 mg in 24 h

NOTES: Use with caution in hepatic impairment; do NOT use in PRG

Zolpidem (Ambien) [C-IV]

COMMON USES: Short-term treatment of insomnia

ACTIONS: Hypnotic agent

DOSAGE: 5–10 mg PO hs PRN

SUPPLIED: Tabs 5, 10 mg

Zonisamide (Zonegran)

COMMON USES: Partial seizures

ACTIONS: Anticonvulsant

DOSAGE: Initial 100 mg/d; may be ↑ to 400 mg/d

SUPPLIED: Caps 100 mg

NOTES: Contra in persons with hypersensitivity to sulfonamides

Aminoglycoside Dosing

Table 22–7 (pages 631–634) gives information on the trough and peak levels of the aminoglycosides gentamicin, tobramycin, and amikacin. Peak levels should be drawn 30 min after the dose is completely infused; trough levels should be drawn 30 min prior to the dose. As a general rule, draw the peak and trough around the fourth maintenance dose. Therapy can be initiated with the recommended guidelines that follow.

Procedure (Adult)

1. Calculate estimated CrCl based on SCr, age, and weight (in kg), or a formal CrCl can also be ordered, if time permits.
2. Select loading dose:

   Gentamicin: 1.5–2.0 mg/kg
   Tobramycin: 1.5–2.0 mg/kg
   Amikacin: 5.0–7.5 mg/kg

3. By using Table 22–8 (page 635), select maintenance dose (as a percentage of the chosen loading dose) most appropriate for the renal function of patient based on the CrCl and dosing interval. Shaded areas are suggested percentages and intervals for any given CrCl. This is only an empiric dose to begin therapy. Monitor serum levels routinely for optimal therapy. Use Table 22–7 (pages 631–634) for the drug levels to follow for each drug.

IMMUNIZATION SCHEDULE (SEE TABLE 22–9, PAGE 636)

Perform active immunization of normal infants and children based on Table 22–9 (page 636). In addition, perform TB tine test at 15–19 mo and again at the entry to school (4–6 y). Hep B = hepatitis B vaccine; DtaP = diphtheria and tetanus toxoids and acellular pertussis vaccine. Td = Tetanus toxoid. Hib = *Haemophilus* influenza type b vaccine. IPV = all-inactivated polio virus vaccine. MMR = measles-mumps-rubella vaccine. Var = varicella. Hep A = hepatitis A vaccine. For additional details refer to *MMWR* Vol 50, No 01; Jan 12, 2001.

TABLE 22-1
Quick Guide to Dosing of Acetaminophen Based on the Tylenol Product Line

	Suspension* Drops and Original Drops 80 mg/0.8 ml Dropperful	Chewable* Tablets 80 mg tabs	Suspension* Liquid and Original Elixir 160 mg/5 ml	Junior* Strength 160 mg Caplets/Chewables	Regular† Strength 325 mg Caplets/Tablets	Extra Strength† 500 mg Caplets/Gelcaps
Q-3 mo/6-11 lb/2.5-5.4 kg	½ dppr‡ (0.4 mL)					
4-11 mo/12-17 lb/5.5-7.9 kg	1 dppr‡ (0.8 mL)					
12-23 mo/18-23 lb/8.0-10.9 kg	1½ dppr‡ (1.2 mL)		½ tsp			
2-3 y/24-35 lb/11.09-15.9 kg	2 dppr‡ (1.6 mL)	2 tab	¾ tsp			
4-5 y/36-47 lb/16.0-21.9 kg		3 tab	1 tsp			
6-8 y/48-59 lb/22.0-26.9 kg		4 tab	1½ tsp	2 cap/tab		
9-10 y/60-71 lb/27.0-31.9 kg		5 tab	2 tsp	2½ cap/tab		
11 y/72-95 lb/32.0-43.9 kg		6 tab	2½ tsp	3 cap/tab		
Adults & children 12 y and over/96 lb and over/44.0 kg and over			4 tsp	4 cap/tab	1 or 2 caps/tabs	2 caps/gel

*Doses should be administered 4 or 5 times daily or as directed by your doctor. Do not exceed 5 doses in 24 h.
†No more than 8 dosage units in any 24-h period. Not to be taken for pain for more than 10 days or for fever for more than 3 days unless directed by a physician.
‡Dropperful.

22

TABLE 22–2
Comparison of Insulins

Type of Insulin	Onset (h)	Peak (h)	Duration (h)
Ultra Rapid			
Humalog (lispro)	Immediate	0.5–1.5	3–5
NovoLog (Insulin aspart)	Immediate	0.5–1.5	3–5
Rapid			
Regular Iletin II	0.25–0.5	2.0–4.0	5–7
Humulin R	0.5	2.5–4.0	6–8
Novolin R	0.5	2.0–5.0	5–8
Velosulin	0.5	2.0–5.0	6–8
Intermediate			
NPH Iletin II	1.0–2.0	6–12	18–24
Lente Iletin II	1.0–2.0	6–12	18–24
Humulin N	1.0–2.0	6–12	14–24
Novulin L	2.5–5.0	7–15	18–24
Novulin 70/30	0.5	7–12	24
Prolonged			
Ultralente	4.0–6.0	14–24	28–36
Humulin U	4.0–6.0	8–20	24–28
Lantus (insulin glargine)	4.0–6.0	No peak	24
Combination Insulins			
Humalog Mix (lispro protamine/ lispro)	0.25–0.5	1–4	24

TABLE 22-3
Some Oral Contraceptives

Drug (Manufacturer)	Estrogen (μg)*	Progestin (mg)†
MONOPHASICS		
Alesse 21, 28 (Wyeth-Ayerst)	Ethinyl estradiol (20)	Desogestrel (0.15)
Brevicon 21, 28 (Watson)‡	Ethinyl estradiol (35)	Norethindrone (0.5)
Demulen 1/35 21 (Searle)‡	Ethinyl estradiol (35)	Ethynodiol diacetate (1)
Demulen 1/50 21 (Searle)‡	Ethinyl estradiol (50)	Ethynodiol diacetate (1)
Desogen (Organon)	Ethinyl estradiol (30)	Desogestrel (0.15)
Genora 1/50 28 (Physicians total care)	Mestranol (50)	Norethindrone (1)
Genora 1/35 21, 28 (Physicians total care)	Ethinyl estradiol (35)	Norethindrone (1)
Levlen 21, 28 (Berlex)	Ethinyl estradiol (30)	Levonorgestrel (0.15)
Levlite 21, 28 (Berlex)	Ethinyl estradiol (20)	Levonorgestrel (0.1)
Levora 21, 28 (Watson)	Ethinyl estradiol (30)	Levonorgestrel (0.15)
Loestrin 1.5/30 21, 28 (Parke-Davis)	Ethinyl estradiol (30)	Norethindrone acetate (1.5)
Loestrin 1/20 21, 28 (Parke-Davis)	Ethinyl estradiol (20)	Norethindrone acetate (1)
Lo/Ovral (Wyeth-Ayerst)‡	Ethinyl estradiol (30)	Norgestrel (0.3)
Low-Ogestrel (Watson)	Ethinyl estradiol (30)	Norgestrel (0.3)
Modicon 28 (Ortho-McNeil)	Ethinyl estradiol (35)	Norethindrone (0.5)
Necon 1/50 21, 28 (Watson)	Mestranol (50)	Norethindrone (1)
Necon 0.5/35E 21, 28 (Watson)	Ethinyl estradiol (35)	Norethindrone (0.5)
Necon 1/35 21, 28 (Watson)	Ethinyl estradiol (35)	Norethindrone (1)
Nelova 0.5/35E 21 (Warner-Chilcott)‡	Ethinyl estradiol (35)	Norethindrone (0.5)
Nelova 1/35 21 (Warner-Chilcott)	Ethinyl estradiol (35)	Norethindrone (1)
Nelova 1/50 21 (Warner-Chilcott)‡	Mestranol (50)	Norethindrone (1)
Nordette-21 (Wyeth-Ayerst)‡	Ethinyl estradiol (30)	Levonorgestrel (0.15)
Norinyl 1/35 21, 28 (Watson)	Ethinyl estradiol (35)	Norethindrone (1)
Norinyl 1/50 21, 28 (Watson)	Mestranol (50)	Norethindrone (1)

(continued)

22

623

TABLE 22-3
(Continued)

Drug	Estrogen (µg)*	Progestin (mg)†
Ogestrel-28 (Watson)	Ethinyl estradiol (50)	Norgestrel (0.5)
Ortho-Cept 21 (Ortho-McNeil)‡	Ethinyl estradiol (30)	Desogestrel (0.15)
Ortho-Cyclen 21 (Ortho-McNeil)‡	Ethinyl estradiol (35)	Norgestimate (0.25)
Ortho-Novum 1/35 21 (Ortho-McNeil)‡	Ethinyl estradiol (35)	Norethindrone (1)
Ortho-Novum 1/50 21 (Ortho-McNeil)‡	Mestranol (50)	Norethindrone (1)
Ovcon 35 21, 28 (Warner Chilcott)	Ethinyl estradiol (35)	Norethindrone (0.4)
Ovcon 50 21, 28 (Warner Chilcott)	Ethinyl estradiol (50)	Norethindrone (1)
Ovral (Wyeth-Ayerst)‡	Ethinyl estradiol (50)	Norgestrel (0.5)
Zovia 1/50E 21, 28 (Watson)	Ethinyl estradiol (50)	Ethynodiol diacetate (1)
Zovia 1/35E 21, 28 (Watson)	Ethinyl estradiol (35)	Ethynodiol diacetate (1)
BIPHASICS		
Jenest-28 (Organon)	Ethinyl estradiol (35)	Norethindrone (0.5, 1)
Necon 10/11 21, 28 (Watson)	Ethinyl estradiol (35)	Norethindrone (0.5, 1)
Nelova 10/11 21 (Warner-Chilcott)	Ethinyl estradiol (35)	Norethindrone (0.5, 1)
Ortho-Novum 10/11 21 (Ortho-McNeil)‡	Ethinyl estradiol (35, 35)	Norethindrone (0.5, 1.0)
TRIPHASICS§		
Estrostep 28 (Parke-Davis)	Ethinyl estradiol (20, 30, 35)	Norethindrone acetate (1)
Mircette 28 (Organon)	Ethinyl estradiol (20, 0, 10),	Desogestrel (0.15)
Ortho Tri-Cyclen (Ortho-McNeil)‡	Ethinyl estradiol (35, 35, 35)	Norgestimate (0.18, 0.215, 0.25)

(continued)

TABLE 22-3
(Continued)

Drug	Estrogen (μg)*	Progestin (mg)†
Ortho-Novum 7/7/7 21 (Ortho-McNeil)‡	Ethinyl estradiol (35, 35, 35)	Norethindrone (0.5, 0.75, 1.0)
Tri-Levlen 21, 28 (Berlex)	Ethinyl estradiol (30, 40, 30)	Levonorgestrel (0.05, 0.075, 0.125)
Tri-Norinyl 21, 28 (Watson)	Ethinyl estradiol (35, 35, 35)	Norethindrone (0.5, 1.0, 0.5)
Triphasil-21 (Wyeth-Ayerst)‡	Ethinyl estradiol (30, 40, 30)	Levonorgestrel (0.05, 0.075, 0.125)
Trivora-28 (Watson)	Ethinyl estradiol (30, 40, 30)	Levonorgestrel (0.05, 0.075, 0.125)
PROGESTIN ONLY		
Micronor (Ortho-McNeil)	None	Norethindrone (0.35)
Nor-QD (Watson)	None	Norethindrone (0.35)
Ovrette (Wyeth-Ayerst)	None	Norgestrel (0.075)

*Ethinyl estradiol and mestranol are not equivalent milligram for milligram; the results of some studies indicate that 35 μg of ethinyl estradiol is equivalent to 50 mg of mestranol.
†Different progestins are not equivalent milligram for milligram.
‡Also available in a 28-day regimen at slightly different cost.
§Estrogen/progesterone dose varies based on the time of the cycle (ie, days 1–7, 8–14, 15–21).

22

TABLE 22-4
Some Common Oral Potassium Supplements (see page 592)

Brand Name	Salt	Form	meq potassium/ Dosing Unit
Glu-K	Gluconate	Tablet	2 meq/tablet
Kaochlor 10%	KCl	Liquid	20 meq/15 mL
Kaochlor S-F 10% (sugar-free)	KCl	Liquid	20 meq/15 mL
Kaochlor Eff	Bicarbonate/KCl/ citrate	Effervescent tablet	20 meq/tablet
Kaon elixir	Gluconate	Liquid	20 meq/mL
Kaon	Gluconate	Tablets	5 meq/tablet
Kaon-Cl	KCl	Tablet, SR	6.67 meq/tablet
Kaon-Cl 20%	KCl	Liquid	40 meq/15 mL
KayCiel	KCl	Liquid	20 meq/15 mL
K-Lor	KCl	Powder	15 or 20 meq/packet
Klorvess	Bicarbonate/KCl	Liquid	20 meq/15 mL
Klotrix	KCl	Tablet, SR	10 meq/tablet
K-Lyte	Bicarbonate/ citrate	Effervescent tablet	25 meq/tablet
K-Tab	KCl	Tablet, SR	10 meq/tablet
Micro-K	KCl	Capsules, SR	8 meq/capsule
Slow-K	KCl	Tablet, SR	8 meq/tablet
Tri-K	Acetate/bicarbonate and citrate	Liquid	45 meq/15 mL
Twin-K	Citrate/gluconate	Liquid	20 meq/5 mL

Abbreviation: SR = sustained release.

TABLE 22-5
Comparison of Systemic Steroids (see page 603)

Drug	Relative Equivalent Dose (mg)	Mineralocorticoid Activity	Duration (h)	Route
Betamethasone	0.75	0	36–72	PO, IM
Cortisone (Cortone)	25.00	2	8–12	PO, IM
Dexamethasone (Decadron)	0.75	0	36–72	PO, IV
Hydrocortisone (Solu-Cortef, Hydrocortone)	20.00	2	8–12	PO, IM, IV
Methylprednisolone acetate (Depo-Medrol)	4.00	0	36–72	PO, IM, IV
Methylprednisolone succinate (Solu-Medrol)	4.00			PO, IM, IV
Prednisone (Deltasone)	5.00	1	12–36	PO
Prednisolone (Delta-Cortef)	5.00	1	12–36	PO, IM, IV

TABLE 22-6
Topical Steroid Preparations (See page 604 for additional information)

Agent	Common Trade Names	Potency	Apply
Aclometasone dipropionate	Aclovate, cream, oint 0.05%	Low	bid/tid
Amcinonide	Cyclocort, cream, lotion, oint 0.1%	High	bid/tid
Betamethasone			
Betamethasone valerate	Valisone cream, lotion 0.01%	Low	qd/bid
Betamethasone valerate	Valisone cream, 0.01, 0.1%, oint, lotion 0.1%	Intermediate	qd/bid
Betamethasone dipropionate	Diprosone cream (0.05%) Diprosone aerosol (0.1%)	High	qd/bid
Betamethasone dipropionate, augmented	Diprolene oint, gel 0.05%	Ultra high	qd/bid
Clobetasol propionate	Temovate cream, gel, oint, scalp, soln 0.05%	Ultra high	bid (2 wk max)
Clocortolone pivalate	Cloderm cream 0.1%	Intermediate	qd–qid
Desonide	DesOwen, cream, oint, lotion 0.05%	Low	bid–qid
Desoximetasone			
Desoximetasone 0.05%	Topicort LP cream, gel 0.05%	Intermediate	
Desoximetasone 0.25%	Topicort cream, oint	High	
Dexamethasone base	Aeroseb-Dex aerosol 0.01% Decadron cream 0.1%	Low	bid–qid
Diflorasone diacetate	Psorcon cream, oint 0.05%	Ultrahigh	bid/qid
Fluocinolone			
Fluocinolone acetonide 0.01%	Synalar cream, soln 0.01%	Low	bid/tid

(continued)

628

TABLE 22-6
(Continued)

Agent	Common Trade Names	Potency	Apply
Fluocinolone acetonide 0.025%	Synalar oint, cream 0.025%	Intermediate	bid/tid
Fluocinolone acetonide 0.2%	Synalar-HP cream 0.2%	High	bid/tid
Fluocinonide 0.05%	Lidex, anhydrous cream, gel, soln 0.05%	High	bid/tid oint
Flurandrenolide	Lidex-E aqueous cream 0.05%		
	Cordran cream, oint 0.025%	Intermediate	bid/tid
	cream, lotion, oint 0.05%	Intermediate	bid/tid
	tape, 4 μg/cm^2		qd
Fluticasone propionate	Activate cream 0.05%, oint 0.005%	Intermediate	bid
Halobetasol	Cultivate cream, oint 0.05%	Intermediate	bid
Halcinonide	Halog cream 0.025%, emollient base 0.1% cream, oint, solution 0.1%	Very High	
		High	qd/tid
Hydrocortisone			
Hydrocortisone	Cortisone, Caldecort, Hycort, Hytone, etc.	Low	tid/qid
	aerosol 1%, cream: 0.5, 1,2.5%, gel 0.5% oint 0.5, 1, 2.5%, lotion 0.5, 1, 2.5% paste 0.5% soln 1%		
Hydrocortisone acetate	Corticaine cream, oint 0.5, 1%	Low	tid/qid
Hydrocortisone butyrate	Locoid oint, soln 0.1%	Intermediate	bid/tid
Hydrocortisone valerate	Westcort cream, oint 0.2% oint, lotion 0.025%	Intermediate	bid/tid

(continued)

22

629

TABLE 22–6
(Continued)

Agent	Common Trade Names	Potency	Apply
Mometasone furoate	Elocon 0.1% cream, oint, lotion	Intermediate	qd
Prednicarbate	Dermatop 0.1% cream	Intermediate	bid
Triamcinolone			
Triamcinolone acetonide 0.025%	Aristocort, Kenalog cream,	Low	tid/qid
Triamcinolone acetonide 0.1%	Aristocort, Kenalog cream, oint, lotion 0.1%	Intermediate	tid/qid
	Aerosol 0.2 mg/2-sec spray		
Triamcinolone acetonide 0.5%	Aristocort, Kenalog cream, oint 0.5%	High	tid/qid

22

TABLE 22-7
Common Drug Levels

Drug	When to Sample	Therapeutic Levels	Usual Half-life	Potentially Toxic Levels
ANTIBIOTICS				
Gentamicin	Peak: 30 min after 30-min infusion (peak level not necessary if extended interval dosing: 6 mg/kg/dose)	Peak: 5–8 µg/mL Trough <2 mg/mL <1.0 µg/mL for extended intervals (6 mg/kg/dose)	2 h	Peak: >12 µg/mL
	Trough: <0.5 h before next dose	Peak levels not needed with extended-interval dosing		
Tobramycin	Same as above	Same as above	Same as above	
Amikacin	Same as above	Peak: 20–30 µg/mL	2 h	Peak: >35 µg/mL
Vancomycin	Peak: 1 h after 1 h-infusion	Peak: 30–40 µg/mL	6–8 h	Peak: >50 µg/mL
	Trough: <0.5 h before next dose			Trough: >15 µg/mL
ANTICONVULSANTS				
Carbamazepine	Trough: just before next oral dose	8–12 µg/mL (monotherapy) 4–8 µg/mL (polytherapy)	15–20 h	Trough: >12 µg/mL
Ethosuximide	Trough: just before next oral dose	40–100 µg/mL	30–60 h	Trough: >100 µg/mL
Phenobarbital	Trough: just before next dose	15–40 µg/mL	40–120 h	Trough: >40 µg/mL
Phenytoin	Use free phenytoin to monitor Trough: just before next dose	5–12 µg/mL	Concentration-dependent	>2 µg/mL

(continued)

22

TABLE 22-7
(Continued)

22

Drug	When to Sample	Therapeutic Levels	Usual Half-life	Potentially Toxic Levels
Primidone	Trough just before next dose (note-primidone is metabolized to phenobarb. Order levels separately)	5–12 µg/mL	10–12 h	>12 µg/mL
Valproic acid	Trough: just before next dose	50–100 µg/mL	5–20 h	>100 µg/mL
BRONCHODILATORS				
Caffeine	Trough: just before next dose	Adults 5–15 µg/mL Neonate 6–11 mg/mL	Adults 3–4 h Neonates 30–140 h	20 µg/mL
Theophylline (IV)	IV: 12–24 h after infusion started	5–15 µg/mL	Nonsmoking adult-8 h Children and smoking adults -4 h	>20 µg/mL
Theophylline (PO)	Peak levels: not recommended Trough level: just before next dose	5–15 µg/mL		
CARDIOVASCULAR AGENTS				
Amiodarone	Trough: just before next dose	1–2.5 µg/mL	30–100 days	>2.5 µg/mL

(continued)

TABLE 22-7
(Continued)

Drug	When to Sample	Therapeutic Levels	Usual Half-life	Potentially Toxic Levels
Digoxin	Trough: just before next dose (levels drawn earlier than 6 h after a dose will be artificially elevated)	0.8–2.0 ng/mL	36 h	>2 ng/mL
Disopyramide	Trough: just before next dose	2–5 µg/mL	4–10 h	>5 µg/mL
Flecainide	Trough: just before next dose	0.2–1.0 µg/mL	11–14 h	>1.0 µg/mL
Lidocaine	Steady-state levels are usually achieved after 6–12 h	1.2–5.0 µg/mL	1.5 h	>6 µg/mL
Procainamide	Trough: just before next oral dose	4–10 µg/mL NAPA + Procain: 5–30 µg/mL	Procaine: 3–5 h NAPA: 6–10 h	>10 µg/mL >30 µg/mL (NAPA + Procain)
Quinidine	Trough: just before next oral dose	2–5 µg/mL	6 h	0.5 µg/mL
OTHER AGENTS				
Amitriptyline plus nortriptyline	Trough: just before next dose	120–250 ng/mL		
Nortriptyline	Trough: just before next dose	50–140 ng/mL		
Lithium	Trough: just before next dose	0.5–1.5 meq/mL	18–20 h	>1.5 meq/mL
Imipramine plus desipramine	Trough: just before next dose	150–300 ng/mL		
Desipramine	Trough: just before next dose	50–300 ng/mL		
Methotrexate	By protocol	<0.5 µmol/L after 48 h		

(continued)

22

TABLE 22-7
(Continued)

Drug	When to Sample	Therapeutic Levels	Usual Half-life	Potentially Toxic Levels
Cyclosporine	Trough: just before next dose	Highly variable Renal: 150–300 ng/mL (RIA) Hepatic: 150–300 ng/mL	Highly variable	
Doxepin	Trough: just before next dose	100–300 ng/mL		
Trazodone	Trough: just before next dose	900–2100 ng/mL		

*Results of therapeutic drug monitoring must be interpreted in light of the complete clinical situation. For information on dosing or interpretation of drug levels contact the pharmacist or an order for a pharmacokinetic consult may be written in the patient's chart. Based on data from Pharmacy and Therapeutics Committee Formulary, 41st edition, Thomas Jefferson University Hospital, Philadelphia, PA.

TABLE 22–8
Percentage of Loading Dose Required for Dosage Interval Chosen for Aminoglycosides (see page 620 for dosing information)

CrCl	Dosing Interval		
(mL/min)	8 h	12 h	24 h
90	90	—	—
90	88	—	—
70	84	—	—
60	79	91	—
50	74	87	—
40	66	80	—
30	57	72	92
25	51	66	88
20	45	54	83
15	37	50	75
10	29	40	64
7	24	33	55
5	20	28	48
2	14	20	35
0	9	13	25

Source: Based on data from Hull JH, Sarubbi FA: Gentamicin serum concentrations: Pharmacokinetic predictions. *Ann Intern Med* 1976;**85:**183–189. Shaded boxes indicate suggested dosage intervals. *Abbreviation:* CrCl = creatinine clearance.

TABLE 22-9
Recommended Childhood Immunization Schedule (United States, January–December 2001)

VACCINE	Birth	1 mo	2 mo	4 mo	6 mo	12 mo	15 mo	18 mo	24 mo	4-6 y	11-12 y	14-18 y
Hepatitis B† (Hep B)	Hep B #1	Hep B #2			Hep B #3						Hep B	
Diphtheria and tetanus toxoids (Td) and pertussis§ (DTaP)			DTaP	DTaP	DTaP		DTaP	DTaP		DTaP	Td	Td
Haemophilus influenzae type b¶ (Hib)			Hib	Hib	Hib	Hib	Hib					
Inactivated polio** (IPV)			IPV	IPV		IPV	IPV			IPV		
Pneumococcal†† conjugate (PCV)			PCV	PCV	PCV	PCV	PCV					
Measles–mumps–rubella§§ (MMR)						MMR	MMR			MMR	MMR	
Varicella¶¶ (Var)						Var	Var				Var	
Hepatitis A*** (Hep A)									Hep A in selected areas		Hep A in selected areas	

Source: MMWR Vol. 50/No. 1, Jan. 12, 2001.

Range of recommended ages for vaccination.

Vaccines to be given if previously recommended doses were missed or were given earlier than the recommended minimum age.

Recommended in selected states and/or regions.

See text for abbreviations.

TABLE 22–10
Oral Anticoagulant Standards of Practice (see Warfarin, page 618)

Thromboembolic Disorder	INR	Duration
Deep Venous Thrombosis		
Prophylaxis (high-risk surgery)	2–3	<3 mo or until ambulatory
Treatment: single episode	2–3	3–6 mo
Recurrent systemic embolism	2–3	Indefinite
Prevention of Systemic Embolism		
Atrial fibrillation (AF)	2–3	Indefinite
AF: cardioversion	2–3	3 wk prior; 4 wk post sinus rhythm
Valvular heart disease	2–3	Indefinite
Cardiomyopathy	2–3	Indefinite
Acute Myocardial Infarction		
Prevention of systemic embolization	2–3	<3 mo
Prevention of recurrence	2.5–3.5	Indefinite
Prosthetic Valves		
Tissue heart valves	2–3	3 mo
Bileaflet mechanical valve in aortic position	2–3	Indefinite
Other mechanical prosthetic valves[a]	2.5–3.5	Indefinite

Source: Based on data published in *Chest* 1998;114 Supplement 439S–769S.
[a]May add aspirin 81 mg to warfarin in patients with ball–cage valves or with additional risk factors.
Abbreviation: INR: international normalized ratio.

APPENDIX

Apgar Scores
Body Surface Area
    Adult
    Children
Body Weights, Desirable
Cancer Screening
    Recommendations
Epidemiology Basics
Glasgow Coma Scale

Measurements
    Equivalents
SI Prefixes and Symbols
Performance Status Scales
Radiation Terminology
Temperature Conversion
TNM and Other Systems of
    Classification for Common Tumors
Weight Conversion

APGAR SCORES

Apgar scores (Table A–1) are a numerical expression of a newborn infant's physical condition. Usually determined 1 min after birth and again at 5 min, the score is the sum of points gained on assessment of color, heart rate, reflex irritability, muscle tone, and respirations.

BODY SURFACE AREA

Adult

Figure A–1 is a nomogram for determining the body surface area of an adult.

Children

Figure A–2 is a nomogram for determining the body surface area of children.

BODY WEIGHTS, DESIRABLE

Table A–2 gives desirable body weights for men and women.

CANCER SCREENING RECOMMENDATIONS

Table A–3 lists the recommendations from the American Cancer Society for cancer screening programs in average risk, asymptomatic people. These are the recommendations of the ACS and may not be supported by other organizations.

EPIDEMIOLOGY BASICS

$$\text{Prevalence} = \frac{\text{Number of persons who have a disease at one point in time}}{\text{Number of persons at risk at that point}}$$

(continued on page 645)

TABLE A-1
Apgar Scores

Sign	Score		
	0	1	2
Appearance (color)	Blue or pale	Pink body with blue extremities	Completely pink
Pulse (heart rate)	Absent	Slow (<100/min)	>100/min
Grimace (reflex irritability	No response	Grimace	Cough or sneeze
Activity (muscle tone)	Limp	Some flexion	Active movement
Respirations	Absent	Slow, irregular	Good, crying

TABLE A-2
Desirable Weights (in lb) for Men and Women*

Height	Age	
	19–34	35 Years and Older
5'0"	97–128	108–138
5'1"	101–132	111–143
5'2"	104–137	115–148
5'3"	107–141	119–152
5'4"	111–146	122–157
5'5"	114–150	126–162
5'6"	118–156	130–167
5'7"	121–160	134–172
5'8"	125–164	138–178
5'9"	129–169	142–183
5'10"	132–174	146–188
5'11"	136–179	151–194
6'0"	140–184	155–199
6'1"	144–189	159–205
6'2"	148–195	164–210

*Weights are based on weighing in without shoes or clothes.
Source: United States Department of Agriculture and United States Department of Health and Human Resources, 1990.

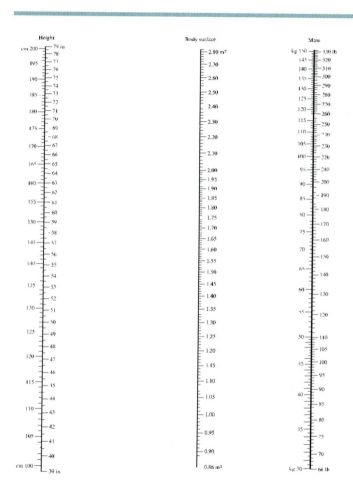

FIGURE A-1 Body surface area: Adult. Use a straight edge to connect the height and mass. The point of intersection on the body surface line gives the body surface area (in m²). (Reprinted, with permission, from: Lentner C [ed]: *Geigy Scientific Tables,* 8th ed. Ciba-Geigy, San Francisco CA, 1981, Vol. 1, p. 226.)

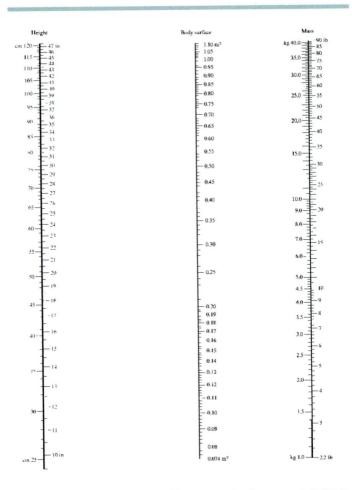

FIGURE A–2 Body surface area: Child. Use a straight edge to connect the height and mass. The point of intersection on the body surface line gives the body surface area (in m²). (Reprinted, with permission, from: Lentner C [ed]: *Geigy Scientific Tables*, 8th ed. Ciba-Geigy, San Francisco CA, 1981, Vol. 1, p. 227.)

TABLE A–3
Recommendations for Cancer Screening for Average Risk, Asymptomatic People

Cancer Site	Population	Test or Procedure	Frequency
Breast	Women, age 20+	Breast self-examination	Monthly, starting at age 20
		Clinical breast examination	Every 3 years, ages 20–39 Annual, starting at age 40*
Colorectal	Men & women, age 50+	Mammography	Annual, starting at age 40
		Fecal occult blood test & flexible sigmoidoscopy†	Annual fecal occult blood test and flexible sigmoidoscopy at age 50; thereafter, fecal occult blood test every year and flexible sigmoidoscopy every 5 years
		-or- Double contrast barium enema†	Double contrast barium enema at age 50; thereafter, every 5–10 y
		-or- Colonoscopy†	Colonoscopy every 10 y starting at age 50
Prostate	Men, age 50+	Digital rectal examination & prostate specific antigen test	Annual digital rectal examination and prostate-specific antigen test should be offered to men starting at age 50‡
Cervix	Women, age 18+	Pap test and pelvic examination	All women who are, or have been, sexually active, or have reached age 18 should have an annual Pap test and pelvic examination. After a woman has had 3 or more consecutive satisfactory normal annual examinations, the Pap test may be performed less frequently at the discretion of the physician.

(continued)

643

TABLE A–3
(Continued)

Cancer Site	Population	Test or Procedure	Frequency
Cancer-related check-up	Men & women age 20+	Examinations every 3 y from ages 20–39 y and annually after age 40. The cancer-related checkup should include examination for cancers of the thyroid, testicles, ovaries, lymph nodes, oral cavity, and skin, as well as health counseling about tobacco, sun exposure, diet and nutrition, risk factors, sexual practices, and environmental and occupational exposures.	

*Beginning at age 40, annual clinical breast examination should be performed prior to mammography.
†Digital rectal examination should be performed at the time of sigmoidoscopy, barium enema, and colonoscopy.
‡Information should be provided to men regarding potential risks and benefits of screening.
Source: Reprinted, with permission, from *Cancer J Clin* 2000:**50:39.**

(continued from page 639)

$$\text{Incidence} = \frac{\text{Number of new cases of a disease over a period of time}}{\text{Number of persons at risk during that period}}$$

Sensitivity = Proportion of subjects with the disease who have a positive test
$$= (a/a + c)$$

Specificity = Proportion of subjects without the disease who have a negative test
$$= (d/b + d)$$

Predictive value = Positive: likelihood of a positive test indicates disease
$$= (a/a + b)$$
= Negative: likelihood of a negative test indicates lack of disease
$$= (d/c + d)$$

		Disease	
		+ (Present)	− (Absent)
Test	(+)	a	b
	(−)	c	d

GLASCOW COMA SCALE

The Glasgow Coma Scale (*EMV* Scale) gives a fairly reliable, objective way to monitor changes in levels of consciousness. It is based on *E*ye opening, *M*otor responses, and *V*erbal responses. A person's EMV score is based on the total of the three responses. The score ranges from 3 (lowest) to 15 (highest) (Table A–4).

TABLE A–4
Glasgow Coma Scale

Parameter	Response		Score
Eyes	Open: Spontaneously		4
		To verbal command	3
		To pain	2
		No response	1
Best motor response	To verbal command	Obeys	6
	To painful stimulus	Localized pain	5
		Flexion-withdrawal	4
		Decorticate (flex)	3
		Decerebrate (extend)	2
		No response	1
Best verbal response		Oriented, converses	5
		Disoriented, converses	4
		Inappropriate responses	3
		Incomprehensible sounds	2
		No response	1

MEASUREMENTS
Equivalents (Approximate)

Length

1 centimeter (cm) = 0.4 in.
1 meter (m) = 39.4 in.

Household

1 teaspoon (tsp) = 5 mL
1 tablespoon (tbsp) = 15 mL
1 ounce (oz) = 30 mL
8 ounces (oz) = 1 cup = 240 mL
1 quart (qt) = 946 mL

Apothecary

1 grain (gr) = 60 mg
30 gram (g) = 1 oz
1 g = 15 gr

SI PREFIXES AND SYMBOLS

Factor	Prefix	Symbol
10^9	giga	G
10^6	mega	M
10^3	kilo	k
10^2	hecto	h
10^1	deka	da
10^{-1}	deci	d
10^{-2}	centi	c
10^{-3}	milli	m
10^{-6}	micro	μ
10^{-9}	nano	n
10^{-12}	pico	p
10^{-15}	femto	f

PERFORMANCE STATUS SCALES

Table A–5 lists the most common performance scales used clinically.

RADIATION TERMINOLOGY

Measure	Old Term	SI Unit
Activity	curie	becquerel (Bq)
Absorbed dose	rad	gray (Gy)

TEMPERATURE CONVERSION

Table A–6 gives information for converting temperature from the Fahrenheit (F) scale to the centigrade, or Celsius (C), scale and vice versa.

(continued on page 649)

TABLE A-5
Performance Status Scales

Karnofsky		ECOG		AJCC	
Functional Status	% Normal Status	Activity Level	Grade	Activity Level	Grade	Activity
Able to carry on normal activity; no special care needed	100	Normal; no complaints; no evidence of disease;	0	Normal activity	H0	Normal activity
	90	Able to carry on normal activity; minor sign or symptoms of disease				
	80	Normal activity with effort; some signs or symptoms of disease	1	Symptoms but ambulatory	H1	Symptomatic and ambulatory; cares for self
Unable to work; able to live at home; cares for most personal needs; varying amount of assistance needed	70	Cares for self; unable to carry on normal activity or progressing rapidly to active work				
	60	Requires occasional assistance but able to care for self	2	In bed 50% of time	H2	Ambulatory 50% of time; occasionally needs assistance
	50	Requires considerable assistance and frequent medical care				

(continued)

TABLE A-5
(Continued)

Karnofsky			ECOG		AJCC	
Functional Status	% Normal Status	Activity Level	Grade	Activity Level	Grade	Activity
Unable to care for self; requires equivalent of needed institutional or hospital care; may be progressing rapidly	40	Disabled; requires special care and assistance	3	In bed 50% of time	H3	Ambulatory 50% of time; nursing care
	30	Severely disabled; hospitalization indicated through death not imminent				
	20	Very sick; hospitalization necessary	4	100% bedridden	H4	Bedridden; may need hospitalization
	10	Moribund; fatal processes				
	0	Dead				

Abbreviations: ECOG = Eastern Cooperative Oncology Group; AJCC = American Joint Committee on Cancer.
Source. Reprinted, with permission, from *Practical Oncology.* Cameron R (ed). Appleton & Lange, Stamford, CT, 1993.

TABLE A–6
Temperature Conversion Table

F	C	C	F
0	-17.7	0	32.0
95.0	35.0	35.0	95.0
96.0	35.5	35.5	95.9
97.0	36.1	36.0	96.8
98.0	36.6	36.5	97.7
98.6	37.0	37.0	98.6
99.0	37.2	37.5	99.5
100.0	37.7	38.0	100.4
101.0	38.3	38.5	101.3
102.0	38.8	39.0	102.2
103.0	39.4	39.5	103.1
104.0	40.0	40.0	104.0
105.0	40.5	40.5	104.9
106.0	41.1	41.0	105.8

$C = (F - 32) \times 5/9$ $F = (C \times 9/5) + 32$

Abbreviations: F = degrees Fahrenheit; C = degrees Celsius.

TNM AND OTHER SYSTEMS OF CLASSIFICATION FOR COMMON TUMORS

TNM stands for "tumor, nodes, metastasis" and is a universally accepted classification system for malignancy staging. The UICC (Union Internationale Contre le Cancer) and the AJCC (American Joint Committee on Cancer) have adopted this system and have published this system in *TNM Classification of Malignant Tumours,* 5th ed John Wiley & Sons, New York, 1997. The following is a highly selected listing of commonly encountered solid tumors (breast, bladder, cervix, colon and rectum, kidney, lung, melanoma, ovary, stomach, thyroid, uterus, and prostate) as well as the classification for lymphomas. Where appropriate, other common staging systems are noted (ie, Duke's classification of colon cancer)

TNM CLASSIFICATION

Breast

Primary Tumor (T)

TX   Primary tumor cannot be assessed

T0   No evidence of primary tumor

Tis   Carcinoma in situ: Intraductal carcinoma, lobular carcinoma in situ, or Paget's disease of the nipple with no tumor. *Note:* Paget disease associated with a tumor is classified according to the size of the tumor.

T1   Tumor 2 cm or less in greatest dimension

     T1mic Microinvasion 0.1 cm or less in greatest dimension

     T1a More than 0.1 cm but not more than 0.5 cm in greatest dimension

	T1b More than 0.5 cm but not more than 1 cm in greatest dimension
	T1c More than 1 cm but not more than 2 cm in greatest dimension
T2	Tumor more than 2 cm but not more than 5 cm in greatest dimension
T3	Tumor more than 5 cm in greatest dimension
T4	Tumor of any size with direct extension to chest wall or skin

    T4a Extension to chest wall

    T4b Edema (including peau d'orange) or ulceration of the skin of breast or satellite skin nodules confined to same breast

  T4c Both T4a and T4b

  T4d Inflammatory carcinoma

Lymph Node (N)

NX	Regional lymph nodes cannot be assessed
N0	No regional lymph node metastasis
N1	Metastasis to movable ipsilateral axillary lymph nodes(s)
N2	Metastasis to ipsilateral axillary lymph node(s) fixed to one another or to other structures
N3	Metastasis to ipsilateral internal mammary lymph node(s)

Distant Metastasis (M)

MX	Presence of distant metastasis cannot be assessed
M0	No distant metastasis
M1	Distant metastasis (includes metastasis to ipsilateral supraclavicular lymph nodes)

Pathologic Classification (pTNM)

Primary Tumor (pT)

The pT categories correspond to the T categories.

Regional Lymph Nodes (pN)

pNX	Regional lymph nodes cannot be assessed
pN0	No regional lymph node metastasis
pN1	Metastasis to movable ipsilateral axillary lymph node(s)

    pN1a Only micrometastasis (none larger than 0.2 cm)

    pN1b Metastasis to lymph nodes, any larger than 0.2 cm

        pN1bi Metastasis in 1–3 lymph nodes, any more than 0.2 cm and all less than 2 cm in greatest dimension

        pN1bii Metastasis to 4 or more lymph nodes, any more than 0.2 cm and all less than 2 cm in greatest dimension

        pN1biii Extension of tumor beyond the capsule of a lymph node metastasis less than 2 cm in greatest dimension

        pN1biv Metastasis to a lymph node 2 cm or more in greatest dimension

pN2	Metastasis to ipsilateral axillary nodes that are fixed
pN3	Metastasis to ipsilateral internal mammary lymph nodes(s)

Pathologic Classification

The pM category corresponds to the M category above.

Bladder

Primary Tumor (T)

TX	Primary tumor cannot be assessed
T0	No evidence of primary tumor

  Tis Carcinoma in situ: "flat tumor"

Ta Noninvasive papillary carcinoma
T1 Tumor invades subepithelial connective tissue
T2 Tumor invades muscle
    T2a Tumor invades superficial muscle (inner half)
    T2b Tumor invades deep muscle (outer half)
T3 Tumor invades perivesical tissue
    T3a Microscopically
    T3b Macroscopically (extravesical mass)
T4 Tumor invades any of the following: prostate, uterus, vagina, pelvic wall, abdominal wall
    T4a Tumor invades prostate or uterus or vagina
    T4b Tumor invades pelvic wall or abdominal wall

Lymph Node (N)

NX Regional lymph nodes cannot be assessed
N0 No regional lymph node metastasis
N1 Metastasis in a single lymph node, 2 cm or less in greatest dimension
N2 Metastasis in a single lymph node, more than 2 cm but not more than 5 cm in greatest dimension, or multiple lymph nodes, none more than 5 cm in greatest dimension
N3 Metastasis in a lymph node more than 5 cm in greatest dimension

Distant Metastasis (M)

MX Presence of distant metastasis cannot be assessed
M0 No distant metastasis
M1 Distant metastasis

Pathologic Classification (pTNM)

The pT, pN, and pM categories correspond to the T, N , and M categories.

Cervix

Primary Tumor (T)

TX Primary tumor cannot be assessed
T0 No evidence of primary tumor
Tis Carcinoma in situ
T1 Cervical carcinoma confined to uterus
    T1a Preclinical invasive carcinoma diagnosed by microscopy only
        T1ai Stromal invasion no greater than 3.0 mm in depth and 7.0 mm or less in horizontal spread
        T1aii Stromal invasion more than 3.0 mm and not more than 5.0 mm with a horizontal spread 7.0 mm or less
    T1b Clinically visible lesion confined to the cervix or microscopic lesion greater than T1a2
        T1bi Clinically visible lesion 4 cm or less in greatest dimension
        T1bii Clinically visible lesion more than 4 cm in greatest dimension
T2 Cervical carcinoma invades beyond uterus but not to pelvic wall or to the lower third of vagina
    T2a Tumor without parametrial invasion
    T2b Tumor with parametrial invasion
T3 Cervical carcinoma extends to pelvic wall and/or involves lower third of vagina and/or causes hydronephrosis or nonfunctioning kidney
    T3a Tumor involves lower third of the vagina, no extension to pelvic wall

T3b   Tumor extends to pelvic wall and/or causes hydronephrosis or nonfunctioning kidney

T4   Tumor invades mucosa of bladder or rectum and/or extends beyond the true pelvis

Note: The presence of bullous edema is not sufficient to classify a tumor as T4.

Lymph Node (N)

NX   Regional lymph nodes cannot be assessed
N0   No regional lymph node metastasis
N1   Regional lymph node metastasis

Distant Metastasis (M)

MX   Presence of distant metastasis cannot be assessed
M0   No distant metastasis
M1   Distant metastasis

Pathologic Classification (pTNM)

The pT, pN and pM categories correspond to the T, N , and M categories.

Colon and Rectum

Primary Tumor (T)

TX   Primary tumor cannot be assessed
T0   No evidence of primary tumor
Tis   Carcinoma in situ: intraepithelial or invasion of lamina propria*
T1   Tumor invades submucosa
T2   Tumor invades muscularis propria
T3   Tumor invades through muscularis propria into subserosa, or into nonperitonealized pericolic or perirectal tissues
T4   Tumor perforates visceral peritoneum or directly invades other organs or structures

Lymph Node (N)

NX   Regional lymph nodes cannot be assessed
N0   No regional lymph node metastasis
N1   Metastasis in 1– 3 pericolic or perirectal lymph nodes
N2   Metastasis in 4 or more pericolic or perirectal lymph nodes

Distant Metastasis (M)

MX   Presence of distant metastasis cannot be assessed
M0   No distant metastasis
M1   Distant metastasis

Pathologic Classification (pTNM)

The pT, pN and pM categories correspond to the T, N , and M categories.

DUKES' CLASSIFICATION (ASTER–COLLER MODIFICATION) OF COLON CANCER

STAGE A:	Into muscularis propria, nodes negative
STAGE B1:	Extends through entire wall, nodes negative
STAGE B2:	Extends into muscularis propria, nodes positive
STAGE C1:	Extends through entire wall, 1–3 nodes positive

*Tis includes cancer cells confined within the glandular basement membrane (intraepithelial) or lamina propria (intramucosal) with no extension through muscularis mucosa into submucosa.

STAGE C2:	≥ 4 nodes positive
STAGE D:	Metastatic disease

Kidney

Primary Tumor (T)
TX Primary tumor cannot be assessed
T0 No evidence of primary tumor
T1 Tumor 7 cm or less in greatest dimension limited to the kidney
T2 Tumor more than 7 cm in greatest dimension limited to the kidney
T3 Tumor extends into major veins or invades adrenal gland or perinephric tissues but not beyond Gerota's fascia
  T3a Tumor invades adrenal gland or perinephric tissues but not beyond Gerota's fascia
  T3b Tumor grossly extends into renal vein(s) or vena cava below diaphragm
  T3c Tumor grossly extends into vena cava above diaphragm
T4 Tumor invades beyond Gerota's fascia

Lymph Node (N)
NX Regional lymph nodes cannot be assessed
N0 No regional lymph node metastasis
N1 Metastasis in a single regional lymph node
N2 Metastasis in more than one regional lymph node

Distant Metastasis (M)
MX Presence of distant metastasis cannot be assessed
M0 No distant metastasis
M1 Distant metastasis

Pathologic Classification (pTNM)
The pT, pN and pM categories correspond to the T, N , and M categories.

Lung

Primary Tumor (T)
TX Primary tumor cannot be assessed, or tumor proven by presence of malignant cells in sputum or bronchial washings but not visualized by imaging or bronchoscopy
T0 No evidence of primary tumor
Tis Carcinoma in situ
T1 Tumor 3 cm or less in greatest dimension, surrounded by lung or visceral pleura, without bronchoscopic evidence of invasion more proximal than the lobar bronchus
T2 Tumor with *any* of the following features of size or extent: More than 3 cm in greatest dimension; involves main bronchus, 2 cm or more distal to the carina; invades the visceral pleura; associated with atelectasis or obstructive pneumonitis that extends to the hilar region but does not involve the entire lung
T3 Tumor of any size that directly invades any of the following: chest wall (including superior sulcus tumors), diaphragm, mediastinal pleura, parietal pericardium; or tumor in the main bronchus less than 2 cm distal to the carina but without involvement of the carina; or associated atelectasis or obstructive pneumonitis of the entire lung
T4 Tumor of any size that invades any of the following: mediastinum, heart, great vessels, trachea, esophagus, vertebral body, carina; or tumor with a malignant pleural effusion

Lymph Node (N)

NX Regional lymph nodes cannot be assessed
N0 No regional lymph node metastasis
N1 Metastasis in ipsilateral peribronchial and/or ipsilateral hilar lymph nodes, including direct extension
N2 Metastasis in ipsilateral mediastinal and/or subcarinal lymph node(s)
N3 Metastasis in contralateral mediastinal, contralateral hilar, ipsilateral or contralateral scalene, or supraclavicular lymph node(s)

Distant Metastasis (M)

MX Presence of distant metastasis cannot be assessed
M0 No distant metastasis
M1 Distant metastasis

Pathologic Classification (pTNM)

The pT, pN and pM categories correspond to the T, N , and M categories.

ANN ARBOR STAGING CLASSIFICATION

Lymphoma (Hodgkin's Disease and Non-Hodgkin's Lymphoma)

STAGE	DEFINITION
I	Limited to one area
II	Involvement of two or more areas on the same side of the diaphragm
III	Involvement of two or more areas on both sides of the diaphragm
	III_1 Upper abdomen, spleen, splenic and hilar nodes
	III_2 Lower abdominal nodes
IV	Extra lymph node involvement

Melanoma of the Skin (Excluding Eyelid)

Primary Tumor (pT)

pTX Primary tumor cannot be assessed
pT0 No evidence of tumor
pTis Melanoma in situ (atypical melanotic hyperplasia, severe melanotic dysplasia), not an invasive lesion (Clark's level I)
pT1 Tumor 0.75 mm or less in thickness and invades the papillary dermis (Clark's level II)
pT2 Tumor more than 0.75 mm but not more than 1.5 mm in thickness and/or invades to papillary–reticular dermal interface (Clark's level III)
pT3 Tumor more than 1.5 mm but not more than 4 mm in thickness and/or invades the reticular dermis (Clark's level IV)
   pT3a Tumor more than 1.5 mm but not more than 3 mm in thickness
   pT3b Tumor more than 3 mm but not more than 4 mm in thickness
pT4 Tumor more than 4 mm in thickness and/or invades the subcutaneous tissue (Clark's level V) and/or satellite(s) within 2 cm of the primary tumor
   pT4a Tumor more than 4 mm in thickness and/or invades the subcutaneous tissue
   pT4b Satellite(s) with 2 cm of primary tumor

Lymph Node (N)

NX Regional lymph nodes cannot be assessed
N0 No regional lymph node metastasis

N1 Metastasis 3 cm or less in greatest dimension in any regional lymph node(s)
N2 Metastasis more than 3 cm in greatest dimension in any regional lymph node(s)
   N2a Metastasis more than 3 cm in greatest dimension in any regional lymph node(s) and/or in-transit metastasis
   N2b In-transit metastasis
   N2c Both (N2a and N2b)

Distant Metastasis (M)

MX Presence of distant metastasis cannot be assessed
M0 No distant metastasis
M1 Distant metastasis
   M1a Metastasis in skin or subcutaneous tissue or lymph node(s) beyond the regional lymph nodes
   M1b Visceral metastasis

Ovary

Primary Tumor (T)

TNM	FIGO*	DEFINITION
TX		Primary tumor cannot be assessed
T0	I	No evidence of primary tumor
T1		Tumor limited to ovaries
T1a	Ia	Tumor limited to one ovary; capsule intact, no tumor on ovarian surface
T1b	Ib	Tumor limited to both ovaries; capsules intact, no tumor on ovarian surface
T1c	Ic	Tumor limited to one or both ovaries with any of the following: capsule ruptured, tumor on ovarian surface, malignant cells in ascites, or peritoneal washings
T2	II	Tumor involves one or both ovaries with pelvic extension
T2a	IIa	Extension or implants on uterus or tubes
T2b	IIb	Extension to other pelvic tissues
T2c	IIc	Pelvic extension (2a or 2b) with malignant cells in ascites or peritoneal washing
T3	III	Tumor involves one or both ovaries with microscopically confirmed and/or N1 peritoneal metastasis outside the pelvis or regional lymph node metastasis
T3a	IIIa	Microscopic peritoneal metastasis beyond pelvis
T3b	IIIb†	Macroscopic peritoneal metastasis beyond pelvis 2 cm or less in greatest dimension
T3c	IIIc	Peritoneal metastasis beyond pelvis more than 2 cm in greatest and/or N1 dimension or regional lymph node metastasis

Lymph Node (N)

NX Regional lymph nodes cannot be assessed
N0 No regional lymph node metastasis
N1 Regional lymph node metastasis

*FIGO = Fédération Internationale de Gynécologie et d'Obstétrique.

†Liver capsule metastasis is T3/stage III, liver parenchymal metastasis M1/stage IV. Pleural effusion must have positive cytology for M1/stage IV.

Distant Metastasis (M)

TNM	FIGO	DEFINITION
MX		Presence of distant metastasis cannot be assessed
M0		No distant metastasis
M1	IV	Distant metastasis (excludes peritoneal metastasis)

Stomach

Primary Tumor (T)

TX	Primary tumor cannot be assessed
T0	No evidence of primary tumor
Tis	Carcinoma in situ: Intraepithelial tumor without invasion of lamina propria
T1	Tumor invades lamina propria or submucosa
T2	Tumor invades muscularis propria or subserosa
T3	Tumor penetrates serosa (visceral peritoneum) without invasion of adjacent structures
T4	Tumor invades adjacent structures

Lymph Node (N)

NX	Regional lymph node(s) cannot be assessed
N0	No regional lymph node metastasis
N1	Metastasis in 1–6 regional lymph node(s)
N2	Metastasis in 7–15 regional lymph nodes(s)
N3	Metastasis in more than 15 regional lymph nodes(s)

Distant Metastasis (M)

MX	Presence of distant metastasis cannot be assessed
M0	No distant metastasis
M1	Distant metastasis

Pathologic Classification (pTNM)

The pT, pN and pM categories correspond to the T, N, and M categories.

Thyroid Gland

Primary Tumor (T)

All categories may be subdivided: (a) solitary; (b) multifocal–measure the largest for classification

TX	Primary tumor cannot be assessed
T0	No evidence of primary tumor
T1	Tumor 1 cm or less in greatest dimension limited to the thyroid
T2	Tumor more than 1 cm but not more than 4 cm in greatest dimension limited to the thyroid
T3	Tumor more than 4 cm in greatest dimension limited to the thyroid
T4	Tumor of any size extending beyond the thyroid capsule

Lymph Node (N)

Regional nodes are the cervical and upper mediastinal lymph nodes

NX	Regional lymph nodes cannot be assessed
N0	No regional lymph node metastasis
N1	Regional lymph node metastasis
	N1a Metastasis in ipsilateral cervical lymph nodes
	N1b Metastasis in bilateral, midline, or contralateral cervical or mediastinal lymph nodes

Distant Metastasis (M)

MX	Presence of distant metastasis cannot be assessed

M0   No distant metastasis
M1   Distant metastasis

Pathologic Classification (pTNM)

The pT, pN, and pM categories correspond to the T, N, and M categories.

Uterus

Primary Tumor (T)

TNM	FIGO	DEFINITION
TX		Primary tumor cannot be assessed
T0		No evidence of primary tumor
Tis	0	Carcinoma in situ
T1	I	Tumor confined to corpus
T1a	Ia	Tumor limited to endometrium
T1b	Ib	Tumor invades up to less than one half of myometrium
T1c	Ic	Tumor invades up to more than one half of myometrium
T2	II	Tumor invades cervix but does not extend beyond uterus
T2a	IIa	Endocervical glandular involvement only
T2b	IIb	Cervical stomal invasion
T3	III	Local and/or regional spread as specified in T3a, b, N1, and FIGO IIIA, B, C.
T3a	IIIa	Tumor involves serosa and/or adnexa (direct extension or metastasis) and/or cancer cells in ascites or peritoneal washings
T3b	IIIb	Vaginal involvement (direct extension or metastasis)
N1	IIIc	Metastasis to pelvic and/or paraaortic lymph nodes
T4*	IVa	Tumor invades bladder mucosa and/or bowel mucosa

Lymph Node (N)

NX   Regional lymph nodes cannot be assessed
N0   No regional lymph node metastasis
N1   Regional lymph node metastasis

Distant Metastasis (M)

TNM	FIGO†	DEFINITION
MX		Presence of distant metastasis cannot be assessed
M0		No distant metastasis
M1	Ivb	Distant metastasis (excluding metastasis to vagina, pelvic serosa, or adnexa, including metastasis to intraabdominal lymph nodes other than paraaortic and/or inguinal nodes)

Pathologic Classification (pTNM)

The pT, pN, and pM categories correspond to the T, N, and M categories.

Prostate

T0   No evidence of primary tumor
T1   Nonpalpable disease (old stage "A")
    T1a   Three or fewer microscopic foci of carcinoma
    T1b   More than 3 microscopic foci of carcinoma
    T1c   No palpable tumor, diagnosed by elevated PSA

---

*The presence of bullous edema is not sufficient evidence to classify a tumor T4.

†FIGO = Fédération Internationale de Gynécologie et d'Obstétrique

T2 Tumor presents clinically or grossly, limited to the gland (old stage "B")
  T2a Tumor involves one lobe
  T2b Tumor involves both lobes
T3 Tumor extends through the prostatic capsule (old stage "C")
  T3a Extracapsular extension (unilateral or bilateral)
  T3b Tumor invades seminal vesical(s)
T4 Tumor is fixed or invades adjacent structures other than seminal vesicles: bladder neck, external sphincter, rectum, levator muscles, and/or pelvic wall.

Regional Lymph Nodes (N)
NX Regional lymph nodes cannot be assessed
N0 No regional lymph node metastasis
N1 Regional lymph node metastasis

Distant Metastasis (M)
MX Distant metastasis cannot be assessed
M0 No distant metastasis
M1 Distant metastasis
  M1a Nonregional lymph node(s)
  M1b Bone(s)
  M1c Other site(s)

Pathologic Classification (pTNM)
The pT, pN and pM categories correspond to the T, N, and M categories. However, there is no pT1 category because there is insufficient tissue to assess the highest pT category.

WEIGHT CONVERSION

Table A–7 gives information for converting weight in pounds (lb) to weight in kilograms (kg) and vice versa.

TABLE A–7
Weight Conversion Table

lb	kg	kg	lb
1	0.5	1	2.2
2	0.9	2	4.4
4	1.8	3	6.6
6	2.7	4	8.8
8	3.6	5	11.0
10	4.5	6	13.2
20	9.1	8	17.6
30	13.6	10	22.0
40	18.2	20	44.0
50	22.7	30	66.0
60	27.3	40	88.0
70	31.8	50	110.0
80	36.4	60	132.0
90	40.9	70	154.0
100	45.4	80	176.0
150	68.2	90	198.0
200	90.8	100	220.9

kg = lb × 0.454   lb = kg × 2.2

INDEX

NOTE: Page numbers followed by *f* indicate figures; those followed by *t* indicate tables.

A

Abacavir (Ziagen), indications, actions, and dosage of, 488

Abbokinase (urokinase), indications, actions, and dosage of, 615

Abciximab (ReoPro)
for emergency cardiac care, 464
indications, actions, and dosage of, 488

Abdominal computed tomography, 330

Abdominal distention, differential diagnosis of, 42

Abdominal magnetic resonance imaging, 332

Abdominal pain, differential diagnosis of, 42

Abdominal paracentesis, 296–297, 298*f*

Abdominal ultrasound, 329

Abdominal x-rays, 326

Abelcet (amphotericin B lipid complex), indications, actions, and dosage of, 497

Abscesses, dental, 470

Absorbable sutures, 345, 346*t*

Acalculous cholecystitis, 434

Acanthocytes, 104

Acarbose (Precose), indications, actions, and dosage of, 488

Accelerations, in fetal heart rate, 276

Accolate (zafirlukast), indications, actions, and dosage of, 619

Accupril (quinapril), indications, actions, and dosage of, 596

Accutane (isotretinoin), indications, actions, and dosage of, 555–556

Acebutolol (Sectral), indications, actions, and dosage of, 488

Aceon (perindopril erbumine), indications, actions, and dosage of, 587–588

Acetaminophen (Datril; Tylenol)
antidote for, 471
indications, actions, and dosage of, 488, 621*t*
route, effects, and dosage for, 321*t*

Acetaminophen + butalbital +/- caffeine (Fioricet; Medigesic; Phrenilin Forte; Repan; Sedapap-10 Two-dyne; Triapin Axocet), indications, actions, and dosage of, 489

Acetaminophen + codeine (Tylenol No. 1, No. 2, No. 4), indications, actions, and dosage of, 489

Acetazolamide (Diamox)
for hyperphosphatemia, 192
indications, actions, and dosage of, 489

Acetic acid + aluminum acetate (Otic Domeboro), indications, actions, and dosage of, 489

Acetoacetate, laboratory diagnosis and, 55

Acetone, laboratory diagnosis and, 55

Acetylcysteine (Mucomyst; Mucosil), 364
indications, actions, and dosage of, 489–490

N-Acetylcysteine, for acetaminophen poisoning, 471

Achromycin V (tetracycline)
indications, actions, and dosage of, 153*t*, 609
interaction with enteral nutrition, 223

Acid-base disorders, 163–175
blood gas interpretation and, 163, 165–166
definition of, 163, 164*t*, 165*f*

Acid-base disorders (*continued*)
hypoxia, 171*f*, 171–172
metabolic acidosis, 164*t*, 166–167
metabolic alkalosis, 164*t*, 167, 169
mixed, 163
respiratory acidosis, 164*t*, 169–170
respiratory alkalosis, 164*t*, 170–171
sample problems involving, 172–175
simple, 163
Acid-fast stain, 121
Acidosis
metabolic, 164*t*, 166–167
respiratory, 164*t*, 169–170
Acid phosphatase, laboratory diagnosis
and, 55
Acinetobacter, Gram stain characteristics
of, 125*t*, 126*t*
Aciphex (rabeprazole), indications,
actions, and dosage of, 597
Aclovate (aclometasone dipropionate),
potency and application of, 628*t*
Acne, organisms responsible and empiric
therapy for, 141*t*
Acne rosacea, organisms responsible and
empiric therapy for, 141*t*
Acquired immunodeficiency syndrome.
See Human immunodeficiency
virus (HIV) infection; Human
immunodeficiency virus (HIV)
testing
ACTH stimulation test, 55–56
Actidose (activated charcoal)
clinical use of, 472
indications, actions, and dosage of, 514
Actimmune (interferon gamma-1B),
indications, actions, and dosage of,
554
Actinomyces, Gram stain characteristics
of, 125*t*
Actiq (fentanyl, transmucosal system),
indications, actions, and dosage of,
538
Activase (alteplase, recombinant)
for emergency cardiac care, 466
indications, actions, and dosage of,
492–493
Activated charcoal (Actidose; Liqui-Char;
Superchar)
clinical use of, 472
indications, actions, and dosage of, 514

Activated clotting time (ACT), 105
Activated partial thromboplastin time
(aPTT), 107
Actonel (risedronate), indications, actions,
and dosage of, 599
Actos (pioglitazone), indications, actions,
and dosage of, 589
Actretin (Soriatane), indications, actions,
and dosage of, 488
Acular (ketorolac, ophthalmic),
indications, actions, and dosage of,
557
Acupuncture, for pain management, 323
Acute abdominal series, 326
Acute coronary syndromes algorithm,
459*f*
Acute intravascular hemolysis, 202
Acute lung injury, transfusions and, 202,
203
Acute renal failure, 432–433
diet for, 207*t*
Acute specimens (titers), 132
Acute tubular necrosis, 432
Acyclovir (Zovirax), indications, actions,
and dosage of, 147*t*, 148*t*, 149*t*,
490
Adalat (nifedipine), indications, actions,
and dosage of, 578
Adalat CC (nifedipine), indications,
actions, and dosage of, 578
Adapin (doxepin)
half-life and therapeutic and toxic levels
of, 634*t*
indications, actions, and dosage of, 530
Adenosine (Adenocard)
for emergency cardiac care, 461
indications, actions, and dosage
of, 490
Adrenalin. *See* Epinephrine (Adrenalin;
Sus-Phrine)
Adrenal masses, differential diagnosis of,
42
Adrenal scans, 333
α_1-Adrenergic blockers, 479
Adrenergic nervous system, 395, 397,
397*t*, 398*t*
Adrenocorticotropic hormone (ACTH),
laboratory diagnosis and, 55
Adriamycin (doxorubicin), indications,
actions, and dosage of, 531

Adrucil (fluorouracil), indications, actions, and dosage of, 540

Adult respiratory distress syndrome (ARDS), 429–431

Advanced cardiac life support (ACLS), 449–468
    algorithms for, 450f–460f
    drugs used in, 449, 461–467
    electrical defibrillation and cardioversion for, 467–468
    transcutaneous pacing for, 468

Advil (Ibuprofen)
    indications, actions, and dosage of, 551
    route, effects, and dosage for, 321t

Aerobid (flunisolide), indications, actions, and dosage of, 540

Aeromonas hydrophilia, Gram stain characteristics of, 126t

Aeroseb-Dex (dexamethasone base), potency and application of, 628t

Aerosol therapy, 363
    topical medications for, 364

AFB smear, 121

Afrinol (pseudoephedrine), indications, actions, and dosage of, 595–596

Afterload, 395
    measurement of, 410

Agenerase (amprenavir), indications, actions, and dosage of, 150t, 498

Aggrastat (tirofiban)
    for emergency cardiac care, 464
    indications, actions, and dosage of, 611

AIDS. *See* Human immunodeficiency virus (HIV) infection; Human immunodeficiency virus (HIV) testing

Air-contrast BE, 328

AK-Beat (levobunolol), indications, actions, and dosage of, 560

AK-DEX Ophthalmic (dexamethasone, ophthalmic), indications, actions, and dosage of, 524

Akne-Mycin Topical (erythromycin, topical), indications, actions, and dosage of, 534

AK-NEO-DEX Ophthalmic (neomycin + dexamethasone), indications, actions, and dosage of, 576

AK Poly Bac Ophthalmic (bacitracin + polymyxin B, ophthalmic), indications, actions, and dosage of, 502

AK Spore HC Ophthalmic (bacitracin, neomycin, polymyxin B, + hydrocortisone, ophthalmic), indications, actions, and dosage of, 502

AK Spore Ophthalmic (bacitracin, neomycin, + polymyxin B, ophthalmic), indications, actions, and dosage of, 502

AK Tob (tobramycin, ophthalmic), indications, actions, and dosage of, 611

AK-Tracin Ophthalmic (bacitracin, ophthalmic), indications, actions, and dosage of, 502

Alanine aminotransferase (ALT; SGPT), laboratory diagnosis and, 57

Albumin, blood levels of, laboratory diagnosis and, 56

Albumin (Albuminar; Albutein; Buminate), indications, actions, and dosage of, 200t, 490

Albumin/globulin ratio (A/G ratio), laboratory diagnosis and, 56

Albalon-A Opthalmic (naphazoline + antazoline), indications, actions, and dosage of, 575

Albendazole, indications for, 153t, 154t

Albuterol (Proventil; Ventolin), 364
    for anaphylaxis, 469
    indications, actions, and dosage of, 490
    nebulized, for asthmatic attacks, 469

Albuterol + ipratropium (Combivent), indications, actions, and dosage of, 490

Aldactazide (hydrochlorothiazide + spironolactone), indications, actions, and dosage of, 549

Aldactone (spironolactone), indications, actions, and dosage of, 603

Aldara (imiquimod), indications, actions, and dosage of, 148t, 552

Aldesleukin [IL-2] (Proleukin), indications, actions, and dosage of, 491

Aldomet (methyldopa), indications, actions, and dosage of, 569

Aldosterone, laboratory diagnosis and, 56

Alendronate (Fosamax), indications, actions, and dosage of, 491

Alesse 21, 28, 623*t*

Aleve (naproxen), indications, actions, and dosage of, 575575

Alfentanil (Alfenta), indications, actions, and dosage of, 491

Alginic acid + aluminum hydroxide and magnesium trisilicate (Gaviscon), indications, actions, and dosage of, 491

Alimentum, 224*t*

Alkaline phosphatase, laboratory diagnosis and, 56–57

Alkalinization, for poisoning, 472

Alkalosis
metabolic, 164*t*, 167, 169
respiratory, 164*t*, 170–171

Alka-Mints (calcium carbonate)
for hypocalcemia, 190
indications, actions, and dosage of, 508

Alkeran (melphalan), indications, actions, and dosage of, 566

Alkylating agents, 478

Allegra (fexofenadine), indications, actions, and dosage of, 538–539

Allergic reactions
to latex, 344
medications for, 476
to transfusions, 202, 203

Allopurinol (Aloprim; Lopurin; Zyloprim), indications, actions, and dosage of, 491

Alomide Ophthalmic (lodoxamide), indications, actions, and dosage of, 562

Alopecia, differential diagnosis of, 42

Aloprim (allopurinol), indications, actions, and dosage of, 491

Alosetran (Iotronex), indications, actions, and dosage of, 491

Alpha-fetoprotein (AFP), laboratory diagnosis and, 57

Alphagan (brimonidine), indications, actions, and dosage of, 506

Alpha-1 receptors, 397

Alprazolam (Xanax), indications, actions, and dosage of, 492

Alprostadil [prostaglandin E₁] (Prostin VR), indications, actions, and dosage of, 492

Alprostadil, intracavernosal (Caverject; Edex), indications, actions, and dosage of, 492

Alprostadil, urethral suppository (Muse), indications, actions, and dosage of, 492

Altace (ramipril)
for emergency cardiac care, 461
indications, actions, and dosage of, 597

Alteplase, recombinant [TPA] (Activase)
for emergency cardiac care, 466
indications, actions, and dosage of, 492–493

AlternaGel (aluminum hydroxide)
for hyperphosphatemia, 192
indications, actions, and dosage of, 493

Altretamine (Hexalen), indications, actions, and dosage of, 493

Alum (ammonium aluminum sulfate), indications, actions, and dosage of, 496

Aluminum carbonate (Basaljel)
for hyperphosphatemia, 192
indications, actions, and dosage of, 493

Aluminum hydroxide (ALternaGel; Amphojel)
for hyperphosphatemia, 192
indications, actions, and dosage of, 493

Aluminum hydroxide + magnesium carbonate (Gaviscon), indications, actions, and dosage of, 493

Aluminum hydroxide + magnesium hydroxide (Maalox), indications, actions, and dosage of, 493–494

Aluminum hydroxide + magnesium trisilicate (Gaviscon; Gaviscon-2), indications, actions, and dosage of, 493

Alupent (metaproterenol), 364
indications, actions, and dosage of, 567

Amantadine (Symmetrel), indications, actions, and dosage of, 148*t*, 494

Amaryl (glimepiride), indications, actions, and dosage of, 545

Ambien (zolpidem), indications, actions, and dosage of, 620

Ambisome (amphotericin B liposomal), indications, actions, and dosage of, 497

Amcil (ampicillin)
indications, actions, and dosage of, 497
for subacute bacterial endocarditis prophylaxis, 158t, 159t

Amcinonide (Cyclocort), potency and application of, 628t

Amebiasis, drugs for treating, 153t

Amenorrhea, differential diagnosis of, 42

Amerge (naratriptan), indications, actions, and dosage of, 575–576

Amicar (aminocaproic acid), indications, actions, and dosage of, 494–495

Amifostine (Ethyol), indications, actions, and dosage of, 494

Amikacin (Amikin)
half-life and therapeutic and toxic levels of, 631t
indications, actions, and dosage of, 494

Amiloride (Midamor), indications, actions, and dosage of, 494

Amino acid solutions, for total parenteral nutrition, 229–230, 230t

Aminocaproic acid (Amicar), indications, actions, and dosage of, 494–495

Amino-Cerv pH 5.5 Cream, indications, actions, and dosage of, 495

Aminoglutethimide (Cytadren), indications, actions, and dosage of, 495

Aminoglycosides, 476
dosing procedure for, 620
levels of, 620, 631t
loading dose required for chosen dosing intervals for, 635t

Aminophylline, indications, actions, and dosage of, 495

Amiodarone (Cordarone; Pacerone)
for emergency cardiac care, 461
half-life and therapeutic and toxic levels of, 632t
indications, actions, and dosage of, 495

Amitriptyline (Elavil)
indications, actions, and dosage of, 495
route, effects, and dosage for, 322t

Amitriptyline + nortriptyline, half-life and therapeutic and toxic levels of, 633t

Amlodipine (Norvasc), indications, actions, and dosage of, 496

Ammonia, laboratory diagnosis and, 57

Ammonium aluminum sulfate (Alum), indications, actions, and dosage of, 496

Ammonium lactate [lactic acid + ammonium hydroxide], indications, actions, and dosage of, 558

Amniotic fluid fern test, 242–243

Amoxapine (Asendin), indications, actions, and dosage of, 496

Amoxicillin (Amoxil; Polymox)
indications, actions, and dosage of, 496
for subacute bacterial endocarditis prophylaxis, 158t, 159t

Amoxicillin + clavulanic acid (Augmentin), indications, actions, and dosage of, 496

Amphojel (aluminum hydroxide)
for hyperphosphatemia, 192
indications, actions, and dosage of, 493

Amphotec (amphotericin B cholesteryl), indications, actions, and dosage of, 497

Amphotericin B (Fungizone), indications, actions, and dosage of, 151t, 496–497

Amphotericin B cholesteryl (Amphotec), indications, actions, and dosage of, 497

Amphotericin B lipid complex (Abelcet), indications, actions, and dosage of, 497

Amphotericin B liposomal (Ambisome), indications, actions, and dosage of, 497

Ampicillin (Amcil; Omnipen)
indications, actions, and dosage of, 497
for subacute bacterial endocarditis prophylaxis, 158t, 159t

Ampicillin-sulbactam (Unasyn), indications, actions, and dosage of, 497

Amprenavir (Agenerase), indications,
        actions, and dosage of, 150*t*, 498
Amrinone (Inocor)
    for emergency cardiac care, 461
    indications, actions, and dosage of, 498
    infusion guidelines for, 439*t*
Amylase, laboratory diagnosis and, 57
Amyl nitrate, for cyanide poisoning, 471
Analgesics
    for migraine headaches, 486
    narcotic, 486
    nonnarcotic, 486
    nonopioid, 320, 321*t*
    nonsteroidal anti-inflammatory agents,
        486
    opioid, 320, 321*t*–322*t*
Anaphylaxis, 468–469
    transfusions and, 203
Anaprox (naproxen), indications, actions,
        and dosage of, 575
Anaspaz (hyoscyamine), indications,
        actions, and dosage of, 551
Anastrozole (Arimidex), indications,
        actions, and dosage of, 498
Anatomic hand scrubs, 341
Ancef (cefazolin)
    indications, actions, and dosage of, 511
    for subacute bacterial endocarditis
        prophylaxis, 158*t*
Ancylostoma duodenale infections, drugs
        for treating, 153*t*
Anectine (succinylcholine), indications,
        actions, and dosage of, 605
Anemia, chronic, red blood cell
        transfusions for, 196
Anergy screen (battery), 304
Anestacon Topical. *See* Lidocaine
        (Anestacon Topical; Xylocaine)
Anesthetics
    local, 320, 348, 349*t*, 486
    systemic, 320
Angiography, 327–328
Angiotensin-converting enzyme (ACE)
        inhibitors, 479
    for emergency cardiac care, 449
Angiotensin II receptor antagonists, 479
Anion gap, 166
Anion gap acidosis, 166
Anistreplase (Eminase)
    for emergency cardiac care, 467

    indications, actions, and dosage of, 498
Ankle, arthrocentesis of, 249, 250*f*
Ankle-Arm Index (AAI), 266
Ankle-brachial (A/B) index, 266
Ann Arbor staging classification, 654
Anogenital warts, drugs of choice for
        treating, 148*t*
Anorexia, differential diagnosis of, 42
Anoscopy, 300
Ansaid (flurbiprofen), indications, actions,
        and dosage of, 541
Antacids, 483
Anthralin (Anthraderm), indications,
        actions, and dosage of, 498
Antianxiety agents, 480
Antiarrhythmic agents, 479
Antibiotics, 476–477
    antineoplastic, 478
    half-life and therapeutic and toxic levels
        of, 631*t*
    ophthalmic, 483
Anticholinergic crisis, 469–470
Anticholinesterases, antidote for, 471
Anticoagulants, 484
    standards of practice for, 637*t*
Anticonvulsants, 480
    half-life and therapeutic and toxic levels
        of, 631*t*–632*t*
    for pain management, 320
Antidepressants, 480
    cyclic, antidote for, 471
    for pain management, 320
Antidiabetic agents, 482
Antidiarrheal agents, 483
Antidiuretic hormone [vasopressin]
        (Pitressin)
    indications, actions, and dosage
        of, 617
    infusion guidelines for, 443*t*
Antidotes, 471, 476
Antiemetic agents, 483
Antifungals, 477
Antiglobulin test
    direct, 105
    indirect, 105, 107
Antigout agents, 485
Antihemophilic factor [AHF; factor VIII]
        (Monoclate)
    indications, actions, and dosage of, 498
    for transfusion, 199*t*

Antihemophilic factor, cryoprecipitated, 198*t*

Antihistamines, 476

Antilirium (physostigmine)
  for anticholinergic crisis, 470
  antidote for, 471
  indications, actions, and dosage of, 589

Antimetabolites, 478

Antimicrobial agents, 476–478. *See also*
  Antibiotics

Antimycobacterials, 477

Antineoplastic agents, 478–479

Antinuclear antibody (ANA; FANA),
  laboratory diagnosis and, 58

Antiparkinson agents, 480

Antiplatelet agents, 484

Antipsychotics, 481

Antiretrovirals, 477

Antistreptolysin O/antistreptococcal O
  (ASO) titer, laboratory diagnosis
  and, 57

Antithrombic agents, 484

Antithrombin-III (AT-III), 105

Antithymocyte globulin [ATG] (Atgam),
  indications, actions, and dosage of,
  499

Antithyroid agents, 482

Antitussives, 487

Antiulcer agents, 483

Antivert (meclizine), indications, actions,
  and dosage of, 564

Antivirals, 477–478

Anturane (sulfinpyrazone), indications,
  actions, and dosage of, 606

Anuria, differential diagnosis of, 43,
  49–50

Anusol Ointment (pramoxine),
  indications, actions, and dosage of,
  592

Anzemet (dolasetron), indications,
  actions, and dosage of, 529–530

Aortic insufficiency (AI), 16*t*

Aortic stenosis (AS), 16*t*

AP films of chest, 325

Apgar scores, 639, 640*t*

Apheresis, 194

Apley's test, 21

Apothecary measurement units, 646

Apraclonidine (Iodipine), indications,
  actions, and dosage of, 499

Apresoline (hydralazine), indications,
  actions, and dosage of, 549

Aprotinin (Trasylol), indications, actions,
  and dosage of, 499

AquaMEPHYTON (phytonadione)
  indications, actions, and dosage of, 589
  in total parenteral nutrition, 231

Ara-C [cytarabine] (Cytosar-U),
  indications, actions, and dosage of,
  522

Aramine (metaraminol), indications,
  actions, and dosage of, 567

Arava (leflunomide), indications, actions,
  and dosage of, 559

Ardeparin (Normiflo), indications,
  actions, and dosage of, 499

Arduan (pipecuronium), indications,
  actions, and dosage of, 590

Aredia (pamidronate)
  for hypercalcemia, 189
  indications, actions, and dosage of,
  584–585

Argyll-Robertson pupil, 21

Arimidex (anastrozole), indications,
  actions, and dosage of, 498

Aristocort (triamcinolone acetonide),
  potency and application of, 630*t*

Artane (trihexyphenidyl), indications,
  actions, and dosage of, 614

Arterial line placement, 243–245, 244*f*

Arterial oxygen content (Ca$_{O_2}$), derivation
  and normal values for, 437*t*

Arterial oxygen saturation (S$_{A_{O_2}}$), for
  cardiac output determination, 413

Arterial puncture, 245–246

Arteriovenous oxygen (A-V$_{O_2}$) difference
  for cardiac output determination,
  410–412, 411*t*
  derivation and normal values for,
  437*t*

Arthritis
  differential diagnosis of, 43
  septic, organisms responsible and
    empiric therapy for, 134*t*
  synovial fluid interpretation and, 250

Arthrocentesis, 246–250
  contraindications to, 246
  indications for, 246
  materials for, 247
  procedures for, 247–250, 248*f*–250*f*

Arthrocentesis (*continued*)
  synovial fluid interpretation and,
    249–250, 251*t*
Artificial tears (Tears Naturale),
    indications, actions, and dosage of,
    499
Asacol (mesalamine), indications, actions,
    and dosage of, 566
Ascariasis, drugs for treating, 153*t*
Ascites, differential diagnosis of, 43
Ascitic fluid, diagnosis of, 297, 299*t*
Ascorbic acid, in total parenteral nutrition,
    231*t*
Asendin (amoxapine), indications, actions,
    and dosage of, 496
Aseptic meningitis, cerebrospinal fluid in,
    287*t*
L-Asparaginase (Elspar), indica-
    tions, actions, and dosage
    of, 499
Aspartate aminotransferase (AST; SGOT),
    laboratory diagnosis and, 58
Aspergillosis, systemic drugs for treating,
    151*t*
Aspiration, with enteral nutrition, 223
Aspirin (sodium salicylate)
  for emergency cardiac care, 461
  indications, actions, and dosage of,
    499–500
  route, effects, and dosage for, 321*t*
Aspirin + butalbital, caffeine and codeine
    (Fiorinal + Codeine), indications,
    actions, and dosage of, 500
Aspirin + butalbital compound (Fiorinal;
    Lanorinal), indications, actions,
    and dosage of, 500
Aspirin + codeine (Empirin No. 2, No. 3,
    No. 4), indications, actions, and
    dosage of, 500
Assist controlled ventilation, 424, 425*f*
Asthmatic attacks, 469
Asystole algorithm, 454*f*
Atacand (candesartan), indications,
    actions, and dosage of, 509
Atarax (hydroxyzine), indications, actions,
    and dosage of, 551
Atenolol (Tenormin)
  for emergency cardiac care, 462
  indications, actions, and dosage
    of, 500

Atenolol + chlorthalidone (Tenoretic),
    indications, actions, and dosage of,
    500
Atgam (antithymocyte globulin),
    indications, actions, and dosage of,
    499
Ativan (lorazepam)
  indications, actions, and dosage of, 563
  for seizures, 472
Atorvastatin (Lipitor), indications, actions,
    and dosage of, 500
Atovaquone (Mepron), indications,
    actions, and dosage of, 500–501
Atracurium (Tracrium), indications,
    actions, and dosage of, 501
Atrial arrhythmias, on electrocardiograms,
    372–374, 373*f*–375*f*
Atrial fibrillation (AF), 373–374, 375*f*
  anticoagulant standard of practice for,
    637*t*
Atrial flutter, 374, 375*f*
Atrial hypertrophy, electrocardiogram and,
    380
Atrial septal defect (ASD), 17*t*
Atrioventricular junctional or nodal
    rhythm, 374–375, 376*f*
Atrophy, of skin, 20
Atropine, 364
  for anticholinesterase poisoning, 471
  indications, actions, and dosage of, 501
Atropine sulfate, for emergency cardiac
    care, 461
Attending physicians, 2
Attending rounds, 3
Auer rods, 104
Aufalglan (benzocaine + antipyrine),
    indications, actions, and dosage of,
    504
Augmentin (amoxicillin + clavulanic
    acid), indications, actions, and
    dosage of, 496
Austin Flint murmur, 21
Autoantibodies, laboratory diagnosis and,
    58
Autoantibody test, 105, 107
Autologous blood donation, 193–194
Avandia (rosiglitazone), indications,
    actions, and dosage of, 599–600
Avapro (irbesartan), indications, actions,
    and dosage of, 555

Avelox (moxifloxacin), indications, actions, and dosage of, 574

Aventyl (nortriptyline)
half-life and therapeutic and toxic levels of, 633*t*
indications, actions, and dosage of, 580

Avita (tretinoin, topical), indications, actions, and dosage of, 613

Avlosulfon (dapsone), indications, actions, and dosage of, 523

Avulsed teeth, 470

Axid (nizatidine), indications, actions, and dosage of, 579

Axis deviation, o electrocardiograms, 369–370, 370*f*

Azactam (aztreonam), indications, actions, and dosage of, 501

Azathioprine (Imuran), indications, actions, and dosage of, 501

Azithromycin (Zithromax)
indications, actions, and dosage of, 501
for subacute bacterial endocarditis prophylaxis, 158*t*

Azopt (brinzolamide), indications, actions, and dosage of, 506

Azotemia, progressive, 432–433

Aztreonam (Azactam), indications, actions, and dosage of, 501

Azulfidine (sulfasalazine), indications, actions, and dosage of, 605–606

B

Babesia microti infections, characteristics and treatment of, 156*t*–157*t*

Babesiosis, characteristics and treatment of, 156*t*–157*t*

Babinski's sign, 24

Baby bilirubin, laboratory diagnosis and, 59

Baciguent (bacitracin, topical), indications, actions, and dosage of, 502

Bacilli anthracis, Gram stain characteristics of, 125*t*

Bacillus, Gram stain characteristics of, 123*f*

Bacillus Calmette-Guérin [BCG], indications, actions, and dosage of, 503

Bacillus fragilis, Gram stain characteristics of, 126*t*

Bacitracin
neomycin, polymyxin B, + hydrocortisone, ophthalmic (AK Spore HC Ophthalmic; Cortisporin Ophthalmic), indications, actions, and dosage of, 502
neomycin, polymyxin B, + hydrocortisone, topical (Cortisporin), indications, actions, and dosage of, 502
neomycin, polymyxin B, + lidocaine, topical (Clomycin), indications, actions, and dosage of, 502
neomycin, + polymyxin B, ophthalmic (AK Spore Ophthalmic; Neosporin Ophthalmic), indications, actions, and dosage of, 502
neomycin, + polymyxin B, topical (Neosporin ointment), indications, actions, and dosage of, 502

Bacitracin, ophthalmic (AK-Tracin Ophthalmic), indications, actions, and dosage of, 502

Bacitracin + polymyxin B, ophthalmic (AK Poly Bac Ophthalmic; Polysporin Ophthalmic), indications, actions, and dosage of, 502

Bacitracin + polymyxin B, topical (Polysporin), indications, actions, and dosage of, 502

Bacitracin, topical (Baciguent), indications, actions, and dosage of, 502

Back pain, differential diagnosis of, 43

Baclofen (Lioresal), indications, actions, and dosage of, 502

Bacterial endocarditis
organisms responsible and empiric therapy for, 136*t*–137*t*
subacute, prophylaxis, 155, 158*t*–159*t*

Bacterial infections. *See also specific infections*
cerebrospinal fluid in, 287*t*
transfusion-associated risk of transmission, 204

Bactocill (oxacillin), indications, actions, and dosage of, 582–583

Bactrim (trimethoprim-sulfamethoxazole), indications, actions, and dosage of, 153*t*, 615

Bactroban (mupirocin), indications, actions, and dosage of, 574

Bainbridge's reflex, 24

Baker tubes, 273

Balloon port, of Swan-Ganz catheter, 399

Band cells, 100

Barium enema (BE), 328

Barium swallow, 328

Basal energy expenditure (BEE), 209

Basaljel (aluminum carbonate)
   for hyperphosphatemia, 192
   indications, actions, and dosage of, 493

Base excess/deficit, laboratory diagnosis and, 59

Basiliximab (Simulect), indications, actions, and dosage of, 502

Basophil(s), laboratory diagnosis and, 101

Basophilia, 100, 104

Basophilic stippling, 104

Battle's sign, 24

Baycol (cerivastatin), indications, actions, and dosage of, 514

BCG [bacillus Calmette-Guérin] (BCG; Thera Cys; TICE), indications, actions, and dosage of, 503

BCNU (carmustine), indications, actions, and dosage of, 510

Beat-to-beat variability, 276

Beau's lines, 24

Becaplermin (Regranex Gel), indications, actions, and dosage of, 503

Beck's triad, 24

Beclomethasone (Beconase; Vancenase Nasal Inhaler), indications, actions, and dosage of, 503

Bedside procedures, 239–314. *See also specific procedures*
   basic equipment for, 240, 240*t*, 241*f*, 242*f*
   notes for, 35

Bedside rounds, 4

Belladonna + opium suppositories (B & O Supprettes), indications, actions, and dosage of, 503

Bell's palsy, 24

Benadryl (diphenhydramine)

for anaphylaxis, 469
   indications, actions, and dosage of, 528

Benazepril (Lotensin), indications, actions, and dosage of, 503

Benemid (probenecid), indications, actions, and dosage of, 593

Benign prostatic hyperplasia, medications for, 487

Bentyl (dicyclomine), indications, actions, and dosage of, 526

Benylin DM (dextromethorphan), indications, actions, and dosage of, 525

Benzamycin (erythromycin + benzoyl peroxide), indications, actions, and dosage of, 534

Benznidazole, indications for, 154*t*

Benzocaine + antipyrine (Aufalglan), indications, actions, and dosage of, 504

Benzonatate (Cogentin), indications, actions, and dosage of, 504

Bepridil (Vascar), indications, actions, and dosage of, 504

Beractant (Survanta), indications, actions, and dosage of, 504

Bergman's triad, 24

Beta blockers, 479–480
   antidote for, 471
   for emergency cardiac care, 461–462

Betadine hand scrub, 340–341

Betagan (levobunolol), indications, actions, and dosage of, 560

Betamethasone, dose, activity, duration, and route for, 627*t*

Betamethasone dipropionate (Diprosone), potency and application of, 628*t*

Betamethasone valerate (Valisone), potency and application of, 628*t*

Betapace (sotalol), indications, actions, and dosage of, 602

Beta-1 receptors, 397

Beta-2 receptors, 397

Betaseron (interferon ß-1B), indications, actions, and dosage of, 554

Betaxolol (Kerlone), indications, actions, and dosage of, 504

Betaxolol, ophthalmic (Betoptic), indications, actions, and dosage of, 504

Bethanechol (Duvoid; Urecholine), indications, actions, and dosage of, 504–505

Betoptic (betaxolol, ophthalmic), indications, actions, and dosage of, 504

Biaxin (clarithromycin) indications, actions, and dosage of, 517 for subacute bacterial endocarditis prophylaxis, 158t

Bicalutamide (Casodex), indications, actions, and dosage of, 505

Bicarbonate. *See also* Potassium bicarbonate; Sodium bicarbonate laboratory diagnosis and, 59, 61–62

Bicillin (penicillin G benzathine), indications, actions, and dosage of, 586

Bicitra (sodium citrate), indications, actions, and dosage of, 602

BiCNU (carmustine), indications, actions, and dosage of, 510

BIDA-scans, 334

Bigeminy, 375, 377f

Bile loss, IV fluid replacement with, 179

Bilirubin neonatal, laboratory diagnosis and, 59 in urine, 111

Biopsy, of skin, 302

Biotin, in total parenteral nutrition, 231t

Biot's breathing, 24

Bisacodyl (Dulcolax), indications, actions, and dosage of, 505

Bisferious pulse, 24

Bismuth subsalicylate (Pepto-Bismol), indications, actions, and dosage of, 505

Bisoprolol (Zebeta), indications, actions, and dosage of, 505

Bite wound (human and animal) infections, organisms responsible and empiric therapy for, 142t

Bitolterol (Tornalate), indications, actions, and dosage of, 505

Bitot's spots, 24

Bladder aspiration, suprapubic, percutaneous, 309, 310f

Bladder cancer, staging of, 650–651

Bladder catheterization, 306–308 contraindications to, 306 indications for, 306 materials for, 307, 307f procedure for, 307–308

Blastomycosis, systemic drugs for treating, 151t

Bleeding scans, 333

Bleeding time, 105

Bleomycin sulfate (Blenoxane), indications, actions, and dosage of, 505–506

Bleph-10 (sulfacetamide), indications, actions, and dosage of, 605

Blephamide (sulfacetamide + prednisolone), indications, actions, and dosage of, 605

Blocadren (timolol), indications, actions, and dosage of, 610

Blood, in urine, 111

Blood alcohol, laboratory diagnosis and, 67

Blood and body fluid precautions, 155

Blood collection, 95 heelstick for, 274, 275f venipuncture for, 309–314

Blood component therapy, 193–204 apheresis for, 194 autologous blood donation for, 193–194 blood banking procedures, 193 blood groups and, 194, 196t donor-restricted blood products for, 194 emergency transfusions, 194 infectious disease risk associated with, 203–204 irradiated blood components for, 194 preoperative blood set up for, 194, 195t procedure for, 201–202 products for, 196, 197t–200t, 201 routine blood donation for, 193 transfusion reactions and, 202–203

Blood cultures, 129–130

Blood gases, 161–163 capillary, 161 determination of, 162–163 interpretation of, 163, 165–166 normal values for, 161, 162t venous, 161

Blood groups, 194, 196t

Blood loss acute, red blood cell transfusions for, 196

Blood loss (*continued*)
allowable, red blood cell transfusions for, 196
Blood pressure guidelines, 14, 20*t*
Blood pressure measurement, of orthostatic pressure, 286–289
Blood smears, 95–97, 96*f*, 97*t*
Blood urea nitrogen (BUN), laboratory diagnosis and, 59
Blood volume, total, 177
Blumberg's sign, 24
Blumer's shelf, 24
Body fluids. *See also* Fluids and electrolytes; *specific fluids and electrolytes*
composition and daily production of, 181*t*
total body water, 177
Body surface area
of adults, 639, 641*f*
of children, 639, 642*f*
Body weight, desirable, 639, 640*t*
Bone infections, organisms responsible and empiric therapy for, 134*t*
Bone marrow aspiration/biopsy, 250, 252–253
Bone scans, 333
Bone turnover, high, hypercalcemia with, 188
Bordetella pertussis, Gram stain characteristics of, 124*f*, 126*t*
Borrelia burgdorferi infections, characteristics and treatment of, 156*t*–157*t*
B & O Supprettes (belladonna + opium suppositories), indications, actions, and dosage of, 503
Bouchard's nodes, 24
Bradycardia, 276, 371
algorithm for, 455*f*
Brain scans, 333
Branhamella catarrhalis, Gram stain characteristics of, 125*t*
Branham's sign, 24
Breast cancer
screening recommendations for, 643*t*
staging of, 649–650
Breast lumps, differential diagnosis of, 43
Brethine (terbutaline), indications, actions, and dosage of, 608

Bretylium
indications, actions, and dosage of, 506
infusion guidelines for, 439*t*
Brevibloc (esmolol)
for emergency cardiac care, 462
indications, actions, and dosage of, 534
infusion guidelines for, 440*t*
Brevicon 21, 28, 623*t*
Bricanyl (terbutaline), indications, actions, and dosage of, 608
Brimonidine (Alphagan), indications, actions, and dosage of, 506
Brinzolamide (Azopt), indications, actions, and dosage of, 506
Broad casts, in urine sediment, 114
Bromocriptine (Parlodel), indications, actions, and dosage of, 506
Bronchiolitis, drug of choice for treating, 148*t*
Bronchitis, organisms responsible and empiric therapy for, 134*t*
Bronchodilators, 487
half-life and therapeutic and toxic levels of, 632*t*
Bronchopulmonary hygiene, 362–364
Brontex (guaifenesin + codeine), indications, actions, and dosage of, 546
Brucella, Gram stain characteristics of, 124*f*, 126*t*
Brudzinski's sign, 24
Brugia malayi infections, drugs for treating, 153*t*
Buclizine (Bucladin-s Softabs), indications, actions, and dosage of, 506
Budesonide (Pulmicort; Rhinocort), indications, actions, and dosage of, 506
Bullae, 20
Bumetanide (Bumex), indications, actions, and dosage of, 506–507
Buminate (albumin), indications, actions, and dosage of, 200*t*, 490
BUN/creatinine ratio (BUN/CR), laboratory diagnosis and, 59–60
Bundle branch block (BBB), 379, 380*f*, 381*f*

Bupivacaine (Marcaine; Sensoricaine)
indications, actions, and dosage of, 507
for suturing, 349*t*

Buprenorphine (Buprenex), indications, actions, and dosage of, 507

Bupropion (Wellbutrin; Zyban), indications, actions, and dosage of, 507

Burn wounds
infections of, organisms responsible and empiric therapy for, 141*t*–142*t*
IV fluid replacement with, 179

Burr cells, 104

Burrows, 20

Buspirone (Buspar), indications, actions, and dosage of, 507

Busulfan (Myleran), indications, actions, and dosage of, 507

Butorphanol (Stadol), indications, actions, and dosage of, 507

Butterfly needles, 280

C

C. diphtheriae, throat culture for, 131

CA 15-3, laboratory diagnosis and, 60

CA 19-9, laboratory diagnosis and, 60

CA-125, laboratory diagnosis and, 60

Caffeine, half-life and therapeutic and toxic levels of, 632*t*

Calan (verapamil)
for emergency cardiac care, 467
indications, actions, and dosage of, 617

Calcipotriene (Davonex), indications, actions, and dosage of, 507–508

Calcitonin, blood levels of, laboratory diagnosis and, 61

Calcitonin (Cibocalcin; Miacalcin)
for hypercalcemia, 189
indications, actions, and dosage of, 508

Calcitriol (Rocaltrol), indications, actions, and dosage of, 508

Calcium
elemental, for hypocalcemia, 190
excess of. *See* Hypercalcemia
requirement for, 178
serum, laboratory diagnosis and, 61
urine, 116

Calcium acetate (Calphron; Phos-Ex; PhosLo), indications, actions, and dosage of, 508

Calcium alginate swab, 129

Calcium carbonate (Alka-Mints; Tums)
for hypocalcemia, 190
indications, actions, and dosage of, 508

Calcium-channel blockers, 479
antidote for, 471

Calcium chloride
for calcium-channel blocker poisoning, 471
for emergency cardiac care, 462
for hyperkalemia, 187
for hypocalcemia, 190
indications, actions, and dosage of, 508–509

Calcium citrate, for hypocalcemia, 190

Calcium glubionate (Neo-calglucon)
for hypocalcemia, 190
indications, actions, and dosage of, 508

Calcium gluceptate, indications, actions, and dosage of, 508–509

Calcium gluconate
for emergency cardiac care, 462
for hypermagnesemia, 190
for hypocalcemia, 190
indications, actions, and dosage of, 508–509

Calcium lactate, for hypocalcemia, 190

Calcium salts (chloride, gluconate, gluceptate), indications, actions, and dosage of, 508–509

CaldeCort (hydrocortisone)
indications, actions, and dosage of, 550
potency and application of, 629*t*

Calfactant (Infasurf), indications, actions, and dosage of, 509

Calgiswab, 129

Caloric requirements
calculation of, 209, 213
in stressed patients, calculation of, 228

Calphron (calcium acetate), indications, actions, and dosage of, 508

Camptosar (irinotecan), indications, actions, and dosage of, 555

Cancer
hypercalcemia with, 188

Cancer (*continued*)
  screening recommendations for, 639,
    643*t*–644*t*
Cancer-related check-ups, 644*t*
Candesartan (Atacand), indications,
    actions, and dosage of, 509
Candidiasis
  cystitis due to, systemic drugs for
    treating, 151*t*
  oral, systemic drugs for treating, 151*t*
  vaginal. *See* Vaginal candidiasis
Cantor tubes, 272
Capillary fingersticks/heelsticks, 95
Capoten (captopril)
  for emergency cardiac care, 449
  indications, actions, and dosage of, 509
Capsaicin (Capsin; Zostrix), indications,
    actions, and dosage of, 509
Captopril (Capoten)
  for emergency cardiac care, 449
  indications, actions, and dosage of, 509
Captopril test, 61
Caraway tubes, 274
Carbamazepine (Tegretol)
  half-life and therapeutic and toxic levels
    of, 631*t*
  indications, actions, and dosage of, 509
  route, effects, and dosage for, 322*t*
Carbidopa + levodopa (Sinemet),
    indications, actions, and dosage of,
    509–510
Carbocaine (mepivacaine), for suturing,
    349*t*
Carbohydrate controlled diet, 207*t*
Carbon dioxide, laboratory diagnosis and,
    61–62
Carbon monoxide
  antidote for, 471
  laboratory diagnosis and, 62
Carboplatin (Paraplatin), indications,
    actions, and dosage of, 510
Carboxyhemoglobin, laboratory diagnosis
    and, 62
Carcinoembryonic antigen (CEA),
    laboratory diagnosis and, 62
Cardene (nicardipine)
  indications, actions, and dosage of, 578
  infusion guidelines for, 441*t*–442*t*
Cardiac angiography, 328
Cardiac care, emergency, 449–468

  algorithms for, 450*f*–460*f*
  drugs used in, 449, 461–467
  electrical defibrillation and
    cardioversion for, 467–468
Cardiac contractility, 395
  measurement of, 410
Cardiac failure, renal failure, 235
Cardiac hypertrophy, on
    electrocardiograms, 380–383,
    381*f*–383*f*
Cardiac index (CI), 395
  derivation and normal values for, 437*t*
Cardiac output (CO), 395
  adrenergic nervous system and, 395,
    397, 397*t*, 398*t*
  derivation and normal values for, 437*t*
  determinants of, 395, 396*f*
  determinations of, 410–413
Cardiac pacing, 468
Cardiac scans, 333–334
Cardiogenic shock, 414, 431
Cardiomyopathy, anticoagulant standard
    of practice for, 637*t*
Cardiopulmonary resuscitation (CPR),
    445–449
  adult, 445–447, 448
  child, 447, 448
  foreign body obstructed airway
    sequence for, 448
  infant, 447, 448
  neonatal, 447–448
  one-rescuer, 445–446
  primary survey for, 447
  recovery position for, 449
  secondary survey for, 447
  two-rescuer, 446–447
Cardiovascular agents, 479–480
  half-life and therapeutic and toxic levels
    of, 632*t*–633*t*
Cardiovascular evaluation, 391–395
  blood pressure in, 392–393
  heart murmurs in, 393–395
  inspection in, 391–392
  mean arterial blood pressure in, 393,
    394*f*
  pulse pressure in, 393
Cardioversion, 468
  DC-synchronized, 374
Cardizem (diltiazem)
  for emergency cardiac care, 462

indications, actions, and dosage of, 528
infusion guidelines for, 439*t*
Cardura (doxazosin), indications, actions, and dosage of, 530
Carisoprodol (Soma), indications, actions, and dosage of, 510
Carmustine (BCNU; BiCNU), indications, actions, and dosage of, 510
Carteolol (Cartrol; Occupress Ophthalmic), indications, actions, and dosage of, 510
Carvedilol (Coreg), indications, actions, and dosage of, 510
Casodex (bicalutamide), indications, actions, and dosage of, 505
Casts, in urine sediment, 114
Cataflam (diclofenac)
indications, actions, and dosage of, 526
route, effects, and dosage for, 321*t*
Catapres (clonidine, oral), indications, actions, and dosage of, 518
Catapres TS (clonidine, transdermal), indications, actions, and dosage of, 518
Catecholamines
fractional serum, laboratory diagnosis and, 62
fractionated, in urine, 117
Cathartics, 483
Catheter(s). *See also* Bladder catheterization; Central venous catheterization; Peripherally inserted central catheter (PICC) lines; Pulmonary artery catheters
French units for, 240, 241*f*
vascular, sepsis of, 435
Catheterization. *See* Peripherally inserted central catheter (PICC) lines
Caverject (alprostadil, intracavernosal), indications, actions, and dosage of, 492
Cavitary lesions, of lungs, 338
CCNU (lomustine), indications, actions, and dosage of, 562
Ceclor (cefaclor), indications, actions, and dosage of, 510–511
Cedax (ceftibutin), indications, actions, and dosage of, 513
CeeNu (lomustine), indications, actions, and dosage of, 562

Cefaclor (Ceclor), indications, actions, and dosage of, 510–511
Cefadroxil (Duricef; Ultracef)
indications, actions, and dosage of, 511
for subacute bacterial endocarditis prophylaxis, 158*t*
Cefadyl (cephapirin), indications, actions, and dosage of, 514
Cefazolin (Ancef; Kefzol)
indications, actions, and dosage of, 511
for subacute bacterial endocarditis prophylaxis, 158*t*
Cefdinir (Omnicef), indications, actions, and dosage of, 511
Cefepime (Maxipime), indications, actions, and dosage of, 511
Cefixime (Suprax), indications, actions, and dosage of, 511
Cefizox (ceftizoxime), indications, actions, and dosage of, 513
Cefmetazole (Zefazone), indications, actions, and dosage of, 511
Cefobid (cefoperazone), indications, actions, and dosage of, 512
Cefonicid (Monocid), indications, actions, and dosage of, 511–512
Cefoperazone (Cefobid), indications, actions, and dosage of, 512
Cefotan (cefotetan), indications, actions, and dosage of, 512
Cefotaxime (Claforan), indications, actions, and dosage of, 512
Cefotetan (Cefotan), indications, actions, and dosage of, 512
Cefoxitin (Mefoxin), indications, actions, and dosage of, 512
Cefpodoxime (Vantin), indications, actions, and dosage of, 512
Cefprozil (Cefzil), indications, actions, and dosage of, 512
Ceftazidime (Ceptaz; Fortaz; Tazicef; Tazidime), indications, actions, and dosage of, 513
Ceftibutin (Cedax), indications, actions, and dosage of, 513
Ceftin (cefuroxime), indications, actions, and dosage of, 513
Ceftizoxime (Cefizox), indications, actions, and dosage of, 513

Ceftriaxone (Rocephin), indications, actions, and dosage of, 513

Cefuroxime (Ceftin; Zinacef), indications, actions, and dosage of, 513

Cefzil (cefprozil), indications, actions, and dosage of, 512

Celecoxib (Celebrex)
indications, actions, and dosage of, 513
route, effects, and dosage for, 321t

Celexa (citalopram), indications, actions, and dosage of, 517

Cellcept (mycophenolate mofetil), indications, actions, and dosage of, 574

Cellulitis, organisms responsible and empiric therapy for, 142t

Celsius/Fahrenheit conversion, 646, 649t

Cenestin (estrogens, conjugated-synthetic), indications, actions, and dosage of, 535–536

Centrally acting antihypertensive agents, 479

Central nervous system agents, 480–481

Central venous catheterization, 253–260
catheter removal and, 260
complications of, 257–258, 260
contraindications to, 254
femoral vein approach for, 259–260
historical background of, 254
indications for, 253
left internal jugular vein approach for, 258–259, 259f
materials for, 254
right internal jugular vein approach for, 256–258, 257f
subclavian approach for, 254–256

Central venous pressure (CVP), 397–399, 398t
derivation and normal values for, 437t

Centrax (prazepam), indications, actions, and dosage of, 593

Cephalexin (Keflex; Keftab)
indications, actions, and dosage of, 513
for subacute bacterial endocarditis prophylaxis, 158t

Cephalosporins, 476

Cephapirin (Cefadyl), indications, actions, and dosage of, 514

Cephradine (Velosef), indications, actions, and dosage for, 514

Cephulac (lactulose), indications, actions, and dosage of, 558

Ceptaz (ceftazidime), indications, actions, and dosage of, 513

Cerebellum, herniation of, with lumbar puncture, 286

Cerebral angiography, 328

Cerebral perfusion pressure (CPP), derivation and normal values for, 438t

Cerebrospinal fluid (CSF), differential diagnosis of, 287t–288t

Cerebryx (fosphenytoin)
indications, actions, and dosage of, 543
for seizures, 473t

Cerivastatin (Baycol), indications, actions, and dosage of, 514

Cerubidine (daunorubicin), indications, actions, and dosage of, 523

Cerumenex (triethanolamine), indications, actions, and dosage of, 614

Cervical cancer
screening recommendations for, 643t
staging of, 651–652

Cervical infections, tests for, 291

Cervicitis, organisms responsible and empiric therapy for, 135t

Cetamide (sulfacetamide), indications, actions, and dosage of, 605

Cetirizine (Zyrtec), indications, actions, and dosage of, 514

Chadwick's sing, 24

Chagas' disease, drugs for treating, 154t

Chancroid, organism responsible and empiric therapy for, 135t

Chandelier sign, 24, 290

Charcot's triad, 24

Chartwork, 33–40

Check-out rounds, 3–4

Chemet (succimer), indications, actions, and dosage of, 604–605

Chemically defined formulas, for enteral nutrition, 217

Chest computed tomography, 331

Chest electrodes, 267, 267f

Chest magnetic resonance imaging, 332

Chest pain, differential diagnosis of, 43

Chest physiotherapy, 363

Chest tube placement, 260–263
complications of, 263

historical background of, 261
indications for, 260–261
materials for, 261
procedure for, 261–263, 262f
Chest x-rays, 325
reading, 335, 336f, 337f, 338
Cheyne-Stokes respirations, 24
Children. *See also* Infant formulas and
feeding
body surface area of, 639, 642f
"rule of sixes" nomogram for
calculating fluids in, 179, 181t
Chills, differential diagnosis of, 43
Chlamydia cultures, 291
Chlamydial infections, organism
responsible and empiric therapy
for, 135t
Chloral hydrate (Noctec), indications,
actions, and dosage of, 514
Chlorambucil (Leukeran), indications,
actions, and dosage of, 514
Chlordiazepoxide (Librium), indications,
actions, and dosage of, 515
Chlorhexidine 6-min hand scrub, 341
Chloride
requirement for, 178
serum, laboratory diagnosis and, 62
spot urine study for, 114
Chloride-insensitive (resistant) metabolic
alkalosis, 169
Chloride-sensitive (responsive) metabolic
alkalosis, 167, 169
Chloroquine phosphate, indications for, 153t
Chlorothiazide (Diuril), indications,
actions, and dosage of, 515
Chlorpheniramine (Chlor-Trimeton),
indications, actions, and dosage of,
515
Chlorpromazine (Thorazine), indications,
actions, and dosage of, 515
Chlorpropamide (Diabinese), indications,
actions, and dosage of, 515
Chlorthalidone (Hygroton), indications,
actions, and dosage of, 515
Chlor-Trimeton (chlorpheniramine),
indications, actions, and dosage of,
515
Chlorzoxazone (Paraflex; Parafon Forte
DSC), indications, actions, and
dosage of, 515–516

Cholangiography, T-tube, 329
Cholangitis, organisms responsible and
empiric therapy for, 137t
Cholecalciferol [vitamin D$_3$],
indications, actions, and dosage
of, 516
Cholecystitis
acalculous, 434
organisms responsible and empiric
therapy for, 137t
Cholestasis, total parenteral nutrition for,
237
Cholesterol, laboratory diagnosis and,
62–63, 63t, 80f
Cholesterol restricted diet, 208t
Cholestyramine (Questran), indications,
actions, and dosage of, 516
Chromic catgut sutures, 346t
Chromium, in total parenteral nutrition,
231, 232t
Chronulac (lactulose), indications, actions,
and dosage of, 558
Chvostek's sign, 24
Chylothorax, 50
Cibocalcin (calcitonin)
for hypercalcemia, 189
indications, actions, and dosage
of, 508
Ciclopirox (Loprox), indications, actions,
and dosage of, 516
Cidofovir (Vistide), indications, actions,
and dosage of, 146t, 516
Ciloxan (ciprofloxacin, ophthalmic),
indications, actions, and dosage of,
517
Cimetidine (Tagamet), indications,
actions, and dosage of, 516
Ciprofloxacin (Cipro), indications,
actions, and dosage of, 516
Ciprofloxacin, ophthalmic (Ciloxan),
indications, actions, and dosage of,
517
Ciprofloxacin, otic (Cipro HC Otic),
indications, actions, and dosage of,
517
Cipro HC Otic (ciprofloxacin, otic),
indications, actions, and dosage of,
517
Cisplatin (Platinol AQ), indications,
actions, and dosage of, 517

13-cis retinoic acid [isotretinoin]
(Accutane), indications, actions,
and dosage of, 555–556

Citalopram (Celexa), indications, actions,
and dosage of, 517

Citrobacter, Gram stain characteristics of,
124*f*

Cladribine (Leustatin), indications,
actions, and dosage of, 517

Claforan (cefotaxime), indications,
actions, and dosage of, 512

Clarithromycin (Biaxin)
indications, actions, and dosage
of, 517
for subacute bacterial endocarditis
prophylaxis, 158*t*

Claritin (loratadine), indications, actions,
and dosage of, 563

Clean catch urine specimens, urine,
308–309

Clear liquid diet, 206*t*–207*t*

Clemastine fumarate (Tavist), indications,
actions, and dosage of, 518

Clindamycin (Cleocin; Cleocin-T)
indications, actions, and dosage of,
153*t*, 518
for subacute bacterial endocarditis
prophylaxis, 158*t*

Clinoril (ulindac), indications, actions, and
dosage of, 606

Clobetasol propionate (Temovate),
potency and application
of, 628*t*

Clocortolone pivalate (Cloderm), potency
and application of, 628*t*

Clofazimine (Lamprene), indications,
actions, and dosage of, 518

Clomycin (bacitracin, neomycin,
polymyxin B, + lidocaine, topical),
indications, actions, and dosage of,
502

Clonazepam (Klonopin), indications,
actions, and dosage of, 518

Clonidine, oral (Catapres), indications,
actions, and dosage of, 518

Clonidine, transdermal (Catapres TS),
indications, actions, and dosage of,
518

Clopidogrel (Plavix), indications, actions,
and dosage of, 519

Clopra (metoclopramide), indications,
actions, and dosage of, 569

Clorazepate (Tranxene), indications,
actions, and dosage of, 519

Clostridium, Gram stain characteristics of,
123*f*, 126*t*

Clostridium difficile assay, 63, 131

Clotrimazole (Lotrimin; Mycelex),
indications, actions, and dosage of,
519

Clotrimazole + betamethasone
(Lotrisone), indications, actions,
and dosage of, 519

Cloxacillin (Cloxapen; Tegopen),
indications, actions, and dosage of,
519

Clozapine (Clozaril), indications, actions,
and dosage of, 519

Clubbing, differential diagnosis of, 43

Coagulation cascade, 106*f*

Cocaine, indications, actions, and dosage
of, 519–520

Coccidioidomycosis, systemic drugs for
treating, 151*t*

Codeine
indications, actions, and dosage of,
520
route, effects, and dosage for, 321*t*

Cogentin (benzonatate), indications,
actions, and dosage of, 504

Cognex (tacrine), indications, actions, and
dosage of, 606

Coin lesions, of lungs, 338

Colace (docusate sodium), indications,
actions, and dosage of, 529

Colchicine, indications, actions, and
dosage of, 520

Cold agglutinins, laboratory diagnosis
and, 63–64

Colesevelam (Welchol), indications,
actions, and dosage of, 520

Colestid (colestipol), indications, actions,
and dosage of, 520

Colfosceril palmitate (Exosurf Neonatal),
indications, actions, and dosage of,
520

Colitis, cytomegalovirus, drugs of choice
for treating, 146*t*

Colloids, composition of, 178

Color, of urine, 110

Colorectal cancer
  screening recommendations for, 643*t*
  staging of, 652
CoLyte (polyethylene glycol [PEG]-
    electrolyte solution), indications,
    actions, and dosage of, 590–591
Coma, 470
  differential diagnosis of, 44
Combivent (albuterol + ipratropium),
    indications, actions, and dosage of,
    490
Combivir (zidovudine + lamivudine),
    indications, actions, and dosage of,
    619
Compazine (prochlorperazine), indica-
    tions, actions, and dosage of, 594
Complement, laboratory diagnosis and, 64
Complete blood cell count (CBC)
  left shift in, 100
  normal values for, 97, 98*t*–99*t*
  normal variations in, 97
Computed tomography (CT), 330–331
Comtan (entacapone), indications, actions,
    and dosage of, 532
Comvax (haemophilus B conjugate
    vaccine), indications, actions, and
    dosage of, 547
Condylox (podophyllin), indications,
    actions, and dosage of, 148*t*,
    590–591
Condylox Gel 0.5% (podophyllin),
    indications, actions, and dosage of,
    148*t*, 590–591
Conjunctivitis, organism responsible and
    empiric therapy for, 135*t*
Consent, informed, 240
Constipation
  differential diagnosis of, 44
  with enteral nutrition, 223
Contact isolation, 155
Contaminants, in urine sediment, 112
Continuous positive airway pressure
    (CPAP), 426
Contrast media, 327
  reactions to, 327
Controlled substances, 475–476
Controlled ventilation, 424, 425*f*
Conus medullaris trauma, with lumbar
    puncture, 286
Convalescent specimens (titers), 132

Coombs' test
  direct, 105
  indirect, 105, 107
Copper, in total parenteral nutrition, 231,
    232*t*
Cordarone (amiodarone)
  for emergency cardiac care, 461
  half-life and therapeutic and toxic levels
    of, 632*t*
  indications, actions, and dosage of, 495
Cordran (flurandrenolide), potency and
    application of, 629*t*
Coreg (carvedilol), indications, actions,
    and dosage of, 510
Corgard (nadolol), indications, actions,
    and dosage of, 574
Corlopam (fenoldopam), indications,
    actions, and dosage of, 537
Corrected reticulocyte count, 100–101
Corrigan's pulse, 24
Corticaine (hydrocortisone acetate)
  indications, actions, and dosage
    of, 603
  potency and application of, 629*t*
Corticosteroids. *See also specific
    corticosteroids*
  for hypercalcemia, 189
  for pain management, 320
  in urine, 118
Cortisol
  free, in urine, 117
  serum, laboratory diagnosis and, 64
Cortisone (Cortone)
  dose, activity, duration, and route for,
    627*t*
  indications, actions, and dosage
    of, 603
Cortisporin (bacitracin, neomycin,
    polymyxin B, + hydrocortisone,
    topical), indications, actions, and
    dosage of, 502
Cortisporin Ophthalmic (bacitracin,
    neomycin, polymyxin B, +
    hydrocortisone, ophthalmic),
    indications, actions, and dosage of,
    502
Cortisporin Ophthalmic and Otic
    (neomycin, polymyxin, +
    hydrocortisone), indications,
    actions, and dosage of, 577

Cortisporin-TC Otic Drops (neomycin, colistin, + hydrocortisone), indications, actions, and dosage of, 576

Cortisporin-TC Otic Suspension (neomycin, colistin, hydrocortisone, + thonzonium), indications, actions, and dosage of, 576

Cortizone (hydrocortisone) indications, actions, and dosage of, 550 potency and application of, 629*t*

Cortone (cortisone) dose, activity, duration, and route for, 627*t* indications, actions, and dosage of, 603

Cortrosyn stimulation test, 55–56

Corvert (ibutilide) for emergency cardiac care, 464 indications, actions, and dosage of, 551

Corynebacterium, Gram stain characteristics of, 123*f*, 126*t*

Cosmegen (dactinomycin), indications, actions, and dosage of, 523

Cosopt (dorzolamide + timolol), indications, actions, and dosage of, 530

Cotazyme (pancreatin + pancrelipase), indications, actions, and dosage of, 585

Co-trimoxazole [trimethoprim-sulfamethoxazole] (Bactrim; Septra), indications, actions, and dosage of, 153*t*, 615

Coudé catheter, 307, 307*f*

Cough, differential diagnosis of, 44

Coumadin (warfarin) indications, actions, and dosage of, 618 interaction with enteral nutrition, 223

Counterimmunoelectrophoresis (CEP; CIEP), laboratory diagnosis and, 64–65

Cozaar (losartan), indications, actions, and dosage of, 563

C-peptide, insulin, laboratory diagnosis and, 60

C-reactive protein (C-RP), laboratory diagnosis and, 60

Creatinine, 115

serum, laboratory diagnosis and, 65

Creatinine clearance, 115–116 determination of, 116

Creatinine phosphokinase (CPK) isoenzymes of, laboratory diagnosis and, 65 laboratory diagnosis and, 65

Creeping eruption, drugs for treating, 153*t*

Creon (pancreatin + pancrelipase), indications, actions, and dosage of, 585

Cricothyrotomy, 263–264

Critical care. *See* Intensive care unit (ICU)

Critical closing volume (CCV), 416*f*, 417

Critical illness, hypocalcemia and, 189

Crixivan (indinavir), indications, actions, and dosage of, 150*t*, 553

Cromolyn sodium (Intal; Nasalcrom; Opticrom), indications, actions, and dosage of, 520–521

Cross-table lateral abdominal x-rays, 326

Crotamiton, indications for, 154*t*

Croup, 131

Crusts, 20

Cryocrit, laboratory diagnosis and, 65

Cryoglobulins, laboratory diagnosis and, 65

Cryoprecipitated antihemophilic factor, 198*t*

Cryptococcosis, systemic drugs for treating, 151*t*

Cryptosporidiosis, drugs for treating, 153*t*

Crystal(s), in urine sediment, 112

Crystalline amino acid solutions, for total parenteral nutrition, 229–230, 230*t*

Crystalloids, composition of, 180*t*

Crystal violet, 122

C-spine x-rays, 326

Culdocentesis, 264–265

Cullen's sign, 24

Curling's ulcers, 433

Cushing's triad, 24

Cushing's ulcers, 433

Cutaneous larva migrans, drugs for treating, 153*t*

Cutivate (fluticasone propionate), potency and application of, 629*t*

Cyanide, antidote for, 471

Cyanocobalamin [vitamin B_{12}]
blood level of, laboratory diagnosis and, 92–93
indications, actions, and dosage of, 521
in total parenteral nutrition, 231*t*
Cyanosis, differential diagnosis of, 44
Cyclic antidepressants, antidote for, 471
Cyclobenzaprine (Flexeril), indications, actions, and dosage of, 521
Cyclocort (amcinonide), potency and application of, 628*t*
Cyclogyl (cyclopentolate), indications, actions, and dosage of, 521
Cyclopentolate (Cyclogyl), indications, actions, and dosage of, 521
Cyclophosphamide (Cytoxan; Neosar), indications, actions, and dosage of, 521
Cyclospora infection, drugs for treating, 153*t*
Cyclosporine (Neoral; Sandimmune)
half-life and therapeutic and toxic levels of, 634*t*
indications, actions, and dosage of, 521–522
Cycrin (medroxyprogesterone), indications, actions, and dosage of, 564
Cyproheptadine (Periactin), indications, actions, and dosage of, 522
Cysteine, in urine, 117
Cysticercosis, drugs for treating, 154*t*
Cysticercus cellulosae infections, drugs for treating, 154*t*
Cystitis, organisms responsible and empiric therapy for, 143*t*
Cystography, 328
Cystospaz (hyoscyamine), indications, actions, and dosage of, 551
Cytadren (aminoglutethimide), indications, actions, and dosage of, 495
Cytarabine [Ara-C] (Cytosar-U), indications, actions, and dosage of, 522
Cytarabine liposome (DepoCyt), indications, actions, and dosage of, 522

CytoGam (cytomegalovirus immune globulin), indications, actions, and dosage of, 522
Cytology, of ascitic or pleural fluid, 299*t*
Cytomegalovirus (CMV)
antibodies to, laboratory diagnosis and, 66
cultures for, 132
drugs of choice for treating infections by, 146*t*
transfusion-associated risk of transmission, 204
Cytomegalovirus immune globulin [CMV-IVIG] (CytoGam), indications, actions, and dosage of, 522
Cytomel (liothyronine), indications, actions, and dosage of, 562
Cytosar-U (cytarabine), indications, actions, and dosage of, 522
Cytotec (misoprostol), indications, actions, and dosage of, 572
Cytovene (ganciclovir), indications, actions, and dosage of, 146*t*, 543–544
Cytoxan (cyclophosphamide), indications, actions, and dosage of, 521

D

Dacarbazine (DTIC), indications, actions, and dosage of, 522
Dacliximab (Zenapax), indications, actions, and dosage of, 522
Dactinomycin (Cosmegen), indications, actions, and dosage of, 523
Dalgan (dezocine), indications, actions, and dosage of, 525
Dalmane (flurazepam), indications, actions, and dosage of, 541
Dalteparin (Fragmin), indications, actions, and dosage of, 523
Dantrolene (Dantrium), indications, actions, and dosage of, 523
Dapsone (Avlosulfon), indications, actions, and dosage of, 523
Darier's sign, 24
Darkfield examination, 122
Darvocet (propoxyphene + acetaminophen), indications, actions, and dosage of, 595

Darvon (propoxyphene), indications, actions, and dosage of, 595

Darvon Compound-65 (propoxyphene + aspirin), indications, actions, and dosage of, indications, actions, and dosage of, 595

Darvon-N + Aspirin (propoxyphene + aspirin), indications, actions, and dosage of, indications, actions, and dosage of, 595

Daunomycin (daunorubicin), indications, actions, and dosage of, 523

Daunorubicin (Cerubidine; Daunomycin), indications, actions, and dosage of, 523

Davonex (calcipotriene), indications, actions, and dosage of, 507–508

Daypro (oxaprozin), indications, actions, and dosage of, 583

Daytril (acetaminophen)
antidote for, 471
indications, actions, and dosage of, 488, 621t
route, effects, and dosage for, 321t

DDAVP (desmopressin), indications, actions, and dosage of, 524

Decadron (dexamethasone base), potency and application of, 628t

Decadron (dexamethasone)
dose, activity, duration, and route for, 627t
indications, actions, and dosage of, 603, 604
route, effects, and dosage for, 322t

Decelerations, in fetal heart rate, 276

Declomycin (demeclocycline), indications, actions, and dosage of, 524

Decongestants, 487

Decubitus abdominal x-rays, 326

Decubitus ulcers, organisms responsible and empiric therapy for, 142t

Deep somatic pain, 315

Deep venous thrombosis (DVT)
anticoagulant standard of practice for, 637t
prevention of, 435

Dehydroepiandrosterone (DHEA), laboratory diagnosis and, 66

Dehydroepiandrosterone sulfate (DHEAS), laboratory diagnosis and, 66

Delavirdine (Rescriptor), indications, actions, and dosage of, 523–524

Delayed hypersensitivity skin testing, 303

Delirium, differential diagnosis of, 44

Delivery notes, 37

Del-Mycin Topical (erythromycin, topical), indications, actions, and dosage of, 534

Delta-Cortef (prednisolone)
dose, activity, duration, and route for, 627t
indications, actions, and dosage of, 603

Deltasone (prednisone)
dose, activity, duration, and route for, 627t
for hypercalcemia, 189
indications, actions, and dosage of, 603

Demadex (torsemide), indications, actions, and dosage of, 613

Demeclocycline (Declomycin), indications, actions, and dosage of, 524

Dementia, differential diagnosis of, 44–45

Demerol (meperidine)
indications, actions, and dosage of, 566
route, effects, and dosage for, 321t

Demser (metyrosine), indications, actions, and dosage of, 570

Demulen 1/35 21, 623t

Demulen 1/50 21, 623t

de Musset's sign, 26

Denavir (penciclovir), indications, actions, and dosage of, 147t, 585

Dennis tubes, 273

Dental emergencies, 470

Dental examination, 14, 17, 19f

Depakene (valproic acid)
half-life and therapeutic and toxic levels of, 632t
indications, actions, and dosage of, 616

Depakote (divalproex), indications, actions, and dosage of, 616

DepoCyt (cytarabine liposome), indications, actions, and dosage of, 522

Depo-Medrol (methylprednisolone acetate)
dose, activity, duration, and route for,
627t
indications, actions, and dosage of, 603
Depo Provera (medroxyprogesterone),
indications, actions, and dosage of,
564
Dermalon (nylon) sutures, 346t
Dermatologic agents, 481
Dermatologic descriptions, 20–21
Dermatome, 22f–23f
Dermatop (prednicarbate), potency and
application of, 630t
Desipramine (Norpramin)
half-life and therapeutic and toxic levels
of, 633t
indications, actions, and dosage of, 524
Desmopressin (DDAVP; Stimate),
indications, actions, and dosage of,
524
Desogen (Organon), 623t
Desonide (DesOwen), potency and
application of, 628t
Desoximetasone (Topicort), potency and
application of, 628t
Desyrel (trazodone)
half-life and therapeutic and toxic levels
of, 634t
indications, actions, and dosage of, 613
Detrol LA (tolterodine), indications,
actions, and dosage of, 612
DEXA, 326
Dexacort Phosphate Turbinaire
(dexamethasone, nasal),
indications, actions, and dosage of,
524
Dexamethasone (Decadron)
dose, activity, duration, and route for,
627t
indications, actions, and dosage of, 603,
604
route, effects, and dosage for, 322t
Dexamethasone base (Aeroseb-Dex;
Decadron), potency and
application of, 628t
Dexamethasone, nasal (Dexacort
Phosphate Turbinaire), indications,
actions, and dosage of, 524
Dexamethasone, ophthalmic (AK-DEX
Ophthalmic; Decadron

Ophthalmic), indications, actions,
and dosage of, 524
Dexamethasone suppression test, 66
Dexferrum (iron dextran), indications,
actions, and dosage of, 555
Dexpanthenol (Ilopan; Ilopan-choline
Oral)
indications, actions, and dosage of, 525
in total parenteral nutrition, 231t
Dexrazoxane (Zinecard), indications,
actions, and dosage of, 525
Dextran 40 (Rheomacrodex), indications,
actions, and dosage of, 525
Dextromethorphan (Benylin DM;
Mediquell; Pediacare 1),
indications, actions, and dosage of,
525
Dey-Drop (silver nitrate), indications,
actions, and dosage of, 601
Dezocine (Dalgan), indications, actions,
and dosage of, 525
Diabeta (glyburide), indications, actions,
and dosage of, 545
Diabetes
insulins for. See Insulins
total parenteral nutrition formulation
for, 235
Diabinese (chlorpropamide), indications,
actions, and dosage of, 515
Diagnostic peritoneal lavage (DPL),
295
Dialose (docusate potassium), indications,
actions, and dosage of, 529
Diamox (acetazolamide)
for hyperphosphatemia, 192
indications, actions, and dosage of, 489
Diaphragm, on chest x-rays, 335, 337f
Diarrhea
differential diagnosis of, 45
with enteral nutrition, 218, 223
IV fluid replacement with, 179
Diastolic heart murmurs, 394–395
Diastolic hypertension, 392
Diazepam (Valium)
indications, actions, and dosage of,
525–526
for seizures, 472, 473t
Diazoxide (Hyperstat; Proglycem),
indications, actions, and dosage of,
526

Dibucaine (Nupercainal), indications, actions, and dosage of, 526

Diclofenac (Cataflam; Voltaren) indications, actions, and dosage of, 526 route, effects, and dosage for, 321t

Dicloxacillin (Dycill; Dynapen), indications, actions, and dosage of, 526

Dicyclomine (Bentyl), indications, actions, and dosage of, 526

Didanosine [DDI] (Videx), indications, actions, and dosage of, 526–527

Didronel (etidronate disodium), indications, actions, and dosage of, 536

Diet(s), hospital, 205, 206t–208t

Dietary supplements, 481

Diethylcarbamazine, indications for, 153t

Diethylenetriamine pentaacetic acid (technetium-99m DTPA), 334

Differential diagnosis, 41–52

Differential WBC, 96–97, 97t

Diflorasone diacetate (Psorcon), potency and application of, 628t

Diflucan (fluconazole), indications, actions, and dosage of, 151t, 539–540

Diflunisal (Dolobid), indications, actions, and dosage of, 527

Digibind (digoxin immune Fab) for emergency cardiac care, 462 indications, actions, and dosage of, 471, 527

Digitalis electrocardiogram and, 386 toxicity of, 386

Digoxin (Lanoxicaps; Lanoxin) antidote for, 471 for emergency cardiac care, 462 half-life and therapeutic and toxic levels of, 633t indications, actions, and dosage of, 527

Digoxin immune Fab (Digibind) for emergency cardiac care, 462 indications, actions, and dosage of, 471, 527

Dihydrohydroxycodeinone [oxycodone] (Oxycontin; OxyIR; Roxicodone), indications, actions, and dosage of, 583

Dilacor (diltiazem) for emergency cardiac care, 462 indications, actions, and dosage of, 528 infusion guidelines for, 439t

Dilantin (phenytoin) half-life and therapeutic and toxic levels of, 631t–632t indications, actions, and dosage of, 589 interaction with enteral nutrition, 223

Dilaudid (hydromorphone), indications, actions, and dosage of, 550

Diltiazem (Cardizem; Dilacor; Tiazac) for emergency cardiac care, 462 indications, actions, and dosage of, 528 infusion guidelines for, 439t

Dimenhydrinate (Dramamine), indications, actions, and dosage of, 528

Dimercaptosuccinic acid (technetium-99m DMSA), 334

Dimethyl sulfoxide [DMSO] (Rimso 50), indications, actions, and dosage of, 528

Diovan (valsartan), indications, actions, and dosage of, 616

Dipentum (olsalazine), indications, actions, and dosage of, 580–581

Diphenhydramine (Benadryl) for anaphylaxis, 469 indications, actions, and dosage of, 528

Diphenoxylate + atropine (Lomotil), indications, actions, and dosage of, 528

Diphyllobothrium latum infections, drugs for treating, 154t

Dipivefrin (Propine), indications, actions, and dosage of, 528

Diplopia, differential diagnosis of, 45

Diprivan (propofol), indications, actions, and dosage of, 594

Diprosone (betamethasone dipropionate), potency and application of, 628t

Dipylidium caninum infections, drugs for treating, 154t

Dirithromycin (Dynabac), indications, actions, and dosage of, 529

Discharge precautions, 156

Discharge summaries/notes, 34–35

Disopyramide (Napamide; Norpace)

half-life and therapeutic and toxic levels of, 633t

indications, actions, and dosage of, 529

Disseminated intravascular coagulation (DIC), 434–435

Distal port, of Swan-Ganz catheter, 400

Ditropan (oxybutynin), indications, actions, and dosage of, 583

Ditropan XL (oxybutynin), indications, actions, and dosage of, 583

Diuretics, 479–480

Diuril (chlorothiazide), indications, actions, and dosage of, 515

Divalproex (Depakote), indications, actions, and dosage of, 616

Diverticulitis, organisms responsible and empiric therapy for, 135t

Dizziness, differential diagnosis of, 45

DNA probes, 132

Dobbhoff tubes, 273

Dobutamine (Dobutrex)
for emergency cardiac care, 462
indications, actions, and dosage of, 398t, 529
infusion guidelines for, 439t–440t

Docetaxel (Taxotere), indications, actions, and dosage of, 529

Docusate calcium (Surfak), indications, actions, and dosage of, 529

Docusate potassium (Dialose), indications, actions, and dosage of, 529

Docusate sodium (Colace; Doss), indications, actions, and dosage of, 529

Döhle's inclusion bodies, 104

Dolasetron (Anzemet), indications, actions, and dosage of, 529–530

Doll's eyes, 24

Dolobid (diflunisal), indications, actions, and dosage of, 527

Dolophine (methadone)
indications, actions, and dosage of, 567–568
route, effects, and dosage for, 321t

Donnatal (hyoscyamine, atropine, scopolamine, + phenobarbital), indications, actions, and dosage of, 551

Donor-directed blood products, 194

Dopamine (Dopastat; Intropin)
for emergency cardiac care, 462
indications, actions, and dosage of, 398t, 530
infusion guidelines for, 440t

Doppler echocardiography, 330

Doppler pressures, 265–266

Doral (quazepam), indications, actions, and dosage of, 596

Dornase alfa (Pulmozyme), indications, actions, and dosage of, 530

Dorzolamide (Trusopt), indications, actions, and dosage of, 530

Dorzolamide + timolol (Cosopt), indications, actions, and dosage of, 530

Doss (docusate sodium), indications, actions, and dosage of, 529

Doxazosin (Cardura), indications, actions, and dosage of, 530

Doxepin (Adapin; Sinequan)
half-life and therapeutic and toxic levels of, 634t
indications, actions, and dosage of, 530

Doxepin, topical (Zonalon), indications, actions, and dosage of, 531

Doxorubicin (Adriamycin; Rubex), indications, actions, and dosage of, 531

Doxycycline (Vibramycin), indications, actions, and dosage of, 153t, 531

Dramamine (dimenhydrinate), indications, actions, and dosage of, 528

Draping patients, for surgery, 343

Drawer sign, 24

Dronabinol (Marinol), indications, actions, and dosage of, 531

Droperidol (Inapsine), indications, actions, and dosage of, 531

Droxia (hydroxyurea), indications, actions, and dosage of, 551

Drug interactions, with enteral nutrition, 223

DSA, 327

DTIC (dacarbazine), indications, actions, and dosage of, 522

Dukes' classification, of colon cancer, 652

Dulcolax (bisacodyl), indications, actions, and dosage of, 505

Duodenal ulcers, organism responsible and empiric therapy for, 144*t*

Duo-Tube, 273

Dupuytren's contracture, 25

Duragesic (fentanyl, transdermal), indications, actions, and dosage of, 538

Duramorph (morphine)
for emergency cardiac care, 465
indications, actions, and dosage of, 573
route, effects, and dosage for, 321*t*

Duricef (cefadroxil)
indications, actions, and dosage of, 511
for subacute bacterial endocarditis prophylaxis, 158*t*

Duroziez's sign, 25

Duvoid (bethanechol), indications, actions, and dosage of, 504–505

Dyazide (hydrochlorothiazide + triamterene), indications, actions, and dosage of, 549

Dycill (dicloxacillin), indications, actions, and dosage of, 526

Dynabac (dirithromycin), indications, actions, and dosage of, 529

Dynacirc (isradipine), indications, actions, and dosage of, 555–556

Dynamic compliance, 417–418

Dynapen (dicloxacillin), indications, actions, and dosage of, 526

Dyrenium (triamterene), indications, actions, and dosage of, 613–614

Dysmorphic red cells, 114–115

Dysphagia, differential diagnosis of, 45

Dyspnea, differential diagnosis of, 45

Dysuria, differential diagnosis of, 46

E

Ear(s), medications for, 482

Earache, differential diagnosis of, 46

Ecchymoses, 20

Echinococcus granulosus infections, drugs for treating, 154*t*

Echocardiography, 330

Echothiophate iodine (Phospholine Ophthalmic), indications, actions, and dosage of, 532

Econazole (Spectazole), indications, actions, and dosage of, 531–532

Edecrin (ethacrynic acid), indications, actions, and dosage of, 536

Edema, differential diagnosis of, 46

Edex (alprostadil, intracavernosal), indications, actions, and dosage of, 492

Edrophonium (Tensilon), indications, actions, and dosage of, 532

Education, assertiveness in obtaining, 3

Efavirenz (Sustiva), indications, actions, and dosage of, 532

Effer-Syllium (psyllium), indications, actions, and dosage of, 596

Effexor (venlafaxine), indications, actions, and dosage of, 617

Efudex (fluorouracil, topical), indications, actions, and dosage of, 541

Ehrlichiosis, characteristics and treatment of, 156*t*–157*t*

Elavil (amitriptyline)
indications, actions, and dosage of, 495
route, effects, and dosage for, 322*t*

Eldepryl (selegiline), indications, actions, and dosage of, 600

Electrical alternans, 25

Electrical defibrillation, 467–468

Electrical stimulation, for pain management, 323

Electrocardiograms (ECGs), 266–268, 367–388, 368*f*, 369*f*
atrial arrhythmias on, 372–374, 373*f*–375*f*
axis deviation in, 369–370, 370*f*
in cardiac hypertrophy, 380–383, 381*f*–383*f*
drug effects on, 386
electrolyte effects on, 385–386, 386*f*
heart blocks on, 377–379, 379*f*–381*f*
heart rate and, 371, 371*f*
hypothermia, 387*f*, 388
in hypothermia, 387*f*, 388
indications for, 266
leads for, 368
materials for, 266
in myocardial infarction, 383*f*–385*f*, 383–384, 385*t*
nodal rhythm on, 374–375, 376*f*

normal ECG complex and, 368f, 368–369
paper for, 368
in pericarditis, 387, 387f
procedure for, 266–268, 267f
sinus rhythms on, 371–372, 372f–373f
standardization for, 367, 368f
ventricular arrhythmias on, 375–377, 376f–378f
in Wolff-Parkinson-White syndrome, 388, 388f
Electrolytes. *See also* Fluids and electrolytes; *specific electrolytes*
electrocardiograms and, 385–386, 386f
spot urine study for, 114
Electromyography, for pain evaluation, 319
Elemental formulas, for enteral nutrition, 217
Elimite (permethrin), indications, actions, and dosage of, 153t, 154t, 588
Elmiron (pentosan polysulfate sodium), indications, actions, and dosage of, 587
Elocon (mometasone furoate), potency and application of, 630t
Elspar (L-asparaginase), indications, actions, and dosage of, 499
Embolism, prevention of, anticoagulant standard of practice for, 637t
Emcyt (estramustine phosphate), indications, actions, and dosage of, 535
Emergency cardiac care (ECC), 449–468
algorithms for, 450f–460f
drugs used in, 449, 461–467
electrical defibrillation and cardioversion for, 467–468
Emergency transfusions, 194
Emesis, IV fluid replacement for, 179
Emgel Topical (erythromycin, topical), indications, actions, and dosage of, 534
Eminase (anistreplase)
for emergency cardiac care, 467
indications, actions, and dosage of, 498
EMLA (lidocaine + prilocaine), indications, actions, and dosage of, 561

Empirin No. 2, No. 3, No. 4 (aspirin + codeine), indications, actions, and dosage of, 500
Empyema, 50
organisms responsible and empiric therapy for, 136t
E-mycin (erythromycin), indications, actions, and dosage of, 533–534
Enalapril (Vasotec)
for emergency cardiac care, 449
indications, actions, and dosage of, 532
Enalaprilat IV, for emergency cardiac care, 449
Encephalitis, herpes simplex virus, drugs of choice for treating, 147t
Endobronchial endoscopic collection, 130
Endocarditis, bacterial
organisms responsible and empiric therapy for, 136t–137t
subacute, prophylaxis of, 155, 158t–159t
Endocrine system, medications for, 482
Endotracheal intubation, 268–270
contraindications to, 268
indications for, 268
materials for, 268, 269t
technique for, 268–270, 270f
Endovaginal ultrasound, 329
Enfamil 20, 224t
Enfamil 24, 224t
Enfamil Premature 20, 225t
Enfamil Special Care 24, 225t
Engerix-B (hepatitis B vaccine), indications, actions, and dosage of, 548
Enoxaparin (Lovenox), indications, actions, and dosage of, 532
Entacapone (Comtan), indications, actions, and dosage of, 532
Entamoeba histolytica infections, drugs for treating, 153t
Enteral nutrition, 213, 214t, 214–223
complications of, 218, 223
initiating tube feedings for, 217–218, 218t–222t
postoperative, 223
products for, 214, 215t–216t, 217
Enteric precautions, 155
Enterobacter, Gram stain characteristics of, 124f

Enterobius vermicularis infections, drugs for treating, 153*t*

Enteroclysis, 328

Enterococcus, Gram stain characteristics of, 123*f*, 125*t*

Entriflex tubes, 273

Entuss-D (hydrocodone + pseudoephedrine), indications, actions, and dosage of, 550

Enzone (pramoxine + hydrocortisone), indications, actions, and dosage of, 592

Enzymes, 484

Eosinophils, laboratory diagnosis and, 101

Ephedrine, indications, actions, and dosage of, 532–533

Epidemiology, 639, 645

Epiglottitis, 131
  organisms responsible and empiric therapy for, 137*t*

Epinephrine, racemic, 364

Epinephrine (Adrenalin; Sus-Phrine)
  actions of, 398*t*
  for anaphylaxis, 468, 469
  for asthmatic attacks, 469
  for emergency cardiac care, 462
  indications, actions, and dosage of, 533
  infusion guidelines for, 440*t*
  for suturing, 348, 349*t*

Epistaxis, differential diagnosis of, 46

Epithelial casts, in urine sediment, 114

Epithelial cells, in urine sediment, 112

Epivir (lamivudine), indications, actions, and dosage of, 146*t*, 558

Epivir-HBV (lamivudine), indications, actions, and dosage of, 146*t*, 558

Epoetin alfa [erythropoietin] (Epogen; Procrit), indications, actions, and dosage of, 533

Epoprostenol (Flolan), indications, actions, and dosage of, 533

Eprosartan (Teveten), indications, actions, and dosage of, 533

Epstein-Barr virus (EBV), 146*t*

Eptifibatide (Integrilin)
  for emergency cardiac care, 464
  indications, actions, and dosage of, 533

Equanil (meprobamate), indications, actions, and dosage of, 566

ERCP (endoscopic retrograde cholangiopancreatography), 328

Erectile dysfunction, differential diagnosis of, 48

Ergamisol (levamisole), indications, actions, and dosage of, 560

Erosions, cutaneous, 20

Erysipelas, organism responsible and empiric therapy for, 142*t*

Erythrocin (erythromycin), indications, actions, and dosage of, 533–534

Erythrocytapheresis, 194

Erythrocytes. *See* Red blood cell(s) (RBCs)

Erythrocyte sedimentation rate (ESR), 108

Erythromycin (E-mycin; Erythrocin; Ilosone), indications, actions, and dosage of, 533–534

Erythromycin + benzoyl peroxide (Benzamycin), indications, actions, and dosage of, 534

Erythromycin, ophthalmic (Ilotycin Ophthalmic), indications, actions, and dosage of, 534

Erythromycin + sulfisoxazole (Eryzole; Pediazole), indications, actions, and dosage of, 534

Erythromycin, topical (Akne-Mycin Topical; Del-Mycin Topical; Emgel Topical; Staticin Topical), indications, actions, and dosage of, 534

Erythropoietin [epoetin alfa] (Epogen; Procrit), indications, actions, and dosage of, 533

Erythropoietin (EPO), laboratory diagnosis and, 66–67

Eryzole (erythromycin + sulfisoxazole), indications, actions, and dosage of, 534

Escherichia coli, Gram stain characteristics of, 124*f*, 126*t*

Esidrix (hydrochlorothiazide), indications, actions, and dosage of, 549

Eskalith (lithium carbonate), indications, actions, and dosage of, 562

Esmolol (Brevibloc)
  for emergency cardiac care, 462
  indications, actions, and dosage of, 534
  infusion guidelines for, 440*t*

Esophageal procedures, subacute bacterial endocarditis prophylaxis for, 158*t*

Esophagitis, cytomegalovirus, drugs of choice for treating, 146*t*

Esophagography, 328

Estazolam (Prosom), indications, actions, and dosage of, 534

Estinyl (ethinyl estradiol), indications, actions, and dosage of, 536

Estrace (estradiol), indications, actions, and dosage of, 535

Estracyte (estramustine phosphate), indications, actions, and dosage of, 535

Estraderm (estradiol, transdermal), indications, actions, and dosage of, 535

Estradiol (Estrace), indications, actions, and dosage of, 535

Estradiol, serum, laboratory diagnosis and, 67

Estradiol, transdermal (Estraderm), indications, actions, and dosage of, 535

Estramustine phosphate (Emcyt; Estracyte), indications, actions, and dosage of, 535

Estratab (estrogens, esterified), indications, actions, and dosage of, 535

Estratest (estrogens, esterified + methyltestosterone), indications, actions, and dosage of, 535

Estrogen(s), conjugated (Premarin), indications, actions, and dosage of, 535

Estrogen(s), conjugated + methylprogesterone (Premarin + Methylprogesterone), indications, actions, and dosage of, 535–536

Estrogen(s), conjugated + methyltestosterone (Premarin + Methyltestosterone), indications, actions, and dosage of, 536

Estrogen(s), conjugated-synthetic (Cenestin), indications, actions, and dosage of, 535–536

Estrogen(s), esterified (Estratab; Menest), indications, actions, and dosage of, 535

Estrogen(s), esterified + methyltestosterone (Estratest), indications, actions, and dosage of, 535

Estrogen receptors, laboratory diagnosis and, 67

Estrogen supplementation, 485

Estrostep 28, 624*t*

Ethacrynic acid (Edecrin), indications, actions, and dosage of, 536

Ethambutol (Myambutol), indications, actions, and dosage of, 536

Ethanol
blood levels of, laboratory diagnosis and, 67
for methanol poisoning, 471

Ethibond (polyester) sutures, 347*t*

Ethilon (nylon) sutures, 346*t*

Ethinyl estradiol (Estinyl; Feminone), indications, actions, and dosage of, 536

Ethmozine (moricizine), indications, actions, and dosage of, 573

Ethosuximide (Zarontin)
half-life and therapeutic and toxic levels of, 631*t*
indications, actions, and dosage of, 536

Ethyol (amifostine), indications, actions, and dosage of, 494

Etidronate disodium (Didronel), indications, actions, and dosage of, 536

Etodolac (Lodine), indications, actions, and dosage of, 536–537

Etoposide [VP-16] (Vepesid), indications, actions, and dosage of, 537

Eubacterium, Gram stain characteristics of, 126*t*

Eulexin (flutamide), indications, actions, and dosage of, 541–542

Eumorphic blood cells, 114

Euvolemic hypernatremia, 184–185

Evening rounds, 3–4

Evista (raloxifene), indications, actions, and dosage of, 597

Ewald tubes, 273

Ewart's sign, 25

Excoriations, 21*t*

Exosurf Neonatal (colfosceril palmitate), indications, actions, and dosage of, 520

Expiratory chest x-rays, 325

Expiratory reserve volume (ERV), 416

Exsel Shampoo (selenium sulfide), indications, actions, and dosage of, 600

Extremity perfusion, 392

Extrinsic factor, laboratory diagnosis and, 92–93

Extubation, from mechanical ventilation, 428–429

ExU (excretory urography), 328

Exudative ascites, 297

Eyes, medications for, 482–483

F

Factor VII, for transfusion, 199t

Factor VIII [antihemophilic factor] (Monoclate)
 indications, actions, and dosage of, 498
 for transfusion, 199t

Factor IX concentrate, 200t

Fahrenheit/celsius conversion, 646, 649t

Failure to thrive, differential diagnosis of, 46

Famciclovir (Famvir), indications, actions, and dosage of, 147t, 148t, 537

Family history, 10

Famotidine (Pepcid), indications, actions, and dosage of, 537

Famvir (famciclovir), indications, actions, and dosage of, 147t, 148t, 537

Fast catgut sutures, 346t

Fat, fecal, laboratory diagnosis and, 67

Fat restricted diet, 208t

Fatty casts, in urine sediment, 114

Febrile reactions, to transfusions, nonhemolytic, 202

Fecal fat, laboratory diagnosis and, 67

Fecal leukocytes, 128

Feeding tubes, 273

Feldene (piroxicam)
 indications, actions, and dosage of, 590
 route, effects, and dosage for, 321t

Fellows, 2

Felodipine (Plendil), indications, actions, and dosage of, 537

Femara (letrozole), indications, actions, and dosage of, 559

Feminone (ethinyl estradiol), indications, actions, and dosage of, 536

Femoral vein, venipuncture using, 313

Fenofibrate (Tricor), indications, actions, and dosage of, 537

Fenoldopam (Corlopam), indications, actions, and dosage of, 537

Fenoprofen (Nalfon), indications, actions, and dosage of, 537–538

Fentanyl (Sublimaze)
 indications, actions, and dosage of, 538
 route, effects, and dosage for, 321t

Fentanyl Oralet (fentanyl, transmucosal system), indications, actions, and dosage of, 538

Fentanyl, transdermal (Duragesic), indications, actions, and dosage of, 538

Fentanyl, transmucosal system (Actiq; Fentanyl Oralet), indications, actions, and dosage of, 538

Fergon (ferrous gluconate), indications, actions, and dosage of, 538

Ferric gluconate complex (Ferrlecit), indications, actions, and dosage of, 538

Ferritin, laboratory diagnosis and, 68

Ferrlecit (ferric gluconate complex), indications, actions, and dosage of, 538

Ferrous gluconate (Fergon), indications, actions, and dosage of, 538

Ferrous sulfate, indications, actions, and dosage of, 538

Fetal heart rate, internal fetal scalp monitoring of, 275–276

Fetal scalp monitoring, internal, 275–276

Fever
 differential diagnosis of, 46
 of unknown origin, differential diagnosis of, 46

Fever work-up, 270–272

Fexofenadine (Allegra), indications, actions, and dosage of, 538–539

Fibrin D-Dimers, 107

Fibrin degradation products (FDPs), 107

Fibrinogen, 107

Fibrin split products (FSPs), 107

FIGO classification, 655, 657

Filariasis, drugs for treating, 153t

Filgrastim [G-CSF] (Neupogen), indications, actions, and dosage of, 539

Finasteride (Propecia; Proscar), indications, actions, and dosage of, 539

Fioricet (acetaminophen + butalbital +/- caffeine), indications, actions, and dosage of, 489

Fiorinal (aspirin + butalbital compound), indications, actions, and dosage of, 500

Fiorinal + Codeine (aspirin + butalbital, caffeine and codeine), indications, actions, and dosage of, 500

First-degree heart block, 377, 379f

Fissures, cutaneous, 21t

Fistulography, 328

Flagyl (metronidazole), indications, actions, and dosage of, 153t, 154t, 570

Flamp (fludarabine phosphate), indications, actions, and dosage of, 540

Flat and upright abdominal x-rays, 326

Flat plates, 326

Flatulence, differential diagnosis of, 47

Flavoxate (Urispas), indications, actions, and dosage of, 539

Flecainide (Tambocor)
  half-life and therapeutic and toxic levels of, 633t
  indications, actions, and dosage of, 539

Fleet's Phospho-soda (sodium phosphate), for hypophosphatemia, 192

Flexeril (cyclobenzaprine), indications, actions, and dosage of, 521

Flexible sigmoidoscopy, 300

Flolan (epoprostenol), indications, actions, and dosage of, 533

Flomax (tamsulosin), indications, actions, and dosage of, 607

Flonase (fluticasone, nasal), indications, actions, and dosage of, 542

Florinef (fludrocortisone acetate), indications, actions, and dosage of, 540

Flovent (fluticasone, oral), indications, actions, and dosage of, 542

Flovent Rotadisk (fluticasone, oral), indications, actions, and dosage of, 542

Floxin (ofloxacin), indications, actions, and dosage of, 580–581

Floxuridine (FUDR), indications, actions, and dosage of, 539

Fluconazole (Diflucan), indications, actions, and dosage of, 151t, 539–540

5-Flucytosine, indications for, 151t

Fludarabine phosphate (Flamp; Fludara), indications, actions, and dosage of, 540

Fludrocortisone, for renal tubular acidosis, 168t

Fludrocortisone acetate (Florinef), indications, actions, and dosage of, 540

Fluids and electrolytes, 177–192. *See also* Intravenous (IV) fluids
  baseline fluid requirement and, 178
  electrolyte abnormality diagnosis and treatment, 184–192
  electrolyte requirements and, 178
  fluid compartments and, 177
  glucose requirements and, 178
  IV rate determination for, 183–184
  maintenance fluids, 179, 181t
  ordering IV fluids, 179–183
  parenteral fluid composition and, 178–179
  red blood cell mass and, 177
  specific replacement fluids, 179, 182f–183f, 183
  total blood volume and, 177
  total body water, 177
  water balance and, 177–178

Flumadine (rimantadine), indications, actions, and dosage of, 148t, 598–599

Flumazenil (Romazicon)
  for benzodiazepine poisoning, 471
  for emergency cardiac care, 462
  indications, actions, and dosage of, 540

Flunisolide (Aerobid; Nasolide), indications, actions, and dosage of, 540

Fluocinolone acetonide (Synalar; Synalar-HP), potency and application of, 628*t*, 629*t*

Fluocinonide (Lidex; Lidex-E), potency and application of, 629*t*

Fluogen (influenza vaccine), indications, actions, and dosage of, 553

Fluorescent treponemal antibody absorbed (FTS-ABS), laboratory diagnosis and, 68

Fluoroquinolones, 477

Fluorouracil [5-FU] (Adrucil), indications, actions, and dosage of, 540

Fluorouracil, topical [5-FU] (Efudex), indications, actions, and dosage of, 541

Fluoxetine (Prozac; Sarafem), indications, actions, and dosage of, 541

Fluoxymesterone (Halotestin), indications, actions, and dosage of, 541

Fluphenazine (Permitil; Prolixin), indications, actions, and dosage of, 541

Flurandrenolide (Cordran), potency and application of, 629*t*

Flurazepam (Dalmane), indications, actions, and dosage of, 541

Flurbiprofen (Ansaid), indications, actions, and dosage of, 541

Flushield (influenza vaccine), indications, actions, and dosage of, 553

Flutamide (Eulexin), indications, actions, and dosage of, 541–542

Fluticasone, nasal (Flonase), indications, actions, and dosage of, 542

Fluticasone, oral (Flovent; Flovent Rotadisk), indications, actions, and dosage of, 542

Fluticasone propionate (Cutivate), potency and application of, 629*t*

Fluvastatin (Lescol), indications, actions, and dosage of, 542

Fluvirin (influenza vaccine), indications, actions, and dosage of, 553

Fluvoxamine (Luvox), indications, actions, and dosage of, 542

Fluzone (influenza vaccine), indications, actions, and dosage of, 553

Folex (methotrexate)
   half-life and therapeutic and toxic levels of, 633*t*
   indications, actions, and dosage of, 568

Foley catheter, 307, 307*f*

Folic acid
   blood levels of, laboratory diagnosis and, 68
   indications, actions, and dosage of, 542
   in total parenteral nutrition, 231*t*

Follicle-stimulating hormone (FSH), laboratory diagnosis and, 68

Fomivirsen (Vitravene), indications and dosage for, 146*t*

Fong lesion/syndrome, 25

Food fibers, in ascitic fluid, 299*t*

Forced expired volume in 1 second (FEV/d1/D), 360, 361*t*

Forced vital capacity (FVC), 360, 361*t*

Fortaz (ceftazidime), indications, actions, and dosage of, 513

Fortovase (saquinavir), indications, actions, and dosage of, 150*t*, 600

Fosamax (alendronate), indications, actions, and dosage of, 491

Foscarnet (Foscavir)
   indications, actions, and dosage of, 542
   indications and dosage for, 146*t*, 147*t*, 149*t*

Fosfomycin (Monurol), indications, actions, and dosage of, 542–543

Fosinopril (Monopril), indications, actions, and dosage of, 543

Fosphenytoin (Cerebryx)
   indications, actions, and dosage of, 543
   for seizures, 473*t*

Fourth heart sound (S_4), 17*t*

Fragmin (dalteparin), indications, actions, and dosage of, 523

Frank's sign, 25

French units, 240, 241*f*

Frequency, urinary, differential diagnosis of, 47

Fresh frozen plasma (FFP), 198*t*–199*t*

FUDR (floxuridine), indications, actions, and dosage of, 539

Full liquid diet, 206*t*

Functional residual capacity (FRC), 360, 361*t*, 416, 416*f*, 417*f*

Fungal infections, systemic drugs for treating, 151t–152t

Fungal serologies, laboratory diagnosis and, 68

Fungizone (amphotericin B), indications, actions, and dosage of, 151t, 496–497

Furadantin Macrobid (nitrofurantoin), indications, actions, and dosage of, 579

Furosemide (Lasix)
for emergency cardiac care, 462–463
indications, actions, and dosage of, 543
for renal tubular acidosis, 168t

Fusobacterium, Gram stain characteristics of, 126t

G

Gabapentin (Neurontin), indications, actions, and dosage of, 543

Gabitril (tiagabine), indications, actions, and dosage of, 610

Galactorrhea, differential diagnosis of, 47

Gallium nitrate (Ganite)
for hypercalcemia, 189
indications, actions, and dosage of, 543

Gallium scans, 334

Gallops, 394

Gamimmune N (immune globulin, intravenous), indications, actions, and dosage of, 552

Gamma globulin, indications and dosage for, 146t

Gamma-glutamyl transpeptidase, serum (SGGT), laboratory diagnosis and, 69

Gammar IV (immune globulin, intravenous), indications, actions, and dosage of, 552

Ganciclovir (Cytovene; Vitrasert), indications, actions, and dosage of, 146t, 543–544

Ganite (gallium nitrate)
for hypercalcemia, 189
indications, actions, and dosage of, 543

Garamycin (gentamicin)
half-life and therapeutic and toxic levels of, 631t

indications, actions, and dosage of, 544
for subacute bacterial endocarditis prophylaxis, 159t

Garamycin (gentamicin, ophthalmic), indications, actions, and dosage of, 544

Garamycin (gentamicin, topical), indications, actions, and dosage of, 545

Gastric cancer, staging of, 656

Gastric loss, IV fluid replacement with, 179

Gastric ulcers, organism responsible and empiric therapy for, 144t

Gastrin, serum, laboratory diagnosis and, 69

Gastroenteritis, organisms responsible and empiric therapy for, 137t–138t

Gastrografin enema, 328

Gastrointestinal agents, 483–484

Gastrointestinal intubation, 272–274
complications of, 274
indications for, 272
materials for, 272
procedure for, 273–274
tubes for, 272–273

Gastrointestinal procedures, subacute bacterial endocarditis prophylaxis for, 158t, 159t

Gatifloxacin (Tequin), indications, actions, and dosage of, 544

Gaviscon (alginic acid + aluminum hydroxide and magnesium trisilicate), indications, actions, and dosage of, 491

Gaviscon (aluminum hydroxide + magnesium carbonate), indications, actions, and dosage of, 493

Gaviscon (aluminum hydroxide + magnesium trisilicate), indications, actions, and dosage of, 493

Gaviscon-2 (aluminum hydroxide + magnesium trisilicate), indications, actions, and dosage of, 493

GC culture, 291

Gemzar (gemcitabine), indications, actions, and dosage of, 544

Genital herpes, drugs of choice for treating, 147t

Genital warts, drugs of choice for treating, 148t

Genitourinary agents, 487

Genitourinary procedures, subacute bacterial endocarditis prophylaxis for, 159t

Genoptic (gentamicin, ophthalmic), indications, actions, and dosage of, 544

Genora 1/35 21, 28, 623t

Genora 1/50 28, 623t

Gentacidin (gentamicin, ophthalmic), indications, actions, and dosage of, 544

Gentak (gentamicin, ophthalmic), indications, actions, and dosage of, 544

Gentamicin (Garamycin)
half-life and therapeutic and toxic levels of, 631t
indications, actions, and dosage of, 544
for subacute bacterial endocarditis prophylaxis, 159t

Gentamicin, ophthalmic (Garamycin; Genoptic; Gentacidin; Gentak), indications, actions, and dosage of, 544

Gentamicin + prednisolone, ophthalmic (Pred-G Ophthalmic), indications, actions, and dosage of, 545

Gentamicin, topical (Garamycin; G-Myticin), indications, actions, and dosage of, 545

Geriatrics, total parenteral nutrition formulation for, 235

Giardiasis, drugs for treating, 153t

Gibbus, 25

Giemsa stain, 122

Glasgow Coma Scale (*EMV* Scale), 645, 645t

Glaucoma agents, 482–483

Glimepiride (Amaryl), indications, actions, and dosage of, 545

Glipizide (Glucotrol), indications, actions, and dosage of, 545

Glitter cells, in urine sediment, 114

Gloving, for operating room, 342–343

Glucagon
for beta blocker poisoning, 471
for emergency cardiac care, 464
indications, actions, and dosage of, 545

Glucophage (metformin), indications, actions, and dosage of, 567

Glucose
laboratory diagnosis and, 69
in pleural fluid, 299t
requirement for, 178
in urine, 111

Glucose tolerance test (GTT), 69–70
oral, 69–70

Glucotrol (glipizide), indications, actions, and dosage of, 545

Glu-K (potassium gluconate), form and dosage of, 626t

Glyburide (Diabeta; Micronase), indications, actions, and dosage of, 545

Glycerin suppositories, indications, actions, and dosage of, 545–546

Glycohemoglobin (GHB), laboratory diagnosis and, 70

Glycoprotein IIb/IIIa inhibitors, for emergency cardiac care, 464

Glyset (miglitol), indications, actions, and dosage of, 571

G-Myticin (gentamicin, topical), indications, actions, and dosage of, 545

GoLYTELY (polyethylene glycol [PEG]-electrolyte solution), indications, actions, and dosage of, 590–591

Gonadorelin (Lutrepulse), indications, actions, and dosage of, 546

Gonococcal antigen assay, 129

Gonorrhea
cultures and smear for, 129
organism responsible and empiric therapy for, 138t

Gonozyme, 129

Goserelin (Zoladex), indications, actions, and dosage of, 546

Gowning, for operating room, 342–343

Gram stain, 122, 291
of common pathogens, 122, 123f–124f, 125t–127t

Granisetron (Kytril), indications, actions, and dosage of, 546

Granulocytes, for transfusion, 197*t*

Granuloma inguinale, organism responsible and empiric therapy for, 138*t*

Granulomatous infection, cerebrospinal fluid in, 287*t*

Gregg's triad, 25

Grey Turner's sign, 25

Grocco's sign, 25

Guaifenesin (Robitussin), indications, actions, and dosage of, 546

Guaifenesin + codeine (Brontex; Robitussin A-C), indications, actions, and dosage of, 546

Guaifenesin + dextromethorphan, indications, actions, and dosage of, 546

Guanabenz (Wytensin), indications, actions, and dosage of, 546–547

Guanadrel (Hylorel), indications, actions, and dosage of, 547

Guanethidine (Ismelin), indications, actions, and dosage of, 547

Guanfacine (Tenex), indications, actions, and dosage of, 547

Guillain-Barré syndrome, cerebrospinal fluid in, 287*t*

Gynecologic agents, 485–486

Gynecomastia, differential diagnosis of, 47

H

Habitrol (nicotine, transdermal), indications, actions, and dosage of, 578

Haemophilus B conjugate vaccine (Comvax; Prohibit), indications, actions, and dosage of, 547

Haemophilus ducreyi, Gram stain characteristics of, 126*t*

Haemophilus influenza, Gram stain characteristics of, 124*f*, 126*t*

Hairworm infection, drugs for treating, 154*t*

Halcinonide (Halog), potency and application of, 629*t*

Halcion (triazolam), indications, actions, and dosage of, 614

Haldol (haloperidol)
indications, actions, and dosage of, 547
route, effects, and dosage for, 322*t*

Halobetasol (Ultravate), potency and application of, 629*t*

Halog (halcinonide), potency and application of, 629*t*

Haloperidol (Haldol)
indications, actions, and dosage of, 547
route, effects, and dosage for, 322*t*

Haloprogin (Halotex), indications, actions, and dosage of, 547

Halotestin (fluoxymesterone), indications, actions, and dosage of, 541

Halotex (haloprogin), indications, actions, and dosage of, 547

Hampton's hump, 436

Hand scrub, surgical, 340–341

Haptoglobin, laboratory diagnosis and, 70

Harris-Benedict BEE, 209

Havrix (hepatitis A vaccine), indications, actions, and dosage of, 548

H-BIG (hepatitis B immune globulin), indications, actions, and dosage of, 548

HDL-C (high-density lipoprotein cholesterol), laboratory diagnosis and, 63

Headache
differential diagnosis of, 47
spinal, 286

Head computed tomography, 330

Head magnetic resonance imaging, 332–333

Healing, of wounds, 345

Health, personal, 2–3

Heart, on chest x-rays, 335, 336*f*, 337*f*

Heart blocks, on electrocardiograms, 377–379, 379*f*–381*f*

Heartburn, differential diagnosis of, 47

Heart murmurs, 16*t*–17*t*, 18*f*, 393–395

Heart rate
on electrocardiograms, 371, 371*f*
measurement of, 408

Heart sounds, extra, 16*t*–17*t*

Heberden's nodes, 25

Heelstick, 274, 275*f*

Hegar's sign, 25

Helical computed tomography, 331

Helicobacter pylori antibody titers, laboratory diagnosis and, 70

Hellenhorst's plaque, 25
Helmet cells, 104
Hematemesis, differential diagnosis of, 47
Hematochezia, differential diagnosis of, 47
Hematocrit, 97, 101
Hematologic agents, 484
Hematuria, differential diagnosis of, 48
Hemoccult test, 89, 300
Hemodialysis, diet for, 207
Hemopoietic stimulants, 484
Hemoptysis, differential diagnosis of, 48
Hemorrhage, synovial fluid interpretation and, 250, 251t
Henderson equation, 162
Henderson-Hasselbalch equation, 162
Heparin
  indications, actions, and dosage of, 548
  low molecular weight, for emergency cardiac care, 464
  for pulmonary embolism, 436
  unfractionated, for emergency cardiac care, 464
Hepatitis
  drugs of choice for treating, 146t–147t
  transfusion-associated risk of transmission, 203
Hepatitis A vaccine (Havrix; Vaqta), indications, actions, and dosage of, 548
Hepatitis B immune globulin (H-BIG; Hyperhep), indications, actions, and dosage of, 548
Hepatitis B vaccine (Engerix-B; Recombivax-HB), indications, actions, and dosage of, 548
Hepatitis testing, 70, 71t–72t, 73f, 74
  for hepatitis A, 72t, 73f, 74
  for hepatitis B, 72t, 73f, 74
  for hepatitis C, 72t, 74
Hepatobiliary scans, 334
Hepatomegaly, differential diagnosis of, 48
Herpes cultures, 291
Herpes simplex virus (HSV)
  cultures for, 132
  drugs of choice for treating infections by, 147t
Herpes zoster. See also Varicella zoster virus (VZV)

drugs of choice for treating, 148t, 149t
Hetastarch (Hespan), indications, actions, and dosage of, 548
Hexalen (altretamine), indications, actions, and dosage of, 493
Hibiclens 6-min hand scrub, 341
Hiccups, differential diagnosis of, 48
HIDA-scans, 334
High-density formulas, for enteral nutrition, 217
High-density lipoprotein cholesterol (HDL), laboratory diagnosis and, 63
Higher osmolality infant formulas, 224t
High-frequency ventilation, 424, 426
Hill's sign, 25
Hilum, on chest x-rays, 335
[131] Hippuran, 334
Hiprex (methenamine), indications, actions, and dosage of, 568
Hirsutism, differential diagnosis of, 48
Histoplasmosis, systemic drugs for treating, 151t
History, 9–11
  psychiatric, 13–14
  written, 5, 28–32
Histussin D (hydrocodone + pseudoephedrine), indications, actions, and dosage of, 550
Hivid (zalcitabine), indications, actions, and dosage of, 619
Hoffmann's sign/reflex, 25
Holoxan (ifosfamide), indications, actions, and dosage of, 552
Homans' sign, 25
Homocysteine, serum, laboratory diagnosis and, 75
Hookworm infections, drugs for treating, 153t
Hormones, 482. See also specific hormones
  antineoplastic, 478
  gynecologic agents, 485
Horner's syndrome, 25
Hospital diets, 205, 206t–208t
Hounsfield units, 330
House diet, 206t
Household measurement units, 646
Howell-Jolly bodies, 104

Humalog (lispro), onset, peak, and duration of effect of, 622*t*

Humalog Mix (lispro protamine/lispro), onset, peak, and duration of effect of, 622*t*

Human chorionic gonadotropin (hCG), serum, laboratory diagnosis and, 75

Human granulocytic ehrlichiosis, characteristics and treatment of, 156*t*–157*t*

Human immunodeficiency virus (HIV) infection
  drugs of choice for treating, 150*t*
  transfusion-associated risk of transmission, 203–204

Human immunodeficiency virus (HIV) testing, 75–77, 76*f*
  HIV antibody and, 75
  HIV antibody by ELISA determination and, 76
  HIV antibody ELISA and, 75–76
  HIV antigen and, 77
  HIV core antigen and, 83
  HIV DNA PCR and, 77
  HIV RNA PCR and, 77
  HIV viral load and, 77
  HIV Western blot and, 76

Human leukocyte antigens (HLA), laboratory diagnosis and, 74–75

Human milk, 224*t*

Human papillomavirus (HPV), drugs of choice for treating infections by, 148*t*

Human T-cell leukemia virus type 1 (HTLV-1), transfusion-associated risk of transmission, 204

Humidity therapy, 362, 363*t*

Humulin N, onset, peak, and duration of effect of, 622*t*

Humulin U, onset, peak, and duration of effect of, 622*t*

Hyaline casts, in urine sediment, 114

Hycamtin (topotecan), indications, actions, and dosage of, 612

Hycodan (hydrocodone + homatropine), indications, actions, and dosage of, 550

Hycomine (hydrocodone, chlorpheniramine, phenylephrine, acetaminophen, + caffeine), indications, actions, and dosage of, 550

Hycort (hydrocortisone)
  indications, actions, and dosage of, 550
  potency and application of, 629*t*

Hycotuss Expectorant (hydrocodone + guaifenesin), indications, actions, and dosage of, 550

Hydralazine (Apresoline), indications, actions, and dosage of, 549

Hydrea (hydroxyurea), indications, actions, and dosage of, 551

Hydrochlorothiazide (Esidrix; Hydrodiuril), indications, actions, and dosage of, 549

Hydrochlorothiazide + amiloride (Moduretic), indications, actions, and dosage of, 549

Hydrochlorothiazide + spironolactone (Aldactazide), indications, actions, and dosage of, 549

Hydrochlorothiazide + triamterene (Dyazide; Maxzide), indications, actions, and dosage of, 549

Hydrocodone + acetaminophen (Lorcet; Vicodin), indications, actions, and dosage of, 549

Hydrocodone + aspirin (Lortab ASA), indications, actions, and dosage of, 549

Hydrocodone, chlorpheniramine, phenylephrine, acetaminophen, + caffeine (Hycomine), indications, actions, and dosage of, 550

Hydrocodone + guaifenesin (Hycotuss Expectorant), indications, actions, and dosage of, 550

Hydrocodone + homatropine (Hycodan), indications, actions, and dosage of, 550

Hydrocodone + ibuprofen (Vicoprofen), indications, actions, and dosage of, 550

Hydrocodone + pseudoephedrine (Entuss-D; Histussin D), indications, actions, and dosage of, 550

Hydrocortisone (CaldeCort; Cortizone; Hycort; Hytone)
  indications, actions, and dosage of, 550
  potency and application of, 629*t*
Hydrocortisone (Hydrocortone; Solu-Cortef)
  dose, activity, duration, and route for, 627*t*
  for hypercalcemia, 189
  indications, actions, and dosage of, 603–604
Hydrocortisone acetate (Corticaine)
  indications, actions, and dosage of, 603
  potency and application of, 629*t*
Hydrocortisone butyrate (Locoid), potency and application of, 629*t*
Hydrocortisone sodium, for asthmatic attacks, 469
Hydrocortisone succinate, indications, actions, and dosage of, 603
Hydrocortisone valerate (Westcort), potency and application of, 629*t*
Hydrocortone (hydrocortisone)
  dose, activity, duration, and route for, 627*t*
  for hypercalcemia, 189
  indications, actions, and dosage of, 603–604
Hydrodiuril (hydrochlorothiazide), indications, actions, and dosage of, 549
Hydromorphone (Dilaudid), indications, actions, and dosage of, 550
Hydrothorax, 50
5-Hydroxyindoleacetic acid (5-HIAA), in urine, 117
Hydroxyurea (Droxia; Hydrea), indications, actions, and dosage of, 551
Hydroxyzine (Atarax; Vistaril), indications, actions, and dosage of, 551
Hygroton (chlorthalidone), indications, actions, and dosage of, 515
Hylorel (guanadrel), indications, actions, and dosage of, 547
Hymenolepis nana infections, drugs for treating, 154*t*
Hyoscyamine (Anaspaz; Cystospaz; Levsin), indications, actions, and dosage of, 551

Hyoscyamine, atropine, scopolamine, + phenobarbital (Donnatal), indications, actions, and dosage of, 551
Hyperalimentation. *See* Total parenteral nutrition (TPN)
Hypercalcemia, 188–189
  electrocardiogram and, 386
Hypercalcemia agents, 482
Hyperchloremic acidosis, 166, 168*t*
Hyperhep (hepatitis B immune globulin), indications, actions, and dosage of, 548
Hyperkalemia, 186–187
  electrocardiogram and, 385, 386*f*
  total parenteral nutrition for, 237
Hypermagnesemia, 190
  total parenteral nutrition for, 237
Hypernatremia, 184–185
Hyperosmolar nonketotic coma, total parenteral nutrition for, 236
Hyperparathyroidism, hypercalcemia with, 188
Hyperphosphatemia, 191–192
Hypersegmentation, of white blood cells, 104
Hyperstat (diazoxide), indications, actions, and dosage of, 526
Hypertension, 392–393
  algorithm for, 460*f*
Hypertensive crisis, 470
Hypertonic hyponatremia, 185
Hypertrophy, on electrocardiogram, 367
Hyperventilation syndrome, 171
Hypervolemic hypernatremia, 184, 185
Hypervolemic hyponatremia, 186
Hypocalcemia, electrocardiogram and, 386
Hypoglycemia, 471
Hypokalemia, 187–188
  electrocardiogram and, 385, 386*f*
Hypomagnesemia, 190–191
Hyponatremia, 185–186
  total parenteral nutrition for, 237
Hypophosphatemia, 192
  total parenteral nutrition for, 236
Hypotonic hyponatremia, 185
Hypovolemic hypernatremia, 184
Hypovolemic hyponatremia, 186
Hypovolemic shock, 414, 431, 472

Hypoxia, 171*f*, 171–172
    differential diagnosis of, 171–172
Hysterosalpingography (HSG), 328
Hytone (hydrocortisone)
    indications, actions, and dosage of, 550
    potency and application of, 629*t*
Hytrin (terazosin), indications, actions, and dosage of, 608

I
Ibuprofen (Advil; Motrin; Rufen)
    indications, actions, and dosage of, 551
    route, effects, and dosage for, 321*t*
Ibutilide (Corvert)
    for emergency cardiac care, 464
    indications, actions, and dosage of, 551
Idarubicin (Idamycin), indications, actions, and dosage of, 551
Ifex (ifosfamide), indications, actions, and dosage of, 552
I^{125} fibrinogen scanning, 334
Ifosfamide (Holoxan; Ifex), indications, actions, and dosage of, 552
Iliopsoas test, 26
Ilopan (dexpanthenol)
    indications, actions, and dosage of, 525
    in total parenteral nutrition, 231*t*
Ilopan-choline Oral (dexpanthenol)
    indications, actions, and dosage of, 525
    in total parenteral nutrition, 231*t*
Ilosone (erythromycin), indications, actions, and dosage of, 533–534
Ilotycin Ophthalmic (erythromycin, ophthalmic), indications, actions, and dosage of, 534
Imaging studies, 325–338
    computed tomography, 330–331
    contrast x-ray studies, 326–329
    magnetic resonance, 331–333
    noncontrast x-ray studies, 325–326
    nuclear scans, 333–335
    preparation for, 325
    reading x-rays, 335, 336*f*, 337*f*, 338
    ultrasound, 329–330
Imdur (isosorbide mononitrate), indications, actions, and dosage of, 555–556
Imipenem-cilastin (Primaxin), indications, actions, and dosage of, 552

Imipramine (Tofranil), indications, actions, and dosage of, 552
Imipramine + desipramine, half-life and therapeutic and toxic levels of, 633*t*
Imiquimod (Aldara), indications, actions, and dosage of, 148*t*, 552
Imitrex (sumatriptan), indications, actions, and dosage of, 606
Immune globulin, intravenous (Gammar IV; Gamimmune N; Sandoglobulin), indications, actions, and dosage of, 552
Immune serum globulin, 200*t*
Immune system agents, 484–485
Immunization schedule, 620, 636*t*
Immunoglobulins, quantitative, laboratory diagnosis and, 77
Immunomodulators, 484
Immunosuppressive agents, 485
Imodium (loperamide), indications, actions, and dosage of, 562–563
Impetigo, organisms responsible and empiric therapy for, 142*t*
Impotence, differential diagnosis of, 48
Imuran (azathioprine), indications, actions, and dosage of, 501
Inapsine (droperidol), indications, actions, and dosage of, 531
Incentive spirometry, 363–364
Incidence, definition of, 645
Indapamide (Lozol), indications, actions, and dosage of, 552
Inderal (propranolol)
    for emergency cardiac care, 462
    indications, actions, and dosage of, 595
India ink preparation, 127
Indinavir (Crixivan), indications, actions, and dosage of, 150*t*, 553
Indium-111 octreotide scans, 334
Indomethacin (Indocin)
    indications, actions, and dosage of, 553
    route, effects, and dosage for, 321*t*
Infant formulas and feeding, 223–226, 224*t*–225*t*, 225–226
    formulas for, 224*t*–225*t*
    initiating, criteria for, 225
    oral rehydration solutions for, 226
    for premature infants, 225*t*, 225–226

Infasurf (calfactant), indications, actions, and dosage of, 509

Infections. *See also specific infections*
  bacterial, 204, 287*t*
  of bone, organisms responsible and empiric therapy for, 134*t*
  cervical, tests for, 291
  common, differential diagnosis and empiric therapy, 133, 134*t*–154*t*, 156*t*
  fungal, systemic drugs for treating, 151*t*–152*t*
  granulomatous, cerebrospinal fluid in, 287*t*
  of joints, organisms responsible and empiric therapy for, 134*t*
  of skin, organisms responsible and empiric therapy for, 141*t*–142*t*
  of soft tissue, organisms responsible and empiric therapy for, 141*t*–142*t*
  total parenteral nutrition for, 236
  transfusion-associated risk of, 202–204
  urinary tract, organisms responsible and empiric therapy for, 143*t*–144*t*
  vaginal, 144*t*–145*t*, 291
  viral, 146*t*–149*t*, 287*t*. *See also specific infections*

Infectious mononucleosis, 146*t*

Infed (iron dextran), indications, actions, and dosage of, 555

Infergen (interferon alfacon-1), indications, actions, and dosage of, 147*t*, 554

Infiltrates, in lungs, 338

Inflammatory arthritis, synovial fluid interpretation and, 250, 251*t*

Inflammatory bowel disease (IBD), total parenteral nutrition formulation for, 235

Infliximab (Remicade), indications, actions, and dosage of, 553

Influenza A virus, drugs of choice for treating infections by, 147*t*–148*t*

Influenza B virus, drugs of choice for treating infections by, 147*t*

Influenza vaccine (Fluogen; Flushield; Fluvirin; Fluzone), indications, actions, and dosage of, 553

Informed consent, 240

INH (isoniazid), indications, actions, and dosage of, 555–556

Inhalers, 365

Injection techniques, 276–277

Innervation, cutaneous, 22*f*–23*f*

Inocor (amrinone)
  for emergency cardiac care, 461
  indications, actions, and dosage of, 498
  infusion guidelines for, 439*t*

Inotropic agents, 480

Inspiratory capacity (IC), 416

Inspiratory reserve volume (IRV), 416

Instrument tie, 357*f*

Insufflation, for sigmoidoscopy, 301

Insulins
  comparison of, 622*t*
  indications, actions, and dosage of, 553
  in total parenteral nutrition, 232, 232*t*

Intal (cromolyn sodium), indications, actions, and dosage of, 520–521

Integrilin (eptifibatide)
  for emergency cardiac care, 464
  indications, actions, and dosage of, 533

Intensive care unit (ICU)
  drug infusions used in, 439*t*–443*t*
  equations used in, 437*t*–438*t*
  progress notes for, 389–391

Interferon alfa-2a (Roferon-A), indications and dosage for, 146*t*, 554

Interferon alfa-2b (Intron A), indications and dosage for, 146*t*, 148*t*, 554

Interferon alfa-2B + ribavirin combination (Robetron), indications, actions, and dosage of, 554

Interferon alfacon-1 (Infergen), indications, actions, and dosage of, 147*t*, 554

Interferon ß-1B (Betaseron), indications, actions, and dosage of, 554

Interferon gamma-1B (Actimmune), indications, actions, and dosage of, 554

Intern(s), 1

Internal fetal scalp monitoring, 275–276

Intestinal decompression tubes, 272

Intracranial pressure (ICP), derivation and normal values for, 438*t*

Intradermal injections, 276, 277

Intramuscular injections, 276, 277

Intrauterine pressure monitoring, 277–278

Intravascular hemolysis, acute, 202

Intravenous (IV) fluids, 179–183
  maintenance fluids, 179, 181*t*
  specific replacement fluids, 179,
    182*f*–183*f*, 183
Intravenous (IV) infusions, rate
    determination for, 183–184
Intravenous pyelography (IVP), 328
Intravenous techniques, 278–280, 279*f*–281*f*
Intraventricular septum rupture, 394
Intron A (interferon alfa-2b), indications
    and dosage for, 146*t*, 148*t*, 554
Intropin (dopamine)
  for emergency cardiac care, 462
  indications, actions, and dosage of,
    398*t*, 530
  infusion guidelines for, 440*t*
Iodine-125 fibrinogen scanning, 334
Iodipine (apraclonidine), indications,
    actions, and dosage of, 499
Iodoquinol, indications for, 153*t*
Ionic contrast media, 327
Iotronex (alosetran), indications, actions,
    and dosage of, 491
Ipecac syrup, indications, actions, and
    dosage of, 554–555
Ipratropium bromide (Atrovent), 364
  for asthmatic attacks, 469
  indications, actions, and dosage of, 555
Irbesartan (Avapro), indications, actions,
    and dosage of, 555
Irinotecan (Camptosar), indications,
    actions, and dosage of, 555
Iron
  laboratory diagnosis and, 77
  in total parenteral nutrition, 231
Iron-binding capacity, total (TIBC),
    laboratory diagnosis and, 78
Iron dextran (Dexferrum; Infed),
    indications, actions, and dosage of,
    555
Irradiation blood components, 194
Ismelin (guanethidine), indications,
    actions, and dosage of, 547
Ismo (isosorbide mononitrate),
    indications, actions, and dosage of,
    555–556
Isoetharine, indications, actions, and
    dosage of, 555
Isolation protocols, 155–156
Isomil, 224*t*

Isoniazid (INH), indications, actions, and
    dosage of, 555–556
Isoosmolar infant formulas, 224*t*, 225*t*
Isoproterenol (Isuprel; Medihaler-Iso)
  for emergency cardiac care, 464
  indications, actions, and dosage of,
    398*t*, 555–556
  infusion guidelines for, 441*t*
Isoptin (verapamil)
  for emergency cardiac care, 467
  indications, actions, and dosage of, 617
Isosorbide dinitrate (Isordil; Sorbitrate),
    indications, actions, and dosage of,
    555–556
Isosorbide mononitrate (Imdur; Ismo),
    indications, actions, and dosage of,
    555–556
Isosporiasis infections, drugs for treating,
    153*t*
Isotonic hyponatremia, 185
Isotretinoin [13-cis retinoic acid]
    (Accutane), indications, actions,
    and dosage of, 555–556
Isovolemic hypernatremia, 184–185
Isovolemic hyponatremia, 186
Isradipine (Dynacirc), indications, actions,
    and dosage of, 555–556
Isuprel (isoproterenol)
  for emergency cardiac care, 464
  indications, actions, and dosage of,
    398*t*, 555–556
  infusion guidelines for, 441*t*
Itraconazole (Sporanox), indications, actions,
    and dosage of, 151*t*, 556–557
Ivermectin, indications for, 153*t*, 154*t*

J
Janeway's lesion, 25
Jaundice, differential diagnosis of, 49
Jenest-28, 624*t*
Joffroy's reflex, 25
Joint infections, organisms responsible
    and empiric therapy for, 134*t*
Jugular venous distention, 391–392

K
Kabikinase (streptokinase)
  for emergency cardiac care, 466
  indications, actions, and dosage of, 604

Kaochlor (potassium supplements)
form and dosage of, 626*t*
indications, actions, and dosage of, 592
Kaochlor 10% (potassium chloride)
form and dosage of, 626*t*
indications, actions, and dosage of, 592
Kaochlor Eff (potassium chloride, potassium citrate, and bicarbonate), form and dosage of, 626*t*
Kaochlor S-F 10% (potassium chloride)
form and dosage of, 626*t*
indications, actions, and dosage of, 592
Kaolin-pectin (Kaodene; Kao-spen; Kapectolin), indications, actions, and dosage of, 557
Kaon (potassium gluconate)
form and dosage of, 626*t*
indications, actions, and dosage of, 592
Kaon-Cl (potassium chloride)
form and dosage of, 626*t*
indications, actions, and dosage of, 592
Kaon-Cl 20% (potassium chloride)
form and dosage of, 626*t*
indications, actions, and dosage of, 592
Kaon elixir (potassium gluconate), form and dosage of, 626*t*
Kao-spen (kaolin-pectin), indications, actions, and dosage of, 557
Kapectolin (kaolin-pectin), indications, actions, and dosage of, 557
Kayexalate (sodium polystyrene sulfonate)
for hyperkalemia, 187
indications, actions, and dosage of, 602
Kayser-Fleischer rings, 25
Kefzol (cefazolin)
indications, actions, and dosage of, 511
for subacute bacterial endocarditis prophylaxis, 158*t*
Kehr's sign, 25
Keloids, 21*t*
Kemadrin (procyclidine), indications, actions, and dosage of, 594
Kenalog (triamcinolone acetonide), potency and application of, 630*t*
Keogh tubes, 273
Keppra (levetiracetam), indications, actions, and dosage of, 560

Keratoconjunctivitis, herpes simplex virus, drugs of choice for treating, 147*t*
Kerley's B lines, 338
Kerlone (betaxolol), indications, actions, and dosage of, 504
Kernig's sign, 25
Ketoconazole (Nizoral), indications, actions, and dosage of, 557
17-Ketogenic steroids (17-KGS), in urine, 118
Ketone(s), in urine, 111
Ketone bodies, laboratory diagnosis and, 55
Ketoprofen (Orudis; Oruvail), indications, actions, and dosage of, 557
Ketorolac (Toradol), indications, actions, and dosage of, 557
Ketorolac, ophthalmic (Acular), indications, actions, and dosage of, 557
17-Ketosteroids (17-KS), total, in urine, 118
Kidney cancer, staging of, 652–653
Kilogram/pound conversion, 658, 658*t*
Kinase, laboratory diagnosis and, 65
Kinyoun stain, 121
Klebsiella, Gram stain characteristics of, 124*f*, 126*t*
Klonopin (clonazepam), indications, actions, and dosage of, 518
K-Lor (potassium chloride)
form and dosage of, 626*t*
indications, actions, and dosage of, 592
Klorvess (potassium chloride)
form and dosage of, 626*t*
indications, actions, and dosage of, 592
Klotrix (potassium chloride)
form and dosage of, 626*t*
indications, actions, and dosage of, 592
Knee, arthrocentesis of, 248, 248*f*
KOH preparation, 127
Koplik's spots, 25
Korotkoff's sounds, 25
K-Phos (potassium phosphate), for hypophosphatemia, 192
K-Tab (potassium chloride)
form and dosage of, 626*t*
indications, actions, and dosage of, 592
KUB x-rays, 326
Kussmaul's respirations, 25

Kussmaul's sign, 25
Kwell (lindane), indications, actions, and dosage of, 561
Kyphosis, 26
Kytril (granisetron), indications, actions, and dosage of, 546

L

Labetalol (Normodyne; Trandate)
  for emergency cardiac care, 462
  for hypertensive crisis, 470
  indications, actions, and dosage of, 557
  infusion guidelines for, 441*t*
Laboratory diagnosis
  chemistry, immunology, and serology in, 53–93
  hematology and, 95–108
  urine studies for, 109–119
Laboratory studies. *See also specific studies*
  before initiating total parenteral nutrition, 233
  for monitoring total parenteral nutrition, 234
  shorthand for values and, 40*f*
Lactate dehydrogenase (LD; LDH)
  isozymes of, laboratory diagnosis and, 78
  laboratory diagnosis and, 78
Lactic acid, laboratory diagnosis and, 78
Lactic acid + ammonium hydroxide [ammonium lactate], indications, actions, and dosage of, 558
Lactinex Granules (lactobacillus), indications, actions, and dosage of, 558
Lactobacillus, Gram stain characteristics of, 126*t*
Lactobacillus (Lactinex Granules), indications, actions, and dosage of, 558
Lactose-free diet, 208*t*
Lactulose (Cephulac; Chronulac), indications, actions, and dosage of, 558
Lamictal (lamotrigine), indications, actions, and dosage of, 558
Lamisil (terbinafine), indications, actions, and dosage of, 608

Lamivudine (Epivir; Epivir-HBV), indications, actions, and dosage of, 146*t*, 558
Lamotrigine (Lamictal), indications, actions, and dosage of, 558
Lamprene (clofazimine), indications, actions, and dosage of, 518
Lanorinal (aspirin + butalbital compound), indications, actions, and dosage of, 500
Lanoxicaps (digoxin)
  antidote for, 471
  for emergency cardiac care, 462
  half-life and therapeutic and toxic levels of, 633*t*
  indications, actions, and dosage of, 527
Lanoxin (digoxin)
  antidote for, 471
  for emergency cardiac care, 462
  half-life and therapeutic and toxic levels of, 633*t*
  indications, actions, and dosage of, 527
Lansoprazole (Prevacid), indications, actions, and dosage of, 558
Lantus (insulin glorgine), onset, peak, and duration of effect of, 622*t*
Large cells, 97, 100
Larva migrans
  cutaneous, drugs for treating, 153*t*
  visceral, drugs for treating, 154*t*
Laryngoscopes, 269, 270*f*
Lasegue's sign, 26
Lasix (furosemide)
  for emergency cardiac care, 462–463
  indications, actions, and dosage of, 543
  for renal tubular acidosis, 168*t*
Latanoprost (Xalatan), indications, actions, and dosage of, 558
Late decelerations, in fetal heart rate, 276
Lateral chest films, reading, 337*f*, 338
Lateral decubitus chest x-rays, 325
Latex allergy, 344
Laxatives, 483
LCTATE, laboratory diagnosis and, 78
Lead, blood, laboratory diagnosis and, 79
Leads, for electrocardiography, 368
Lee-White clotting time, 107
Leflunomide (Arava), indications, actions, and dosage of, 559

Left atrial enlargement (LAE),
        electrocardiogram and, 380, 382*f*
Left bundle branch block (LBBB), 379,
        381*f*
Left shift, 100
Left ventricular end-diastolic pressure
        (LVEDP), 407–408
Left ventricular hypertrophy (LVH),
        electrocardiogram and, 382–383,
        383*f*
Legionella antibody, laboratory diagnosis
        and, 79
Legionella pneumophila, Gram stain
        characteristics of, 126*t*
Lente Iletin II, onset, peak, and duration
        of effect of, 622*t*
Leonard tubes, 273
Lepirudin (Refludan), indications, actions,
        and dosage of, 559
Leptocytes, 104
Lescol (fluvastatin), indications, actions,
        and dosage of, 542
Letrozole (Femara), indications, actions,
        and dosage of, 559
Leucovorin (Wellcovorin), indications,
        actions, and dosage of, 559
Leukapheresis, 194
Leukeran (chlorambucil), indications,
        actions, and dosage of, 514
Leukine (sargramostim), indications,
        actions, and dosage of, 600
Leukocyte alkaline phosphatase (LAP)
        score/stain, laboratory diagnosis
        and, 78
Leukocyte esterase, in urine, 112
Leukocyte-poor (reduced) red cells, 197*t*
Leuprolide (Lupron), indications, actions,
        and dosage of, 559
Leustatin (cladribine), indications, actions,
        and dosage of, 517
Levalbuterol (Xopenex), indications,
        actions, and dosage of, 559
Levamisole (Ergamisol), indications,
        actions, and dosage of, 560
Levaquin (levofloxacin), indications,
        actions, and dosage of, 560
Levatol (penbutolol), indications, actions,
        and dosage of, 585
Levelen 21, 28, 623*t*
Levelite 21, 28, 623*t*

Levetiractam (Keppra), indications,
        actions, and dosage of, 560
Levine's sign, 26
Levin tubes, 272
Levobunolol (A-K Beta; Betagan),
        indications, actions, and dosage of,
        560
Levocabastine (Livostin), indications,
        actions, and dosage of, 560
Levo-Dromoran (levorphanol),
        indications, actions, and dosage of,
        560
Levofloxacin (Levaquin), indications,
        actions, and dosage of, 560
Levonorgestrel implant (Norplant),
        indications, actions, and dosage of,
        560
Levophed (norepinephrine)
    actions of, 398*t*
    for emergency cardiac care, 466
    indications, actions, and dosage
        of, 580
    infusion guidelines for, 442*t*
Levora 21, 28, 623*t*
Levorphanol (Levo-Dromoran),
        indications, actions, and dosage of,
        560
Levothyroxine (Synthroid), indications,
        actions, and dosage of, 560–561
Levsin (hyoscyamine), indications,
        actions, and dosage of, 551
Lhermitte's sign, 26
Librium (chlordiazepoxide), indications,
        actions, and dosage of, 515
Lice, drugs for treating, 153*t*
Lichenification, 21*t*
Lidex (fluocinonide), potency and
        application of, 629*t*
Lidex-E (fluocinonide), potency and
        application of, 629*t*
Lidocaine (Anestacon Topical; Xylocaine)
    for emergency cardiac care, 465
    half-life and therapeutic and toxic levels
        of, 633*t*
    indications, actions, and dosage
        of, 561
    infusion guidelines for, 441*t*
    for premature ventricular contractions,
        376
    for suturing, 348, 349*t*

Lidocaine + prilocaine (EMLA), indications, actions, and dosage of, 561

Limb electrodes, 267

Lindane (Kwell), indications, actions, and dosage of, 561

Line sepsis, 435

Linezolid (Xyvox), indications, actions, and dosage of, 561

Linolenic acid, 233

Linton tubes, 273

Lioresal (baclofen), indications, actions, and dosage of, 502

Liothyronine (Cytomel), indications, actions, and dosage of, 562

Lipase, laboratory diagnosis and, 79

Lipid emulsions, 232–233

Lipid-lowering agents, 480

Lipid profile, laboratory diagnosis and, 79, 80f, 81t

Lipitor (atorvastatin), indications, actions, and dosage of, 500

Lipoprotein profile/analysis, laboratory diagnosis and, 79, 80f, 81t

Liqui-Char (activated charcoal)
    clinical use of, 472
    indications, actions, and dosage of, 514

Liquid diets, 206t–207t

Lisinopril (Prinivil; Zestril)
    for emergency cardiac care, 461
    indications, actions, and dosage of, 562

List, definition of, 26

Listeria, Gram stain characteristics of, 123f

Listeria monocytogenes, Gram stain characteristics of, 126t

Lithium, half-life and therapeutic and toxic levels of, 633t

Lithium carbonate (Eskalith), indications, actions, and dosage of, 562

Liver disease
    diet for, 208t
    total parenteral nutrition formulation for, 235

Liver function tests, elevated, total parenteral nutrition for, 237

Liver-spleen scans, 334

Livostin (levocabastine), indications, actions, and dosage of, 560

Loa loa, drugs for treating, 153t

Local anesthetics
    for suturing, 348, 349t
    systemic, 320

Locoid (hydrocortisone butyrate), potency and application of, 629t

Lodine (etodolac), indications, actions, and dosage of, 536–537

Lodoxamide (Alomide Ophthalmic), indications, actions, and dosage of, 562

Löffler methylene blue stain, 128

Lomefloxacin (Maxaquin), indications, actions, and dosage of, 562

Lomotil (diphenoxylate + atropine), indications, actions, and dosage of, 528

Lomustine (CCNU; CeeNu), indications, actions, and dosage of, 562

Loniten (minoxidil), indications, actions, and dosage of, 572

Lo/Ovral, 623t

Loperamide (Imodium), indications, actions, and dosage of, 562–563

Lopid (gemfibrozil), indications, actions, and dosage of, 544

Lopressor (metoprolol)
    for emergency cardiac care, 462
    indications, actions, and dosage of, 569

Loprox (ciclopirox), indications, actions, and dosage of, 516

Lopurin (allopurinol), indications, actions, and dosage of, 491

Loracarbef (Lorabid), indications, actions, and dosage of, 563

Loratadine (Claritin), indications, actions, and dosage of, 563

Lorazepam (Ativan)
    indications, actions, and dosage of, 563
    for seizures, 472

Lorcet (hydrocodone + acetaminophen), indications, actions, and dosage of, 549

Lordosis, 26

Lordotic chest x-rays, 325

Lortab ASA (hydrocodone + aspirin), indications, actions, and dosage of, 549

Losartan (Cozaar), indications, actions, and dosage of, 563

Lotensin (benazepril), indications, actions, and dosage of, 503

Lotrimin (clotrimazole), indications, actions, and dosage of, 519

Lotrisone (clotrimazole + betamethasone), indications, actions, and dosage of, 519

Louvel's sign, 26

Lovastatin (Mevacor), indications, actions, and dosage of, 563

Lovenox (enoxaparin), indications, actions, and dosage of, 532

Low-fiber diet, 207*t*

Low lactose diet, 208*t*

Low-Ogestrel, 623*t*

Low osmolality infant formulas, 224*t*

Lowsium (magaldrate), indications, actions, and dosage of, 564

Low-sodium diet, 208*t*

Lozol (indapamide), indications, actions, and dosage of, 552

L-PAM (melphalan), indications, actions, and dosage of, 566

Ludiomil (maprotiline), indications, actions, and dosage of, 564

Lumbar cistern, 282

Lumbar puncture, 280, 282–286
complications of, 286
contraindications to, 282
historical background of, 282–283, 283*f*
indications for, 280
materials for, 282
technique for, 284, 285*f*, 286, 287*t*–288*t*

Lumens, of Swan-Ganz catheters, 399–400

Lung(s), on chest x-rays, 335, 336*f*, 337*f*, 338

Lung cancer, staging of, 653–654

Lung capacity, 416, 416*f*, 417*f*

Lung compliance, 417–418, 418*f*

Lung scans, 334

Lupron (leuprolide), indications, actions, and dosage of, 559

Lupus erythematosus (LE) preparation, laboratory diagnosis and, 78

Luteinizing hormone (LH), serum, laboratory diagnosis and, 79, 82

Lutrepulse (gonadorelin), indications, actions, and dosage of, 546

Luvox (fluvoxamine), indications, actions, and dosage of, 542

Lyme disease
characteristics and treatment of, 156*t*–157*t*
serology in, laboratory diagnosis and, 82

Lyme disease vaccine (Lymerix), indications, actions, and dosage of, 563–564

Lymphadenopathy, differential diagnosis of, 49

Lymphangiography, 328

Lymphocytes
atypical, laboratory diagnosis and, 102
laboratory diagnosis and, 101–102
subsets of, laboratory diagnosis and, 103–104

Lymphogranuloma venereum, organism responsible and empiric therapy for, 135*t*

Lymphoma, staging of, 654

Lysodren (mitotane), indications, actions, and dosage of, 572

M

Maalox (aluminum hydroxide + magnesium hydroxide), indications, actions, and dosage of, 493–494

McBurney's point/sign, 26

McGill Pain Questionnaire (MPQ), 319

McMurray's test, 26

Macrodantin (nitrofurantoin), indications, actions, and dosage of, 579

Macrolides, 477

Macules, 21*t*

MAG3 (technetium-99m mercaptoacetylthiglycine), 334

Magaldrate (Lowsium; Riopan), indications, actions, and dosage of, 564

Magnesium
deficiency of, 190–191
excess of, 190, 237
laboratory diagnosis and, 82
requirement for, 178
total parenteral nutrition for excess of, 237

Magnesium citrate, indications, actions, and dosage of, 564

Magnesium hydroxide (Milk of Magnesia), indications, actions, and dosage of, 564

Magnesium oxide (Mag-Ox 400)
  for hypomagnesemia, 191
  indications, actions, and dosage of, 564

Magnesium sulfate
  for emergency cardiac care, 465
  for hypomagnesemia, 191
  indications, actions, and dosage of, 564

Magnetic resonance imaging (MRI), 331–333
  reading, 331–332
  uses of, 332–333

Magnetic resonance spectroscopy (MRS), 332–333

Mag-Ox 400 (magnesium oxide)
  for hypomagnesemia, 191
  indications, actions, and dosage of, 564

Malaria
  drugs for treating, 153t
  prevention of, 153t

Malathion, indications for, 153t

Malignancies
  classification systems for, 646, 649–658
  hypercalcemia with, 188

Malnutrition, identification of, 209, 210t–212t

Mammography, 326

Manganese, in total parenteral nutrition, 231, 232t

Mannitol
  for emergency cardiac care, 465
  indications, actions, and dosage of, 564

Mantoux test, 303–304

Maprotiline (Ludiomil), indications, actions, and dosage of, 564

Marcaine (bupivacaine)
  indications, actions, and dosage of, 507
  for suturing, 349t

Marcus-Gunn pupils, 26

Marinol (dronabinol), indications, actions, and dosage of, 531

Mastitis, organism responsible and empiric therapy for, 134t

Mastoiditis, organisms responsible and empiric therapy for, 135t

Matulane (procarbazine), indications, actions, and dosage of, 593–594

Mavik (trandolapril), indications, actions, and dosage of, 613

Maxair (pirbuterol), indications, actions, and dosage of, 590

Maxalt (rizatriptan), indications, actions, and dosage of, 599

Maxaquin (lomefloxacin), indications, actions, and dosage of, 562

Maxipime (cefepime), indications, actions, and dosage of, 511

Maxitrol (neomycin, polymyxin B, + dexamethasone), indications, actions, and dosage of, 577

Maxon (polyglyconate) sutures, 346t

Maxzide (hydrochlorothiazide + triamterene), indications, actions, and dosage of, 549

Mean arterial blood pressure (MAP), 393, 394f
  derivation and normal values for, 437t

Mean cellular (corpuscular) hemoglobin (MCH), laboratory diagnosis and, 102

Mean cell (corpuscular) volume (MCV), laboratory diagnosis and, 102

Mean pulmonary arterial pressure (MPAP), derivation and normal values for, 437t

Measles virus, drug of choice for treating infections by, 148t

Measurement units, 645–646

Mebendazole, indications for, 153t

Mechanical soft diet, 206t

Mechanical ventilation, 423–429
  extubation and, 428–429
  indications for, 423, 424t
  orders for, 426
  ventilator classes for, 423–424
  ventilator modes for, 424, 425f, 426
  ventilator setting changes for, 426–427
  weaning from, 427–429, 428t

Mechlorethamine (Mustargen), indications, actions, and dosage of, 564

Meclizine (Antivert), indications, actions, and dosage of, 564

Mediastinal computed tomography, 331

Mediastinum, on chest x-rays, 335

Medical history, 9–10

Medigesic (acetaminophen + butalbital +/- caffeine), indications, actions, and dosage of, 489

Medihaler-Iso (isoproterenol)
for emergency cardiac care, 464
indications, actions, and dosage of, 398*t*, 555–556
infusion guidelines for, 441*t*

Mediquell (dextromethorphan), indications, actions, and dosage of, 525

Medroxyprogesterone (Cycrin; Depo Provera; Provera), indications, actions, and dosage of, 564

Medulla, herniation of, with lumbar puncture, 286

Mefaxin (cefoxitin), indications, actions, and dosage of, 512

Mefloquine, indications for, 153*t*

Megestrol acetate (Megace), indications, actions, and dosage of, 564

Melanoma, staging of, 654–655

Melena, differential diagnosis of, 47

Mellaril (thioridazine), indications, actions, and dosage of, 609–610

Meloxicam (Mobic), indications, actions, and dosage of, 564

Melphalan (Alkeran; L-PAM), indications, actions, and dosage of, 566

Menest (estrogens, esterified), indications, actions, and dosage of, 535

Meningitis
aseptic, cerebrospinal fluid in, 287*t*
organisms responsible and empiric therapy for, 138*t*–139*t*

Meperidine (Demerol)
indications, actions, and dosage of, 566
route, effects, and dosage for, 321*t*

Mepivacaine (Carbocaine), for suturing, 349*t*

Meprobamate (Equanil; Miltown), indications, actions, and dosage of, 566

Mepron (atovaquone), indications, actions, and dosage of, 500–501

Mercaptopurine [6-MP] (Purinethol), indications, actions, and dosage of, 566

Meridia (sibutramine), indications, actions, and dosage of, 601

Meropenem (Merrem), indications, actions, and dosage of, 566

Mesalamine (Asacol; Pentasa; Rowasa), indications, actions, and dosage of, 566

Mesna (Mesnex), indications, actions, and dosage of, 567

Mesoridazine (Serentil), indications, actions, and dosage of, 567

Metabolic acidosis, 164*t*, 166–167
differential diagnosis of, 17B, 167*f*, 168*t*
treatment of, 167

Metabolic alkalosis, 164*t*, 167, 169
differential diagnosis of, 167, 169, 169*f*
total parenteral nutrition for, 237
treatment of, 169

Metamucil (psyllium), indications, actions, and dosage of, 596

Metanephrines, in urine, 117

Metaproterenol (Alupent; Metaprel), 364
indications, actions, and dosage of, 567

Metaraminol (Aramine), indications, actions, and dosage of, 567

Metastron, 334

Metaxalone (Skelaxin), indications, actions, and dosage of, 567

Metered-dose inhalers, 365

Metformin (Glucophage), indications, actions, and dosage of, 567

Methadone (Dolophine)
indications, actions, and dosage of, 567–568
route, effects, and dosage for, 321*t*

Methanol, antidote for, 471

Methenamine (Hiprex; Urex), indications, actions, and dosage of, 568

Methergine (methylergonovine), indications, actions, and dosage of, 569

Methimazole (Tapazole), indications, actions, and dosage of, 568

Methocarbamol (Robaxin), indications, actions, and dosage of, 568

Methotrexate (Folex; Rheumatrex)
half-life and therapeutic and toxic levels of, 633*t*
indications, actions, and dosage of, 568

Methoxamine (Vasoxyl), indications, actions, and dosage of, 568–569

Methyldopa (Aldomet), indications, actions, and dosage of, 569

Methylergonovine (Methergine), indications, actions, and dosage of, 569

Methylprednisolone
for anaphylaxis, 469
for asthmatic attacks, 469
indications, actions, and dosage of, 603

Methylprednisolone acetate (Depo-Medrol)
dose, activity, duration, and route for, 627t
indications, actions, and dosage of, 603

Methylprednisolone sodium succinate (Solu-Medrol)
dose, activity, duration, and route for, 627t
indications, actions, and dosage of, 603

Metoclopramide (Clopra; Octamide; Reglan), indications, actions, and dosage of, 569

Metolazone (Diulo; Zaroxolyn), indications, actions, and dosage of, 569

Metopirone (metyrapone), indications, actions, and dosage of, 570

Metoprolol (Lopressor; Toprol XL)
for emergency cardiac care, 462
indications, actions, and dosage of, 569

Metronidazole (Flagyl; Metrogel), indications, actions, and dosage of, 153t, 154t, 570

Metyrapone (Metopirone), indications, actions, and dosage of, 570

Metyrosine (Demser), indications, actions, and dosage of, 570

Mevacor (lovastatin), indications, actions, and dosage of, 563

Mexiletine (Mexitil), indications, actions, and dosage of, 570

Mezlocillin (Mezlin), indications, actions, and dosage of, 570

Miacalcin (calcitonin)
for hypercalcemia, 189
indications, actions, and dosage of, 508

MIBG, 333

Micardis (telmisartan), indications, actions, and dosage of, 607

Miconazole (Monistat), indications, actions, and dosage of, 571

Microalbumin, spot urine study for, 115

Microbiology, 121–159
blood cultures, 129–130
differential diagnosis of common infections and empiric therapy, 133, 134t–154t, 156t
gonorrhea cultures and smear, 129
isolation protocols, 155–156
molecular, 132
nasopharyngeal cultures, 129
SBE prophylaxis, 155, 158t–159t
Scotch tape test, 132
sputum culture, 130
staining techniques for, 121–128
stool cultures, 130–131
susceptibility testing, 133
throat cultures, 131
urine cultures, 131–132
viral cultures and serology, 132

β_2-Microglobulin
laboratory diagnosis and, 82
spot urine study for, 114

Microhemagglutination, *Treponema pallidum* (MHA-TP), laboratory diagnosis and, 82

Micro-K (potassium chloride)
form and dosage of, 626t
indications, actions, and dosage of, 592

Micronase (glyburide), indications, actions, and dosage of, 545

Micronor, 625t

Midamor (amiloride), indications, actions, and dosage of, 494

Midazolam (Versed)
indications, actions, and dosage of, 571
for seizures, 472

Middle cells, 97, 100

Mifepristone [RU 486] (Mifeprex), indications, actions, and dosage of, 571

Miglitol (Glyset), indications, actions, and dosage of, 572

Migraine headache agents, 486

Milk of Magnesia (magnesium hydroxide), indications, actions, and dosage of, 564

Miller-Abbott tubes, 272

Milrinone (Primacor), indications, actions, and dosage of, 571

Miltown (meprobamate), indications, actions, and dosage of, 566

Mineral oil, indications, actions, and dosage of, 571

Mini mental status examination, 13–14, 15*t*

Minimum bactericidal concentration (MBC), 133

Minimum inhibitory concentration (MIC), 133

Minipress (prazosin), indications, actions, and dosage of, 593

Minnesota tubes, 273

Minoxidil (Loniten; Rogaine), indications, actions, and dosage of, 572

Mirapex (pramipexole), indications, actions, and dosage of, 592

Mircette 28, 624*t*

Mirtazapine (Remeron), indications, actions, and dosage of, 572

Misoprostol (Cytotec), indications, actions, and dosage of, 572

Mithracin (plicamycin)
for hypercalcemia, 189
indications, actions, and dosage of, 590–591

Mitomycin C (Mutamycin), indications, actions, and dosage of, 572

Mitotane (Lysodren), indications, actions, and dosage of, 572

Mitotic inhibitors, 478

Mitoxantrone (Novantrone), indications, actions, and dosage of, 572–573

Mitral insufficiency (MI), 16*t*

Mitral stenosis (MS), 16*t*

Mivacurium (Mivacron), indications, actions, and dosage of, 573

Mixed acid-base disorders, 163

Mixed venous oxygen content (C_{VO2}), derivation and normal values for, 437*t*

M-mode echocardiography, 330

Moban (molindone), indications, actions, and dosage of, 573

Mobic (meloxicam), indications, actions, and dosage of, 564

Mobitz type I heart block, 377–378, 379*f*

Mobitz type II heart block, 378

Möbius' sign, 26

Modicon 28, 623*t*

Moduretic (hydrochlorothiazide + amiloride), indications, actions, and dosage of, 549

Moexipril (Univasc), indications, actions, and dosage of, 573

Molecular microbiology, 132

Molindone (Moban), indications, actions, and dosage of, 573

Mometasone furoate (Elocon), potency and application of, 630*t*

Monistat (miconazole), indications, actions, and dosage of, 571

Monocid (cefonicid), indications, actions, and dosage of, 511–512

Monoclate (antihemophilic factor)
indications, actions, and dosage of, 498
for transfusion, 199*t*

Monocryl (poliglecaprone) sutures, 346*t*

Monocytes, laboratory diagnosis and, 102–103

Monopril (fosinopril), indications, actions, and dosage of, 543

Monospot, laboratory diagnosis and, 83

Montelukast (Singulair), indications, actions, and dosage of, 573

Monurol (fosfomycin), indications, actions, and dosage of, 542–543

Moraxella catarrhalis, Gram stain characteristics of, 125*t*

Morganella morganii, Gram stain characteristics of, 126*t*

Moricizine (Ethmozine), indications, actions, and dosage of, 573

Morning rounds, 3

Moro's reflex, 26

Morphine (Duramorph; MS Contin; Roxanol)
for emergency cardiac care, 465
indications, actions, and dosage of, 573
route, effects, and dosage for, 321*t*

Motrin (Ibuprofen)
indications, actions, and dosage of, 551
route, effects, and dosage for, 321*t*

Moxifloxacin (Avelox), indications, actions, and dosage of, 574

MS Contin (morphine)
for emergency cardiac care, 465

indications, actions, and dosage
of, 573
route, effects, and dosage for, 321*t*
Mucomyst (acetylcysteine), 364
indications, actions, and dosage of,
489–490
Mucormycosis, systemic drug for treating,
152*t*
Mucosil (acetylcysteine), 364
indications, actions, and dosage of,
489–490
Mucus, in urine sediment, 114
MUGA scans, 333–334
Multifocal atrial tachycardia (MAT), 373,
374*f*
Multiple sclerosis, cerebrospinal fluid in,
288*t*
Mupirocin (Bactroban), indications,
actions, and dosage of, 574
Muromonab-CD3 (Orthoclone OKT3),
indications, actions, and dosage of,
574
Murphy's sign, 26
Muscle relaxants, 485
Musculoskeletal agents, 485
Musculoskeletal magnetic resonance
imaging, 333
Muse (alprostadil, urethral suppository),
indications, actions, and dosage of,
492
Musset's sign, 26
Mustargen (mechlorethamine),
indications, actions, and dosage of,
564
Mutamycin (mitomycin C), indications,
actions, and dosage of, 572
Myambutol (ethambutol), indications,
actions, and dosage of, 536
Mycelex (clotrimazole), indications,
actions, and dosage of, 519
Mycobacterium, Gram stain
characteristics of, 126*t*
Mycobutin (rifabutin), indications,
actions, and dosage of, 598
Mycolog-II (triamcinolone + nystatin),
indications, actions, and dosage of,
613
Mycophenolate mofetil (Cellcept),
indications, actions, and dosage of,
574

Mycostatin (nystatin), indications, actions,
and dosage of, 580
Myelography, 329
Myleran (busulfan), indications, actions,
and dosage of, 507
Mylicon (simethicone), indications,
actions, and dosage of, 601
Myocardial infarction (MI)
anticoagulant standard of practice for,
637*t*
on electrocardiograms, 367, 383*f*–385*f*,
383–384, 385*t*
Myocardial ischemia
on electrocardiogram, 367
electrocardiogram and, 383*f*–385*f*, 384
Myoglobin
laboratory diagnosis and, 83
spot urine study for, 115

N

Nabumetone (Relafen), indications,
actions, and dosage of, 574
Nadolol (Corgard), indications, actions,
and dosage of, 574
Nafcillin (Nallpen), indications, actions,
and dosage of, 574
Naftifine (Naftin), indications, actions,
and dosage of, 574
Nalbuphine (Nubain)
indications, actions, and dosage of, 575
route, effects, and dosage for, 322*t*
Nalfon (fenoprofen), indications, actions,
and dosage of, 537–538
Nalidixic acid (Neggram), indications,
actions, and dosage of, 575
Nallpen (nafcillin), indications, actions,
and dosage of, 574
Naloxone (Narcan)
for emergency cardiac care, 465
indications, actions, and dosage
of, 575
for opiate overdose, 471
Naltrexone (Revia), indications, actions,
and dosage of, 575
Napamide (disopyramide)
half-life and therapeutic and toxic levels
of, 633*t*
indications, actions, and dosage of, 529

Naphazoline + antazoline (Albalon-A
Ophthalmic), indications, actions,
and dosage of, 575
Naphazoline + pheniramine acetate
(Naphcon A), indications, actions,
and dosage of, 575
Naphcon A (naphazoline + pheniramine
acetate), indications, actions, and
dosage of, 575
Naprosyn (naproxen), indications, actions,
and dosage of, 575
Naproxen (Aleve; Anaprox; Naprosyn),
indications, actions, and dosage of,
575
Naratriptan (Amerge), indications, actions,
and dosage of, 575–576
Narcan (naloxone)
for emergency cardiac care, 465
indications, actions, and dosage of, 575
for opiate overdose, 471
Narcotics, 486
analgesics, 320, 321*t*–322*t*
overdose of, 471
Nardil (phenelzine), indications, actions,
and dosage of, 588
Narrow complex SVT algorithm, 457*f*
Nasalcrom (cromolyn sodium),
indications, actions, and dosage of,
520–521
Nasogastric intubation
IV fluid replacement with, 179
procedure for, 273–274
tubes for, 272
Nasolide (flunisolide), indications,
actions, and dosage of, 540
Nasopharyngeal cultures, 129
Nausea, differential diagnosis of, 49
Navane (thiothixene), indications, actions,
and dosage of, 610
Navelbine (vinorelbine), indications,
actions, and dosage of, 618
NAVEL mnemonic, 313
for arterial puncture, 246
Nebcin (tobramycin)
half-life and therapeutic and toxic levels
of, 631*t*
indications, actions, and dosage of, 611
Nebulizer therapy, 363
topical medications for, 364

Nebupent (pentamidine), indications,
actions, and dosage of, 153*t*, 585
Necator americanus infections, drugs for
treating, 153*t*
Neck computed tomography, 331
Necon 1/35 21, 28, 623*t*
Necon 1/50 21, 28, 623*t*
Necon 10/11 21, 28, 624*t*
Necon 0.5/35E 21, 28, 623*t*
Nedocromil (Tilade), indications, actions,
and dosage of, 576
Needle(s)
French units for, 240, 241*f*
for suturing, 345
Needle cricothyrotomy, 263–264
Nefazodone (Serzone), indications,
actions, and dosage of, 576
Negative nitrogen balance, 229
Neggram (nalidixic acid), indications,
actions, and dosage of, 575
Neisseria gonorrhoeae
Gram stain characteristics of, 124*f*, 125*t*
throat culture for, 131
Neisseria meningitides, Gram stain
characteristics of, 124*f*, 125*t*
Nelfinavir (Viracept), indications, actions,
and dosage of, 150*t*, 576
Nelova 1/35 21, 623*t*
Nelova 1/50 21, 623*t*
Nelova 10/11 21, 624*t*
Nelova 0.5/35E 21, 623*t*
Nembutal (pentobarbital), indications,
actions, and dosage of, 587
Neo-calglucon (calcium glubionate)
for hypocalcemia, 190
indications, actions, and dosage of, 508
Neodecadron Ophthalmic (neomycin +
dexamethasone), indications,
actions, and dosage of, 576
Neomycin, colistin, hydrocortisone, +
thonzonium (Cortisporin-TC Otic
Suspension), indications, actions,
and dosage of, 576
Neomycin, colistin, + hydrocortisone
(Cortisporin-TC Otic Drops),
indications, actions, and dosage of,
576
Neomycin + dexamethasone (AK-NEO-
DEX Ophthalmic; Neodecadron

Ophthalmic), indications, actions, and dosage of, 576

Neomycin + polymyxin B (Neosporin Cream), indications, actions, and dosage of, 576

Neomycin, polymyxin B, + dexamethasone (Maxitrol), indications, actions, and dosage of, 577

Neomycin, polymyxin bladder irrigant, indications, actions, and dosage of, 577

Neomycin, polymyxin, + hydrocortisone (Cortisporin Ophthalmic and Otic), indications, actions, and dosage of, 577

Neomycin, polymyxin-B, + prednisolone (Poly-Pred Ophthalmic), indications, actions, and dosage of, 577

Neomycin sulfate, indications, actions, and dosage of, 577

Neonatal ophthalmia, organism responsible and empiric therapy for, 135*t*

Neoplasms. *See also* Malignancies
adrenal, differential diagnosis of, 42
cerebrospinal fluid in, 288*t*
classification systems for, 646, 649–658
cutaneous, 21*t*

Neoral (cyclosporine)
half-life and therapeutic and toxic levels of, 634*t*
indications, actions, and dosage of, 521–522

Neosar (cyclophosphamide), indications, actions, and dosage of, 521

Neosporin Cream (neomycin + polymyxin B), indications, actions, and dosage of, 576

Neosporin ointment (bacitracin, neomycin, + polymyxin B, topical), indications, actions, and dosage of, 502

Neosporin Ophthalmic (bacitracin, neomycin, + polymyxin B, ophthalmic), indications, actions, and dosage of, 502

Neo-Synephrine (phenylephrine)

indications, actions, and dosage of, 398*t*, 588–589
infusion guidelines for, 443*t*

Nephrostography, percutaneous, 329

Nephrotomography, 328

Nerve blocks, 320

Nerve conduction testing, for pain evaluation, 319

Nerve root trauma, with lumbar puncture, 286

Neumega (oprelvekin), indications, actions, and dosage of, 582

Neupogen (filgrastim), indications, actions, and dosage of, 539

Neural blockade, for pain management, 319

Neurogenic shock, 414, 431

Neuroleptics, for pain management, 320

Neurologic examination, 12

Neurolysis, 320

Neuromuscular blockers, 485

Neurontin (gabapentin), indications, actions, and dosage of, 543

Neutra-Phos (sodium-potassium phosphate)
for hypercalcemia, 189
for hypophosphatemia, 192

Neutrexin (trimetrexate), indications, actions, and dosage of, 615

Neutrophils. *See* Polymorphonuclear neutrophils (PMNs)

Nevirapine (Viramune), indications, actions, and dosage of, 577

Niacin (Nicolar)
indications, actions, and dosage of, 577
in total parenteral nutrition, 231*t*

Nicardipine (Cardene)
indications, actions, and dosage of, 578
infusion guidelines for, 441*t*–442*t*

Nicoderm (nicotine, transdermal), indications, actions, and dosage of, 578

Nicolar (niacin)
indications, actions, and dosage of, 577
in total parenteral nutrition, 231*t*

Nicorette (nicotine gum), indications, actions, and dosage of, 578

Nicorette D5 (nicotine gum), indications, actions, and dosage of, 578

Nicotine, transdermal (Habitrol; Nicoderm; Nicotrol; Prostep), indications, actions, and dosage of, 578

Nicotine gum (Nicorette; Nicorette D5), indications, actions, and dosage of, 578

Nicotine nasal spray (Nicotrol NS), indications, actions, and dosage of, 578

Nicotrol (nicotine, transdermal), indications, actions, and dosage of, 578

Nicotrol NS (nicotine nasal spray), indications, actions, and dosage of, 578

Nifedipine (Adalat; Adalat CC; Procardia; Procardia XL), indications, actions, and dosage of, 578

Night of surgery notes, 36–37

Nilandron (nilutamide), indications, actions, and dosage of, 578

Nilstat (nystatin), indications, actions, and dosage of, 580

Nilutamide (Nilandron), indications, actions, and dosage of, 578

Nimodipine (Nimotop), indications, actions, and dosage of, 578–579

Nipent (pentostatin), indications, actions, and dosage of, 587

Nipride (nitroprusside)
for emergency cardiac care, 465–466
for hypertensive crisis, 470
indications, actions, and dosage of, 579
infusion guidelines for, 442t

Nisoldipine (Sular), indications, actions, and dosage of, 579

Nitrite, in urine, 111

Nitro-Bid IV (nitroglycerin)
for emergency cardiac care, 465
indications, actions, and dosage of, 579

Nitro-Bid Ointment (nitroglycerin)
for emergency cardiac care, 465
indications, actions, and dosage of, 579

Nitrodisc (nitroglycerin)
for emergency cardiac care, 465
indications, actions, and dosage of, 579

Nitrofurantoin (Furadantin Macrobid; Macrodantin), indications, actions, and dosage of, 579

Nitrogen balance, 229

Nitrogen mustards, 478

Nitroglycerin (Nitro-Bid IV; Nitro-Bid Ointment; Nitrodisc; Nitrolingual; Transderm-Nitro)
for emergency cardiac care, 465
indications, actions, and dosage of, 579

Nitroglycerin (Tridil), infusion guidelines for, 442t

Nitrolingual (nitroglycerin)
for emergency cardiac care, 465
indications, actions, and dosage of, 579

Nitroprusside (Nipride; Nitropress)
for emergency cardiac care, 465–466
for hypertensive crisis, 470
indications, actions, and dosage of, 579
infusion guidelines for, 442t

Nitrosoureas, 478

Nix (permethrin), indications, actions, and dosage of, 153t, 154t, 588

Nizatidine (Axid), indications, actions, and dosage of, 579

Nizoral (ketoconazole), indications, actions, and dosage of, 557

Nocardia, Gram stain characteristics of, 126t

Nocardiosis, organism responsible and empiric therapy for, 139t

Noctec (chloral hydrate), indications, actions, and dosage of, 514

Nodal rhythm, on electrocardiograms, 374–375, 376f

Nodules, cutaneous, 21t

Nolvadex (tamoxifen), indications, actions, and dosage of, 606–607

Nonanion gap acidosis, 166, 168t

Nonhemolytic febrile reactions, 202, 203

Noninflammatory arthritis, synovial fluid interpretation and, 250, 251t

Nonionic contrast media, 327

Nonsteroidal anti-inflammatory agents, 486

Norcuron (vecuronium), indications, actions, and dosage of, 617

Nordette-21, 623t

Norepinephrine (Levophed)
actions of, 398t
for emergency cardiac care, 466
indications, actions, and dosage of, 580
infusion guidelines for, 442t

Norflex (orphenadrine), indications, actions, and dosage of, 582

Norfloxacin (Noroxin), indications, actions, and dosage of, 580

Norgestrel (Ovrette), 625*t*
indications, actions, and dosage of, 580

Norinyl 1/35 21, 28, 623*t*

Norinyl 1/50 21, 28, 623*t*

Normal compensatory response, 163

Normiflo (ardeparin), indications, actions, and dosage of, 499

Normodyne (labetalol)
for emergency cardiac care, 462
for hypertensive crisis, 470
indications, actions, and dosage of, 557
infusion guidelines for, 441*t*

Noroxin (norfloxacin), indications, actions, and dosage of, 580

Norpace (disopyramide)
half-life and therapeutic and toxic levels of, 633*t*
indications, actions, and dosage of, 529

Norplant (levonorgestrel implant), indications, actions, and dosage of, 560

Norpramin (desipramine)
half-life and therapeutic and toxic levels of, 633*t*
indications, actions, and dosage of, 524

Nor-QD, 625*t*

Nortriptyline (Aventyl; Pamelor)
half-life and therapeutic and toxic levels of, 633*t*
indications, actions, and dosage of, 580

Norvasc (amlodipine), indications, actions, and dosage of, 496

Norvir (ritonavir), indications, actions, and dosage of, 150*t*, 599

Novafed (pseudoephedrine), indications, actions, and dosage of, 595–596

Novantrone (mitoxantrone), indications, actions, and dosage of, 572–573

Novocain (procaine), for suturing, 349*t*

NovoLog (insulin aspart), onset, peak, and duration of effect of, 622*t*

Novulin 70/30, onset, peak, and duration of effect of, 622*t*

Novulin L, onset, peak, and duration of effect of, 622*t*

NPH Iletin II, onset, peak, and duration of effect of, 622*t*

Nubain (nalbuphine)
indications, actions, and dosage of, 575
route, effects, and dosage for, 322*t*

Nuclear scans, 333–335

Nucleated RBCs, 104

5′-Nucleotidase, laboratory diagnosis and, 83

Numorphan (oxymorphone), indications, actions, and dosage of, 584

Nupercainal (dibucaine), indications, actions, and dosage of, 526

Nurolong (nylon) sutures, 347*t*

Nursoy, 224*t*

Nutramigen, 224*t*

Nutrition, 205–226. *See also* Nutritional support; Total parenteral nutrition (TPN)
assessment of, 205, 209, 210*t*–212*t*
for critically ill patents, 434
hospital diets and, 205, 206*t*–208*t*
requirements for, 209, 213

Nutritional support
enteral, 213, 214*t*, 214–223
parenteral, 213–214

Nylon (Dermalon; Ethilon) sutures, 346*t*

Nylon (Nurolon) sutures, 347*t*

Nystagmus, differential diagnosis of, 49

Nystatin (Mycostatin; Nilstat), indications, actions, and dosage of, 580

O

Obesity, medication for, 482

Obstetric agents, 485–486

Obstruction series, 326

Obturator sign, 26

Occupress Ophthalmic (carteolol), indications, actions, and dosage of, 510

Octamide (metoclopramide), indications, actions, and dosage of, 569

OctreoScans, 334

Octreotide (Sandostatin), indications, actions, and dosage of, 580–581

Ocuflox Ophthalmic (ofloxacin), indications, actions, and dosage of, 580–581

Off-service notes, 35

Ofloxacin (Floxin; Ocuflox Ophthalmic), indications, actions, and dosage of, 580–581

Olanzapine (Zyprexa), indications, actions, and dosage of, 580–581

Oligoclonal banding, CSF, laboratory diagnosis and, 83

Oliguria, 432–433
differential diagnosis of, 49–50

Olsalazine (Dipentum), indications, actions, and dosage of, 580–581

Omeprazole (Prilosec), indications, actions, and dosage of, 580–581

Omnicef (cefdinir), indications, actions, and dosage of, 511

Omnipen (ampicillin)
indications, actions, and dosage of, 497
for subacute bacterial endocarditis prophylaxis, 158*t*, 159*t*

Oncovin (vincristine), indications, actions, and dosage of, 617–618

Ondansetron (Zofran), indications, actions, and dosage of, 580–581

On-service notes, 35

Operating room, 339–344
draping patients for, 343
entering, 339–340
gowning and gloving for, 342–343
hand scrub for, 340–341
patient preparation for, 341–342
position in, 343–344
sterile technique for, 339
universal precautions in, 344

Operative notes, 36

Ophthalmia, neonatal, organism responsible and empiric therapy for, 135*t*

Ophthalmic agents, 482–483

Opioids, 486
analgesics, 320, 321*t*–322*t*
overdose of, 471

Oprelvekin (Neumega), indications, actions, and dosage of, 582

Opticrom (cromolyn sodium), indications, actions, and dosage of, 520–521

Oral cholecystography (OCG), 329

Oral contraceptives, 485
composition of, 623*t*–625*t*

indications, actions, and dosage of, 582

Oral herpes, drugs of choice for treating, 147*t*

Oral procedures, subacute bacterial endocarditis prophylaxis for, 158*t*

Oral supplements, 217

Orders, 6
writing, 33–34

Organon (desogen), 623*t*

Organophosphates, antidote for, 471

Orgestrel-28, 624*t*

Orinase (tolbutamide), indications, actions, and dosage of, 612

Orphenadrine (Norflex), indications, actions, and dosage of, 582

Ortho-Cept 21, 624*t*

Orthoclone OKT3 (muromonab-CD3), indications, actions, and dosage of, 574

Ortho-Cyclen 21, 624*t*

Ortho-Novum 1/35 21, 624*t*

Ortho-Novum 1/50 21, 624*t*

Ortho-Novum 7/7/7 21, 625*t*

Ortho-Novum 10/11 21, 624*t*

Orthostatic blood pressure measurement, 286–289

Ortho Tri-Cyclen, 624*t*

Ortolani's test/sign, 26

Orudis (ketoprofen), indications, actions, and dosage of, 557

Oruvail (ketoprofen), indications, actions, and dosage of, 557

Oseltamivir (Tamiflu), indications, actions, and dosage of, 147*t*, 582

Osler's nodes, 26

Osmolality
serum, laboratory diagnosis and, 83
spot urine study for, 115

Osteomyelitis, organisms responsible and empiric therapy for, 134*t*

Osteoporosis, medications for, 482

Otic agents, 482

Otic Domeboro (acetic acid + aluminum acetate), indications, actions, and dosage of, 489

Otitis externa, organisms responsible and empiric therapy for, 135*t*–136*t*

Otitis media, organisms responsible and empiric therapy for, 136*t*

Otobiotic Otic (polymyxin B + hydrocortisone), indications, actions, and dosage of, 590–591

Outpatient prescriptions, writing, 37–39, 38*f*

Ova, stool for, 131

Ovarian cancer, staging of, 655

Ovral, 624*t*

Ovrette (norgestrel), 625*t* indications, actions, and dosage of, 580

Oxacillin (Bactocill; Prostaphlin), indications, actions, and dosage of, 582–583

Oxaprozin (Daypro), indications, actions, and dosage of, 583

Oxazepam (Serax), indications, actions, and dosage of, 583

Oxcarbazepine (Trileptal), indications, actions, and dosage of, 583

Oxiconazole (Oxistat), indications, actions, and dosage of, 583

Oximetric PA catheters, 401

Oxistat (oxiconazole), indications, actions, and dosage of, 583

Oxybutynin (Ditropan; Ditropan XL), indications, actions, and dosage of, 583

Oxycodone [dihydrohydroxycodeinone] (Oxycontin; OxyIR; Roxicodone), indications, actions, and dosage of, 583

Oxycodone + acetaminophen (Percocet; Tylox), indications, actions, and dosage of, 583–584

Oxycodone + aspirin (Percodan; Percodan-Demi), indications, actions, and dosage of, 584

Oxycontin (oxycodone), indications, actions, and dosage of, 583

Oxygen, for carbon monoxide poisoning, 471

Oxygenation, 418–423, 420*f*–422*f*

Oxygen carrying capacity, derivation and normal values for, 437*t*

Oxygen consumption, derivation and normal values for, 438*t*

Oxygen delivery, 419

Oxygen supplements, 362*t*

OxyIR (oxycodone), indications, actions, and dosage of, 583

Oxymorphone (Numorphan), indications, actions, and dosage of, 584

Oxytocin (Pitocin; Syntocinon), indications, actions, and dosage of, 584

P

Pacerone (amiodarone) for emergency cardiac care, 461 half-life and therapeutic and toxic levels of, 632*t* indications, actions, and dosage of, 495

Pacing, transcutaneous, 468

Pacing Swans, 401

Pacis (BCG [bacillus Calmette-Guérin]), indications, actions, and dosage of, 503

Packed red cells (PRBCs), 197*t*

Paclitaxel (Taxol), indications, actions, and dosage of, 584

Pain acute, 315–316 chronic, 316 differential diagnosis of, 42

Pain management, 315–323. *See also* Analgesics adverse physiologic effects of pain and, 316, 317*t*–318*t* classification of pain and, 315–316 evaluation for, 317 nonpharmacologic, 320, 323 pain measurement and, 316, 319 patient controlled analgesia for, 323 pharmacologic, 319–320, 321*t*–322*t* terminology for, 315

Pamelor (nortriptyline) half-life and therapeutic and toxic levels of, 633*t* indications, actions, and dosage of, 580

Pamidronate (Aredia) for hypercalcemia, 189 indications, actions, and dosage of, 584–585

Panacryl sutures, 346*t*

Pancoast's syndrome, 26

Pancrease (pancreatin + pancrelipase), indications, actions, and dosage of, 585

Pancreatic disease, total parenteral nutrition formulation for, 235

Pancreatic loss, IV fluid replacement with, 179

Pancreatin + pancrelipase (Cotazyme; Creon; Pancrease; Ultrase), indications, actions, and dosage of, 585

Pancuronium (Pavulon), indications, actions, and dosage of, 585

P-24 antigen, laboratory diagnosis and, 77, 83

Pantoprazole (Protonix), indications, actions, and dosage of, 585

Papanicolaou smear, 290–291

Paper, for electrocardiography, 368

Papillary muscle rupture, 393–394

Papules, 21*t*

Paracentesis, peritoneal (abdominal), 296–297, 298*f*

Paracoccidioidomycosis, systemic drug for treating, 152*t*

Paradoxical pulse, 393, 394*f*

Paraflex (hlorzoxazone), indications, actions, and dosage of, 515–516

Parafon Forte DSC (hlorzoxazone), indications, actions, and dosage of, 515–516

Paraldehyde, for seizures, 473*t*

Paranasal sinus radiographs, 326

Paraplatin (carboplatin), indications, actions, and dosage of, 510

Parasites
    drugs for treating infections by, 153*t*–154*t*
    stool for, 131
    transfusion-associated risk of transmission, 204
    in urine sediment, 112

Parathyroid hormone (PTH)
    deficiency of, hypocalcemia and, 189
    hypocalcemia and, 189
    laboratory diagnosis and, 84

Paregoric, indications, actions, and dosage of, 585

Parenteral fluids, composition of, 178–179

Parenteral nutrition, 213–214, 434. *See also* Total parenteral nutrition (TPN)

Parlodel (bromocriptine), indications, actions, and dosage of, 506

Paromomycin, indications for, 153*t*

Paromycin, indications for, 153*t*

Paroxetine (Paxil), indications, actions, and dosage of, 585

Paroxysmal atrial tachycardia (PAT), 372–373, 374*f*

Partial thromboplastin time (PTT), 107

Pasteurella, Gram stain characteristics of, 124*f*

Pastia's lines, 26

Patches, cutaneous, 21*t*

Patient controlled analgesia (PCA), 323

Patient preparation, for surgery, 341–342

Pavulon (pancuronium), indications, actions, and dosage of, 585

Paxil (paroxetine), indications, actions, and dosage of, 585

Pediacare 1 (dextromethorphan), indications, actions, and dosage of, 525

Pediazole (erythromycin + sulfisoxazole), indications, actions, and dosage of, 534

Pediculus capitis, drugs for treating, 153*t*

Pediculus humanus infections, drugs for treating, 153*t*

PEG tubes, 214

Pelvic drug therapy, 330

Pelvic examination, 289–291
    indications for, 289
    materials for, 289
    procedures for, 289–291

Pelvic inflammatory disease (PID), organisms responsible and empiric therapy for, 139*t*

Pelvic magnetic resonance imaging, 333

Pelvic ultrasound, 330

Penbutolol (Levatol), indications, actions, and dosage of, 585

Penciclovir (Denavir), indications, actions, and dosage of, 147*t*, 585

Penicillin(s), 477
    for dental abscesses, 470

Penicillin G, aqueous (potassium or sodium) (Pentids; Pfizerpen), indications, actions, and dosage of, 586

Penicillin G benzathine (Bicillin), indications, actions, and dosage of, 586

Penicillin G procaine (Wycillin), indications, actions, and dosage of, 585

Penicillin V (Pen-Vee K; Veetids), indications, actions, and dosage of, 585

Pentam 300 (pentamidine), indications, actions, and dosage of, 153*t*, 585

Pentamidine (Nebupent; Pentam 300), indications, actions, and dosage of, 153*t*, 585

Pentasa (mesalamine), indications, actions, and dosage of, 566

Pentazocine (Talwin), indications, actions, and dosage of, 586–587

Pentids [penicillin G, aqueous (potassium or sodium)], indications, actions, and dosage of, 586

Pentobarbital (Nembutal), indications, actions, and dosage of, 587

Pentosan polysulfate sodium (Elmiron), indications, actions, and dosage of, 587

Pentostatin (Nipent), indications, actions, and dosage of, 587

Pentoxifylline (Trental), indications, actions, and dosage of, 587

Pen-Vee K (penicillin V), indications, actions, and dosage of, 585

Pepcid (famotidine), indications, actions, and dosage of, 537

Peptic ulcer disease, organism responsible and empiric therapy for, 144*t*

Pepto-Bismol (bismuth subsalicylate), indications, actions, and dosage of, 505

Peptostreptococcus, Gram stain characteristics of, 125*t*

Percocet (oxycodone + acetaminophen), indications, actions, and dosage of, 583–584

Percodan (oxycodone + aspirin), indications, actions, and dosage of, 584

Percodan-Demi (oxycodone + aspirin), indications, actions, and dosage of, 584

Percutaneous nephrostography, 329

Percutaneous suprapubic bladder aspiration, 309

Percutaneous transhepatic cholangiography (PTHC), 329

Performance status scales, 646, 647*t*–648*t*

Pergolide (Permax), indications, actions, and dosage of, 587

Periactin (cyproheptadine), indications, actions, and dosage of, 522

Pericardial friction rub, 394–395

Pericardiocentesis, 291–292, 293*f*

Pericarditis, on electrocardiograms, 387, 387*f*

Perindopril erbumine (Aceon), indications, actions, and dosage of, 587–588

Peripherally inserted central catheter (PICC) lines, 292–295
complications of, 295
contraindications to, 293
historical background of, 294
indications for, 292
materials for, 293
procedure for, 294
removal of, 294–295

Peritoneal dialysis, diet for, 208*t*

Peritoneal lavage, 295–296, 296*t*

Peritoneal paracentesis, 296–297, 298*f*
complications of, 297
contraindications to, 296–297
diagnosis of ascitic fluid and, 297, 299*t*
indications for, 296
materials for, 297
procedure for, 297, 298*f*

Peritonitis, organisms responsible and empiric therapy for, 139*t*

Permax (pergolide), indications, actions, and dosage of, 587

Permethrin (Elimite; Nix), indications, actions, and dosage of, 153*t*, 154*t*, 588

Permitil (fluphenazine), indications, actions, and dosage of, 541

Perphenazine (Trilafon), indications, actions, and dosage of, 588

Petechiae, 21*t*

Pfizerpen [penicillin G, aqueous (potassium or sodium)], indications, actions, and dosage of, 586

pH
of pleural fluid, 299*t*
of urine, 110–111

Phalen's test, 26

Pharyngitis, organisms responsible and empiric therapy for, 140*t*

Phenazopyridine (Pyridium), indications, actions, and dosage of, 588

Phenelzine (Nardil), indications, actions, and dosage of, 588

Phenergan (promethazine), indications, actions, and dosage of, 594

Phenobarbital
half-life and therapeutic and toxic levels of, 631*t*
indications, actions, and dosage of, 588
for seizures, 473*t*

Phenylephrine (Neo-Synephrine)
indications, actions, and dosage of, 398*t*, 588–589
infusion guidelines for, 443*t*

Phenytoin (Dilantin)
half-life and therapeutic and toxic levels of, 631*t*–632*t*
indications, actions, and dosage of, 589
interaction with enteral nutrition, 223

Phlebotomy, 309–314
materials for, 309, 311*t*–312*t*
procedure for, 310, 313–314

Phos-Ex (calcium acetate), indications, actions, and dosage of, 508

PhosLo (calcium acetate), indications, actions, and dosage of, 508

Phosphate
deficiency of, 192
excess of, 191–192

Phospholine Ophthalmic (echothiophate iodine), indications, actions, and dosage of, 532

Phosphorus, laboratory diagnosis and, 84

Phrenilin Forte (acetaminophen + butalbital +/- caffeine), indications, actions, and dosage of, 489

Phthirus pubis infections, drugs for treating, 153*t*

Physical examination, 11–12

example of, 28–32
written, 5

Physical therapy, for pain management, 320

Physostigmine (Antilirium)
for anticholinergic crisis, 470
antidote for, 471
indications, actions, and dosage of, 589

Phytonadione [vitamin K] (AquaMEPHYTON)
indications, actions, and dosage of, 589
in total parenteral nutrition, 231

Pindolol (Visken), indications, actions, and dosage of, 589

Pinworm infections, drugs for treating, 153*t*

Pinworm preparation, 132

Pioglitazone (Actos), indications, actions, and dosage of, 589

Pipecuronium (Arduan), indications, actions, and dosage of, 590

Piperacillin (Pipracil), indications, actions, and dosage of, 590

Piperacillin-tazobactam (Zosyn), indications, actions, and dosage of, 590

Pipracil (piperacillin), indications, actions, and dosage of, 590

Pirbuterol (Maxair), indications, actions, and dosage of, 590

Piroxicam (Feldene)
indications, actions, and dosage of, 590
route, effects, and dosage for, 321*t*

Pitocin (oxytocin), indications, actions, and dosage of, 584

Pitressin (vasopressin)
indications, actions, and dosage of, 617
infusion guidelines for, 443*t*

Plain catgut sutures, 346*t*

Plaques, cutaneous, 21*t*

Plasmanate (plasma protein fraction), 200*t*

Plasma protein fraction (Plasmanate), 200*t*
indications, actions, and dosage of, 590

Plasmodium falciparum infections, drugs for treating, 153*t*

Plasmodium malariae infections, drugs for treating, 153*t*

Plasmodium ovale infections, drugs for treating, 153*t*

Plasmodium vivax infections, drugs for treating, 153*t*

Platelet(s)
  laboratory diagnosis and, 103
  for transfusion, 198*t*
  transfusions of, 201

Plateletpheresis, 194

Platinol AQ (cisplatin), indications, actions, and dosage of, 517

Plavix (clopidogrel), indications, actions, and dosage of, 519

Plendil (felodipine), indications, actions, and dosage of, 537

Pleural effusion, differential diagnosis of, 50

Pleural fluid, differential diagnosis of, 299*t*, 306

Plicamycin (Mithracin)
  for hypercalcemia, 189
  indications, actions, and dosage of, 590–591

Pneumococcal vaccine, polyvalent (Pneumovax-23), indications, actions, and dosage of, 590–591

Pneumococcal 7-valent conjugate vaccine (Prevnar), indications, actions, and dosage of, 590–591

Pneumocystis carinii pneumonia
  diagnosis of, 130
  drugs for treating, 153*t*

Pneumonia, organisms responsible and empiric therapy for, 135*t*, 140*t*–141*t*

Pneumovax-23 (pneumococcal vaccine, polyvalent), indications, actions, and dosage of, 590–591

Podocon-25 (podophyllin), indications, actions, and dosage of, 148*t*, 590–591

Podofilox, indications and dosage for, 148*t*

Podophyllin (Condylox; Condylox Gel 0.5%; Podocon-25), indications, actions, and dosage of, 148*t*, 590–591

Poisoning, 471–472

Poliglecaprone 25 (Monocryl) sutures, 346*t*

Polychromasia, 104

Polycitra-K (potassium citrate + citric acid), indications, actions, and dosage of, 592

Polydioxanone (PDS) sutures, 345, 346*t*

Polyester (Ethibond; Tycron) sutures, 347*t*

Polyethylene glycol [PEG]-electrolyte solution (CoLyte; GoLYTELY), indications, actions, and dosage of, 590–591

Polyglactin 910 (Vicryl) sutures, 346*t*

Polyglycolic acid 910 (Vicryl Rapide) sutures, 346*t*

Polyglyconate (Maxon) sutures, 346*t*

Polymerase chain reaction (PCR), 132

Polymorphonuclear neutrophils (PMNs)
  bands or stabs, 100
  laboratory diagnosis and, 103
  left shift and, 100

Polymox (amoxicillin)
  indications, actions, and dosage of, 496
  for subacute bacterial endocarditis prophylaxis, 158*t*, 159*t*

Polymyxin B + hydrocortisone (Otobiotic Otic), indications, actions, and dosage of, 590–591

Poly-Pred Ophthalmic (neomycin, polymyxin-B, + prednisolone), indications, actions, and dosage of, 577

Polypropylene (Prolene) sutures, 347*t*

Polysporin (bacitracin + polymyxin B, topical), indications, actions, and dosage of, 502

Polysporin Ophthalmic (bacitracin + polymyxin B, ophthalmic), indications, actions, and dosage of, 502

Portable chest x-rays, 325

Portagen, 224*t*

Positive end-expiratory pressure (PEEP), 417, 417*f*, 426

Posteroanterior (PA) chest films, reading, 335, 336*f*, 338

Postop notes, 36–37

Postrenal renal failure, 433

Potassium
  deficiency of. *See* Hypokalemia
  excess of. *See* Hyperkalemia
  requirement for, 178

Potassium (*continued*)
serum, laboratory diagnosis and, 84
spot urine study for, 114
Potassium acetate, potassium citrate, +
bicarbonate (Tri-K), form and
dosage of, 626*t*
Potassium bicarbonate, for renal tubular
acidosis, 168*t*
Potassium chloride (Kaochlor 10%;
Kaochlor S-F 10%; Kaon-Cl;
Kaon-Cl 20%; K-Lor; Klorvess;
Klotrix; K-Tab; Micro-K; Slow-
K), form and dosage of, 626*t*
indications, actions, and dosage of, 592
Potassium chloride, potassium citrate, and
bicarbonate (Kaochlor Eff), form
and dosage of, 626*t*
Potassium citrate (Urocit-K), indications,
actions, and dosage of, 590–591
Potassium citrate + citric acid (Polycitra-
K), indications, actions, and
dosage of, 592
Potassium citrate + potassium gluconate
(Twin-K), form and dosage of,
626*t*
Potassium gluconate (Glu-K; Kaon; Kaon
elixir)
form and dosage of, 626*t*
indications, actions, and dosage of, 592
Potassium hydroxide preparation, 291
Potassium phosphate (K-Phos), for
hypophosphatemia, 192
Pound/kilogram conversion, 658, 658*t*
Povidone-iodine hand scrub, 340–341
PPD test, 303–304
Pramipexole (Mirapex), indications,
actions, and dosage of, 592
Pramoxine (Anusol Ointment;
Proctofoam-NS), indications,
actions, and dosage of, 592
Pramoxine + hydrocortisone (Enzone;
Proctofoam-HC), indications,
actions, and dosage of, 592
Prandin (repaglinide), indications, actions,
and dosage of, 598
Pravastatin (Pravachol), indications,
actions, and dosage of, 592–593
Prazepam (Centrax), indications, actions,
and dosage of, 593
Praziquantel, indications for, 154*t*

Prazosin (Minipress), indications, actions,
and dosage of, 593
Precordial contusion, 392
Precordial electrodes, 267, 267*f*
Precose (acarbose), indications, actions,
and dosage of, 488
Pred-G Ophthalmic (gentamicin +
prednisolone, ophthalmic),
indications, actions, and dosage of,
545
Predictive value, definition of, 645
Prednicarbate (Dermatop), potency and
application of, 630*t*
Prednisolone (Delta-Cortef)
dose, activity, duration, and route for,
627*t*
indications, actions, and dosage of, 603
Prednisone (Deltasone)
dose, activity, duration, and route for,
627*t*
for hypercalcemia, 189
indications, actions, and dosage of, 603
Preemie SMA 20, 225*t*
Preemie SMA 24, 225*t*
Pregnancy precautions, 156
Preload, 395, 396*f*
measurement of, 408, 410
Premarin (estrogens, conjugated),
indications, actions, and dosage of,
535
Premarin + Methylprogesterone
(estrogens, conjugated +
methylprogesterone), indications,
actions, and dosage of, 535–536
Premarin + Methyltestosterone (estrogens,
conjugated + methyltestosterone),
indications, actions, and dosage of,
536
Premature atrial contractions (PACs), 372,
373*f*
Premature infant(s), feeding, 225–226
formulas for, 225*t*
Premature ventricular contractions
(PVCs), 375–376, 376*f*, 377*f*
Preoperative notes, 36
Prerenal renal failure, 433
Prescriptions
safe, tips for, 39
writing, 37–39, 38*f*
Presentation, 5

Present illness, history of, 9

Pressor agents, 480

Pressure-limited ventilators, 423

Pressure regulated volume control ventilation, 426

Pressure support ventilation (PSV), 425f, 426

Prevacid (lansoprazole), indications, actions, and dosage of, 558

Prevalence, definition of, 639

Prevnar (pneumococcal 7-valent conjugate vaccine), indications, actions, and dosage of, 590–591

Priftin (rifapentine), indications, actions, and dosage of, 598

Prilosec (omeprazole), indications, actions, and dosage of, 580–581

Primacor (milrinone), indications, actions, and dosage of, 571

Primaxin (imipenem-cilastin), indications, actions, and dosage of, 552

Primidone, half-life and therapeutic and toxic levels of, 632t

Prinivil (lisinopril)
 for emergency cardiac care, 461
 indications, actions, and dosage of, 562

PR interval, 367, 369f

Priscoline (tolazoline), indications, actions, and dosage of, 612

Pro-Banthine (propantheline), indications, actions, and dosage of, 594

Probenecid (Benemid), indications, actions, and dosage of, 593

Problem-oriented progress notes, 34

Procainamide (Procan; Pronestyl)
 electrocardiogram and, 386
 for emergency cardiac care, 466
 half-life and therapeutic and toxic levels of, 633t
 indications, actions, and dosage of, 593
 infusion guidelines for, 443t

Procaine (Novocain), for suturing, 349t

Procan (procainamide)
 electrocardiogram and, 386
 for emergency cardiac care, 466
 half-life and therapeutic and toxic levels of, 633t
 indications, actions, and dosage of, 593
 infusion guidelines for, 443t

Procarbazine (Matulane), indications, actions, and dosage of, 593–594

Procardia (nifedipine), indications, actions, and dosage of, 578

Procardia XL (nifedipine), indications, actions, and dosage of, 578

Prochlorperazine (Compazine), indications, actions, and dosage of, 594

Procrit (epoetin alfa), indications, actions, and dosage of, 533

Proctitis, organism responsible and empiric therapy for, 135t

Proctofoam-HC (pramoxine + hydrocortisone), indications, actions, and dosage of, 592

Proctofoam-NS (pramoxine), indications, actions, and dosage of, 592

Proctoscopy, 300

Procyclidine (Kemadrin), indications, actions, and dosage of, 594

Progesterone, laboratory diagnosis and, 84

Progesterone receptors, laboratory diagnosis and, 67

Progestimil, 224t

Proglycem (diazoxide), indications, actions, and dosage of, 526

Prograf (tacrolimus), indications, actions, and dosage of, 606

Progress notes
 ICU, 389–391
 problem-oriented, 34

Prohibit (haemophilus B conjugate vaccine), indications, actions, and dosage of, 547

Prokine (sargramostim), indications, actions, and dosage of, 600

Prolactin, laboratory diagnosis and, 85

Prolastin (α_1-Protease inhibitor), indications, actions, and dosage of, 492

Proleukin (aldesleukin), indications, actions, and dosage of, 491

Prolixin (fluphenazine), indications, actions, and dosage of, 541

Proloprim (trimethoprim), indications, actions, and dosage of, 615

Promethazine (Phenergan), indications, actions, and dosage of, 594

Pronestyl (procainamide)
 electrocardiogram and, 386
 for emergency cardiac care, 466
 half-life and therapeutic and toxic levels
  of, 633*t*
 indications, actions, and dosage
  of, 593
 infusion guidelines for, 443*t*
Propafenone (Rhythmol), indications,
 actions, and dosage of, 594
Propantheline (Pro-Banthine), indications,
 actions, and dosage of, 594
Propecia (finasteride), indications, actions,
 and dosage of, 539
Propine (dipivefrin), indications, actions,
 and dosage of, 528
Propionibacterium acne, Gram stain
 characteristics of, 126*t*
Propofol (Diprivan), indications, actions,
 and dosage of, 594
Propoxyphene (Darvon), indications,
 actions, and dosage of, 595
Propoxyphene + acetaminophen
  (Darvocet), indications, actions,
  and dosage of, 595
Propoxyphene + aspirin (Darvon
  Compound-65; Darvon-N +
  Aspirin), indications, actions, and
  dosage of, 595
Propranolol (Inderal)
 for emergency cardiac care, 462
 indications, actions, and dosage
  of, 595
Propylthiouracil [PTU], indications,
 actions, and dosage of, 595
Proscar (finasteride), indications, actions,
 and dosage of, 539
ProSobee, 224*t*
Prosom (estazolam), indications, actions,
 and dosage of, 534
Prostaglandin E$_1$ [alprostadil] (Prostin
  VR), indications, actions, and
  dosage of, 492
Prostaphlin (oxacillin), indications,
 actions, and dosage of, 582–583
Prostate cancer
 screening recommendations for, 643*t*
 staging of, 657–658
Prostate-specific antigen (PSA),
 laboratory diagnosis and, 85

Prostatic acid phosphatase (PAP),
 laboratory diagnosis and, 55
Prostatitis, organisms responsible and
 empiric therapy for, 144*t*
Prostep (nicotine, transdermal),
 indications, actions, and dosage of,
 578
Prosthetic joint infections, organisms
 responsible and empiric therapy
 for, 134*t*
Prosthetic valves, anticoagulant standard
 of practice for, 637*t*
Prostin VR (alprostadil), indications,
 actions, and dosage of, 492
Protamine sulfate, indications, actions,
 and dosage of, 595
α$_1$-Protease inhibitor (Prolastin),
 indications, actions, and dosage of,
 492
Protein
 needs for, 213
 serum, laboratory diagnosis and, 87–88
 spot urine study for, 115
 in urine, 112, 117–118
Protein electrophoresis
 serum, laboratory diagnosis and, 85,
  86*f*, 87*t*
 urine, laboratory diagnosis and,
  85, 86*f*
Protein hydrosylate infant formulas, 224*t*
Proteus, Gram stain characteristics of,
 124*f*
Proteus mirabilis, Gram stain
 characteristics of, 126*t*
Proteus vulgaris, Gram stain
 characteristics of, 126*t*
Prothrombin complex, 200*t*
Prothrombin time (PT), 107–108
Protonix (pantoprazole), indications,
 actions, and dosage of, 585
Proventil (albuterol), 364
 for anaphylaxis, 469
 indications, actions, and dosage of, 490
 nebulized, for asthmatic attacks, 469
Provera (medroxyprogesterone),
 indications, actions, and dosage of,
 564
Providencia, Gram stain characteristics of,
 127*t*
Proximal port, of Swan-Ganz catheter, 399

Prozac (fluoxetine), indications, actions, and dosage of, 541

Pruritus, differential diagnosis of, 50

Pseudoephedrine (Afrinol; Novafed; Sudafed), indications, actions, and dosage of, 595–596

Pseudo-hyponatremia, 185

Pseudomonas, Gram stain characteristics of, 124*f*

Pseudomonas aeruginosa, Gram stain characteristics of, 127*t*

Pseudotumor cerebri, cerebrospinal fluid in, 288*t*

Psoas sign, 26

Psorcon (diflorasone diacetate), potency and application of, 628*t*

Psychiatric history and physical, 13–14

Psychiatric mental status examination, 13

Psychologic examination, for pain evaluation, 319

Psychologic intervention, for pain management, 320

Psychosocial history, 10

Psyllium (Effer-Syllium; Metamucil; Serutan), indications, actions, and dosage of, 596

Pulmicort (budesonide), indications, actions, and dosage of, 506

Pulmonary angiography, 328

Pulmonary artery catheters, 399–410, 400*f*
  catheterization procedure with, 402–404, 403*f*–405*f*, 406, 407*t*
  catheters for, 399–402, 401*f*, 402*f*
  clinical applications of, 408, 410
  complications of, 406–407
  differential diagnosis using, 408, 409*t*
  indications for, 399
  measurements using, 407–408

Pulmonary artery occlusion pressure, 407

Pulmonary artery pressure, 407

Pulmonary artery pressure, systolic/diastolic (PAS/PAD), derivation and normal values for, 437*t*

Pulmonary capillary wedge pressure (PCWP), derivation and normal values for, 437*t*

Pulmonary disease, total parenteral nutrition formulation for, 235

Pulmonary embolism, 435–436

algorithm for, 460*f*

Pulmonary function tests (PFTs), 359–361, 360*f*
  differential diagnosis of, 361, 361*t*

Pulmonary vascular resistance (PVR), derivation and normal values for, 437*t*

Pulmonic insufficiency (PI), 16*t*

Pulmonic stenosis (PS), 16*t*

Pulmozyme (dornase alfa), indications, actions, and dosage of, 530

Pulseless electrical activity algorithm, 453*f*

Pulseless ventricular tachycardia algorithm, 452*f*

Pulse oximetry, for cardiac output determination, 413

Pulse pressure, 393

Pulsus alternans, 26

Pulsus paradoxus measurement, 298–300

Pureed diet, 206*t*

Purinethol (mercaptopurine), indications, actions, and dosage of, 566

Purpura, 21*t*

Pustules, 21*t*

P wave, 368

Pyelonephritis, organisms responsible and empiric therapy for, 144*t*

Pyrantel pamoate, indications for, 153*t*, 154*t*

Pyrazinamide, indications, actions, and dosage of, 596

Pyridium (phenazopyridine), indications, actions, and dosage of, 588

Pyridoxine [vitamin B$_6$]
  indications, actions, and dosage of, 596
  in total parenteral nutrition, 231*t*

Pyrimethamine, indications for, 154*t*

Pyrimethamine-sulfadoxine, indications for, 153*t*

Pyrosis, differential diagnosis of, 47

Q

QRS axis, 370

QRS complex, 369

QRS interval, 367, 369*f*

QT interval, 367, 369*f*

Quazepam (Doral), indications, actions, and dosage of, 596

Queckenstedt's test, 26
Quelicin (succinylcholine), indications, actions, and dosage of, 605
Questran (cholestyramine), indications, actions, and dosage of, 516
Quetiapine (Seroquel), indications, actions, and dosage of, 596
Quinaglute (quinidine)
  electrocardiogram and, 386
  half-life and therapeutic and toxic levels of, 633*t*
  indications, actions, and dosage of, 596–597
Quinapril (Accupril), indications, actions, and dosage of, 596
Quinidine (Quinaglute; Quinidex)
  electrocardiogram and, 386
  half-life and therapeutic and toxic levels of, 633*t*
  indications, actions, and dosage of, 596–597
Quinine dihydrochloride, indications for, 153*t*
Quinine gluconate, indications for, 153*t*
Quinine sulfate, indications for, 153*t*
Quinke's sign, 27
Quinupristin + dalfopristin (Synercid), indications, actions, and dosage of, 597
Q waves, 369
  in myocardial infarction, 384, 385*f*

R
Rabeprazole (Aciphex), indications, actions, and dosage of, 597
Racemic epinephrine, 364
Radiation, for pain management, 320
Radiation terminology, 646
Radovici's sign, 27
RA latex test, laboratory diagnosis and, 88
Raloxifene (Evista), indications, actions, and dosage of, 597
Ramipril (Altace)
  for emergency cardiac care, 461
  indications, actions, and dosage of, 597
Random urine studies, 114–115
Ranitidine (Zantac)
  for anaphylaxis, 469
  indications, actions, and dosage of, 597

Rapamycin [sirolimus] (Rapamune), indications, actions, and dosage of, 602
Rapid plasma reagin (RPR), laboratory diagnosis and, 92
Raynaud's phenomenon/disease, 27
Reading, 4–5
Rebetron (ribavirin), indications, actions, and dosage of, 146*t*, 148*t*, 598
Recombivax-HB (hepatitis B vaccine), indications, actions, and dosage of, 548
Rectovaginal examination, 290
Red blood cell(s) (RBCs)
  abnormalities of, differential diagnosis of, 104
  laboratory diagnosis and, 68
  mass of, 177
  morphologic abnormalities of, spot urine study for, 114–115
  nucleated, 104
  transfusions of, 196, 197*t*, 201
  in urine sediment, 112
  washed, 197*t*
Red blood cell (RBC) casts, in urine sediment, 114
Red cell distribution width (RDW), laboratory diagnosis and, 103
Red rubber catheter, 307
Reducing substances, in urine, 112
Refludan (lepirudin), indications, actions, and dosage of, 559
Reglan (metoclopramide), indications, actions, and dosage of, 569
Regranex Gel (becaplermin), indications, actions, and dosage of, 503
Regular diet, 206*t*
Regular Iletin II, onset, peak, and duration of effect of, 622*t*
Relafen (nabumetone), indications, actions, and dosage of, 574
Relenza (zanamivir), indications, actions, and dosage of, 147*t*, 619
Remeron (mirtazapine), indications, actions, and dosage of, 572
Remicade (infliximab), indications, actions, and dosage of, 553
Renal cancer, staging of, 652–653
Renal failure
  acute, 207*t*, 432–433

diet for, 207t
hypercalcemia with, 188
renal, 433
total parenteral nutrition formulation
for, 235–236
Renal scans, 334
Renal tubular acidosis, diagnosis and
management of, 168t
Renin, laboratory diagnosis and, 88
ReoPro (abciximab)
for emergency cardiac care, 464
indications, actions, and dosage of, 488
Repaglinide (Prandin), indications,
actions, and dosage of, 598
Repan (acetaminophen + butalbital +/-
caffeine), indications, actions, and
dosage of, 489
Rescriptor (delavirdine), indications,
actions, and dosage of, 523–524
Residents, 1–2
Residual volume (RV), 361, 361t, 416
Resin uptake, laboratory diagnosis and, 90
Respiratory acidosis, 164t, 169–170
differential diagnosis of, 169–170
treatment of, 170
Respiratory agents, 487
Respiratory alkalosis, 164t, 170–171
differential diagnosis of, 170
treatment of, 170–171
Respiratory inhalants, 487
Respiratory isolation, 155
Respiratory procedures, subacute bacterial
endocarditis prophylaxis for, 158t
Respiratory syncytial virus (RSV), drug of
choice for treating infections by,
148t
Respiratory therapy, 359
Responsibility, 5–6
Restoril (temazepam), indications, actions,
and dosage of, 607
Reteplase (Retavase), indications, actions,
and dosage of, 598
Reticulocyte count, 100–101
Retin-A (tretinoin, topical), indications,
actions, and dosage of, 613
Retinitis, cytomegalovirus, drugs of
choice for treating, 146t
Retinoic acid [tretinoin, systemic]
(Vesanoid), indications, actions,
and dosage of, 613

Retinoic acid [tretinoin, topical] (Avita;
Retin-A), indications, actions, and
dosage of, 613
Retinol-binding protein (RBP), laboratory
diagnosis and, 88
Retrograde pyelography (RPG), 329
Retrograde urethrography (RUG), 329
Retroperitoneal computed tomography,
330
Revia (naltrexone), indications, actions,
and dosage of, 575
Review of systems (ROS), 10–11
Rheomacrodex (dextran 40), indications,
actions, and dosage of, 525
Rheumatoid factor, laboratory diagnosis
and, 88
Rheumatrex (methotrexate)
half-life and therapeutic and toxic levels
of, 633t
indications, actions, and dosage
of, 568
Rhinocort (budesonide), indications,
actions, and dosage of, 506
Rho Gam, 199t
Rhythmol (propafenone), indications,
actions, and dosage of, 594
Rib(s), x-rays of, 325
Ribavirin (Rebetron; Virazole),
indications, actions, and dosage of,
146t, 148t, 598
Riboflavin, in total parenteral nutrition,
231t
Rickettsia rickettsii infections,
characteristics and treatment of,
156t–157t
Rifabutin (Mycobutin), indications,
actions, and dosage of, 598
Rifampin (Rifadin), indications, actions,
and dosage of, 598
Rifapentine (Priftin), indications,
actions, and dosage of, 598
Right atrial enlargement (RAE),
electrocardiogram and, 380, 381f
Right atrial pressure (RAP), derivation
and normal values for, 437t
Right bundle branch block (RBBB), 379,
380f
Right shift, 100
Right ventricular ejection catheters, 401
Right ventricular ejection fraction, 408

Right ventricular end-diastolic volume index, 408

Right ventricular hypertrophy (RVH), electrocardiogram and, 381, 382*f*

Right ventricular pressure (RVP), derivation and normal values for, 437*t*

Rimantadine (Flumadine), indications, actions, and dosage of, 148*t*, 598–599

Rimexolone (Vexol Ophthalmic), indications, actions, and dosage of, 597–598

Rimso 50 (dimethyl sulfoxide), indications, actions, and dosage of, 528

Ringworm, organisms responsible and empiric therapy for, 142*t*

Riopan (magaldrate), indications, actions, and dosage of, 564

Risedronate (Actonel), indications, actions, and dosage of, 599

Risperidone (Risperdal), indications, actions, and dosage of, 599

Ritonavir (Norvir), indications, actions, and dosage of, 150*t*, 599

Rivastigmine (Exelon), indications, actions, and dosage of, 599

Rizatriptan (Maxalt), indications, actions, and dosage of, 599

Robaxin (methocarbamol), indications, actions, and dosage of, 568

Robetron (interferon alfa-2B + ribavirin combination), indications, actions, and dosage of, 554

Robinson catheter, 307

Robitussin (guaifenesin), indications, actions, and dosage of, 546

Robitussin A-C (guaifenesin + codeine), indications, actions, and dosage of, 546

Rocaltrol (calcitriol), indications, actions, and dosage of, 508

Rocephin (ceftriaxone), indications, actions, and dosage of, 513

Rocky Mountain spotted fever (RMSF) antibodies to, laboratory diagnosis and, 88
characteristics and treatment of, 156*t*–157*t*

Rofecoxib (Vioxx) indications, actions, and dosage of, 599
route, effects, and dosage for, 321*t*

Roferon-A (interferon alfa-2a), indications and dosage for, 146*t*, 554

Rogaine (minoxidil), indications, actions, and dosage of, 572

Romazicon (flumazenil)
for benzodiazepine poisoning, 471
for emergency cardiac care, 462
indications, actions, and dosage of, 540

Romberg's test, 27

Rosiglitazone (Avandia), indications, actions, and dosage of, 599–600

Roth's spots, 27

Rounds, 3–4

Roundworm infections, drugs for treating, 153*t*

Rovsing's sign, 27

Rowasa (mesalamine), indications, actions, and dosage of, 566

Roxanol (morphine)
for emergency cardiac care, 465
indications, actions, and dosage of, 573
route, effects, and dosage for, 321*t*

Roxicodone (oxycodone), indications, actions, and dosage of, 583

Rubex (doxorubicin), indications, actions, and dosage of, 531

Rufen (Ibuprofen)
indications, actions, and dosage of, 551
route, effects, and dosage for, 321*t*

"Rule of nines," for calculating extent of burns, 182*f*, 183

"Rule of sixes," for calculating fluids in children, 179, 181*t*

"Rule of thumb" method, for calculating caloric needs, 213

R wave, 369

S

Salem-sump tubes, 272

Salmeterol (Serevent), indications, actions, and dosage of, 600

Salmonella, Gram stain characteristics of, 124*f*, 127*t*

Sandimmune (cyclosporine)
half-life and therapeutic and toxic levels of, 634*t*

indications, actions, and dosage of, 521–522

Sandoglobulin (immune globulin, intravenous), indications, actions, and dosage of, 552

Sandostatin (octreotide), indications, actions, and dosage of, 580–581

Saquinavir (Fortovase), indications, actions, and dosage of, 150*t*, 600

Sarafem (fluoxetine), indications, actions, and dosage of, 541

Sarcoptes scabiei infections, drugs for treating, 154*t*

Sargramostim [GM-CSF] (Leukine; Prokine), indications, actions, and dosage of, 600

Scabies, drugs for treating, 154*t*

Scales, cutaneous, 21*t*

Scalpels, 240, 242*f*

Scalp vein needles, 280

Scars, 21*t*

Schedules of controlled substances, 475–476

Schistocytes, 104

Schlichter test, 133

Schmorl's nodes, 27

Scoliosis, 27

Scopolamine, indications, actions, and dosage of, 600

Scopolamine, transdermal (Transderm Scop), indications, actions, and dosage of, 600

Scotch tape test, 132

Scout films, 326

Screen film mammography, 326

Secobarbital (Seconal), indications, actions, and dosage of, 600

Second-degree heart block, 377–378, 379*f*

Secretion precautions, 156

Sectral (acebutolol), indications, actions, and dosage of, 488

Sedapap-10 Two-dyne (acetaminophen + butalbital +/− caffeine), indications, actions, and dosage of, 489

Sedative hypnotics, 481

Sedimentation rate, 108

Segs, 100

Seizures, 472, 473*t*

differential diagnosis of, 50

Seldinger technique, for femoral artery cannulation, 245

Selegiline (Eldepryl), indications, actions, and dosage of, 600

Selenium, in total parenteral nutrition, 232*t*

Selenium sulfide (Exsel Shampoo; Selsun Blue Shampoo; Selsun Shampoo), indications, actions, and dosage of, 600

Selsun Blue Shampoo (selenium sulfide), indications, actions, and dosage of, 600

Selsun Shampoo (selenium sulfide), indications, actions, and dosage of, 600

Semen analysis, laboratory diagnosis and, 88–89

Sengstaken-Blakemore tubes, 273

Sensitivity, definition of, 645

Sensoricaine (bupivacaine)
indications, actions, and dosage of, 507
for suturing, 349*t*

Sentinel loop, 27

Sepsis
total parenteral nutrition for, 236
total parenteral nutrition formulation for, 236
transfusions and, 202, 203

Septic arthritis
organisms responsible and empiric therapy for, 134*t*
synovial fluid interpretation and, 250, 251*t*

Septic shock, 414, 431

Septra (trimethoprim-sulfamethoxazole), indications, actions, and dosage of, 153*t*, 615

Serax (oxazepam), indications, actions, and dosage of, 583

Serentil (mesoridazine), indications, actions, and dosage of, 567

Serevent (salmeterol), indications, actions, and dosage of, 600

Seroquel (quetiapine), indications, actions, and dosage of, 596

Serratia, Gram stain characteristics of, 124*f*, 127*t*

Serratia marcescens, Gram stain characteristics of, 127*t*

Sertraline (Zoloft), indications, actions, and dosage of, 601

Serum(s), 485

Serum bactericidal level, 133

Serutan (psyllium), indications, actions, and dosage of, 596

Serzone (nefazodone), indications, actions, and dosage of, 576

Shigella, Gram stain characteristics of, 124*f,* 127*t*

Shock, 413–414, 431
    algorithm for, 460*f*

Shock lung, 429–431

Shunt fraction (Qs/Qt), 419–423, 420*f*–422*f*
    derivation and normal values for, 438*t*

Sibutramine (Meridia), indications, actions, and dosage of, 601

Sickling, 104

Sigmoidoscopy, 300–302
    complications of, 302
    indications for, 300
    materials for, 300
    procedure for, 200–201, 201*f*

Signal sentinel sign, 27

Sildenafil (Viagra), indications, actions, and dosage of, 601

Silent heart algorithm, 454*f*

Silk sutures, 347*f*

Silvadene (silver sulfadiazine), indications, actions, and dosage of, 601

Silver nitrate (Dey-Drop), indications, actions, and dosage of, 601

Silver sulfadiazine (Silvadene), indications, actions, and dosage of, 601

Simethicone (Mylicon), indications, actions, and dosage of, 601

Similac 13, 224*t*

Similac 20, 224*t*

Similac 24, 224*t*

Similac 27, 224*t*

Similac PM 60/40, 224*t*

Similac Special Care 20, 225*t*

Similac Special Care 24, 225*t*

Simple acid-base disorders, 163

Simulect (basiliximab), indications, actions, and dosage of, 502

Simvastatin (Zocor), indications, actions, and dosage of, 601

Sinemet (carbidopa + levodopa), indications, actions, and dosage of, 509–510

Sinequan (doxepin)
    half-life and therapeutic and toxic levels of, 634*t*
    indications, actions, and dosage of, 530

Single donor plasma, 199*t*

Single-photon emission computed tomography (SPECT), 335

Singulair (montelukast), indications, actions, and dosage of, 573

Singultus, differential diagnosis of, 48

Sinography, 328

Sinus arrhythmia, 372

Sinus bradycardia, 371–372, 375*f*

Sinus films, 326

Sinusitis, organisms responsible and empiric therapy for, 141*t*

Sinusoidal pattern, 276

Sinus rhythms, on electrocardiograms, 371–372, 372*f*–373*f*

Sinus tachycardia, 371, 375*f*

SI prefixes and symbols, 646

Sirolimus [rapamycin] (Rapamune), indications, actions, and dosage of, 602

Sister Mary Joseph's sign/node, 27

Skelaxin (metaxalone), indications, actions, and dosage of, 567

Skin
    innervation of, 22*f*–23*f*
    melanoma of, staging of, 654–655

Skin biopsy, 302

Skin infections, organisms responsible and empiric therapy for, 141*t*–142*t*

Skin precautions, 155

Skin staples, 252, 258*f*

Skin testing, 303–304

Skull films, 326

Slow-K (potassium chloride)
    form and dosage of, 626*t*
    indications, actions, and dosage of, 592

SMA 20, 224*t*

Small bowel follow-through (SBFT), 329

Small cells, 97, 100

SOAP, 34

Social history, 10

Sodium
  deficiency of, 185–186, 237
  excess of, 184–185
  requirement for, 178
  serum, laboratory diagnosis and, 89
  spot urine study for, 114
  total parenteral nutrition for deficiency
    of, 237
Sodium bicarbonate
  for cyclic antidepressant poisoning, 471
  for emergency cardiac care, 466
  for hyperkalemia, 187
  indications, actions, and dosage of, 602
  pediatric, for emergency cardiac care,
    466
  for renal tubular acidosis, 168t
Sodium citrate (Bicitra), indications,
    actions, and dosage of, 602
Sodium nitroprusside (Nipride;
    Nitropress)
  for emergency cardiac care, 465–466
  for hypertensive crisis, 470
  indications, actions, and dosage of, 579
  infusion guidelines for, 442t
Sodium phosphate (Fleet's Phospho-soda),
    for hypophosphatemia, 192
Sodium polystyrene sulfonate
    (Kayexalate)
  for hyperkalemia, 187
  indications, actions, and dosage of, 602
Sodium-potassium phosphate (Neutra-
    Phos)
  for hypercalcemia, 189
  for hypophosphatemia, 192
Sodium salicylate (aspirin)
  for emergency cardiac care, 461
  indications, actions, and dosage of,
    499–500
  route, effects, and dosage for, 321t
Sodium Sulamyd (sulfacetamide),
    indications, actions, and dosage of,
    605
Soft diet, mechanical, 206t
Soft tissue infections, organisms
    responsible and empiric therapy
    for, 141t–142t
Solu-Cortef (hydrocortisone)
  dose, activity, duration, and route for,
    627t
  for hypercalcemia, 189

  indications, actions, and dosage of,
    603–604
Solu-Medrol (methylprednisolone sodium
    succinate)
  dose, activity, duration, and route for,
    627t
  indications, actions, and dosage of, 603
Soma (carisoprodol), indications, actions,
    and dosage of, 510
Somatic pain, deep, 315
Somophyllin (theophylline)
  half-life and therapeutic and toxic levels
    of, 632t
  indications, actions, and dosage
    of, 609
Sonata (zaleplon), indications, actions,
    and dosage of, 619
Sorbitol
  for hyperkalemia, 187
  indications, actions, and dosage of, 602
  for poisoning, 472
Sorbitrate (isosorbide dinitrate),
    indications, actions, and dosage of,
    555–556
Soriatane (actretin), indications, actions,
    and dosage of, 488
Sotalol (Betapace), indications, actions,
    and dosage of, 602
Soy infant formulas, 224t
Specific gravity, of urine, 111
Specificity, definition of, 645
Spectazole (econazole), indications,
    actions, and dosage of, 531–532
Speculum examination
  bimanual examination, pelvic, 290
  pelvic, 290
Spermatozoa, in urine sediment, 112
Spherocytes, 104
Spinal headache, 286
Spine computed tomography, 331
Spine magnetic resonance imaging, 333
Spiral computed tomography, 331
Spirometry, incentive, 363–364
Spironolactone (Aldactone), indications,
    actions, and dosage of, 603
Splenomegaly, differential diagnosis of,
    49
Sporanox (itraconazole), indications,
    actions, and dosage of, 151t,
    556–557

Sporotrichosis, systemic drug for treating, 152*t*

Spot urine studies, 114–115

Sputum, Gram stain of, 122

Sputum culture, 130

Square knots, 355*f*, 356*f*

Stab cells, 100

Stadol (butorphanol), indications, actions, and dosage of, 507

Staining techniques, 121–128

Stainless steel sutures, 347*t*

Staphylococcus, Gram stain characteristics of, 123*f*, 125*t*

Staphylococcus agalactiae, Gram stain characteristics of, 125*t*

Staphylococcus aureus, Gram stain characteristics of, 123*f*, 125*t*

Staphylococcus epidermidis, Gram stain characteristics of, 123*f*, 125*t*

Staphylococcus saphrophyticus, Gram stain characteristics of, 123*f*, 125*t*

Staples, skin, 252, 258*f*

Startle reflex, 26

Staticin Topical (erythromycin, topical), indications, actions, and dosage of, 534

Status epilepticus, 472, 473*t*

Stavudine (Zerit), indications, actions, and dosage of, 603

Stelazine (trifluoperazine), indications, actions, and dosage of, 614

Stellwag's sign, 27

Stentrophomonas maltophilia, Gram stain characteristics of, 127*t*

Sterile technique, 339

Steroids, systemic. *See also specific steroids*

  dose, activity, duration, and route for, 627*t*

  indications, actions, and dosage of, 603–604

Steroids, topical. *See also specific steroids*

  indications, actions, and dosage of, 604

  potency and application of, 628*t*–630*t*

Stimate (desmopressin), indications, actions, and dosage of, 524

Stomach cancer, staging of, 656

Stool cultures, 130–131

Stool for occult blood, laboratory diagnosis and, 89

Stool for ova and parasites, 131

Stool leukocyte stain, 128

Straight-leg-raising sign, 26

Strep screen, 131

Streptase (streptokinase)

  for emergency cardiac care, 466

  indications, actions, and dosage of, 604

Streptococcus, Gram stain characteristics of, 123*f*, 125*t*

Streptococcus agalactiae, Gram stain characteristics of, 123*f*

Streptococcus bovis, Gram stain characteristics of, 125*t*

Streptococcus faecalis, Gram stain characteristics of, 125*t*

Streptococcus mutans, Gram stain characteristics of, 123*f*

Streptococcus pneumoniae, Gram stain characteristics of, 123*f*, 125*t*

Streptococcus pyogenes, Gram stain characteristics of, 123*f*, 125*t*

Streptococcus viridans, Gram stain characteristics of, 125*t*

Streptokinase (Kabikinase; Streptase)

  for emergency cardiac care, 466

  indications, actions, and dosage of, 604

Streptomycin, indications, actions, and dosage of, 604

Streptozocin (Zanosar), indications, actions, and dosage of, 604

Streptozyme, laboratory diagnosis and, 57

Stress ulcers, 433

Strict isolation, 155

Stroke volume, measurement of, 408, 410

Strongyloidiasis, drugs for treating, 154*t*

Strontium-89, 334

Subacute bacterial endocarditis (SBE), prophylaxis of, 155, 158*t*–159*t*

Subarachnoid hemorrhage, 286

  cerebrospinal fluid in, 288*t*

Subcutaneous injections, 276, 277

Sublimaze (fentanyl)

  indications, actions, and dosage of, 538

  route, effects, and dosage for, 321*t*

Succimer (Chemet), indications, actions, and dosage of, 604–605

Succinylcholine (Anectine; Quelicin; Sucostrin), indications, actions, and dosage of, 605

Sucostrin (succinylcholine), indications, actions, and dosage of, 605

Sucralfate (Sufenta), indications, actions, and dosage of, 605

Sudafed (pseudoephedrine), indications, actions, and dosage of, 595–596

Sudan stain, of pleural fluid, 299*t*

Sufenta (sucralfate), indications, actions, and dosage of, 605

Sular (nisoldipine), indications, actions, and dosage of, 579

Sulfacetamide (Bleph-10; Cetamide; Sodium Sulamyd), indications, actions, and dosage of, 605

Sulfacetamide + prednisolone (Blephamide), indications, actions, and dosage of, 605

Sulfadiazine, indications for, 154*t*

Sulfasalazine (Azulfidine), indications, actions, and dosage of, 605–606

Sulfinpyrazone (Anturane), indications, actions, and dosage of, 606

Sulindac (Clinoril), indications, actions, and dosage of, 606

Sumatriptan (Imitrex), indications, actions, and dosage of, 606

Sumycin (tetracycline)
    indications, actions, and dosage of, 153*t*, 609
    interaction with enteral nutrition, 223

Superchar (activated charcoal)
    clinical use of, 472
    indications, actions, and dosage of, 514

Superficial pain, 315

Suprapubic bladder aspiration, percutaneous, 309, 310*f*

Supraventricular tachycardia algorithms
    for narrow complex SVT, 457*f*
    for stable SVT, 458*f*

Suprax (cefixime), indications, actions, and dosage of, 511

Surfak (docusate calcium), indications, actions, and dosage of, 529

Surgery, nutritional support following, 223

Surgical cricothyrotomy, 263–264

Surgical hand scrub, 340–341

Surmontil (trimipramine), indications, actions, and dosage of, 615

Survanta (beractant), indications, actions, and dosage of, 504

Susceptibility testing, microbiologic, 133

Sus-Phrine. *See* Epinephrine (Adrenalin; Sus-Phrine)

Sustiva (efavirenz), indications, actions, and dosage of, 532

Suturing, 345–358
    materials for, 345, 346*t*–347*t*
    patterns for, 348, 350, 351*f*–354*f*
    procedure for, 345, 348, 349*t*, 350*t*
    surgical knots for, 350, 355*f*–357*f*
    suture removal and, 350, 353, 358*f*

Swan-Ganz catheters, 399–402, 401*f*, 402*f*

S wave, 369

Sweat chloride, laboratory diagnosis and, 89–90

Symmetrel (amantadine), indications, actions, and dosage of, 148*t*, 494

Sympathetic nervous system, 395, 397, 397*t*, 398*t*

Sympathomimetic drugs, actions of, 398*t*

Synalar (fluocinolone acetonide), potency and application of, 628*t*, 629*t*

Synalar-HP (fluocinolone acetonide), potency and application of, 628*t*, 629*t*

Synchronous intermittent mandatory ventilation (SIMV), 424, 425*f*

Syncope, differential diagnosis of, 51

Synercid (quinupristin + dalfopristin), indications, actions, and dosage of, 597

Synovial fluid, interpretation of, 249–250, 251*t*

Synthroid (levothyroxine), indications, actions, and dosage of, 560–561

Syntocinon (oxytocin), indications, actions, and dosage of, 584

Syphilis, organism responsible and empiric therapy for, 143*t*

Systemic inflammatory response syndrome (SIRS), 414

Systemic vascular resistance (SVR), derivation and normal values for, 437*t*

Systolic heart murmurs, 393–394

Systolic hypertension, 392

T

Tabloid (6-thioguanine), indications, actions, and dosage of, 609

Tachycardia, 276, 371
    algorithm for, 456*f*

Tacrine (Cognex), indications, actions, and dosage of, 606

Tacrolimus [FK 506] (Prograf), indications, actions, and dosage of, 606

Taenia saginata infections, drugs for treating, 154*t*

Taenia solium infections, drugs for treating, 154*t*

Tagamet (cimetidine), indications, actions, and dosage of, 516

Talwin (pentazocine), indications, actions, and dosage of, 586–587

Tambocor (flecainide)
half-life and therapeutic and toxic levels of, 633*t*
indications, actions, and dosage of, 539

Tamiflu (oseltamivir), indications, actions, and dosage of, 147*t*, 582

Tamoxifen (Nolvadex), indications, actions, and dosage of, 606–607

Tamsulosin (Flomax), indications, actions, and dosage of, 607

Tapazole (methimazole), indications, actions, and dosage of, 568

Tapeworms, drugs for treating, 154*t*

Target cells, 104

Tavist (clemastine fumarate), indications, actions, and dosage of, 518

Taxol (paclitaxel), indications, actions, and dosage of, 584

Taxotere (docetaxel), indications, actions, and dosage of, 529

Tazarotene (Tazorac), indications, actions, and dosage of, 607

Tazicef (ceftazidime), indications, actions, and dosage of, 513

Tazidime (ceftazidime), indications, actions, and dosage of, 513

Tazorac (tazarotene), indications, actions, and dosage of, 607

Teamwork, 2

Tears Naturale (artificial tears), indications, actions, and dosage of, 499

Technetium-99-labeled red cell scans, 333

Technetium-99m DMSA (dimercaptosuccinic acid), 334

Technetium-99m DTPA (diethylenetriamine pentaacetic acid), 334

Technetium-99m glucoheptonate, 334

Technetium-99m mercaptoacetylthiglycine (MAG3), 334

Technetium-99m pyrophosphate cardiac scans, 333

Technetium-99m sulfur colloid scans, 333

Technetium-99m ventriculography, 333–334

Teeth
emergencies involving, 470
eruption of, 17, 19*f*

Tegopen (cloxacillin), indications, actions, and dosage of, 519

Tegretol (carbamazepine)
half-life and therapeutic and toxic levels of, 631*t*
indications, actions, and dosage of, 509
route, effects, and dosage for, 322*t*

Telangiectasia, 21*t*

Telmisartan (Micardis), indications, actions, and dosage of, 607

Temazepam (Restoril), indications, actions, and dosage of, 607

Temovate (clobetasol propionate), potency and application of, 628*t*

Temperature conversion, 646, 649*t*

Tenecteplase (Tnkase), indications, actions, and dosage of, 607

Tenex (guanfacine), indications, actions, and dosage of, 547

Teniposide [VM-26] (Vumon), indications, actions, and dosage of, 607–608

Tenoretic (atenolol + chlorthalidone), indications, actions, and dosage of, 500

Tenormin (atenolol)
for emergency cardiac care, 462
indications, actions, and dosage of, 500

Tensilon (edrophonium), indications, actions, and dosage of, 532

Tequin (gatifloxacin), indications, actions, and dosage of, 544

Terazol (terconazole), indications, actions, and dosage of, 608

Terazosin (Hytrin), indications, actions, and dosage of, 608

Terbinafine (Lamisil), indications, actions, and dosage of, 608

Terbutaline (Brethine; Bricanyl), indications, actions, and dosage of, 608

Terconazole (Terazol), indications, actions, and dosage of, 608

TESPA (triethylenetriphosphoramide), indications, actions, and dosage of, 614

Testosterone, laboratory diagnosis and, 90

Tetanus immune globulin, indications, actions, and dosage of, 608

Tetanus prophylaxis, 350t

Tetanus toxoid, indications, actions, and dosage of, 608–609

Tetracycline (Achromycin V; Sumycin) indications, actions, and dosage of, 153t, 477, 609
   interaction with enteral nutrition, 223

Teveten (eprosartan), indications, actions, and dosage of, 533

Thallium-201 cardiac scans, 333

Thayer-Martin medium, 129, 291

Theophylline (Somophyllin; Theo-Dur; Theolair)
   half-life and therapeutic and toxic levels of, 632t
   indications, actions, and dosage of, 609

Thera Cys (BCG [bacillus Calmette-Guérin]), indications, actions, and dosage of, 503

Therapeutic apheresis, 194

Thermal dilution technique, for cardiac output determination, 410

Thermistor, of Swan-Ganz catheter, 400

Thermography, for pain evaluation, 319

Thiabendazole, indications for, 153t

Thiamine [vitamin B₁]
   indications, actions, and dosage of, 609
   for seizures, 472
   in total parenteral nutrition, 231t

Thiethylperazine (Torecan), indications, actions, and dosage of, 609

6-Thioguanine [6-TG] (Tabloid), indications, actions, and dosage of, 609

Thioridazine (Mellaril), indications, actions, and dosage of, 609–610

Thio-Tepa (triethylenetriphosphoramide), indications, actions, and dosage of, 614

Thiothixene (Navane), indications, actions, and dosage of, 610

Third-degree heart block, 378–379

Third heart sound (S₃), 17t

Thoracentesis, 304–306
   complications of, 306
   contraindications to, 304
   differential diagnosis of pleural fluid and, 299t, 306
   indications for, 304
   materials for, 304
   procedure for, 305f, 305–306

Thoracic catheters, 261

Thoracostomy, closed (tube). See Chest tube placement

Thorazine (chlorpromazine), indications, actions, and dosage of, 515

Three-cell differential count, 97, 100

Throat cultures, 131

Thrombin time, 108

Through-and-through technique, for arterial line placement, 244

Thyrocalcitonin, laboratory diagnosis and, 61

Thyroglobulin, laboratory diagnosis and, 90

Thyroid agents, 482

Thyroid cancer, staging of, 656–657

Thyroid scans, 335

Thyroid-stimulating hormone (TSH), laboratory diagnosis and, 90

Thyroid ultrasound, 330

Thyroxine, laboratory diagnosis and, 90–91

Thyroxine-binding globulin (TBG), laboratory diagnosis and, 91

Thyroxine-binding globulin ratio, laboratory diagnosis and, 90

Thyroxine index, free (FTI), laboratory diagnosis and, 91

Tiagabine (Gabitril), indications, actions, and dosage of, 610

Tiazac (diltiazem)
for emergency cardiac care, 462
indications, actions, and dosage of, 528
infusion guidelines for, 439*t*
TIBC (iron-binding capacity, total),
laboratory diagnosis and, 78
Ticarcillin (Ticar), indications, actions,
and dosage of, 610
Ticarcillin + potassium clavulanate
(Timentin), indications, actions,
and dosage of, 610
TICE (BCG [bacillus Calmette-Guérin]),
indications, actions, and dosage of,
503
Tick-borne diseases. *See also specific
diseases*
characteristics and treatment of,
156*t*–157*t*
Ticlodipine (Ticlid), indications, actions,
and dosage of, 610
Tidal volume (TV), 360, 361*t*, 415
Tigan (trimethobenzamide), indications,
actions, and dosage of, 615
Tilade (nedocromil), indications, actions,
and dosage of, 576
Timed hand scrubs, 340–341
Time management, 6–7
Timentin (ticarcillin + potassium
clavulanate), indications, actions,
and dosage of, 610
Timolol (Blocadren), indications, actions,
and dosage of, 610
Timolol, ophthalmic (Timoptic),
indications, actions, and dosage of,
611
Tinactin (tolnaftate), indications, actions,
and dosage of, 612
Tinea capitis, organisms responsible and
empiric therapy for, 142*t*
Tinea corporis, organisms responsible and
empiric therapy for, 142*t*
Tinea unguium, organisms responsible and
empiric therapy for, 142*t*
Tinel's sign, 27
Tine test, 303
Tinidazole, indications for, 153*t*, 154*t*
Tioconazole (Vagistat), indications,
actions, and dosage of, 611
Tirofiban (Aggrastat)
for emergency cardiac care, 464

indications, actions, and dosage of, 611
Tissue adhesives, 358
^{201}Tl cardiac scans, 333
Tnkase (tenecteplase), indications,
actions, and dosage of, 607
TNM classification system, 646, 649–658
Tobradex (tobramycin + dexamethasone,
ophthalmic), indications, actions,
and dosage of, 611
Tobramycin (Nebcin)
half-life and therapeutic and toxic levels
of, 631*t*
indications, actions, and dosage
of, 611
Tobramycin + dexamethasone, ophthalmic
(Tobradex), indications, actions,
and dosage of, 611
Tobramycin, ophthalmic (AK Tob;
Tobrex), indications, actions, and
dosage of, 611
Tobrex (tobramycin, ophthalmic),
indications, actions, and dosage of,
611
Tocainide (Tonocard), indications, actions,
and dosage of, 611
α Tocopherol, in total parenteral nutrition,
231*t*
Tofranil (imipramine), indications,
actions, and dosage of, 552
Tolazamide (Tolinase), indications,
actions, and dosage of, 611
Tolazoline (Priscoline), indications,
actions, and dosage of, 612
Tolbutamide (Orinase), indications,
actions, and dosage of, 612
Tolectin (tolmetin), indications, actions,
and dosage of, 612
Tolinase (tolazamide), indications, actions,
and dosage of, 611
Tolmetin (Tolectin), indications, actions,
and dosage of, 612
Tolnaftate (Tinactin), indications, actions,
and dosage of, 612
Tolterodine (Detrol; Detrol LA),
indications, actions, and dosage of,
612
Tonocard (tocainide), indications, actions,
and dosage of, 611
Toothaches, 470
Tooth emergencies, 470

Topamax (topiramate), indications, actions, and dosage of, 612

Topicort (desoximetasone), potency and application of, 628t

Topiramate (Topamax), indications, actions, and dosage of, 612

Topotecan (Hycamtin), indications, actions, and dosage of, 612

Toprol XL (metoprolol)
for emergency cardiac care, 462
indications, actions, and dosage of, 569

Toradol (ketorolac), indications, actions, and dosage of, 557

Torch battery, laboratory diagnosis and, 91

Torecan (thiethylperazine), indications, actions, and dosage of, 609

Tornalate (bitolterol), indications, actions, and dosage of, 505

Torsemide (Demadex), indications, actions, and dosage of, 613

Total blood volume, 177

Total body water, 177

Total CO_2, laboratory diagnosis and, 59, 61–62

Total lung capacity (TLC), 360, 361t

Total parenteral nutrition (TPN), 227–237, 434
additives for, 231t, 231–232, 232t
assessing, 234
calculation of caloric requirements in stressed patients and, 228
complications of, 236–237
disease-specific formulations for, 235–236
fat emulsions for, 232–233
indications for, 227
nitrogen balance and, 229
nutritional components in, 228
peripheral, 230–231
solutions for, 229–230, 230t
starting, 233–234
stopping, 234

Toxic granulation, of white blood cells, 104

Toxocara canis infections, drugs for treating, 154t

Toxoids, 485

Toxoplasma gondii infections, drugs for treating, 154t

Toxoplasmosis, drugs for treating, 154t

Trace elements, for total parenteral nutrition, 231, 232t

Tracrium (atracurium), indications, actions, and dosage of, 501

Tramadol (Ultram), indications, actions, and dosage of, 613

Trandate (labetalol)
for emergency cardiac care, 462
for hypertensive crisis, 470
indications, actions, and dosage of, 557
infusion guidelines for, 441t

Trandolapril (Mavik), indications, actions, and dosage of, 613

Transcutaneous electrical nerve stimulation (TENS), 323

Transcutaneous pacing, 468

Transderm-Nitro (nitroglycerin)
for emergency cardiac care, 465
indications, actions, and dosage of, 579

Transderm Scop (scopolamine, transdermal), indications, actions, and dosage of, 600

Transferrin, laboratory diagnosis and, 91

Transfusion reactions, 202–203

Transfusion therapy. *See* Blood component therapy

Transgrow medium, 129

Transrectal ultrasound, 330

Transtracheal aspirate, 130

Transudative ascites, 297

Tranxene (clorazepate), indications, actions, and dosage of, 519

Trasylol (aprotinin), indications, actions, and dosage of, 499

Traube's sign, 27

Trauma, total parenteral nutrition formulation for, 236

Traumatic tap, 286
cerebrospinal fluid in, 288t

Trazodone (Desyrel)
half-life and therapeutic and toxic levels of, 634t
indications, actions, and dosage of, 613

Tremors, differential diagnosis of, 51

Trendelenburg's test, 27

Trental (pentoxifylline), indications, actions, and dosage of, 587

Tretinoin, systemic [retinoic acid] (Vesanoid), indications, actions, and dosage of, 613

Tretinoin, topical [retinoic acid] (Avita; Retin-A), indications, actions, and dosage of, 613

Triamcinolone acetonide (Aristocort; Kenalog), potency and application of, 630*t*

Triamcinolone + nystatin (Mycolog-II), indications, actions, and dosage of, 613

Triamterene (Dyrenium), indications, actions, and dosage of, 613–614

Triapin Axocet (acetaminophen + butalbital +/- caffeine), indications, actions, and dosage of, 489

Triazolam (Halcion), indications, actions, and dosage of, 614

Trichinosis, drugs for treating, 154*t*

Trichomonas infection
  drugs for treating, 154*t*
  organism responsible and empiric therapy for, 145*t*
  test for, 291
  vaginal, 145*t*, 291

Trichostrongylus colubriformis infections, drugs for treating, 154*t*

Trichuriasis, drugs for treating, 154*t*

Tricor (fenofibrate), indications, actions, and dosage of, 537

Tricuspid insufficiency (TI), 16*t*

Tridil (nitroglycerin), infusion guidelines for, 442*t*

Triethanolamine (Cerumenex), indications, actions, and dosage of, 614

Triethylenetriphosphoramide (TESPA; Thio-Tepa; TSPA), indications, actions, and dosage of, 614

Trifluoperazine (Stelazine), indications, actions, and dosage of, 614

Trifluridine (Viroptic), indications, actions, and dosage of, 147*t*, 614

Trigeminy, 375

Triglycerides
  laboratory diagnosis and, 91–92
  in pleural fluid, 299*t*

Trihexyphenidyl (Artane), indications, actions, and dosage of, 614

Triiodothyronine (T₃ RIA), laboratory diagnosis and, 92

Trilafon (perphenazine), indications, actions, and dosage of, 588

Trileptal (oxcarbazepine), indications, actions, and dosage of, 583

Tri-Levlen 21, 28, 625*t*

Trimethobenzamide (Tigan), indications, actions, and dosage of, 615

Trimethoprim (Proloprim; Trimpex), indications, actions, and dosage of, 615

Trimethoprim-sulfamethoxazole [co-trimoxazole] (Bactrim; Septra), indications, actions, and dosage of, 153*t*, 615

Trimetrexate (Neutrexin), indications, actions, and dosage of, 615

Trimipramine (Surmontil), indications, actions, and dosage of, 615

Trimpex (trimethoprim), indications, actions, and dosage of, 615

Tri-Norinyl 21, 28, 625*t*

Triphasil-21, 625*t*

Trivora-28, 625*t*

Troponin, cardiac-specific, laboratory diagnosis and, 92

Trousseau's sign, 27

T₃ RU, laboratory diagnosis and, 90

Trusopt (dorzolamide), indications, actions, and dosage of, 530

Trypanosoma cruzi infections, drugs for treating, 154*t*

Trypanosomiasis, drugs for treating, 154*t*

TSPA (triethylenetriphosphoramide), indications, actions, and dosage of, 614

T₄ total, laboratory diagnosis and, 90–91

T-tube cholangiography, 329

Tube feeding, 213, 214–223
  complications of, 218, 223
  contraindications to, 214*t*
  enteral products for, 214, 215*t*–216*t*, 217
  initiating, 217–218, 218*t*–222*t*

Tuberculin skin testing (TST), 303–304

Tuberculosis, organism responsible and empiric therapy for, 143*t*

Tube thoracostomy. *See* Chest tube placement

Tubular casts, in urine sediment, 114

Tucks Pads (witch hazel), indications, actions, and dosage of, 618
Tumors. *See* Malignancies; Neoplasms
Tums (calcium carbonate)
  for hypocalcemia, 190
  indications, actions, and dosage of, 508
Turner's sign, 27
T wave, 369
24-hour urine studies, 116–118
Twin-K (potassium citrate + potassium gluconate), form and dosage of, 626t
Two-dimensional echocardiography, 330
Tycron (polyester) sutures, 347t
Tylenol (acetaminophen)
  antidote for, 471
  indications, actions, and dosage of, 488, 621t
  route, effects, and dosage for, 321t
Tylenol No. 1, No. 2, No. 4 (acetaminophen + codeine), indications, actions, and dosage of, 489
Tylox (oxycodone + acetaminophen), indications, actions, and dosage of, 583–584
Tzanck smear, 128

U
Ulcers
  cutaneous, 21t
  gastrointestinal, organism responsible and empiric therapy for, 144t
  stress, 433
Ultracef (cefadroxil)
  indications, actions, and dosage of, 511
  for subacute bacterial endocarditis prophylaxis, 158t
Ultralente, onset, peak, and duration of effect of, 622t
Ultram (tramadol), indications, actions, and dosage of, 613
Ultrase (pancreatin + pancrelipase), indications, actions, and dosage of, 585
Ultrasound, 329–330
Ultravate (halobetasol), potency and application of, 629t

Unasyn (ampicillin-sulbactam), indications, actions, and dosage of, 497
Univasc (moexipril), indications, actions, and dosage of, 573
Universal/international advanced cardiac life support algorithm, 450f
Universal Pedi-Packs, 197t
Universal precautions, 239–240, 344
Upper gastrointestinal (UGI) series, 329
Urate, laboratory diagnosis and, 92
Urecholine (bethanechol), indications, actions, and dosage of, 504–505
Urethritis
  organism responsible and empiric therapy for, 135t
  organisms responsible and empiric therapy for, 143t–144t
Urex (methenamine), indications, actions, and dosage of, 568
Uric acid, laboratory diagnosis and, 92
Urinalysis
  differential diagnosis for, 110–112
  normal values for, 110
  procedure for, 109–110
Urinary agents, 487
Urinary incontinence, differential diagnosis of, 48
Urinary tract infections, organisms responsible and empiric therapy for, 143t–144t
Urine
  bilirubin in, 111
  blood in, 111
  clean catch specimens of, 308–309
  color of, 110
  glucose in, 111
  in-and-out catheterized, 308
  ketones in, 111
  leukocyte esterase in, 112
  nitrite in, 111
  output of, 119
  pH of, 110–111
  protein electrophoresis of, 119
  protein in, 112
  reducing substances in, 112
  specific gravity of, 111
  urobilinogen in, 112
Urine cultures, 131–132
Urine sediment, 112, 113f, 114

Urine studies, 109–119
  creatinine and creatinine clearance,
    115–116
  drug abuse screen, 118
  indices useful in diagnosing oliguria,
    119*t*
  spot (random), 114–115
  24-hour, 116–118
  urinalysis, 109–112
  urine sediment, 112, 113*f*, 114
  xylose tolerance test, 118–119
Urispas (flavoxate), indications, actions,
    and dosage of, 539
Urobilinogen, in urine, 112
Urocit-K (potassium citrate), indications,
    actions, and dosage of,
    590–591
Urokinase (Abbokinase), indications,
    actions, and dosage of, 615
Uterine cancer, staging of, 657
UUN levels, 228

V

Vaccines, 485
Vacutainer system, 313
  tubes for, 311*t*–312*t*
Vaginal bleeding, differential diagnosis of,
    51
Vaginal candidiasis
  organisms responsible and empiric
    therapy for, 144*t*
  systemic drugs for treating, 151*t*
Vaginal discharge, differential diagnosis
    of, 51
Vaginal infections
  organisms responsible and empiric
    therapy for, 144*t*–145*t*
  tests for, 291
Vaginal preparations, 485
Vaginal saline (wet) preparation, 291
Vaginosis, bacterial, organism responsible
    and empiric therapy for, 145*t*
Vagistat (tioconazole), indications,
    actions, and dosage of, 611
Valacyclovir (Valtrex), indications,
    actions, and dosage of, 147*t*, 148*t*,
    616
Valisone (betamethasone valerate),
    potency and application of, 628*t*

Valium (diazepam)
  indications, actions, and dosage of,
    525–526
  for seizures, 472, 473*t*
Valproic acid (Depakene)
  half-life and therapeutic and toxic levels
    of, 632*t*
  indications, actions, and dosage of, 616
Valrubicin (Valstar), indications, actions,
    and dosage of, 616
Valsartan (Diovan), indications, actions,
    and dosage of, 616
Valstar (valrubicin), indications, actions,
    and dosage of, 616
Valtrex (valacyclovir), indications, actions,
    and dosage of, 147*t*, 148*t*, 616
Valvular heart disease, anticoagulant
    standard of practice for, 637*t*
Vancenase Nasal Inhaler
    (beclomethasone), indications,
    actions, and dosage of, 503
Vancomycin (Vancocin; Vancoled)
  half-life and therapeutic and toxic levels
    of, 631*t*
  indications, actions, and dosage of, 616
  for subacute bacterial endocarditis
    prophylaxis, 159*t*
Vanillylmandelic acid, in urine, 118
Vantin (cefpodoxime), indications,
    actions, and dosage of, 512
Vaqta (hepatitis A vaccine), indications,
    actions, and dosage of, 548
Variable decelerations, in fetal heart rate,
    276
Varicella, drugs of choice for treating,
    148*t*
Varicella immune globulin (VZIG),
    indications and dosage for, 148*t*
Varicella virus vaccine (Varivax),
    indications, actions, and dosage of,
    616
Varicella zoster virus (VZV)
  cultures for, 132
  drugs of choice for treating infections
    by, 148*t*–149*t*
Varivax (varicella virus vaccine),
    indications, actions, and dosage of,
    616
Vascar (bepridil), indications, actions, and
    dosage of, 504

Vascular catheters. *See also* Central venous catheterization; Peripherally inserted central catheter (PICC) lines; Pulmonary artery catheters
sepsis of, 435
Vasodilators, 480
Vasopressin [antidiuretic hormone] (Pitressin)
indications, actions, and dosage of, 617
infusion guidelines for, 443*t*
Vasotec (enalapril)
for emergency cardiac care, 449
indications, actions, and dosage of, 532
Vasoxyl (methoxamine), indications, actions, and dosage of, 568–569
Vecuronium (Norcuron), indications, actions, and dosage of, 617
Veetids (penicillin V), indications, actions, and dosage of, 585
Veillonella, Gram stain characteristics of, 125*t*
Velban (vinblastine), indications, actions, and dosage of, 617
Velbe (vinblastine), indications, actions, and dosage of, 617
Velosef (cephradine), indications, actions, and dosage of, 514
Velosulin, onset, peak, and duration of effect of, 622*t*
Venereal Disease Research Laboratory (VDRL) test, 92
Venipuncture, 309–314
materials for, 309, 311*t*–312*t*
procedure for, 310, 313–314
Venlafaxine (Effexor), indications, actions, and dosage of, 617
Venography, peripheral, 329
Venous oxygen saturation (S_{VO2}), for cardiac output determination, 412, 413*f*
Ventilation, 414–416, 415*f*–417*f*
mechanical. *See* Mechanical ventilation
Ventolin (albuterol), 364
for anaphylaxis, 469
indications, actions, and dosage of, 490
nebulized, for asthmatic attacks, 469
Ventricular arrhythmias, on electrocardiograms, 375–377, 376*f*–378*f*

Ventricular fibrillation, 377, 378*f*
algorithm for, 452*f*
Ventricular septal defect (VSD), 17*t*
Ventricular tachycardia, 376–377, 378*f*
algorithm for, 452*f*
Ventriculography, technetium-99m, 333–334
Vepesid (etoposide), indications, actions, and dosage of, 537
Verapamil (Calan; Isoptin)
for emergency cardiac care, 467
indications, actions, and dosage of, 617
Versed (midazolam)
indications, actions, and dosage of, 571
for seizures, 472
Vertebral radiography, 326
Vertigo, differential diagnosis of, 51
Vesanoid (tretinoin, systemic), indications, actions, and dosage of, 613
Vesicles, 21*t*
Vexol Ophthalmic (rimexolone), indications, actions, and dosage of, 597–598
Viadar, 559
Viagra (sildenafil), indications, actions, and dosage of, 601
Vibramycin (doxycycline), indications, actions, and dosage of, 153*t*, 531
Vibrio cholerae, Gram stain characteristics of, 127*t*
Vicodin (hydrocodone + acetaminophen), indications, actions, and dosage of, 549
Vicoprofen (hydrocodone + ibuprofen), indications, actions, and dosage of, 550
Vicryl Rapide (polyglycolic acid 910) sutures, 346*t*
Vicryl (polyglactin 910) sutures, 346*t*
Videx (didanosine), indications, actions, and dosage of, 526–527
Vinblastine (Velban; Velbe), indications, actions, and dosage of, 617
Vincasar PFS (vincristine), indications, actions, and dosage of, 617–618
Vincristine (Oncovin; Vincasar PFS), indications, actions, and dosage of, 617–618
Vinorelbine (Navelbine), indications, actions, and dosage of, 618

Vioxx (rofecoxib)
  indications, actions, and dosage of, 599
  route, effects, and dosage for, 321*t*
Viracept (nelfinavir), indications, actions,
    and dosage of, 150*t*, 576
Viral cultures and serology, 132
Viral infections. *See also specific*
    infections
  cerebrospinal fluid in, 287*t*
  pathogens and drugs of choice for
    treating, 146*t*–149*t*
Viramune (nevirapine), indications,
    actions, and dosage of, 577
Virazole (ribavirin), indications, actions,
    and dosage of, 146*t*, 148*t*, 598
Virchow's node, 27
Viroptic (trifluridine), indications, actions,
    and dosage of, 147*t*, 614
Visceral larva migrans, drugs for treating,
    154*t*
Visceral pain, 316
Visken (pindolol), indications, actions,
    and dosage of, 589
Vistaril (hydroxyzine), indications,
    actions, and dosage of, 551
Vistide (cidofovir), indications, actions,
    and dosage of, 146*t*, 516
Visual Analogue Scale (VAS), 319
Vital capacity (VC), 361, 361*t*, 416, 416*f*
Vitamin(s), for total parenteral nutrition,
    231, 231*t*
Vitamin A, in total parenteral nutrition,
    231*t*
Vitamin B₁
  indications, actions, and dosage of, 609
  for seizures, 472
  in total parenteral nutrition, 231*t*
Vitamin B₆
  indications, actions, and dosage of, 596
  in total parenteral nutrition, 231*t*
Vitamin B₁₂
  blood level of, laboratory diagnosis and,
    92–93
  indications, actions, and dosage of, 521
  laboratory diagnosis and, 92–93
  in total parenteral nutrition, 231*t*
Vitamin C, in total parenteral nutrition,
    231*t*
Vitamin D
  deficiency of, hypocalcemia and, 189

  indications, actions, and dosage of, 516
  intoxication by, hypercalcemia with,
    188
  in total parenteral nutrition, 231*t*
Vitamin E, in total parenteral nutrition,
    231*t*
Vitamin K
  indications, actions, and dosage of, 589
  in total parenteral nutrition, 231
Vitrasert (ganciclovir), indications,
    actions, and dosage of, 146*t*,
    543–544
Vitravene (fomivirsen), indications and
    dosage for, 146*t*
Vitrobacter, Gram stain characteristics of,
    126*t*
Vivonex tubes, 273
Voiding cystourethrography (VCUG), 329
Voltaren (diclofenac)
  indications, actions, and dosage of, 526
  route, effects, and dosage for, 321*t*
Volume expanders, 484
Volume limited ventilators, 423
Volume overload, transfusions and, 202,
    203
Vomiting, differential diagnosis of, 49
von Graefe's sign, 27
V/Q scans, 334
Vumon (teniposide), indications, actions,
    and dosage of, 607–608

W

Warfarin (Coumadin)
  indications, actions, and dosage of, 618
  interaction with enteral nutrition, 223
Washed red blood cells, 197*t*
Water balance, 177–178
Water loss, hypernatremia and, 184–185
Waxy casts, in urine sediment, 114
Wayson stain, 128
Weaning, from mechanical ventilation,
    427–429, 428*t*
Weber-Rinne test, 27
Weight conversion, 658, 658*t*
Weight loss, differential diagnosis of, 52
Welchol (colesevelam), indications,
    actions, and dosage of, 520
Wellbutrin (bupropion), indications,
    actions, and dosage of, 507

Wellcovorin (leucovorin), indications, actions, and dosage of, 559

Wenckebach heart block, 377–378, 379f

Westcort (hydrocortisone valerate), potency and application of, 629t

Whaid's maneuver, 280

Wheals, 21t

Wheezing, differential diagnosis of, 52

Whipple's triad, 27

White blood cell(s) (WBCs)
  differential, 96–97, 97t
  morphologic changes in, 104
  three-cell differential count, 97, 100
  transfusions of, 201
  in urine sediment, 112

White blood cell (WBC) casts, in urine sediment, 114

Whole blood, for transfusion, 197t

Witch hazel (Tucks Pads), indications, actions, and dosage of, 618

Wolff-Parkinson-White syndrome, on electrocardiograms, 388, 388f

Wound care, medications for, 487

Wound healing, 345

Wound precautions, 155

Wright's stain, 95, 96

Wrist, arthrocentesis of, 248, 249f

Written history and physical, 5
  example of, 28–32

Wuchereria bancrofti infections, drugs for treating, 153t

Wycillin (penicillin G procaine), indications, actions, and dosage of, 585

Wytensin (guanabenz), indications, actions, and dosage of, 546–547

X

Xalatan (latanoprost), indications, actions, and dosage of, 558

Xanax (alprazolam), indications, actions, and dosage of, 492

Xanthochromia, 286

Xanthomonas maltophilia, Gram stain characteristics of, 127t

Xeromammography, 326

Xopenex (levalbuterol), indications, actions, and dosage of, 559

X-ray studies
  contrast, 326–329
  noncontrast, 325–326, 335–338

Xylocaine. *See* Lidocaine (Anestacon Topical; Xylocaine)

Xyvox (linezolid), indications, actions, and dosage of, 561

Y

Yeast, in urine sediment, 112

Yersinia enterocolitica, Gram stain characteristics of, 127t

Yersinia pestis, Gram stain characteristics of, 127t

Z

Zafirlukast (Accolate), indications, actions, and dosage of, 619

Zalcitabine (Hivid), indications, actions, and dosage of, 619

Zaleplon (Sonata), indications, actions, and dosage of, 619

Zanamivir (Relenza), indications, actions, and dosage of, 147t, 619

Zanosar (streptozocin), indications, actions, and dosage of, 604

Zantac (ranitidine)
  for anaphylaxis, 469
  indications, actions, and dosage of, 597

Zarontin (ethosuximide)
  half-life and therapeutic and toxic levels of, 631t
  indications, actions, and dosage of, 536

Zaroxolyn (metolazone), indications, actions, and dosage of, 569

Zebeta (bisoprolol), indications, actions, and dosage of, 505

Zefazone (cefmetazole), indications, actions, and dosage of, 511

Zenapax (dacliximab), indications, actions, and dosage of, 522

Zerit (stavudine), indications, actions, and dosage of, 603

Zestril (lisinopril)
  for emergency cardiac care, 461
  indications, actions, and dosage of, 562

Ziagen (abacavir), indications, actions, and dosage of, 488

Zidovudine (Retrovir), indications, actions, and dosage of, 619

Zidovudine + lamivudine (Combivir), indications, actions, and dosage of, 619

Zileuton (Zyflo), indications, actions, and dosage of, 619

Zinacef (cefuroxime), indications, actions, and dosage of, 513

Zinc
    laboratory diagnosis and, 93
    in total parenteral nutrition, 231, 232*t*

Zinecard (dexrazoxane), indications, actions, and dosage of, 525

Zithromax (azithromycin)
    indications, actions, and dosage of, 501
    for subacute bacterial endocarditis prophylaxis, 158*t*

Zocor (simvastatin), indications, actions, and dosage of, 601

Zofran (ondansetron), indications, actions, and dosage of, 580–581

Zoladex (goserelin), indications, actions, and dosage of, 546

Zolmitriptan (Zomig), indications, actions, and dosage of, 620

Zoloft (sertraline), indications, actions, and dosage of, 601

Zolpidem (Ambien), indications, actions, and dosage of, 620

Zomig (zolmitriptan), indications, actions, and dosage of, 620

Zonalon (doxepin, topical), indications, actions, and dosage of, 531

Zonisamide (Zonegran), indications, actions, and dosage of, 620

Zoster. *See also* Varicella zoster virus (VZV)
    drugs of choice for treating, 148*t*, 149*t*

Zostrix (capsaicin), indications, actions, and dosage of, 509

Zosyn (piperacillin-tazobactam), indications, actions, and dosage of, 590

Zovia 1/35E 21, 28, 624*t*

Zovia 1/50E 21, 28, 624*t*

Zovirax (acyclovir), indications, actions, and dosage of, 147*t*, 148*t*, 149*t*, 490

Zyban (bupropion), indications, actions, and dosage of, 507

Zyflo (zileuton), indications, actions, and dosage of, 619

Zyloprim (allopurinol), indications, actions, and dosage of, 491

Zyprexa (olanzapine), indications, actions, and dosage of, 580–581

Zyrtec (cetirizine), indications, actions, and dosage of, 514